STRATEGIC APPROACHES

IN

CORONARY INTERVENTION

SECOND EDITION

STRATEGIC APPROACHES IN CORONARY INTERVENTION

Second Edition

EDITORS

STEPHEN G. ELLIS, M.D.

DIRECTOR, SONES CARDIAC CATHETERIZATION LABORATORIES
DEPARTMENT OF CARDIOLOGY
THE CLEVELAND CLINIC FOUNDATION
CLEVELAND, OHIO

PROFESSOR OF MEDICINE
OHIO STATE UNIVERSITY
COLUMBUS, OHIO

DAVID R. HOLMES, JR., M.D.

CONSULTANT, DIVISION OF CARDIOVASCULAR DISEASES AND INTERNAL MEDICINE
MAYO CLINIC AND MAYO FOUNDATION

PROFESSOR OF MEDICINE
MAYO MEDICAL SCHOOL
ROCHESTER, MINNESOTA

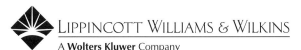

LIPPINCOTT WILLIAMS & WILKINS
A **Wolters Kluwer** Company
Philadelphia · Baltimore · New York · London
Buenos Aires · Hong Kong · Sydney · Tokyo

Acquisitions Editor: Ruth W. Weinberg
Developmental Editor: Michael J. D. Standen
Manufacturing Manager: Kevin Watt
Supervising Editor: Mary Ann McLaughlin
Production Service: Colophon
Cover Designer: Laura Duprey
Compositor: Maryland Composition, Inc.
Printer: Maple Press

© **2000 by LIPPINCOTT WILLIAMS & WILKINS**
227 East Washington Street
Philadelphia, PA 19106-3780 USA
LWW.com

Printed in the USA

Library of Congress Cataloging-in-Publication Data
Strategic approaches in coronary intervention/editors, Stephen G.
  Ellis, David R. Holmes, Jr.—2nd ed.
  p. cm.
  Includes bibliographical references and index.
  ISBN 0-683-30729-0 (alk. paper)
  1. Coronary heart disease—Treatment. 2. Endarterectomy. 3. Coronary heart
disease—Surgery—Complications. I. Ellis, Stephen G. (Stephen Geoffrey), 1951-
II. Holmes, David R., 1945-
  [DNLM: 1. Coronary Disease—therapy. WG 300 S8977 1999]
RD598.35.M95S77 1999
 617.4′12—dc21
 DNLM/DLC
 for Library of Congress
                99-33460
                CIP

10 9 8 7 6 5 4 3 2 1

To my family (Sandy, Jessica, and Gary)
and my mentors (the late Andreas Gruentzig, Spencer King II, and John Douglas),
without whose help and understanding this book would not have been possible.

STEPHEN G. ELLIS

To my family and wife, who, because of their support and tolerance,
have given me the opportunity to work on this
and the myriad of other fascinating activities.

DAVID R. HOLMES, JR.

Contents

SECTION III.

ADJUNCTIVE THERAPIES

SECTION IV.
RELATED ISSUES

SECTION V.
SUMMARY AND FUTURE DIRECTIONS

Preface

In 1996 when the first edition of this textbook was published, we sought to provide a clinically oriented, yet comprehensive, approach to interventional cardiology focusing in particular on the management of specific clinical-anatomical problems. In many ways, this is still how the experienced interventionalist thinks. Yet the available tools, and our appraisal of the benefit of these tools, continue to change with dizzying speed with the rapid introduction of new devices and adjunctive therapies. Three to four years ago, the safety of newer anti-platelet regimens as sole treatment following stent implantation, rather than Coumadin with stents, was just being recognized. This has now become standard. Few stents were available, all seeming ridiculously deficient in one or more characteristics that seem important today. Accordingly, they were used infrequently in less than 20 percent of cases. The relative merits of different stents for certain anatomic situations were largely unknown. Since then, they have become standard for care, used in approximately 80 percent of cases. The benefit of glycoprotein IIb/IIIa antagonists was becoming widely recognized when they were used in conjunction with balloon angioplasty, but they seemed associated with considerable vascular complications. The benefit of these agents for patients receiving stents was unknown. Newer therapies such as brachytherapy for instent restenosis, use of ADP inhibitors, angiogenesis, and direct myocardial revascularization had barely reached the clinical investigation stage. From a diagnostic standpoint, measurement of pressure gradients (in the form of fractional flow reserve) had yet to make a comeback. In addition to adding new approaches, some older approaches have declined, such as directional coronary atherectomy, which while once used frequently, is uncommon today.

The second edition collates the experience of many of the leaders in interventional cardiology to try to make sense of these changes, especially as they apply to the clinical problems of individual patients. Chapters 1 through 5 deal with the technique and application, the merits and the shortcomings, of today's "tools." Chapters 6 through 30 review, in detail, management of most of the challenging clinical problems facing us on a day-to-day basis. Chapters 31 through 34 review the proper use of the increasingly important different anti-platelet agents and also of the thrombin inhibitors. Finally, Chapter 35 deals with the important issue of assessing and then improving quality in the laboratory.

Again, the editors are tremendously indebted to the numerous authors who contributed to the text, who not only reworked previous chapters or prepared new ones, but did so in a timely fashion so as to keep this textbook exceptionally up to date. We would further like to thank the editorial and production staff at Lippincott Williams & Wilkins, particularly Mike Standen and Ruth Weinberg, without whose help and dedication the timely publication of this textbook would not have been possible.

We hope that this text serves as a highly informative and interesting update of the appropriate management of patients undergoing coronary interventional procedures for the interventionalists and noninterventionalists, cardiologists, internists and trainees, who take care of them.

The focus of the chapters is to give the reader the experience of the writer. In many cases, practice patterns have changed in advance of well-grounded scientific studies. In most cases, selection of an optimal strategy takes into consideration clinical experience, published data, sometimes albeit scanty, and if possible, randomized trials, so that the outcome can be optimized.

Stephen G. Ellis
David R. Holmes

Contributing Authors

Janah I. Aji, M.D.
The Center for Cardiovascular Intervention
Cooper University Medical Center
One Cooper Plaza, 4th Floor
Camden, New Jersey 08103

Christoph Altmann, M.D.
Division of Internal Medicine
Department of Cardiology
University-Gesamthochschule-Essen
Hufelandstrasse 55
D-45122 Essen, Germany

Brian H. Annex, M.D.
Assistant Professor of Medicine
Division of Cardiology
Department of Medicine
Duke University Medical Center
Durham, North Carolina 27710

Nelson A. Araujo, M.D.
Cardiovascular Division
Mayo Clinic
200 First Street, S.W.
Rochester, Minnesota 55905

Richard G. Bach, M.D.
Assistant Professor
Department of Internal Medicine
Division of Cardiology
St. Louis University Health Sciences Center
3635 Vista Avenue
St. Louis, Missouri 63110

Steven R. Bailey, M.D., F.A.C.C.
Professor of Medicine and Radiology
University of Texas Health Science Center at
  San Antonio
7703 Floyd Curl Drive
Cardiac Catheterization Laboratories
University Hospital
4502 Medical Drive
San Antonio, Texas 78229-4493

Donald S. Baim, M.D.
Chief, Interventional Cardiology Section
Beth Israel Deaconess Medical Center
Professor of Medicine
Harvard Medical School
330 Brookline Avenue L-453
Boston, Massachusetts 02215

Gregory W. Barsness, M.D.
Department of Cardiology
Mayo Medical School
Division of Cardiovascular Diseases and
  Internal Medicine
Mayo Clinic
200 First Street, S.W.
Rochester, Minnesota 55905

Dietrich Baumgart, M.D.
Division of Internal Medicine
Department of Cardiology
University-Gesamthochschule-Essen
Hufelandstrasse 55
D-45122 Essen, Germany

Heidi N. Benneau, R.N.
Division of Cardiovascular Medicine
Stanford University School of Medicine
300 Pasteur Drive, H-3554
Stanford, California 94305

Michel Bertrand, M.D.
Professor of Medicine (Cardiology)
Chief, Division of Cardiology
Universite de Lille
Service de Cardiologie B
Hopital Cardiologique
59037 Lille, France

Rafael Beyar, M.D., DSc
Technion-Israel Institute of Technology
Head, Heart System Research Center
Professor of Biomedical Engineering and
  Medicine
The Julius Silver Institute
Department of Biomedical Engineering
Technion City, Haifa, 32000, Israel

Sorin J. Brener, M.D.
Department of Medicine
Ohio State University
370 West 9th Avenue
270 Meiling Hall
Columbus, Ohio 43210
Department of Cardiology
The Cleveland Clinic Foundation
9500 Euclid Avenue
Cleveland, Ohio 44195-5066

Joseph R. Califano, M.D., F.A.C.C.
Department of Cardiology
Naval Medical Center San Diego
34800 Bob Wilson Drive
San Diego, California 92134-5000

Charles R. Cannan, M.D.
Cardiovascular Division
Mayo Clinic
200 First Street, S.W.
Rochester, Minnesota 55905

Christakis Christodoulou, M.D.
University of Southern California School of
    Medicine
Division of Cardiology
1355 San Pablo Street, Suite 117
Los Angeles, California 90033

Mauricio G. Cohen, M.D.
Interventional Cardiology Fellow
Cardiac Catheterization Laboratory
Division of Cardiology
Department of Medicine
Duke University Medical Center
Durham, North Carolina 27710

Antonio Colombo, M.D.
Director, Cardiac Catheterization Laboratory
Centro Cuore Columbus
Via M. Buonarroti 48
20145 Milano, Italy

Patrick Coussement, M.D.
Department of Cardiology
University Hospital Gasthuisberg
Herestraat 49
B-3000 Leuven, Belgium

Larry S. Dean, M.D.
Professor
Division of Cardiovascular Diseases
University of Alabama at Birmingham
UAB Station–BDB 373
Birmingham, Alabama 35294-0001

Ivan De Scheerder, M.D., Ph.D.
University Hospital Gasthuisberg
Department of Cardiology
Herestraat 49
B-3000 Leuven, Belgium

Carlo Di Mario, M.D., Ph.D., F.E.S.C.,
    F.A.C.C.
Associate Director
Cardiac Catheterization Laboratory
Columbus Clinic and San Raffaele Hospital
Via M. Buonarroti 48
20145 Milano, Italy

John S. Douglas, Jr., M.D.
Associate Professor of Medicine
Division of Cardiology
Emory University School of Medicine
Co-Director, Cardiac Catheterization
    Laboratory
Emory University Hospital
Room C-430
1364 Clifton Road, N.E.
Atlanta, Georgia 30322-1104

Daniel L. Dries, M.D., M.P.H.
Division of Cardiology
Georgetown University Medical Center
3800 Reservoir Road N.W.
Washington, DC 20007-2197

Eric Eeckhout, M.D.
Cardiologist
Division of Cardiology BH-10
University Hospital
1011 Lausanne, Switzerland

Neal L. Eigler, M.D.
Co-Director, Cardiovascular Intervention
    Center
Cedars-Sinai Medical Center
8700 Beverly Boulevard
Associate Professor
Department of Medicine
U.C.L.A. School of Medicine
Los Angeles, California 90048-1869

Stephen G. Ellis, M.D.
Director, Sones Cardiac Catheterization
    Laboratories
Department of Cardiology
The Cleveland Clinic Foundation
9500 Euclid Avenue
Cleveland, Ohio 44195-5066
Professor of Medicine
Ohio State University
Columbus, Ohio 43210

Raimund Erbel, M.D., F.A.C.C, F.E.S.C.
Director of the Department of Cardiology
Division of Internal Medicine
University-Gesamthochschule-Essen
Hufelandstrasse 55
D-45122 Essen, Germany

Jean Fajadet, M.D.
UCI
Clinique Pasteur
45, Avenue de Lombez
31076 Toulouse, France

David P. Faxon, M.D.
Professor of Medicine
University of Southern California School of
* Medicine*
Chief, Division of Cardiology
1355 San Pablo Street, Suite 117
Los Angeles, California 90033

Tim A. Fischell, M.D.
Professor of Medicine
Heart Institute at Borgess Medical Center
Michigan State University
1521 Gull Road
Kalamazoo, Michigan 49001

David L. Fischman, M.D.
Associate Professor of Medicine
Co-Director, Cardiac Catheterization
* Laboratory*
Director, Interventional Cardiovascular
* Research*
Department of Cardiology
Thomas Jefferson University Hospital
410 College Building
1025 Walnut Street, Suite 410
Philadelphia, Pennsylvania 19107

Peter J. Fitzgerald, M.D., Ph.D.
Assistant Professor of Medicine
Division of Cardiovascular Medicine
Stanford University School of Medicine
300 Pasteur Drive, H-3554
Stanford, California 94305

David P. Foley, M.B., Ph.D., M.R.C.P.I.,
  F.E.S.C.
Clinical Director, Interventional Cardiology
Thoraxcenter
University Hospital Rotterdam
3015 GD Rotterdam, The Netherlands

Kirk N. Garratt, M.D.
Associate Professor of Medicine
Mayo Graduate School of Medicine
Division of Cardiovascular Diseases and
* Internal Medicine*
Consultant, Adult Cardiac Catheterization
* Laboratory*
St. Mary's Hospital
Mayo Clinic and Foundation
Department of Medicine
Rochester, Minnesota 55905

Junbo Ge, M.D.
Division of Internal Medicine
Department of Cardiology
University-Gesamthochschule-Essen
Hufelandstrasse 55
D-45122 Essen, Germany

Bernard J. Gersh, M.B., Ch.B., D.Phil.,
  F.R.C.P.
Chairman, Division of Cardiology
Georgetown University Medical Center
3800 Reservoir Road N.W.
Washington, DC 20007-2197

Sheldon Goldberg, M.D.
The Center for Cardiovascular Intervention
Cooper University Medical Center
One Cooper Plaza, 4th Floor
Camden, New Jersey 08103

J.-J. Goy, M.D.
Associate Professor
Division of Cardiology
University Hospital
1011 Lausanne, Switzerland

Navin Gupta, M.D.
Phoenix Heart Center
1901 East Thomas Road, Suite 107
Phoenix, Arizona 83106

Jaap N. Hamburger, M.D.
Clinical Co-Director
Department of Interventional Cardiology
Erasmus University, BD 416
Heartcenter Rotterdam
PO Box 1738
3000 Dr Rotterdam, The Netherlands

David Hasdai, M.D.
Department of Cardiology
Rabin Medical Center
Beilinson Campus
49100 Petah Tikva, Israel

Michael Haude, M.D.
Division of Internal Medicine
Department of Cardiology
University-Gesamthochschule-Essen
Hufelandstrasse 55
D-45122 Essen, Germany

Richard R. Heuser, M.D.
Phoenix Heart
1901 East Thomas Road, Suite 107
Phoenix, Arizona 83106

Stuart T. Higano, M.D.
Cardiovascular Division
Mayo Clinic
200 First Street, S.W.
Rochester, Minnesota 55905

David R. Holmes, Jr., M.D.
Professor of Medicine
Consultant, Division of Cardiovascular
   Diseases and Internal Medicine
Mayo Clinic and Mayo Foundation
Department of Medicine
Mayo Medical School
200 First Street, S.W.
Rochester, Minnesota 55905

Alice K. Jacobs, M.D.
Professor of Medicine
Director, Cardiac Catheterization Laboratory
   and Interventional Cardiology
Boston University Medical Center
Section of Cardiology
88 East Newton Street
Boston, Massachusetts 02118

James G. Jollis, M.D.
Assistant Professor of Medicine
Division of Cardiology
Duke University Medical Center
2400 Pratt Street DUMC 3254
Durham, North Carolina 27708-3485

Thierry Joseph, M.D.
UCI
Clinique Pasteur
45, Avenue de Lombez
31076 Toulouse, France

Morton J. Kern, M.D.
Director, Catheterization Laboratory
St. Louis University Medical Center
3635 Vista Avenue
St. Louis, Missouri 63110

Ferdinand Kiemeneij, M.D., Ph.D.
Amsterdam Department of Interventional
   Cardiology, Onze Lieve Vrouwe Gasthuis
1e Oosterparkstraat 279
1090 HM Amsterdam, The Netherlands

Thomas Konorza
Division of Internal Medicine
Department of Cardiology
University-Gesamthochschule-Essen
Hufelandstrasse 55
D-45122 Essen 1, Germany

Michael J.B. Kutryk, M.D., Ph.D.
Department of Cardiology
Saint Michael's Hospital
30 Bond Street
Toronto, M5B 1W8 Canada

Warren K. Laskey, M.D.
Director of Cardiac Catheterization
   Laboratories
Division of Cardiology
University of Maryland
22 South Greene Street, Room S3B316
Baltimore, Maryland 21201

David P. Lee, M.D.
Division of Cardiovascular Medicine
Stanford University Medical Center
300 Pasteur Drive, H-2321
Stanford, California 94305-5246

Martin B. Leon, M.D.
The Cardiac Catheterization Laboratory
Washington Hospital Center and
The Cardiovascular Research Foundation
110 Irving Street, N.W., Suite 4B1
Washington, DC 20010-2975

Jane A. Leopold, M.D.
Assistant Professor of Medicine
Department of Cardiology
Boston Medical Center
88 East Newton Street
Boston, Massachusetts 02118

Amir Lerman, M.D.
Division of Cardiovascular Diseases
Mayo Clinic
200 First Street, S.W.
Rochester, Minnesota 55905

A. Michael Lincoff, M.D.
Department of Cardiology
Center of the Ohio State University
The Cleveland Clinic Foundation
9500 Euclid Avenue
Cleveland, Ohio 44195-5066

Frank Litvack, M.D.
Co-Director, Catheterization Laboratory
Cedars-Sinai Medical Center
8700 Beverly Blvd., #5347
Los Angeles, California 90048-1865

Fengqi Liu, M.D.
Division of Internal Medicine
Department of Cardiology
University-Gesamthochschule-Essen
Hufelandstrasse 55
D-45122 Essen, Germany

Sidney T.H. Lo, M.D.
Division of Cardiovascular Medicine
Stanford University Medical Center
300 Pasteur Drive, H-2321
Stanford, California 94305-5246

Alejandro N. Lopez, M.D.
Phoenix Heart
1901 East Thomas Road, Suite 107
Phoenix, Arizona 83106

Jean Marco, M.D.
UCI
Clinique Pasteur
45, Avenue de Lombez
31076 Toulouse, France

Daniel B. Mark, M.D., M.P.H.
Professor
Department of Medicine
Division of Cardiology
Duke University Medical Center
2400 Pratt Street
Durham, North Carolina 27705

Steven P. Marso, M.D.
Chief Cardiology Fellow
Department of Cardiology
The Cleveland Clinic Foundation
9500 Euclid Avenue
Cleveland, Ohio 44195-5066

Roxana Mehran, M.D.
The Cardiac Catheterization Laboratory
Washington Hospital Center and
The Cardiovascular Research Foundation
110 Irving Street, N.W.
Washington DC 20010-2975

Bernhard Meier, M.D.
Professor and Head of Cardiology
Department of Cardiology
University Hospital
Murtenstrasse 11
Hallerstrasse 12
CH-3012 Bern, Switzerland

Giuliana Menegatti, M.D.
Division of Cardiology
University Hospital
University of Verona
P. Le Stefani, 1
37126 Verona, Italy

Jonata Molinari, M.D.
Division of Cardiology
University Hospital
University of Verona
P. Le Stefani, 1
37126 Verona, Italy

Jeffery Moses, M.D.
Department of Clinical Research
Interventional Cardiology
Lenox Hill Hospital
130 East 77th Street, 9th Floor
New York, New York 10021

Issam Moussa, M.D.
Director, Clinical Research
Interventional Cardiology
Lenox Hill Hospital
130 East 77th Street, 9th Floor
New York, New York 10021

Craig R. Narins, M.D.
Department of Cardiology
New Mexico Heart Institute
Presbyterian Medical Plaza
1001 Coal Avenue SE
Albuquerque, New Mexico 87106

Stephen N. Oesterle, M.D.
Associate Professor of Medicine
Department of Medicine
Harvard Medical School
Department of Cardiology
Massachusetts General Hospital
55 Fruit Street, Bulfinch 106
Boston, Massachusetts 02114

Hiroyuki Okura, M.D.
Division of Cardiovascular Medicine
Stanford University School of Medicine
300 Pasteur Drive, H-3554
Stanford, California 94305

Michael A. Peterson, M.D.
The Cardiac Catheterization Laboratory
Washington Hospital Center and
The Cardiovascular Research Foundation
110 Irving Street, N.W., Suite 4B1
Washington, DC 20010-2975

Stephen R. Ramee, M.D.
Director, Cardiac Catheterization Laboratory
Department of Cardiology
Alton Ochsner Medical Institution
1514 Jefferson Highway
New Orleans, Louisiana 70121

Guy S. Reeder, M.D.
Cardiovascular Division
Mayo Clinic
200 First Street, S.W.
Rochester, Minnesota 55905

Bernhard Reimers, M.D.
Cardiac Catheterization Laboratory
Centro Cuore Columbus
Via M. Buonarroti 48
20145 Milano, Italy

Expedito E. Ribeiro, M.D.
2900 Whipple Ave., Suite 230
Redwood City, California 94062

Charanjit S. Rihal, M.D.
Consultant, Division of Cardiovascular
* Diseases and Internal Medicine*
Mayo Clinic and Mayo Foundation
Assistant Professor of Medicine
Mayo Medical School
200 First Street, S.W.
Rochester, Minnesota 55905

Ariel Roguin, M.D.
Technion-Israel Institute of Technology
Heart System Research Center
Department of Biomedical Engineering
The Julius Silver Institute
Technion City, Haifa 32000, Israel

Uri Rosenschein, M.D.
Catheterization Laboratory
Department of Cardiology
The Tel Aviv Sourasky Medical Center
6 Weizman Street
Tel Aviv 64239, Israel

Robert D. Safian, M.D.
Director, Interventional Cardiology
William Beaumont Hospital
3601 West Thirteen Mile Road
Royal Oak, Michigan 48073

Michael P. Savage, M.D.
Associate Professor of Medicine
Director, Cardiac Catheterization Laboratory
Director, Interventional Cardiovascular
* Research*
Department of Cardiology
Thomas Jefferson University Hospital
410 College Building
1025 Walnut Street, Suite 410
Philadelphia, Pennsylvania 19107

Martin J. Sebastian, M.B.B.S.
Research Associate
Cardiovascular Intervention Center
Cedars-Sinai Medical Center
Los Angeles, California 90048-1865

Sigmund Silber, M.D., F.A.C.C.
Professor of Medicine
Department of Cardiology
University of Munich
Dr. Mueller Hospital
Am Isarkanal 36
81379 Munich, Germany

Jose A. Silva, M.D.
Fellow in Interventional Cardiology
Cardiac Catheterization Laboratory
Department of Cardiology
Alton Ochsner Medical Institution
1514 Jefferson Highway
New Orleans, Louisiana 70121

Charles Simonton III, M.D.
The Sanger Clinic, P.A.
1001 Blythe Boulevard, Suite 300
Charlotte, North Carolina 28203-5866

Mandeep Singh, M.D.
SMH Cardiac Catheterization Laboratory
Mayo Clinic
200 First Street, S.W.
Rochester, Minnesota 55905

Michael H. Sketch, Jr., M.D.
Associate Professor of Medicine
Director, Diagnostic and Interventional
* Cardiac Catheterization Laboratories*
Department of Medicine, Division of
* Cardiology*
Duke University Medical Center
Durham, North Carolina 27710

Maj. Steven R. Steinhubl, M.D.
Department of Cardiology/PSMC
Wilford Hall Medical Center
2200 Bergquist Drive, Suite 1
Lackland AFB, Texas 78236-5300

Paul S. Teirstein, M.D.
Director, Interventional Cardiology
Department of Cardiology
Scripps Clinic
10666 North Torrey Pines Road
La Jolla, California 92037

Daniel J. Tiede, M.D.
Cardiovascular Division
Mayo Clinic
200 First Street, S.W.
Rochester, Minnesota 55905

Steven B.H. Timmis, M.D.
Consultant in Cardiology, F.C.
Division of Cardiology
William Beaumont Hospital
3601 West Thirteen Mile Road
Royal Oak, Michigan 48073

Eric J. Topol, M.D.
Chairman and Professor
Department of Cardiology
Director, Joseph J. Jacobs Center for
  Thrombosis and Vascular Biology
Ohio State University School of Medicine
The Cleveland Clinic Foundation
F25 9500 Euclid Avenue
Cleveland, Ohio 44195

Corrado Vassanelli, M.D., F.E.S.C.
Department of Medical Sciences
University "A. Avogadro"
V. Solaroli, 17
Division of Cardiology
Azienda "Maggiore Dellacarita"
C. S. Mazzini, 18
28100 Novara, Italy

Arun Venkat, M.D.
The Center for Cardiovascular Intervention
Cooper University Medical Center
One Cooper Plaza, 4th Floor
Camden, New Jersey 08103

James W. Vetter, M.D.
2900 Whipple Avenue, Suite 230
Redwood City, California 94062

Ron Waksman, M.D.
Director of Experimental Angioplasty and
  Vascular Brachytherapy
Cardiology Research Foundation
Washington Hospital Center
110 Irving Street, N.W.
Washington, DC 20010

Patrick L. Whitlow, M.D., F.A.C.C.
Director, Interventional Cardiology
Department of Cardiology, F25
The Cleveland Clinic Foundation
9500 Euclid Avenue
Cleveland, Ohio 44195

Paul G. Yock, M.D.
Professor
Division of Cardiovascular Medicine
Stanford University School of Medicine
300 Pasteur Drive, H-3554
Stanford, California 94305

Felix Zijlstra
Department of Cardiology
Hospital De Weezenlanden
Groot Wezenland 20
8011 JW Zwolle, The Netherlands

SECTION I

Techniques of Coronary Revascularization and Imaging

1

Balloon Angioplasty and Provisional Stenting

David R. Holmes, Jr.

*Division of Cardiovascular Diseases and Internal Medicine, Mayo Clinic and Mayo Foundation,
Department of Medicine, Mayo Medical School, Rochester, Minnesota 55905*

Stents have revolutionized interventional cardiology and are currently used in 60 to 80% of all interventional procedures. They have been documented to improve both angiographic and clinical outcome in multiple patient subsets. There are, however, some relatively unique problems associated with stent implantation. Some of these may be solved or at least improved by technical advances or adjunctive therapy. Others are apt to remain.

These problems include the following.

1. In-stent restenosis, which may either be focal and relatively easy to treat or diffuse and a major problem. Although for single discrete lesions treated with stent implantation, restenosis rates are very low, for more complex and particularly long lesions, restenosis rates with stents are significantly higher. Diffuse in-stent restenosis refractory to treatment may result in the need for coronary artery bypass surgery even in patients with single vessel disease. This may become more of a problem as longer stents are used.

2. Side branch compromise. This problem has been documented from the early days of angioplasty and is related to the location of the side branch relative to the target lesion as well as the presence or absence of stenosis at its origin. With stent implantation, access is more difficult; in addition, compromise of small branches may be one reason for the CPK evaluation seen with interventional procedures.

3. Subacute closure. This was a major problem with early stent experiences but has been much less of a problem since the development of better adjunctive therapy and high-pressure deployment. It does remain an issue for the very uncommon patient in whom it occurs. When it occurs, it is associated with a marked increase in morbidity and even mortality.

4. Cost. Typically 1.7 to 1.8 stents are used per patient. This increases the cost of the interventional procedure markedly, particularly when multiple balloons are required for pre and post dilatation. The economics of stenting are complex. Initial costs are clearly higher because of the stent cost; however, because of the lower need for subsequent procedures, there may be cost savings over the entire course of patient care. Depending upon the degree of reduction in repeat procedures, there may be valuable cost reductions. Vaitkus et al. analyzed 421 consecutive interventional cases from 1996 using actual cost data to study the misalignment between financial and clinical incentives using the DRG based system in the interventional cardiology arena. They found that the addition of DRG 116 will have a positive effect and will facilitate more equitable reimbursement, allowing hospitals to address the initial higher capital costs of stenting. It must be kept in mind that in subsets of patients at increased risk of restenosis after stenting—e.g. those with long, diffusely diseased small segments >30 mm—there may not be a dramatic reduction in restenosis. This may impact on the cost effectiveness of the procedure.

For these reasons, there has been substantial interest in identifying patients who might uniquely benefit from stents and those who could be treated instead with conventional angioplasty, with stents in the latter group reserved for treatment of restenosis. It has been well known that the most important determinant of long-term angiographic outcome is the immediate post treatment minimum lumen diameter (MLD). This relationship has been found to be independent of device type. This observation has formed the basis for the concept of provisional stenting—i.e., if an ideal result is obtained with conventional percutaneous transluminal coronary angioplasty, then a stent is not deployed. Such a strategy would avoid the need for stents in patients who would be expected to do well without them, thus avoiding the potential problems and issues documented above.

There are several issues with the concept of provisional stenting.

1. How is a "stent-like" result with conventional percutaneous transluminal coronary angioplasty defined? This is crucial. A stent-like result can be defined angiographically; however, it must be remembered that angiographers tend to overestimate the severity of stenosis prior to intervention and underestimate it afterward. A stent-like result should be judged objectively with QCA if possible. It should be a residual stenosis <20%. A stent-like result can also be judged physiologically, defined as restoration of normal flow. There are two major approaches which can be used. A. Doppler flow assessment with measurement of coronary flow reserve (CFR). Normal CFR should be greater than 2.5. If following dilatation the CFR is substantially less than that, perhaps 1.6 or 1.8, despite an excellent angiographic result, it should raise consideration of inadequate dilatation or residual dissection, which should be treated with repeat PTCA or stent implantation. B. Fractional flow reserve (FFR). This is a technique which has been evaluated as an approach to studying indeterminate lesions as well as the results of intervention. FFR is calculated by measuring the transluminal pressure under maximal flow conditions. A normal FFR would be 1; abnormal FFR has been found to be ≤0.75. An ideal result with conventional percutaneous transluminal coronary angioplasty should be >0.85–90. Where an ideal result is obtained with conventional PTCA, the long-term results have been found to be excellent. In the DEBATE study, 225 patients with an angiographically successful PTCA underwent interrogation of the lesion with a Doppler guidewire to measure basal and maximal hyperemia flow proximal and distal to the lesion. Symptoms and/or ischemia were assessed at 1 and 6 months; in addition, restenosis was evaluated. Predictors of these clinical events were diameter stenosis of 35% and CFR of 2.5. In patients with a residual diameter stenosis of ≤35% and a distal CFR of >2.5, there was a lower rate of adverse events including low restenosis rate (16% versus 41% $p = .002$) and a low rate of repeat reintervention (16% versus 34%, $p = .024$). Other series have also found that a stent-like result is associated with an excellent long-term outcome.

2. How often is a stent-like result obtained and how can this percentage be increased? The frequency of obtaining a stent-like result depends in part upon the definition of such a result. In a recent evaluation, Narins et al. summarized the balloon arm of three recent randomized clinical trials involving 4,608 patients: BENESTENT-II, EPILOG, and BOAT. In patients in this balloon arm, what was believed to be an optimal result was achieved in 86% and only 14% required crossover to a stent. If a truly "stent-like" result is the goal, the frequency of achieving this is probably significantly less. In some experiences, only approximately 40% of patients have an optimal result with conventional PTCA, which would be considered stent-like. There are approaches which can be taken to optimize the result of conventional PTCA. It must be kept in mind that these approaches may obviate the potential cost savings seen with avoiding stent implantation. Intravascular ultrasound can be used to select the optimal size balloon. In the Clinical

Outcomes with Ultrasound Trial (CLOUT), the investigators performed intravascular ultrasound in 102 patients immediately after conventional angioplasty, which had used what was believed to be an appropriate balloon size based on the angiographic estimation of vessel diameter. The investigators found that even larger balloons could be used in 73% of cases and achieved an average balloon-artery ratio of 1.3:1. When these larger balloons (which traditionally would have been regarded as oversized) were used, there was a significant increase in the minimal lumen diameter from 1.95 ± 0.49 to 2.21 ± 0.47 mm, with no increase in the frequency of angiographic dissection. Such an increase in MLD should translate into improved longer-term angiographic outcome.

3. Changing adjunctive pharmacologic therapy. Adjunctive therapy is changing rapidly. The most important recent addition has been the widespread use of platelet glycoprotein IIb/IIIa blockade. The EPISTENT trial has now been reported, which randomized 2,399 patients and lesions to stenting plus placebo (N = 809), stenting plus abciximab (N = 794), and PTCA plus abciximab (N = 796). The primary endpoint was death, infarction, or need for urgent revascularization at 30 days. This composite endpoint occurred in 10.8% of the stent plus placebo group, 5.3% in the stent plus abciximab group, and 6.9% in the PTCA plus abciximab group. Longer-term outcomes are being assessed. They have now been reported in abstract form to show improved 6-month outcome in patients treated with stenting plus abciximab, particularly in diabetic patients. The extent to which this will affect the concept of provisional stenting is unclear. It certainly has cost implications because combined therapy is usually more costly. If stenting plus abciximab results in markedly improved outcome compared to PTCA, then attempts to achieve a stent-like result with PTCA may be limited.

4. Effect of brachytherapy. Application of local radiation, either gamma or beta, is the subject of intense investigation with multiple trials involving both ratio lesions as well as in-stent restenosis. At the present time, gamma radiation appears promising for treatment of in-stent restenosis. Depending on the results of the other trials, the role of provisional stenting may change dramatically; e.g., if radiation plus conventional PTCA yields a result as good as with stent implantation, there may be more intense efforts made to optimize the initial result. Alternatively, if stent implantation plus primary radiation gives the best result, then provisional stenting as a concept may decrease in importance.

SUMMARY

Coronary stenting remains a field in rapid evolution. Based upon the known importance of geometry on outcome, the goal of interventional therapy should be to achieve as large a final MLD as is possible safely. Based on the available data, this is the most important determinant of longer-term outcome. If that goal can be achieved with conventional PTCA, leaving a residual stenosis measured of ≤20% measured objectively, then the outcome is apt to be excellent and stent implantation is not required. If such an optimal result cannot be achieved, then stenting should be considered.

From a practical standpoint, we assess the potential of achieving a stent-like result prior to beginning the procedure. Lesion characteristics which lend themselves to that goal are those initially described as Type A lesions: being proximal, noncalcified, discrete, single concentric, and not involving major side branches. In these lesions, we try to pick an optimal balloon/artery ratio of 1 to 1 or 1:1 to 1, using an appropriate nondiseased reference segment. During balloon inflation, we monitor the inflation pressure very closely. If a pressure greater than 10 to 12 atmospheres is required, usually a strategy of proximal stenting does not look promising. Following balloon deflation, we assess the lesion carefully to document that an ideal result has been obtained. If not, the decision must be made between increasing the balloon size or stenting. Those lesions which do not appear reasonable are ostial lesions, bifurcation disease, or heavily calcified lesions. In these circumstances, PTCA rarely gives an excellent angiographic result. If a question arises as to the adequacy of PTCA and stent implantation is not an option, then either intravascular ultrasound or a physiologic assessment should be performed to assess the results.

SUGGESTED READINGS

1. Serruys PW, Di Mario C, Piek S, et al. Prognostic value of intracoronary flow velocity and diameter stenosis in assessing the short- and long-term outcomes of coronary balloon angioplasty: the DEBATE Study (Doppler Endpoints Balloon Angioplasty Trail Europe). *Circulation* 1997;96:3369–3377.
2. Kern MJ, Dupouy P, Drury JH et al. Role of coronary artery lumen enlargement in improving coronary blood flow after balloon angioplasty and stenting: a combined intravascular ultrasound, Doppler flow, and imaging study. *J Am Coll Cardiol* 1997;29:1520–1527.
3. Narins CR, Holmes DR, Topol EJ. A call for provisional stenting. The balloon is back. *Circulation* 1998;97: 1298–1305.
4. Stone G, Hodgson J, St Goar F et al. Improved procedural results of coronary angioplasty with intravascular ultrasound-guided balloon sizing: the CLOUT pilot trial. *Circulation* 1997;95:2044–2052.
5. Holmes DR, Bell M, Holmes D III et al. Interventional cardiology and intracoronary stents: a changing practice approved versus nonapproved indications. *Cathet Cardiovasc Diag* 1997;40:133–138.
6. Topol EJ for the EPISTENT Investigators. Randomized placebo controlled and balloon angioplasty controlled trial to assess safety of coronary stenting with use of platelet glycoprotein IIb/IIIa blockade. *Lancet* 1998;352: 87–92.
7. Holmes DR, Hirshfeld J, Faxon D et al. ACC expert consensus statement: coronary artery stents. *J Am Coll Cardiol* 1998;32(5):1471–1482.
8. Vaitkus PT. The impact of reimbursement changes for intracoronary stents on providers and medicare. Am J Man Care 1998;4:1097–1102.
9. Vaitkus PT, Witmer WT, Brandenburg RG et al. Economic impact of angioplasty salvage techniques with an emphasis on coronary stents: a method incorporating costs, revenues, clinical effectiveness, and payor mix. *J Am Coll Cardiol* 1997;30:894–900.

dures. Coronary perforation occurred in 0.5% of lesions treated. Multivariable analysis showed that Q-wave myocardial infarction was more frequent in lesions >10 mm long, $p = .05$ (15).

Prospective Randomized Clinical Trial Results

The Excimer Rotational Balloon Angioplasty Comparison (ERBAC) trial was a single-center prospective randomized trial of 685 patients with complicated (ACC/AHA type B or C) lesions. Lesions were randomized to receive excimer laser, rotational atherectomy, or standard balloon angioplasty. Two-hundred-thirty-two patients received excimer-laser assisted angioplasty using a 308-nm xenon chloride excimer laser system with catheters 1.3 mm to 2.2 mm. By study design, maximum catheter-to-artery ratio was 0.66, followed by adjunctive balloon angioplasty. Two hundred thirty-one patients were randomized to receive rotational atherectomy with a maximal burr-to-artery ratio of 0.66 by study design. Adjunctive balloon angioplasty was utilized if residual stenosis remained >50%. Two-hundred-twenty-two patients were randomized to receive balloon dilatation alone by standard PTCA techniques.

Moderate to severe calcification was found in 39% of lesions, and 46% of lesions were longer than 10 mm. Reference vessel diameter was 2.9 mm. Procedural success without major complications was higher for rotational atherectomy (89.2%) than for laser or balloon angioplasty (77.2% and 79.7%, respectively, $p = .002$). However, follow-up target vessel revascularization was significantly higher for rotational atherectomy (42.4%) and laser (46.0%) than PTCA (31.9%, $p = .013$) (16).

The Study To determine Rotablator And Transluminal Angioplasty Strategy (STRATAS) was a 497 patient, multicenter, prospective, randomized trial of patients undergoing rotational atherectomy. Patients were randomized to an aggressive Rotablator strategy (≥70% burr-to-artery ratio, either stand alone or with adjunctive balloon angioplasty <1 atm) versus a routine Rotablator strategy (burr-to-artery ratio <70%, followed by routine balloon angioplasty

≥4 atm). Patients enrolled in the trial had rather complicated lesions, with 63% of lesions being classified either Type B2 or C. Lesion length was 12.6 mm versus 12.2 mm for the aggressive and routine Rotablator strategies respectively. Thirty-three percent to 35% of lesions were heavily calcified, and 14% of lesions occurred in a major bifurcation. Angiographic success was documented by the core lab in 96% of lesions utilizing both strategies, and clinical success was reported in 92% of the routine strategy and 94% of the aggressive strategy. Major complications occurred in 2.0% of the aggressive strategy patients and 3.6% of the routine strategy patients (17). On preliminary analysis, rpm drop >5,000 from baseline for a cumulative period >10 seconds was the strongest multivariable predictor of both major adverse clinical events and CKMB elevation (18,19).

Rotablator Strategy

Rotational atherectomy should be viewed as one of the tools used by the interventional cardiologist to obtain the largest lumen diameter safely possible. The idea of utilizing rotational atherectomy alone to obtain a moderate increase in lumen diameter without damaging the deep wall structure and theoretically minimizing late loss has no support from clinical trials. Burr-to-artery ratios from the 0.6 to 0.80 range have been reported to produce very high success rates with acceptable complications, and balloon-to-artery ratios in this range are recommended. Aggressive adjunctive balloon dilatation or stenting should be used to obtain the largest lumen diameter possible at the end of the procedure. Data from both the STRATAS trial (17) and Warth et al.(15), confirm that the most important multivariable predictor of restenosis after rotational atherectomy is final procedural MLD, just as after PTCA, directional atherectomy, and stenting (20,21).

Safian and coworkers have shown that rotational atherectomy predictably enhances the results of balloon angioplasty by reducing the amount of elastic recoil with final balloon inflation (9,13). By this mechanism, rotational atherectomy would be expected to enhance the final

MLD compared to balloon angioplasty, though this result has not yet been confirmed in randomized trials. Data have been collected from the multicenter Dilation versus Ablation Randomized Trial (DART) of Rotablator versus PTCA, but QCA data from this trial have yet to be reported (22).

Whether rotational atherectomy can enhance the results of coronary stenting is a hypothesis that is being tested in the multicenter Stent Implantation Post Rotational atherectomy Trial (SPORT). Theoretically, removing the most fibrous and inelastic atherosclerotic plaque would yield improved MLD with stent placement versus balloon angioplasty, and data from the Washington Hospital Center suggest that this concept may be correct (23). However, confirmation of these single-center data await the completion of the SPORT trial.

Complications

Slow reflow has been reported in 1.8% to 9.5% of Rotablator cases, complicated by Q-wave myocardial infarction in 9% and non-Q-wave MI in 33% of the cases with sustained slow flow (24,25). Slow flow is more likely to occur when there is a large plaque burden, where distal runoff is limited, and in severely calcified long lesions. Multivariate analysis has shown that the incidence of slow reflow was highest when MI had occurred in the territory supplied by the target lesion within 2 weeks, in patients with a history of hypertension, and in long lesions and following prolonged total burr activation time. The precise etiology of slow flow is not clear, but it may be due to plugging of the distal capillary bed by microparticulate debris, arteriolar spasm, platelet activation (26), or microcavitation. Microcavitation, or the formation of minute bubbles within blood at the tip of the rotating burr, has been demonstrated *in vitro,* but its clinical significance is uncertain (27).

Coronary artery dissection and perforation have been reported following rotational atherectomy. Data from the multicenter registry reported dissection in 13% of treated lesions, 73% of which were caused by the passage of the burr (the remainder were visible only after adjunctive PTCA). Dissection was seen more frequently in tortuous, eccentric, and longer lesions and resulted in acute closure in 14% of dissections (1.8% of all treated lesions) (28). Acute closure was relatively infrequent following rotational atherectomy, the reported incidence ranging from 1.4% to 7.8% (14,15,25,28,29). It was more frequent in hinge lesions and long lesions and was seen less frequently when lesions were treated with a small burr first. Coronary perforation was reported in 1.4% of treated lesions (29); of five patients reported by Ellis and coworkers, three required urgent bypass surgery and two died. Perforation was more frequent in lesions located on a bend (25). If a significant perforation occurs, the heparin should be reversed with protamine and an angioplasty balloon inflated across the site to seal the leak. Further management will depend on the size of the perforation, whether the perforation seals, and the patient's hemodynamic condition. Small perforations can be managed conservatively, but patients must be monitored for evidence of delayed tamponade (30).

Restenosis

Angiographic restenosis rates reported with rotational atherectomy have varied between series, from 38% (15) to 57% (16). These results are similar to the restenosis rates reported with PTCA in reference vessels of the same diameter. Five-hundred-forty-seven lesions in the Multicenter Rotablator Registry (MRR) completed angiographic follow-up (64% of those eligible). Dichotomous restenosis occurred in 37.7% of lesions. Restenosis rate for diabetic patients appeared to be higher (55.6%) than for non-diabetic patients (33.7%, $p < .05$) (15). Angiographic dichotomous restenosis rates in STRATAS and ERBAC were both >50% (11,16). At present there is no evidence that the restenosis rate following rotational atherectomy is lower than it is following PTCA (Table 2.1), with the possible exception of diffuse in-stent restenosis lesions (31–34). However, if plaque burden is reduced by rotational atherectomy with burr/artery ratios 70% to 80% followed by aggressive adjunctive PTCA and/or stenting,

TABLE 2.1. *Rotablator versus PTCA randomized trials*

	ERBAC (PTCA/Roto)	COBRA (PTCA/Roto)	DART (PTCA/Roto)
N	222/231	228/209	222/225
Procedural success	80%/89%[a]	78%/85%	89%/91%
# of burrs	NA/1.3	NA/1.7	NA/2.0
Largest burr	NA/1.66 mm	NA/1.64 mm	NA/1.92 mm
Major complications	3.1%/3.2%	3.6%/4.4%	1.4%/0.99%
Residual stenosis	30%/31%	36%/36%	30%/28%
Ref vessel diameter(mm)	2.81/2.87	NAV	2.53 mm/2.45 mm
B_2/C	73%/79%	100%/100%	54%/54%
TVR	32%/42%[b]	29%/25%	18%/22%
Restenosis	47%/57%	29%/39%	NAV/NAV

[a] $p = 0.002$.
[b] $p = 0.01$; N, number of patients; #, number; NA, not applicable; NAV, not available; Ref, reference; TVR, target vessel revascularization.

lower restenosis rates may be achieved in the future.

INDICATIONS FOR ROTATIONAL ATHERECTOMY

The following lesion types should be considered for rotational atherectomy (Table 2.2).

Undilatable Lesions

Brogan and coworkers reported their experience with rotational atherectomy in a group of consecutive patients in whom PTCA had been unsuccessful. Rotational atherectomy was performed in 41 patients in whom balloon angioplasty failed because of lesion rigidity (inability to dilate), inability to cross the lesion with a balloon, or elastic recoil. After high-speed rotational atherectomy with adjunctive PTCA, the angiographic success rate was 49 of 50 lesions reattempted (98%). Procedural success was obtained in 90% of cases. Restenosis occurred in 35% of the patients who had follow-up angiography, and 24% of the group developed recurrent symptoms (35).

There is general consensus that lesions failing dilatation are successfully treated with rotational atherectomy. Therefore, rotational atherectomy enables the successful treatment of selected lesions that previously were not amenable to percutaneous interventions. Failure to cross with a

balloon and failure to dilate a lesion represent the most clear-cut indications for rotational atherectomy.

Calcified Lesions

MacIsaac et al. reported data from 2,161 procedures on 1,078 calcified and 1,083 noncalcified lesions. The patients with calcified lesions had a mean age of 65.9 years, which was significantly older than the group with noncalcified lesions, whose mean age was 60.5 years ($p = .001$). The calcified lesions were located in tortuous vessels more frequently (27% versus 22%; $p = .02$), were more often eccentric (75% versus 64%; $p = .0001$), were longer (32% versus 27%; ≥ 10 mm in length; $p = .001$), were more frequently AHA/ACC lesion classification type C (26% versus 11%; $p = .0001$), and were more frequently located in the left anterior descending coronary artery (51% versus 44%; $p = .001$). There was no difference in procedural success between the two groups: 94.3% for calcified and 95.2% for noncalcified lesions. Complication rates were also similar in the two lesion subsets: 4.1% major complications for the calcified group and 3.1% in the noncalcified lesions (14).

Intravascular ultrasound has also demonstrated that the Rotablator effectively ablates calcified lesions, reducing the extent of the calcium arc within the lesion. In contrast, conventional PTCA and directional atherectomy are associated with reduced success and increased complications in moderately to heavily calcified lesions (36–40). Because of the reported high success rates and general clinical experience, rotational atherectomy has become the treatment of choice for moderate to heavily calcified lesions.

Ostial Lesions

Percutaneous balloon angioplasty has lower success rates and high restenosis rates for ostial lesions (41–43). Goudreau and coworkers reported a 97% success rate in the 31 ostial lesions they treated with rotational atherectomy. Complication rates were low, and the acute angiographic result was not influenced by lesion morphology (44). Kent and coworkers reported the registry data on 147 ostial lesions treated with rotational atherectomy. Procedural success was achieved in 93% of lesions, coronary artery bypass surgery was required in 3.4%, 2.1% died, and none had a Q-wave MI. Angiographic restenosis occurred in 47% of the patients (45). These results compare favorably with those of percutaneous balloon angioplasty, which has been reported to have a success rate of 75% to 88% in ostial lesions with a 10% to 13% major complication rate (41–43). The Rotablator is highly effective in treating ostial lesions, even when they are calcified.

Motwani et al. reported the results of rotational atherectomy in 111 consecutive patients with ostial right coronary artery lesions. The mean age of the patients was 66 ± 3 years, and 59% of the lesions had moderate to severe calcification. In 54% of the patients >1 lesion site was treated (mean 1.9 lesions per patient). Maximum burr-to-artery ratio was 64%, and adjunctive PTCA was utilized in 94% of lesions. Adjunctive stenting was used in only 5% of cases. Procedural success (<50% stenosis without death, QMI, or emergency bypass surgery) was 97.3%. In 1.8% of patients, there was an uncomplicated and unsuccessful procedure. One patient (0.9%) developed a Q-wave myocardial infarction. No patients died, and no patients had emergency bypass surgery. Final percent diame-

ter stenosis was 16 ± 10%. Clinical follow-up at 6.3 ± 0.6 months showed that only 12.9% of patients had recurrent angina due to angiographic restenosis (46).

Although data from prospective randomized trials in patients with ostial lesions is not available, rotational atherectomy has become one of the preferred treatment options for aorto-ostial calcified lesions and ostial lesions of side branches in vessels <3 mm in diameter (47–48). Figure 2.1 shows an example of a patient with an ostial diagonal artery lesion treated with rotational atherectomy.

Complex/Bifurcation Lesions

The Rotablator has a high success rate in complex lesions, as confirmed in the core-laboratory controlled, prospective randomized trials ERBAC (16) and STRATAS (11). In order to assess the influence of multiple angiographic risk factors on procedural success, we analyzed data on 874 lesions in the multicenter registry. The angiographic risk factors considered were lesion calcification, lesion eccentricity, lesion length >10 mm, stenosis severity >90%, the presence of a bifurcation location of the lesion, and proximal vessel tortuosity. The overall success rate was 95%. Individually, these angiographic risk factors did not reduce the success rate. Furthermore, success was not reduced by increasing lesion complexity. When no angiographic risk factor was present, the success rate was 96%. With one factor the success rate was 95%, with two factors 95%, and three factors 97% (p = NS) (28). These data suggest that the presence of one or more angiographic risk factors does not reduce procedural success, and that use of the Rotablator should be considered in complex lesions. Figure 2.2 shows Rotablation and stenting of a complex lesion in a high risk patient.

Bifurcation lesions are problematic for PTCA because plaque frequently shifts from one branch to the other, leaving suboptimal initial results and a high restenosis risk (49). Stenting has improved restenosis compared to PTCA in many lesion types, but restenosis with stenting of bifurcation lesions has remained high. Baim

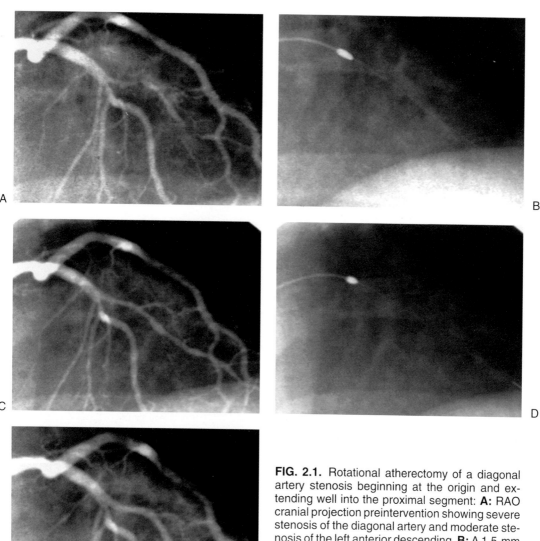

FIG. 2.1. Rotational atherectomy of a diagonal artery stenosis beginning at the origin and extending well into the proximal segment: **A:** RAO cranial projection preintervention showing severe stenosis of the diagonal artery and moderate stenosis of the left anterior descending. **B:** A 1.5-mm Rotablator burr is passed through the diagonal stenosis. **C:** An angiogram after the 1.5-mm Rotablator burr shows improvement in the stenosis. **D:** A 2.0-mm Rotablator burr is passed through the stenosis. **E:** The final angiogram shows good angiographic result without balloon dilatation.

(50) and Colombo (51) have recently advised debulking as the preferred treatment for bifurcation lesions.

Sequential rotablation of the two limbs of the bifurcation, followed by "kissing balloon" inflation, has become a common treatment in our laboratory. The most important limb of the bifurcation is approached first and generally treated with two sequential burr sizes. The Rotawire is then repositioned in the branch, and 1 to 2 burrs are used sequentially. The burr is removed, and a customary PTCA wire is then inserted into the major vessel along with an appropriately sized PTCA balloon. PTCA on the major branch is completed, and then a second PTCA balloon is passed over the Rotawire into the side branch.

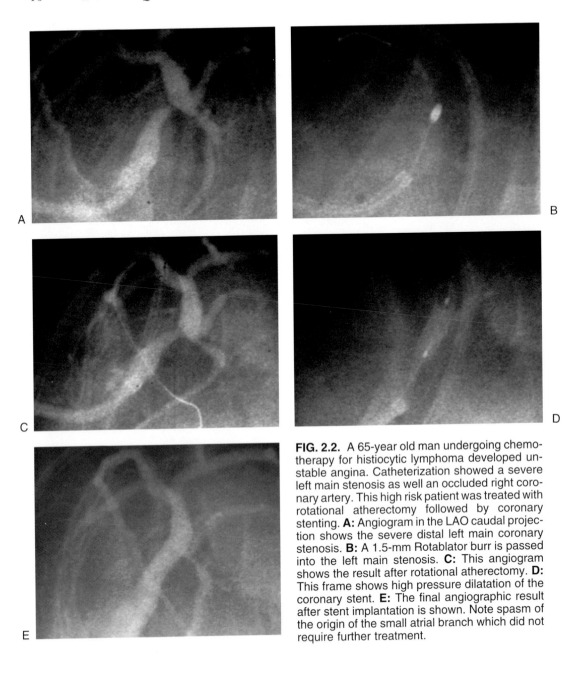

FIG. 2.2. A 65-year old man undergoing chemotherapy for histiocytic lymphoma developed unstable angina. Catheterization showed a severe left main stenosis as well an occluded right coronary artery. This high risk patient was treated with rotational atherectomy followed by coronary stenting. **A:** Angiogram in the LAO caudal projection shows the severe distal left main coronary stenosis. **B:** A 1.5-mm Rotablator burr is passed into the left main stenosis. **C:** This angiogram shows the result after rotational atherectomy. **D:** This frame shows high pressure dilatation of the coronary stent. **E:** The final angiographic result after stent implantation is shown. Note spasm of the origin of the small atrial branch which did not require further treatment.

PTCA is performed on the branch until a satisfactory result is obtained. Then a final inflation is made in both balloons simultaneously at 2 to 4 atm. Care is taken to deflate the balloons simultaneously, and a good result (<20% residual of both limbs) is expected. Figure 2.3 shows a bifurcation lesion treated with rotational atherectomy and adjunctive PTCA.

Diffuse In-Stent Restenosis

As coronary stenting has become the widely utilized treatment in most interventional laboratories, in-stent restenosis has emerged as a frequent and difficult clinical problem. Long areas of restenosis inside a stent have a notoriously high restenosis rate after PTCA (31). Debulking

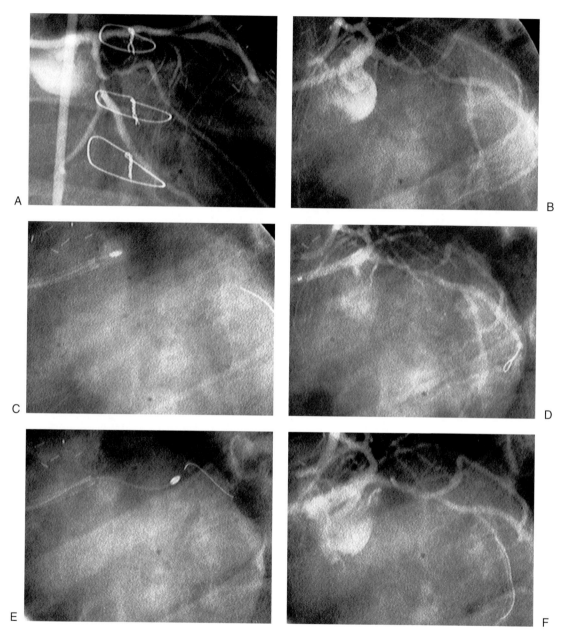

FIG. 2.3. Rotational atherectomy of a complex bifurcation lesion in the circumflex artery. **A:** RAO caudal view of the circumflex lesion. **B:** LAO caudal view of the circumflex bifurcation lesion. **C:** Rotational atherectomy with a 1.5-mm burr being directed down the AV portion of the left circumflex artery. **D:** Angiogram after rotablation of the AV circumflex artery with a 1.5-mm burr. **E:** 1.5-mm burr is next passed down the obtuse marginal branch. Note that the Rotablator wire is pulled back near the lesion in order to minimize guidewire bias. **F:** Angiogram after rotational atherectomy of both limbs of the bifurcation with 1.5-mm burr. *(Figure continues.)*

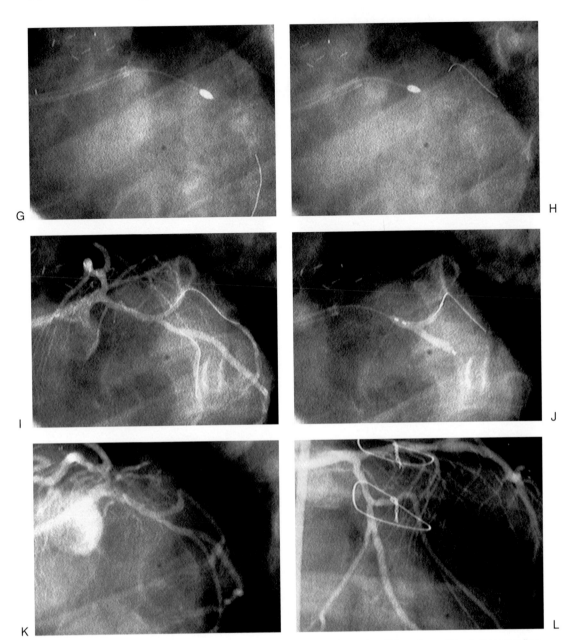

FIG. 2.3. *Continued.* **G:** A 2-mm Rotablator burr is passed down the AV portion of the left circumflex. **H:** The same 2-mm Rotablator burr is passed down the obtuse marginal branch. **I:** Angiogram after the 2.0-mm Rotablator burr is passed down both limbs of the bifurcation and another traditional angioplasty wire is passed into the AV portion of the circumflex in preparation for balloon dilatation. **J:** Kissing balloon dilatation of the bifurcation lesion. **K:** Final angiographic result in the LAO caudal projection. **L:** Final angiographic result in the RAO caudal projection.

TABLE 2.2. *Indications/contra-indications for rotational atherectomy*

Common indications	Relative contra-indications
Undilatable lesions	Ulcerated, thrombotic lesions
Calcified lesions	Spiral dissection lesions
Ostial lesions	Degenerated saphenous vein graft lesions
Complex/bifurcation lesions	De novo diffuse coronary lesions
Diffuse in-stent restenosis	Extremely angulated lesions
Debulking complex lesions before stenting	Lesions in patients with severely depressed left ventricular function

these lesions often gives an excellent angiographic result, and several single-center reports suggest a re-restenosis rate of approximately 30% (32,33). This 30% rate is better than expected for PTCA alone. Therefore, rotational atherectomy has become an accepted treatment for diffuse in-stent restenosis. However, the ultimate impact of rotational atherectomy on re-restenosis of coronary stents has yet to be confirmed in a randomized trial.

Rota/Stenting

Clinical experience has shown that pretreating calcified or complex lesions with the Rotablator prior to stenting provides easy stent placement and optimal stent expansion. Whether debulking with the Rotablator prior to stenting reduces restenosis, complications, and is cost-effective compared to PTCA and stenting is the subject of an ongoing randomized trial, Stent Implantation Post Rotational Atherectomy Trial (SPORT).

CONTRAINDICATIONS FOR ROTATIONAL ATHERECTOMY

Both theoretical concerns regarding the mechanical action of the rotating burr as well as early clinical experience have shown that specific lesion types should generally be avoided when using rotational atherectomy.

Lesions in Patients with Acute MI/ Ulcerated Plaque/Thrombus

Patients with acute coronary ischemic syndromes generally have an ulcerated plaque with overlying thrombus. The soft nature of an ulcer-

ated plaque might cause the lesion to deflect away from the rotating burr, and micro-pulverization of thrombus might release vasoactive materials and expose clot bound thrombin. Thus, rotational atherectomy might theoretically worsen the thrombotic process and exacerbate slow flow. Therefore thrombotic ulcerated lesions were excluded from the multicenter registry and most randomized trials using the Rotablator. If the culprit lesion in a patient with an acute coronary syndrome proves difficult to dilate or cannot be crossed with a balloon, then consideration could be given to using rotational atherectomy with adjunctive abciximab.

Although rotational atherectomy has been shown to activate platelets *in vitro,* platelet activation is significantly inhibited by abciximab (52,53). Theoretically, glycoprotein IIb/IIIa inhibitors might remove thrombus containing lesions from the list of exclusions with the Rotablator. However, clinical experience in this setting is scant and there is no obvious clinical benefit in using rotational atherectomy on thrombus containing lesions unless the lesion fails conventional dilatation attempts. In general, rotational atherectomy is best avoided in acute ischemic syndromes with ulcerated plaque and thrombus.

Lesions with Spiral Dissection

Theoretically, the rotating burr could entwine a dissection flap, extending and complicating the problem. Even though there are no case reports of such a phenomenon, and worsening of a dissection has never been seen by this observer, rotational atherectomy should be avoided in the presence of a spiral dissection.

Degenerated Saphenous Vein Graft Lesions

Embolization of debris from vein grafts is an important problem with PTCA, and was reported to be even higher with directional coronary atherectomy (54). Because of the loosely adherent material present in saphenous vein graft disease, rotational atherectomy might be expected to increase distal embolization as well. Because of this concern, rotational atherectomy is contraindicated in patients with diffuse saphenous vein graft lesions.

Lesions with Extreme Angulation

As discussed previously, the principle of differential cutting might be overwhelmed by guidewire and Rotablator drive shaft bias in cases of extreme angulation. This biased ablation may cause deep wall cutting or even coronary perforation. In order to minimize complications, lesions with extreme angulation should be avoided when using rotational atherectomy.

Diffuse Disease

Early in the clinical experience with Rotablator, lesions with diffuse disease were associated with a high rate of complications and the frequent occurrence of slow flow (55). However, evolution of Rotablator technique has made the approach to longer and longer lesions practical. Particular attention to short run times (<15 seconds), long waits between runs to allow for normalization of ST segments/chest pain, careful attention to not allow RPM drops <5,000 from baseline, a stepped burr approach, and addition of vasodilators to the Rotablator flush solution have helped make rotational atherectomy a safer procedure even in lesions 15 mm to 20 mm. However, for very long lesions (>30 mm), rotablation should be avoided because of an increased risk of slow flow (14,56). When approaching long (15 mm–25 mm) and calcified lesions, rotational atherectomy should be undertaken with focused attention to procedural details and only by an experienced operator.

Lesions in Patients with Depressed Left Ventricular Function

Williams et al. have documented worsening left ventricular regional wall motion in some patients undergoing rotational atherectomy (57). Because of the possibility of transient worsening of wall motion, patients with severe left ventricular dysfunction should be approached with great caution when using rotational atherectomy. Monitoring pulmonary artery pressure and intra-aortic balloon pump counterpulsation should be considered whenever the Rotablator is used in this clinical situation (58).

SUMMARY

Rotational coronary atherectomy with the Rotablator ablates coronary artery lesions, leaving a polished smooth lumen. The effectiveness and safety of the Rotablator have been proven by numerous studies. Indications for the use of the Rotablator include discrete lesions, especially those that are calcified; ostial, bifurcation, and complex lesions; and lesions unyielding to balloon dilation. The Rotablator is also useful in lesions with diffuse in-stent restenosis.

The Rotablator has widened the indications and improved the success of percutaneous coronary interventions. However, in the absence of randomized trials, its benefit over conventional therapy except in cases of PTCA failure has not been definitively proven. Several issues remain to be resolved, in particular the correct balance between the degree of high-speed rotational atherectomy required to facilitate balloon angioplasty or stenting, and the long-term cost-effectiveness of pre-stenting PTCA versus rotational atherectomy. The answer to these issues and the precise role of high-speed rotational atherectomy in coronary intervention will be defined in a series of ongoing and planned randomized clinical trials.

REFERENCES

1. Hansen DD, Auth DC, Vracko R, Ritchie JL. Rotational atherectomy in atherosclerotic rabbit iliac arteries. *Am Heart J* 1988;115(1 Pt 1):160–165.
2. Ahn SS, Auth D, Marcus DR, Moore WS. Removal of

focal atheromatous lesions by angioscopically guided high-speed rotary atherectomy. Preliminary experimental observations. *J Vasc Surg* 1988;7(2)**:**292–300.

3. MacIsaac AI, Whitlow PW. Rotablator. In: Topol EJ, Serruys PW, eds. *Current review of interventional cardiology.* 2nd ed. Philadelphia: *Current Medicine*, 1995: 147–158.

4. Dussaillant GR, Mintz GS, Pichard AD et al. Effect of rotational atherectomy in noncalcified atherosclerotic plaque: a volumetric intravascular ultrasound study. *J Am Coll Cardiol* 1996;28(4)**:**856–860.

5. Braden GA, Bailey RJ, Fitzgerald DM, Young T, Utley L, Applegate RJ. Mechanisms of bradyarrhythmias associated with rotational atherectomy. *J Am Coll Cardiol* 1996;27**:**168a.

6. Reisman M, DeVore LJ, Ferguson M, Kirkman T, Shuman B. Analysis of heat generation during high-speed rotational ablation: technical implications. *J Am Coll Cardiol* 1996;27**:**292.

7. Reisman M. Technique and strategy of rotational atherectomy. *Cath Cardiovasc Diag* 1996;(Suppl)(3)**:**2–14.

8. Reisman M, Harms V. Guidewire bias: potential source of complications with rotational atherectomy. *Cath Cardiovasc Diag* 1996;(Suppl)(3)**:**64–68.

9. Safian RD, Freed M, Lichtenberg A et al. Are residual stenoses after excimer laser angioplasty and coronary atherectomy due to inefficient or small devices? Comparison with balloon angioplasty. *J Am Coll Cardiol* 1993;22(6)**:**1628–1634.

10. Safian RD, Niazi KA, Strzelecki M et al. Detailed angiographic analysis of high-speed mechanical rotational atherectomy in human coronary arteries. *Circulation* 1993;88(3)**:**961–968.

11. Bass TA, Whitlow PL, Moses JW et al. Acute complications related to coronary rotational atherectomy strategy: a report from the STRATAS trial. *J Am Coll Cardiol* 1997;29(Suppl A)**:**314.

12. Whitlow PL, Buchbinder M, Kent K, Kipperman R, Bass T, Cleman M. Coronary rotational atherectomy: angiographic risk factors and their relation to success/ complications. *J Am Coll Cardiol* 1992;19**:**334A.

13. Safian RD, Freed M, Reddy V et al. Do excimer laser angioplasty and rotational atherectomy facilitate balloon angioplasty? Implications for lesion-specific coronary intervention. *J Am Coll Cardiol* 1996;27(3)**:**552–529.

14. MacIsaac AI, Bass TA, Buchbinder M et al. High speed rotational atherectomy: outcome in calcified and noncalcified coronary artery lesions. *J Am Coll Cardiol* 1995;26(3)**:**731–736.

15. Warth DC, Leon MB, W ON, Zacca N, Polissar NL, Buchbinder M. Rotational atherectomy multicenter registry: acute results, complications and 6-month angiographic follow-up in 709 patients. *J Am Coll Cardiol* 1994;24(3)**:**641–648.

16. Reifart N, Vandormael M, Krajcar M et al. Randomized comparison of angioplasty of complex coronary lesions at a single center. Excimer Laser, Rotational Atherectomy, and Balloon Angioplasty Comparison (ERBAC) Study. *Circulation* 1997;96(1)**:**91–98.

17. Whitlow PW, Cowley MJ, Kuntz RE, Williams DO, Bass TA, Kipperman RM. Study to determine Rotablator and transluminal angioplasty strategy (STRATAS). *Circulation* 1996;94(Suppl 1)**:**435.

18. Eccleston DS, M.C. H, M.J. C, Kuntz RE, Williams DO, Whitlow PL. Is there a role for strip chart recording to guide rotational atherectomy? *J Am Coll Cardiol* 1996; 27(Suppl A)**:**292A.

19. Horrigan MC, Eccleston DS, Williams DO, Lasorda DM, Moses JW, Whitlow PL. Technique dependence of CKMB elevation after rotational atherectomy. 94. 1996;94(Suppl 1)**:**560.

20. Kuntz RE, Gibson CM, Nobuyoshi M, Baim DS. A generalized model of restenosis after conventional balloon angioplasty, stenting, and directional atherectomy. *J Am Coll Cardiol* 1993;21**:**15–25.

21. Kuntz RE, Safian RD, Carrozza JP, Fishman RF, Mansour M, Baim DS. The importance of acute luminal diameter in determining restenosis after coronary atherectomy or stenting. *Circulation* 1992;86(6)**:**1827–1835.

22. Brener S, Reifart N, Whitlow PL. The status of three randomized trials: STRATAS, DART, ERBAC. In: Serruys PW, Holmes DL, eds. *Current review of interventional cardiology.* Philadelphia: Current Medicine, 1997:13–21 (vol 3).

23. Hong MK, Mintz GS, Popma JJ et al. Safety and efficacy of elective stent implantation following rotational atherectomy in large calcified coronary arteries. *Cath Cardiovasc Diag* 1996;(Suppl)(3)**:**50–54.

24. Stertzer SH, Pomerantsev EV, Fitzgerald PJ et al. Effects of technique modification on immediate results of high speed rotational atherectomy in 710 procedures on 656 patients. *Cathet Cardiovasc Diagn* 1995;36**:** 304–310.

25. Ellis SG, Popma JJ, Buchbinder M et al. Relation of clinical presentation, stenosis morphology, and operator technique to the procedural results of rotational atherectomy and rotational atherectomy-facilitated angioplasty. *Circulation* 1994;89**:**882–892.

26. Reisman M, Shuman B, Fei R, Dillard D, Nguyen S, Gordon L. Analysis and comparison of platelet aggregation with high-speed rotational atherectomy. *J Am Coll Cardiol* 1997;29(Suppl A)**:**186A.

27. Zotz RJ, Erbel R, Philipp A et al. High-speed rotational angioplasty-induced echo contrast in vivo and in vitro optical analysis. *Cath Cardiovasc Diag* 1992;26(2)**:** 98–109.

28. MacIsaac AI, Whitlow PL, Cowley MJ, Buchbinder M. Angiographic predictors of outcome of coronary rotational atherectomy from the completed multicenter registry. *J Am Coll Cardiol* 1994**:**353A.

29. Ellis SE, Franco I, Satler LF, Whitlow PL. Slow reflow and coronary perforation after Rotablator therapy-incidence, clinical, angiographic and procedural predictors. *Circulation* 1992;86**:**I-652.

30. Sutton J, Raymond R, Ellis S. Coronary artery perforation: risk factors and management. In: Topol EJ, ed. *Textbook of Interventional Cardiology.* Philadelphia: WB Saunders, 1993:576–599.

31. Yokoi H, Kimura T, Nagakawa Y, Nosaka H, Nobuyoshi M. Long-term clinical and quantitative angiographic follow-up after the Palmaz-Schatz stent restenosis. *J Am Coll Cardiol* 1996;27**:**224A.

32. Stone GW. Rotational atherectomy for treatment of in-stent restenosis: role of intracoronary ultrasound guidance. *Cath Cardiovasc Diag* 1996;(Suppl)(3)**:**73–77.

33. Bottner RK, Hardigan KR. High-speed rotational ablation for in-stent restenosis. *Cath Cardiovasc Diag* 1997; 40(2)**:**144–149.

34. Belli G, Whitlow PL. Should we spark interest in rota-

tional atherectomy for in-stent restenosis? *Cath Cardiovasc Diag* 1997;40(2):150–151.

35. Brogan WCd, Popma JJ, Pichard AD et al. Rotational coronary atherectomy after unsuccessful coronary balloon angioplasty. *Am J Cardiol* 1993;71(10):794–798.

36. Ellis SG, Vandormael MG, Cowley MJ et al. Coronary morphologic and clinical determinants of procedural outcome with angioplasty for multivessel coronary disease: implications for patient selection. *Circulation* 1990;82:1193–1202.

37. Myler RK, Shaw RE, Stertzer SH et al. Lesion morphology and coronary angioplasty: current experience and analysis. *J Am Coll Cardiol* 1992;19(7):1641–1652.

38. Ellis SG, De Cesare NB, Pinkerton CA et al. Relation of stenosis morphology and clinical presentation to the procedural results of directional coronary atherectomy (see comments). *Circulation* 1991;84:644–653.

39. Lee RT, Loree HM, Cheng GC, Lieberman EH, Jaramillo N, Schoen FJ. Computational structural analysis based on intravascular ultrasound imaging before in vitro angioplasty: prediction of plaque fracture locations. *J Am Coll Cardiol* 1993;21(3):777–782.

40. Fitzgerald PJ, Ports TA, Yock PG. Contribution of localized calcium deposits to dissection after angioplasty. An observational study using intravascular ultrasound (see comments). *Circulation* 1992;86(1):64–70.

41. Topol EJ, Ellis SG, Fishman J et al. Multicenter study of percutaneous transluminal angioplasty for right coronary artery ostial stenosis. *J Am Coll Cardiol* 1987;9(6):1214–1218.

42. Mathias DW, Mooney JF, Lange HW, Goldenberg IF, Gobel FL, Mooney MR. Frequency of success and complications of coronary angioplasty of a stenosis at the ostium of a branch vessel. *Am J Cardiol* 1991;67(6):491–495.

43. Bedotto JB, McConahay DR, Rutherford BD. Balloon angioplasty of aortoostial coronary stenosis revised. *Circulation* 1991;84(Suppl II):251.

44. Goudreau E, Cowley MJ, DiSciascio G, DeBottis D, Vetrovec GW, Sabri N. Rotational atherectomy for aorto-ostial and branch-ostial lesions. *J Am Coll Cardiol* 1993;21:31A.

45. Kent KM, Stertzer S, Bass T, Cowley M. High-speed rotational ablation in patients with ostial lesions. *Circulation* 1992;86:I-512.

46. Motawni JG, Raymond RE, Franco I et al. Rotational atherectomy of right coronary ostial stenosis: procedure of choice based on long-term clinical outcome? *J Am Coll Cardiol* 1997;29(Suppl A):498A.

47. Koller PT, Freed M, Grines CL, WW ON. Success, complications, and restenosis following rotational and transluminal extraction atherectomy of ostial stenoses. *Cath Cardiovasc Diag* 1994;31(4):255–260.

48. Zimarino M, Corcos T, Favereau X et al. Rotational coronary atherectomy with adjunctive balloon angioplasty for the treatment of ostial lesions. *Cath Cardiovasc Diag* 1994;33(1):22–27.

49. Whitlow PL. Ostial and Bifurcation Lesions. In: Topol EJ, ed. *Textbook of Interventional Cardiology*. Philadelphia: WB Saunders, 1999:317–334. vol 3).

50. Baim DS. Is bifurcation stenting the answer? *Cath Cardiovasc Diag* 1996;37(3):314–316.

51. DiMario C, Colombo A. Trouser-stents: how to choose the right size and shape? *Cath Cardiovasc Diag* 1997;41:197–199.

52. Reisman M, Shuman B, Fei R, Dillard D, Nguyen S, Gordon L. Analysis and comparison of platelet aggregation with high-speed rotational atherectomy. *J Am Coll Cardiol* 1997;29(Suppl A):186A.

53. Williams MS, Coller BS, Vaananen HJ, Scudder LE, Sharma SK, Marmur JD. Activation of platelets in platelet-rich plasma by rotablation is speed-dependent and can be inhibited by abciximab (c7E3 Fab; ReoPro). *Circulation* 1998;98(8):742–748.

54. Holmes DRJ, Topol EJ, Califf RM et al. A multicenter, randomized trial of coronary angioplasty versus directional atherectomy for patients with saphenous vein bypass graft lesions. *Circulation* 1995;91:1966–1974.

55. Teirstein PS, Warth DC, Haq N et al. High speed rotational coronary atherectomy for patients with diffuse coronary artery disease (see comments). *J Am Coll Cardiol* 1991;18(7):1694–1701. 56. Whitlow PL. Rotablator technique and complications? *Cathet Cardiovasc Diagn* 1995;36:311–312.

57. Williams MJ, Dow CJ, Newell JB, Palacios IF, Picard MH. Prevalence and timing of regional myocardial dysfunction after rotational coronary atherectomy. *J Am Coll Cardiol* 1996;28(4):861–869.

58. O'Murchu B, Foreman RD, Shaw RE, Brown DL, Peterson KL, Buchbinder M. Role of intraaortic balloon pump counterpulsation in high risk coronary rotational atherectomy. *J Am Coll Cardiol* 1995;26(5):1270–1275.

3

Stents

A. The Gianturco-Roubin II (GR-II) Intracoronary Stent

Larry S. Dean

Division of Cardiovascular Diseases, University of Alabama at Birmingham,
Birmingham, Alabama 35294-0001

In the early years following the introduction of coronary angioplasty by Gruentzig in 1977 (1), the procedure was plagued by a relatively high technical failure rate, both from design limitations of early guide catheters, guide wires, and PTCA balloons as well as acute closure of the coronary lesion due to coronary dissection. The incidence of acute vessel closure varies from 5%–10%, depending primarily on lesion characteristics (2–4).

Although there were several novel approaches intended to address the problem of acute closure following coronary angioplasty, none were highly successful until the advent of intracoronary stenting for this indication.

Animal studies begun in the mid-1980's culminated in the first implantations of the Gianturco-Roubin stent in 1987 in a small group of patients destined to undergo coronary artery bypass grafting following failed angioplasty (5). This study was designed to evaluate the feasibility of stenting in patients with failed PTCA. Subsequently, a registry was begun to evaluate the efficacy of intracoronary stenting for the treatment of acute or threatened closure. This led to the approval by the Food and Drug Administration (FDA) of the original Gianturco-Roubin coil stent (GR-I) in June 1993.

Despite advances in the treatment of compli-cations following coronary stenting (6) and a better understanding of appropriate stent placement technique and post stent patient management (7,8,9), all stents have potential drawbacks.

There were several limitations noted with the GR-I stent (Table 3.1). The GR-II stent was designed to improve profile, trackability, visibility (Fig. 3.1), and surface area coverage compared to the GR-I stent (Table 3.1). There were also improvements in the stent delivery system, including a semi-compliant balloon and improved profile. The device was also now compatible with 6 Fr guiding catheters.

This led to a large, multi-center, randomized trial and several registries sponsored by Cook, Inc. (Bloomington, NJ), which ultimately included over 2,000 patients. The GR-II stent was approved by the FDA for acute or threatened closure in June 1996.

PRIOR CLINICAL EXPERIENCE WITH THE GR-II STENT

Cook, Inc. began clinical trials of the GR-II stent in early 1993. This included a randomized trial comparing the GR-II stent to the Palmaz-Schatz (Johnson and Johnson, Cordis, Miami, FL) stent. This trial enrolled 755 patients divided equally between the GR-II and the Palmaz-

TABLE 3.1. *Comparison of GR-I and GR-II stents*

Stent property	GR-I	GR-II
Material	316L stainless steel	316L stainless steel
Coating	No	Yes
Radiopacity	+	+ + + with markers
Stent design	Round wire	Flat sheet
Stent thickness (in)	0.006	0.005
Surface area	13%	16%
Flexibility	+	+ + + +
Guide catheter	8 Fr	6 Fr, 7 Fr
Guide wire (in.)	0.018 extra support	0.014 floppy (0.18 compatible)
Diameter	2.5–4.0 mm	2.5–4.0 mm
Lengths	12 and 20 mm	20 and 40 mm

+, minimal; + + +, maximal.

Schatz stent. The lesions randomized were generally very complex. Included in this study were patients with very long lesions and patients with multi-vessel disease. Multiple stents were allowed and analysis of this trial has been difficult and somewhat controversial.

Although the angiographic restenosis rate in the GR-II stent in the overall randomized trial was significantly higher than the Johnson and Johnson stent (10), there were several issues that make interpretation of the randomized trial difficult. Despite the manufacturer recommending that the GR-II stent placed be 0.5 mm larger than the proximal reference vessel diameter, approximately two-thirds of stents placed in this trial were undersized by this definition. Combined with a greater degree of stent recoil, a higher

restenosis rate could have been expected. In addition, the incidence of target lesion revascularization varied widely among the centers involved in the trial, making combining of and analysis of the data problematic. Although the overall trial showed superiority of the Johnson and Johnson stent to the GR-II stent for reduction of restenosis, subgroup analysis of appropriately sized stents (0.5 mm larger than the visually estimated proximal reference vessel diameter) showed equivalent TLR rates in follow-up (Figs. 3.2, 3.3). The company elected not to pursue the

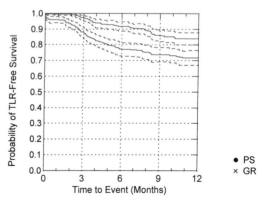

FIG. 3.2. Kaplan-Meier estimates of the probability of target lesion revascularization (TRL) in the GR-II randomized trial. Ninety-five percent confidence limits are indicated by the *dashed lines.* There is clear separation of TLR-free survival at 6 and 12 months. *The upper line* represents the TLR-free survival in the Palmaz-Schatz arm of the trial and the *lower line* represents the GR-II arm.

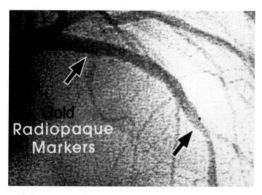

FIG. 3.1. An RAO projection of a GR-II stent placed in the left anterior descending coronary artery. Note the gold stent markers at the proximal and distal ends of the stent.

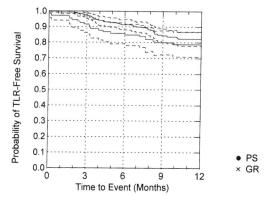

FIG. 3.3. The probability of TLR survival in patients in which a correctly sized GR-II stent has been placed. The *upper solid line* represents the Palmaz-Schatz arm and the *lower line* represents the "correctly sized" GR-II arm. See text for details regarding correct sizing of the GR-II stent. There is clear overlap of the 95% confidence intervals throughout follow-up ($p = .30$). This suggests, in appropriately-sized GR-II stents, that TLR rates are similar to the Palmaz-Schatz stent in follow-up out to 12 months.

indication of reduction of restenosis for the GR-II stent. Several registries also examined the use of this stent in small vessels, vein grafts, restenotic lesions, and in acute/threatened closure.

The focus of this paper is with regard to the indications for use of the GR-II stent in the treatment of acute or threatened closure. A registry of 249 patients with acute or threatened closure led to the approval of this stent in June 1996. As seen with the original GR-I stent, the GR-II resulted in a marked improvement, over historical controls, in the incidence of acute myocardial infarction, and in the need for emergency bypass surgery in patients with acute or threatened closure. Emergency CABG and acute Q-wave MI occurred in 0.8 and 1.3%, respectively. Death occurred in 0.8% at 30 days (11). Acute thrombosis of the stented vessel occurred in 2.9%. Bleeding requiring transfusion occurred in only 2.1% at 30 days, a substantial improvement over the GR-I experience for this indication.

CURRENT IMPLANTATION TECHNIQUE

In the setting of acute or threatened closure, the use of the GR-II stent is quite straight-forward. All devices, including the 4-mm-diameter device, can be placed with a 7 Fr guiding catheter. The 3.5-mm and smaller diameter devices can be placed through currently available 6 Fr guiding catheters. The GR-II stent can be placed over standard 0.014-inch flexible guide wires without difficulty. It does not require extra support guide wires unless severe tortuosity is present. The presence of radiopaque markers at the proximal and distal ends of the stent helps in the accurate placement of the stent. The markers allow very accurate and precise placement, avoiding residual uncovered dissection flaps. Because of the low profile of the delivery catheter, coronary injection during placement is also facilitated with this stent.

This device, as with the previous GR-I stent, should not be undersized. The GR-II is a coil-design flat wire with a clam shell configuration (Fig. 3.4), as previously described (12). If the stent is undersized, subsequent balloon inflation with appropriately-sized balloons may open the clam shell, allowing prolapse of dissection flaps into the lumen of the stented vessel. Although this is generally not catastrophic, in that additional stents can be placed within the previously placed stent, appropriate sizing will avoid this potential problem. Although stent recoil with this device is lower than with the GR-I stent, nonetheless, there is proximally 18% recoil with the GR-II stent. Therefore, in addition to the concerns about undersizing and opening of the clam shell design, it is also critically important to appropriately size this device at approximately one-half millimeter larger than a proximal refer-

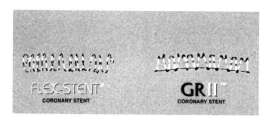

FIG. 3.4. The first-generation GR-I stent in comparison to the GR-II stent. Note the clamshell configuration common to both stents and the flat wire design with a spine running the length of the GR-II stent. This yields improved stent integrity.

ence vessel diameter to compensate for recoil and to avoid undersizing. As seen in Fig. 3.3, proper placement of this device results in TLR rates at 12 months similar to those of the Palmaz-Schatz stent. Undersizing the device will result in excessive TLR rates in follow-up.

Generally, the stent delivery balloon is used only to place the device. Approximately 4 atm to 6 atm should be used. Because of the length of the underlying balloon, it is important not to overinflate it, because this may result in proximal or distal tears in the stented vessel. Following placement of the stent, the delivery balloon is removed and subsequent higher pressure inflations are performed (approximately 12 atm to 16 atm). This should result in complete expansion of the device. We have seen (13), as have others (14), that there is continued increase in cross sectional lumen area with higher balloon pressures.

Following placement of the GR-II stent, patients are managed with aspirin and ticlopidine (Ticlid). Ticlid is discontinued at approximately 4 weeks and aspirin is continued indefinitely. There is only limited experience with this stent using clopidogrel (Plavix). Patients are typically discharged the following day.

CURRENT CLINICAL USE—ACUTE OR THREATENED CLOSURE

The GR-II stent is particularly useful in patients with diffuse disease where significant dissections have occurred. Because it is available in 20- and 40-mm lengths, it is possible to place a single long stent in a severe spiral-type dissection. This allows speedy treatment for long dissections. It is also potentially cost effective, because a single device can be used in long dissections, rather than several multiple shorter stents.

With significant dissections in bifurcation lesions such as the left anterior descending/diagonal or circumflex/marginal, this stent tends to preserve side branch access more readily than stents of the slotted tube design (e.g., the Johnson and Johnson Crown stent). Following placement of the stent in the primary and dissected vessel, the side branch can usually be reaccessed

if additional interventional work is required. If dissections extend into the bifurcation, this stent is useful because it can be precisely placed into the side branch using the stent markers, which are highly visible.

Because of the excellent flexibility of this device, it is particularly useful in situations where significant dissections have occurred in very distal and tortuous locations. This is particularly helpful in patients who are unstable, where rapid correction of significant dissections is important.

Since this stent is available in dimensions of 2.5 mm diameter by 20 mm length, it is also useful in smaller vessels where significant dissections have occurred. It remains one of the few stents available in this diameter and the only one approved for use in acute or threatened vessel closure. Despite concerns over increased restenosis rates in small vessels (15) faced with a significant acute dissection, restenosis becomes secondary to reestablishment of appropriate flow in smaller diameter but critical coronary vessels.

Although the device should not be used in ostial lesions, the combination of a more rigid stent (e.g., Johnson and Johnson Crown) with the GR-II is sometimes helpful in spiral dissections that originate in an ostial location. Likewise, it should not be used in vessels larger than 4.0 mm because undersizing will allow opening of the "clamshell," leaving dissected areas potentially uncovered.

FUTURE DIRECTIONS

Although both the GR-I and the GR-II stent have had a profound impact on the treatment of significant dissection following PTCA, these devices nonetheless represent initial steps in the direction toward the perfect device for all indications. To date, this device does not exist.

With this in mind, Cook, Inc., will shortly be embarking on the evaluation of a next generation stent, the Supra [3]. This is a departure from previous coil designs and represents the first slotted-tube design from Cook, Inc. Trials using this device are scheduled to begin in early 1999. It will offer significant advantages over the coil stent design, with maintenance of flexibility, trackability, low profile, and less recoil.

REFERENCES

1. Gruentzig AR, Senning A, Siegenthaler WE. Non-operative dilatation of coronary artery stenoses. *New Eng J Med* 1979; 301:61.
2. Ellis SG, Vandormael MG, Cowley MJ et al. The Multi-Vessel Angioplasty Prognosis Study Group. Coronary morphologic and clinical determinants, procedural outcome with angioplasty for multi-vessel coronary disease. Implications for patient selection. *Circulation* 1990;82:1193.
3. Deitre KE, Holmes DR, Jr., Holubakov R et al. Incidence and consequence of peri-procedural occlusion. The 1985–1986 NHLB PTCA Registry. *Circulation* 1990;82:839.
4. Ellis SG, Roubin GS, King SB, III et al. In hospital cardiac mortality after acute closure after coronary angioplasty. Analysis of risk factors from 8,207 procedures. *J Am Coll Cardio* 1988;11:211.
5. Roubin GS, Douglas JS, Jr, Lembo NJ et al. Intra-coronary stenting for acute closure following percutaneous transluminal coronary angioplasty. *Circulation* 1998; 78(Suppl 1):407.
6. Agarwal R, Agrawal SK, Roubin GS et al. Clinically guided closure of femoral artery pseudoaneurysms complicating cardiac catheterization and coronary angioplasty. *Cathet Cardiovasc Diagn* 1993;30:96.
7. Goods CM, Al-Shaibi KF, Yadav SS et al. Utilization of coronary balloon expandable coil stent without anti-coagulation or intravascular ultrasound. *Circulation* 1996;93:1803.
8. Albiero R, Rau T, Schluter M et al. Comparison of immediate and intermediate term results of intravascular ultrasound versus angiography-guided Palmaz-Schatz stent implantation in matched lesions. *Circulation* 1997; 96:2997.
9. Schomig A, Neumann FJ, Kastrati A et al A Randomized comparison of anti-platelet and anti-coagulant therapy after the placement of coronary artery stents. *New Eng J Med* 1996;334:1084.
10. Dean LS, Holmes DR, Roubin GS et al. One year Follow-up: the effect of proper stent size on clinical outcome. *Am J Cardiol* 1998;82(Suppl 7A):69S.
11. George BS, Yakubov SJ, O'Shaughnessy CD et al. Early and late outcome following treatment of acute or threatened closure with the GR-II coronary stent. *Am J Cardiol* 1997;80:7A.
12. Rodriguez A, Roubin GS. The Gianturco-Roubin II (GR-II) stent. In: Serruys PW, Kutryk MJB, eds. *Handbook of coronary stents*. 2nd ed. :Martin Dunitz Ltd. 1998.
13. Jain SP, Liu MW, Iyer SS et al. Do high pressure balloon inflations improve acute gain within flexible metallic coil stents? An intravascular ultrasound assessment. *J Am Coll Cardio* 1995; February Special Issue:49A.
14. Colombo A, Hall P, Nakamura S et al. Intra-coronary stenting without anticoagulation accomplished with intravascular ultrasound guidance. *Circulation* 1995;91: 1676.
15. Zidar JP, O'Shaughnessy CD, Dean LS et al. Elective GR-II stenting in small vessels: multi-center results. *J Am Coll Cardio* 1998;31(A):274A.

B. The Medtronic Wiktor Coronary Stent

Kirk N. Garratt

Adult Cardiac Catheterization Laboratory, St. Mary's Hospital, Mayo Clinic and Mayo Foundation, Department of Medicine, Rochester, Minnesota 55905

The utility of coronary stents in the treatment of failed coronary angioplasty and to reduce restenosis has been established, and high stent utilization rates reflect the enthusiasm for these devices today. However, stent use was initially hampered by several technical factors. The relatively large profile of first-generation (and even some second-generation) coronary stents limited their ability to advance smoothly through small-caliber guide catheters and tortuous coronary segments proximal to the target vascular segment. Accurate positioning within a coronary segment was problematic owing to poor stent visibility with routine fluoroscopy for some stent designs. Also, most coronary stents (including all those approved for use in the United States so far) have been constructed of stainless steel or other metals, which are known to have significant thrombogenicity. Although the issue of stent thrombosis has been addressed satisfactorily through refinement in medical therapies (1) use of stents constructed of materials with less thrombogenic potential may be beneficial.

Today, stent design refinements and advances in adjunctive medical therapies have resolved most of the concerns raised initially about stent use. Second- and third-generation stents, now available, offer superior performance and demonstrate improved clinical outcomes relative to earlier stents. However, the history of coronary stent use, albeit short, is enlightening with respect to the direction and focus of current stent design and handling issues. This chapter will review the course of a first-generation stent to examine not just the utility of the product, but also how advanced stent designs have been (and presumably will continue to be) affected by the successes and failures of first-generation stent designs.

WIKTOR STENT DESIGN AND CONSTRUCTION

The History of the Wiktor Stent Concept

In the mid-1980's, a successful engineer named Dominic Wiktor experienced acute abdominal pain and was found to have an abdominal aortic dissection. He was advised to have it repaired promptly, and so underwent vascular surgical repair. The surgery was successful, but the experience left him wondering if there wasn't an easier way to resolve what seemed to be a straightforward mechanical problem. He learned about the earlier efforts to develop endoluminal prosthetic devices, and after a short while he had a design for what he envisioned would be a practical alternative to abdominal vascular surgery for aortic dissections. He formed a partnership with Medtronic, Inc (Minneapolis, MN) to develop a functional product. Noting the much larger population of patients requiring treatment of coronary artery disease, and the limitations posed by abrupt vascular closure and restenosis for patients treated with balloon angioplasty, a decision was made to pursue a smaller version of Dominic Wiktor's endo-

prosthesis aimed at coronary use. The Medtronic Wiktor stent was created.

Design Characteristics

The Medtronic Wiktor stent design is a balloon-expandable, single filament, flexible coil stent. The stent is constructed by forming a single metallic strand into a sinusoidal wave, then forming a helical cylinder from this wave (Fig. 3.5). The only anchoring points are at the ends of the stent, where the ends of the filament are looped loosely around the body of the stent. Thus, the stent represents a relatively free helical three-dimensional geometry. Compression of the sinusoidal waves (increasing the "frequency" of the waveform) allows the stent to be compressed onto a delivery balloon, while distention with the delivery balloon expands the stent by widening these waves (decreasing the "frequency" of the waveform).

The metallic filament used in construction of the Medtronic Wiktor stent (Medtronic Inc., Minneapolis, MN) is a 0.005-inch (0.127-mm) thickness strand of tantalum, a non-ferromagnetic element with physical properties similar to tungsten. Its malleability, high plasticity, and low elasticity are desirable properties for stent formation. Furthermore, and most distinctively, tantalum has high density, which attenuates X-ray significantly. Consequently, even thin filaments of tantalum are easily visible under low-intensity fluoroscopy. To date, tantalum is the best material identified for manufacturing when a highly radio-opaque thin structure is desired. The first Medtronic Wiktor stents were manufactured in 1987 and used in animal experiments (2). The original Medtronic Wiktor stent was constructed such that there were between 3 and 3.5 sinusoidal waves per turn of the helix (i.e., once around the delivery balloon). In the

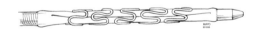

FIG. 3.5. Illustration of the Medtronic Wiktor stent. A sinusoidal wave of tantalum is wrapped in a helical fashion around a deployment balloon catheter.

United States, this stent was mounted on an existing Medtronic angioplasty balloon catheter, the Prime Balloon (Medtronic). This standard over-the-wire balloon catheter was designed in the early 1980s, and so reflected an older style of angioplasty balloon catheter. Nonetheless, the catheter proved to have desirable characteristics as a stent delivery chassis despite its relatively larger profile and bulk. A 16-mm length of Medtronic Wiktor stent mounted onto a 23-mm-long Prime balloon catheter served as the stent delivery system used in the North American studies of this stent. The stent was available in diameters between 3.0 mm and 4.5 mm.

Two modifications to this system followed quickly. In view of the rising use of rapid-exchange/single operator systems in European and Asian markets, Medtronic mounted the Wiktor stent onto an early generation Medtronic rapid-exchange balloon catheter, the GX. This catheter also had a lower profile than the Prime balloon, which meant it had superior handling characteristics and could be advanced through smaller guide catheters. The Medtronic Wiktor GX has been used extensively in Europe and Japan. The other modification was in the density of sinusoidal waves, which was increased to approximately four per turn on the delivery balloon. This version of the Wiktor stent design, designated the Wiktor-*i*, covered approximately 8 to 9.5% of the luminal surface as compared with the original Wiktor design, which covered between 7 and 9%. The Wiktor-*i*, also known as the "dense wave" Wiktor, is available in 10-, 15-, 20-, and 30-mm lengths in diameters ranging from 2.5 mm to 4.0 mm (2).

Following approval of the Medtronic Wiktor Prime stent in North America in 1994, Medtronic responded to complaints about the "clunky" nature of the old balloon delivery chassis (by this time, the balloon catheter reflected a 10-year-old technology) by offering the 16-mm Wiktor stent on a much improved delivery balloon catheter—the Rival (Medtronic). The 23-mm-long Rival balloon catheter has a significantly lower profile, is more easily tracked than the Prime balloon, and can be used to deliver 3.0-mm Wiktor stents through 6 Fr guide catheters. Larger stents require 7 Fr

guides. The Wiktor Rival stent is the version of this stent available commercially in the United States at the time of this writing.

All Medtronic Wiktor stents are available only as unsheathed, pre-mounted delivery systems. Although some operators have reported anecdotally on the use of hand-mounted Wiktor stents (achieved by stripping the stent from its intended delivery catheter and re-mounting on a different balloon catheter), this stent design is easily deformed and does not lend itself to much manipulation.

The free helical design of this stent permits it to track well, thus increasing its ability to pass into distal, tortuous vascular beds. However, the trade-off is in the inherent delicacy this design entails; the free-floating (i.e., unanchored) helical structure allows the stent to be damaged easily, especially by shortening of the stent along its long axis. The principal handling complaint regarding this stent is the ease with which it can be damaged, by impacting delivery catheter components, atheromatous plaque, or other stents already in position. A silver lining in this cloud is that the excellent radio-opacity of this stent permits any problem to be recognized easily, and if stent retrieval is necessary, the stent can be visualized easily.

Some operators speculated that the "flimsy" design of the Wiktor stent must mean that the stent has poor radial strength; i.e., the stent must be easily deformed when a collapsing pressure is applied around its short axis. We have conducted radial collapsing pressure tolerance experiments with the Medtronic Wiktor stent and a variety of other stent types, and have found that the helical sinusoidal wave configuration provides this stent with excellent radial collapse pressure resistance. In fact, the Wiktor stent's ability to resist collapsing forces matches or exceeds that of the Johnson and Johnson Interventional System (JJIS) stent (3).

CLINICAL TRIALS

In the late 1980's, there was great uncertainty about how coronary stents might best be used, if used at all. Richard Schatz and Julio Palmaz formed a partnership with Johnson and Johnson to develop a stent for the purpose of reducing restenosis. This bold decision was made without the benefit of knowledge now available regarding mechanisms of restenosis (4). Intimal hyperplasia was believed to be the sole explanation for restenosis, vascular remodeling was a developing concept, and the early animal experiments indicated that flexible stent placement might result in less intimal hyperplasia (5). However, many clinician-scientists believed abrupt closure would prove to be the most sensible indication for stent placement. This patient population, representing 5 to 8% of angioplasty patients, accounted for the significant majority of adverse clinical events and expense related to catheter-based intervention, and the problem of abrupt closure had few effective therapies other than emergency surgery. Gary Roubin and Cesare Gianturco were working with engineers from Cook, Inc. to design the FlexStent to treat failed angioplasty.

Medtronic was interested initially in evaluating the Wiktor stent for both the restenosis and failed angioplasty indications. In 1991, a pair of studies were initiated in North America to evaluate the Wiktor Prime stent for these two indications. Since the FDA had no mandate for controlled device trial designs at the time, these studies were not randomized controlled trials but rather registries of patient outcomes after stent placement. After a few months, the restenosis study was stopped. Enrollment into the study was slower than anticipated, and preliminary data indicated that 6-month angiographic restenosis rates were higher after stent placement than expected. To best support what appeared to be the more promising and important study, Medtronic discontinued the restenosis study and directed its resources into the failed angioplasty study. As will be discussed later, this may have been an unfortunate decision, since subsequent studies from Europe suggest that restenosis rates after Wiktor stent placement may be as low as or lower than those reported for most other stent designs.

The following section will review the results of several studies regarding Wiktor stent placement for failed angioplasty, including the North American Medtronic Wiktor Prime stent study

completed in 1994. Since the data from this study have never been reported in full, I will review them in some depth here.

North American Failed Angioplasty Study

Purpose and Design

The purposes of the failed angioplasty study were to determine: (a) the short-term (in-hospital) safety and efficacy of the Medtronic Wiktor Prime stent; (b) the intermediate-term (one year) clinical outcome of patients receiving Medtronic Wiktor Prime stents; and (c) performance limitations of the Medtronic Wiktor Prime stent and factors associated with stent failure. The study was designed as a phase 3, open-label, multicenter clinical registry operated under an investigational device exemption held by Medtronic. Eighteen American hospital centers with expertise in coronary angioplasty were enlisted to participate. At the opening of the study, experience with coronary stent use was variable between centers. By the close of the registry (1994), all centers had experience with a variety of coronary stent designs. Stent placement technique was permitted to evolve during the early phases of the registry. Refinements in stent use were discussed at periodic investigator meetings and recommendations for practice changes, if any, were reported to the investigators.

Patients were considered to have had a failed angioplasty if they experienced abrupt closure, threatened closure, or a non-ischemic suboptimal intervention during percutaneous transluminal angioplasty of a native coronary arterial or saphenous vein bypass graft lesion, and they were free of contraindication to participation. Abrupt closure was defined as sudden cessation of anterograde blood flow (TIMI grade 0-1) (6) within the dilated vessel, or NHLBI grade F dissection (7) (corroborated by angiographic core laboratory). Threatened closure was defined as delayed anterograde blood flow (TIMI grade 2, corroborated as an increase of >50% in the number of cineangiographic frames to complete vessel opacification by core laboratory analysis), or NHLBI grade E dissection with persisting luminal filling defects (validated by the core laboratory). A non-ischemic suboptimal intervention

and a large myocardial territory was at risk. Stent thrombosis occurred in ten patients (17%) of the 59 patients with initially successful stent placement and no early bypass surgery; two of these patients died.

In the end, just 65% of the patients treated were dismissed from hospital without a major complication. Clinical follow-up at 6 months demonstrated that the outcome of this group was excellent however, with just 9% of patients experiencing recurrent angina. Angiographic follow-up studies indicated a binary restenosis rate (>50% diameter stenosis) of 27%. The aggressive anticoagulation program used led to high bleeding rates, as were seen commonly for other stents used in other settings.

The investigators concluded that use of the Wiktor stent represented a reasonable alternative to surgery for the treatment of failed angioplasty, although the early outcomes were less than perfect. Certainly these early results, representing patients treated between 1990 and 1991, reflected to a large degree the newness of stent utilization.

Restenosis Studies

As mentioned, no definitive randomized restenosis study has been completed for this stent design. The usual collection of institutional reports and small, uncontrolled series are found in the literature, with variable angiographic follow-up rates and similarly variable restenosis rates. Table 3.5 summarizes representative published restenosis reports.

The most recent study published on this topic comes from Turkey. In this retrospective, case-controlled study by Semiz and colleagues (12), the clinical and angiographic results of elective Wiktor stent implantation in 56 patients treated over a 1-year interval (April 1995 to April 1996) were compared to outcomes among 42 patients matched for important baseline clinical and angiographic characteristics and treated with balloon angioplasty alone. They found a significantly higher procedural success rate with Wiktor stent use (100 versus 92%, $p < .05$) and none of the Wiktor stent-treated patients experienced an early major adverse clinical event. By comparison, one patient required urgent bypass surgery and four others experienced subacute occlusions after angioplasty alone. Angiographic restenosis (>50% diameter stenosis) occurred in 25% of the Wiktor stent-treated patients and in 43% of those treated with angioplasty alone ($p < .05$). At 18 months after therapy, 91% of patients receiving Wiktor stents were asymptomatic and free of ischemia on exercise radionuclide stress testing, whereas only 79% of the angioplasty-alone patients were angina-free and 74% were free of ischemia on radionuclide imaging stress studies. The authors conclude that Wiktor stent implantation provides a more favorable procedural and long-term clinical and angiographic outcome than angioplasty alone. Aside from the study design considerations, an important factor to consider in this study is that 7% of the patients receiving Wiktor stents had reference segment diameters of less than 3 mm, whereas 17% of the

TABLE 3.5. *Published restenosis reports for the Medtronic Wiktor stent*

Author	Year	No. pts	Rest. rate	Comment
Akira	1995	21	24%	Randomized comparison
Colombo	1995	68	23%	9% chronic total occlusion
Hosokawa	1996	162	23%	Small vessels
Kyo	1996	128	23%	Suboptimal PTCA results
Mitsudo	1996	495	26%	Nonrandomized comparison
Fr registry	1996	272	23.6%	Native vessels and grafts
Carrie	1997	21	12.2%	Bifurcation lesions
Anzuini	1997	89	15%	Single stent only
Leguizamon	1997	90	11.6%	Acute ischemic syndromes
Semiz	1998	56	25%	Case-control study
Glogar	1997	187	12–14%	No effect of high-pressure angioplasty

angioplasty-treated patients had small vessels treated.

An interesting and provocative study has been completed by H. Dietmar Glogar in Vienna (13). Conventional wisdom maintains that routine use of high-pressure angioplasty, which is of demonstrated benefit in several stent designs, should be employed universally to optimize final vascular dimensions and thereby reduce the risk of restenosis as much as possible. However, it is far from clear that this strategy is of benefit universally; for example, in the SCORES study of the self-expanding Radius stent (SCIMED, division of Boston Scientific, Boston, MA), high-pressure angioplasty was associated with increased vascular injury, increased intimal hyperplasia, and no angiographic restenosis benefit (14). In a modestly sized study, Glogar allocated patients randomly to receive Wiktor stents followed by routine low-pressure angioplasty (to a target of 8 atm of pressure), or to routine high-pressure angioplasty (to a target of >12 atm of pressure). All patients were evaluated with intravascular ultrasound. Indeed, high-pressure angioplasty did improve ultrasonic vascular dimensions, but did not reduce restenosis rates. Perhaps the most significant finding reported by Glogar was the remarkably low restenosis rate for patients regardless of the Wiktor stent implantation strategy: 12% with adjunctive low-pressure angioplasty and 14% with high-pressure ballooning.

In contrast, there are some reports suggesting that the Wiktor stent may not be placed optimally without high-pressure dilatation. The most significant of these is by Buchwald and associates (15). They reported that high-pressure post-dilatation of Wiktor stents resulted in insignificant improvements in minimal luminal diameters and residual stenoses (by intravascular ultrasound), but did reduce the incidence of incomplete strut apposition and other placement quality concerns.

In the absence of a definitive restenosis endpoint trial, the preponderance of clinical data suggest that restenosis rates following Medtronic Wiktor stent placement should compare favorably with those of other stent designs.

Treatment of Chronic Total Occlusions

Recurrent closure is common after balloon angioplasty of chronic total occlusions. Factors contributing to this are not well understood, but early recoil and adverse remodeling have been proposed as principal mechanisms of treatment failure. Placement of Medtronic Wiktor stents has been used in attempts to improve early and late results.

Anzuini and colleagues from Milan, Italy reported on results of a multicenter registry study of elective Wiktor stent placement following successful balloon dilatation of 91 chronic total occlusions in 89 patients between 1993 and 1996 (16). Roughly half the patients were treated with aspirin plus warfarin (early patients) and half were treated with aspirin plus ticlodipine (later patients). Stent placement was successful in 98% of attempts. Other than subacute stent thrombosis, which occurred in 6% of patients within 30 days of treatment and was associated with Coumadin (Du Pont Pharmaceuticals, Wilmington, DE) use, adverse event rates were low. Six-month angiographic follow-up (obtained in 93% of eligible patients) revealed a restenosis rate of 32%, with a reocclusion rate of 4%. Multiple logistic regression analysis identified multiple stent placement (adjusted odds ratio [OR] 27.67, 95% confidence interval [CI] 4.25 to 79.95, $p = .0008$) and occlusion length (adjusted OR 1.23, 95% CI 1.09 to 1.39, $p = .001$) as independent correlates of increased restenosis risk. Freedom from death, myocardial infarction, or target lesion revascularization was 87% and 72% at 1 and 3 years. The investigators concluded that the short- and long-term clinical and angiographic outcomes were favorable among patients undergoing Wiktor stent implantation for treatment of chronic total occlusions, but that further work was needed to reduce restenosis rates for patients with long lesions treated with multiple stents.

FUTURE WIKTOR STENT USES

It is becoming apparent that the marketplace is outpacing Wiktor stent development. The liabilities of an unsheathed flexible coil stent design are being underscored by the development of many new, ultra-low-profile, highly flexible slotted-tube stent designs, available with or without protective sheaths. The reliability of stent delivery for such new stent designs is difficult to match with the more flexible and more easily damaged flexible coil design. Without significant design reworking, the Medtronic Wiktor stent will likely vanish. The recent partnership leading to the development of the slotted-tube derivative beStent (Medtronic) design, and the acquisition of Advanced Vascular Engineering (AVE) by Medtronic, Inc suggests that Medtronic anticipates its future stent product lines will lean more toward highly flexible self-reinforcing designs than helical coil designs.

There may be future uses for the Wiktor chassis though, in the delivery of expandable stent coverings. Investigators in Germany experimented with polyethylacrylate/polymethacrylate (PEM) coated Wiktor stents that were placed into the infra-renal aortas of New Zealand rabbits (17). They found that the Wiktor stent provided a satisfactory chassis for the deployment of a coated stent device, but they were plagued by a high incidence of early thrombosis over the PEM material.

A technique for coating Wiktor stents with a continuous film of fibrin has been developed (18). Polymerized fibrin causes very little activation of thrombin or platelets, and has sufficient plasticity that a coating sheet placed over a compressed stent can be expanded to 4.0 mm without tearing. However, a key consideration seems to be the ability of the sheet to stretch without being anchored at pivot point, which can create significant tearing damage to the sheet. The continuous free helical configuration of the Medtronic Wiktor stent makes it an ideal chassis for use as a polymer sleeve delivery device, including a fibrin sleeve. Animal experiments have demonstrated the feasibility of fibrin-coated Wiktor stent placement, a low rate of neointimal tissue development, and benign incorporation of the fibrin sleeve into the vessel wall within a few months. Clinical trials are ongoing at Mayo Clinic to evaluate this promising approach further.

CONCLUSIONS

The Medtronic Wiktor stent is a low-mass, radio-opaque flexible metallic stent with demonstrated utility in the treatment of unsuccessful or suboptimal coronary angioplasty, and probable utility in limiting restenosis. It is available on several different delivery balloon chassis and is manufactured in a variety of lengths (although only the 16-mm length mounted on the Rival balloon catheter is available in the United States). The strengths of this stent are its flexibility and accuracy of placement owing to the radio-opacity of the tantalum material of which it is made. Its weaknesses lie in the relative delicacy of a free helical stent design.

Wiktor stent utilization is low in North America. Although the value of radio-opacity with respect to accuracy and quality of stent placement was demonstrated with the Wiktor stent, its undesirable handling characteristics have limited Wiktor stent acceptance in North America. Nonetheless, the experience with the Medtronic Wiktor stent has been of value in defining the relative role of differing stent designs in clinical practice and in determining improved stent designs. The future of this stent may rest with its ability to serve newer niche applications, such as delivery of expandable endoluminal coats or sleeves.

REFERENCES

1. Schomig A, Neumann FJ, Castrate A et al. A randomized comparison of antiplatelet and anticoagulant therapy after the placement of coronary-artery stents. *N Engl J Med* 1996;334:1084–1089.
2. White C. The Wiktor and Wiktor-*i* stents. In: Serruys PW and Kutryk MJB, eds. *Handbook Of Coronary Stents*, 2nd ed. St Louis: Mosby 1998:31–44.
3. Gregoire J, Smith DG, Ragheb A et al. Stent collapse resistance to external pressures: comparison between coil and slotted tube designs. *J Am Coll Cardiol* 1998; 31[Suppl A]:414A(abst).
4. Schwartz, RS. Pathophysiology of restenosis: interaction of thrombosis, hyperplasia, and/or remodeling. *Am J Cardiol* 1998;81:14E–17E.
5. Fontaine AB, Spigos DG, Eaton G et al. Stent-induced intimal hyperplasia: are there fundamental differences

between flexible and rigid stent designs? *J Vasc Intervent Radiol* 1994;5:739–744.

6. Rogers WJ, Baim DS, Gore JM et al. Comparison of immediate invasive, delayed invasive, and conservative strategies after tissue-type plasminogen activator. Results of the Thrombolysis in Myocardial Infarction (TIMI) Phase II-A trial. *Circulation* 1990;81: 1457–1476.

7. Cowley MJ, Dorros G, Kelsey SF, Van Raden M, Detre KM. Emergency coronary bypass surgery after coronary angioplasty: the National Heart, Lung, and Blood Institute's Percutaneous Transluminal Coronary Angioplasty Registry experience. *Am J Cardiol* 1984;53(12): 22C–26C.

8. Fishman NW, Kennard ED, Steenkiste AR, Popma JJ, Baim DS, Detre KM. New Approaches to Coronary Intervention (NACI) registry: history and methods. *Am J Cardiol* 1997;80:10K–18K.

9. Eeckhout E, Stauffer JC, Vogt P, Debbas N, Kappenberger L, Goy JJ. Unplanned use of intracoronary stents for the treatment of a suboptimal angiographic result after conventional balloon angioplasty. *Am Heart J* 1995;130:1164–1167.

10. Goy JJ, Eeckhout E, Stauffer JC, Vogt P, Kappenberger L. Emergency endoluminal stenting for abrupt vessel closure following coronary angioplasty: a randomized comparison of the Wiktor and Palmaz-Schatz stents. *Cathet Cardiovasc Diagn* 1995;34:128–132.

11. Vrolix M, Piessens J. Usefulness of the Wiktor stent for treatment of threatened or acute closure complicating coronary angioplasty. The European Wiktor Stent Study Group. *Am J Cardiol* 1994;73(11):737–741.

12. Semiz E, Sancaktar O, Yalcinkaya S, Ege H, Deger N. Comparative clinical and angiographic analysis of the initial efficacy and long-term follow-up of Wiktor stent implantation with conventional balloon angioplasty. *Jpn Heart J* 1997;38:625–635.

13. Glogar D, Yang P, Hassan A et al. Does high-pressure balloon post-dilation improve long-term results of Wiktor coil stent? (Austrian Wiktor Stent Trial). *J Am Coll Cardiol* 1997;29 [Suppl A]:313A(abst).

14. Kobayashi Y, Mukai S, Brown CL et al. Geometric expansion in a self-expandable stent and a balloon expandable stent: interim results from the IVUS substudy of the SCORES trial. *Circulation* 1997;96[Suppl I]: I–584(abst).

15. Buchwald AB, Werner GS, Moller K, Unterberg C. Expansion of Wiktor stents by oversizing versus high-pressure dilatation: a randomized, intracoronary ultrasound-controlled study. *Am Heart J* 1997;133(2):190–196.

16. Anzuini A, Rosanio S, Legrand V et al. Wiktor stent for treatment of chronic total coronary artery occlusions: short- and long-term clinical and angiographic results from a large multicenter experience. *J Am Coll Cardiol* 1998;31(2):281–288.

17. Tepe G, Duda SH, Hanke H et al. Claussen CD. Covered stents for prevention of restenosis. Experimental and clinical results with different stent designs. *Invest Radiol* 1996;31(4):223–229.

18. McKenna CJ, Camrud AR, Sangiorgi G et al. Fibrin-film stenting in a porcine coronary injury model: efficacy and safety compared with uncoated stents. *J Am Coll Cardiol* 1998;31:1434–1438.

C. The ACS Multi-Link and Duet Stents

Donald S. Baim

Interventional Cardiology Section, Beth Israel Deaconess Medical Center, Harvard Medical School, Boston, Massachusetts 02215

Despite the tremendous success of the Johnson and Johnson Interventional System (JJIS) Palmaz-Schatz Coronary Stent following its commercial release in 1994, its use was complicated by performance issues relating to the rigidity of the stent and delivery sheath that made passage around tortuous vessels difficult, uneven expansion of stent "diamonds," and residual stenosis at the articulation site. It was also limited by availability only in a single, 15-mm length, and radiographic invisibility. In an effort to overcome these limitations, a number of second-generation stents were developed. The first such second-generation stent to be released (October 1997) was the ACS Multi-Link (Guidant Corporation, Santa Clara, CA).

The multi-link stent is cut from 316 stainless steel tubing to form a series of corrugated rings, nested and interconnected by bridging struts to provide excellent lateral flexibility. As such, it is comprised of a series of "u-," "y-," and "w-" shaped complexes, whose geometry and thickness have been engineered to provide even cell expansion at diameters between 3 and 4.0 mm. The large perimeter length of the individual cells allows easy access and dilatation of side branches up to 3.5 mm diameter. Animal data with this device show better lateral flexibility, more even expansion, and slightly greater crush resistance than seen with the current Palmaz-Schatz design (1). Data from the chronic pig model also suggested that the Multi-Link design might have lower thrombogenicity and less late neointimal response.

Clinical trials of this device began in Europe in July 1993, and progressed to two small European trials (WEST I and WEST II) conducted in 1995 and 1996 (2,3). The stent was released for commercial sale in Europe in November 1995. The bulk of the clinical data on the Multi-Link, however, came from a series of U.S. trials. The first U.S. implants were performed in late August 1995, as part of a 50-patient pilot trial (conducted between August 1995 and February 1996) which utilized serial IVUS Intravascular Vascular Ultrasound Sound to evaluate stent expansion and the response to post-dilatation (4). This showed 100% delivery success, progressively greater expansion from deployment at 8 atm, to postdilatation at 12 atm and 16 atm (minimum lumen diameter 2.72 mm, 7% stenosis), with no acute or sub-acute thromboses on an aspirin/Coumadin (Du Pont Pharmaceuticals, Wilmington, DE) regimen.

The 1,000-patient (ASCENT) multi-center randomized trial compared the 15-mm sheathed Multi-Link stent to the JJIS Palmaz-Schatz stent in focal *de novo* native vessel lesions, at 42 U.S. sites and four Canadian sites (5). It used routine high pressure (14 atm) post-dilatation, and an aspirin/Ticlid regimen (as supported by the findings of the Stent Antithrombotic Regimen Study [STARS] trial). The same sites completed a 200-patient registry of Multi-Link stents placed in patients with restenosis after one prior PTCA. A registry of stents placed for abrupt closure or threatened closure (RECREATE) was also performed. Enrollment in ASCENT was completed between March 1996 and August 1996. The primary endpoint was to demonstrate that the Multi-Link had clinical restenosis (8 month target vessel failure [TVF] = target site revascularization [TSR], death, or MI) that was not inferior to (i.e., was equivalent to or better than) the Palmaz-Schatz stent. Secondary endpoints included delivery failure, 30-day major adverse cardiac event (MACE), and angiographic follow-up in a subset of 500 consecutive patients. Acute results show a tendency toward fewer delivery failures (ACS 2.5 % versus PS 4.2%), slightly lower post-treatment residual stenosis (8% versus 10%), and a tendency toward fewer 30-day major adverse clinical events (4.0% versus 8.2%), including trends toward a lower mortality (0% versus 1.2%) and sub-acute thrombosis rates (0.6% versus 1.9%). With angiographic follow-up in 75 % of the restudy cohort, the angiographic restenosis rate also tended to be lower (16% versus 21%) for the Multi-Link, with no difference in the magnitude of the late proliferative response (loss index 0.45 versus 0.43). This demonstrates that the small restenosis benefit is a result of the larger acute lumen diameter, rather than a reduction in proliferative response (as the animal data had suggested). There were non-significant trends for lower clinical restenosis (TSR 8.8% versus 11.3%, TVF 17.3% versus 19.6%). These findings established that the Multi-Link was equivalent to or better than (not inferior to) the Palmaz-Schatz stent (*p* value of .001 for equivalence) for the primary endpoint of TVF at 9 months. Presentation of these trial data to the FDA led to device approval on October 2, 1997.

The Multi-Link was mounted on a PE-600 delivery balloon over which an elastic membrane was placed to protect the delivery balloon and promote even stent expansion. As tested in ASCENT, the 15-mm Multi-Link stent was mounted within a delivery system in which the stent was covered by a 5 Fr (0.068-inch) retractable sleeve that was withdrawn prior to stent delivery. Based on registry testing (6), however, the stent was released in lengths of 15 mm and 25 mm, bare-mounted on a rapid-exchange balloon capable of 8 atm delivery. A high-pressure delivery balloon was also released, but proved stiff during delivery. Within months of release, the Rx Multi-Link became the dominant stent in the U.S. market, virtually eliminating the Palmaz-Schatz design. In clinical use for more challenging anatomic situations than those tested in ASCENT, several limitations became apparent. The bare-mounted stent was virtually invisible by fluoroscopy, and could move up the shaft of the delivery catheter during forceful advancement. Alternatively, when the stent failed to cross a target lesion, it could move forward on the delivery balloon or even strip off that balloon (<1% of attempted placements). Rare instances were also reported in which the C-flex membrane over the delivery balloon detached or became partially entrapped in the deployed stent. The low pressure limit of the delivery balloon required high pressure postdilatation for full expansion, and the fact that the delivery balloon was 5 mm longer than the stent (i.e., balloon lengths of 20 mm and 30 mm) meant that aggressive sizing or higher pressure inflation might lead to edge dissection, particularly in tapered or diffusely diseased vessels. With the approval of other second-generation devices in early 1998, use of the original Multi-Link declined somewhat in favor of the highly-deliverable and radio-opaque stents (AVE Micro II and gfx Arterial Vascular Engineering, Santa Rosa, [CA]), and the NIR (Medinol/Boston Scientific, Jerusalem, Isreal) stent. The NIR stent, though no more deliverable or radio-opaque than the Multi-Link, was available in more lengths (9, 16, 25, and 32 mm), a wider range of diameters (2.5 mm–4.0 mm), on a high pressure balloon whose length was closer matched to the stent, and from which stent movement was prevented by a textured inner member or end-caps.

The Multi-Link design, however, was recently modified in the Duet design (released in November 1998) which had thicker stent walls (0.005 inch versus 0.002 inch) for increased visibility, but retained flexibility due to an alternating pattern of three and two struts connecting consecutive corrugated rings. Approval was based on a 269-patient registry, which looked at acute success and 30-day complications (7) whose results compared favorably with the original Multi-Link arm of ASCENT. The Duet has a larger maximum expanded diameter (4.5 mm),

a broader range of lengths (8, 13, 18, 23, and 28mm), and a higher-pressure (16 atm) delivery balloon whose length is more closely matched to the stent length (balloons 10, 15, and 20 mm, etc.). Both over-the-wire and rapid-exchange formats are available, and the C-flex balloon covering has been eliminated with enhancement in stent retention on the balloon. Although the reduction in the number of struts may slightly reduce the quality of scaffolding (more plaque intrusion, particularly in bulky lesions within curves), the Duet Multi-Link has proven to be an excellent work-horse stent. Future modifications of the Multi-Link family will continue, including the release of a 2.5-mm Duet in February 1999 and a MegaLink stent designed for larger (4–7 mm) vessels.

In summary, the ACS Multi-Link stent design has emerged as competitive second-generation tubular stent that offers improvements in delivery, scaffolding, thrombogenicity, side-branch access, and potentially restenosis, compared to first-generation stents.

REFERENCES

1. Rogers C, Edelman ER. Endovascular stent design dictates experimental restenosis and thrombosis. *Circulation* 1995; 91:2995–3001.
2. Emanuelsson H, Serruys PW, van der Giessen W et al. Clinical and angiographic results with the Multi-Link coronary stent system—the West European Stent Trial (WEST). *J Invas Cardiol* 1998;10:12–19B.
3. Serruys PW, van der Giessen W, Garcia E, Macaya C et al. Clinical and angiographic results with the Multi-Link stent implanted under ultrasound guidance (WEST-2 Study). *J Invas Cardiol* 1998;10:20–27B.
4. Carrozza JPJ, Hermiller JBJ, Linnemeier TJ et al. Quantitative coronary angiographic and intravascular ultrasound assessment of a new nonarticulated stent: Report from the Advanced Cardiovascular Systems Multi-Link Stent Pilot Study. *J Am Coll Cardiol* 1998;31:50–56.
5. Baim DS, Midei M, Linnemeier T et al., for the ASCENT Investigators. A randomized trial comparing the Multi-Link stent to the Palmaz-Schatz Stent in *de novo* lesions. *J Am Coll Cardiol* (in press).
6. Linnemeier TJ. The Rx Multi-Link stent parallel registries to the ASCENT trial. *J Invas Cardiol* 1998;10: 55–56B.
7. Kereiakes DJ, Hermiller J, Schlofmitz R et al. Procedural and late outcomes following the Multi-Link DUET coronary stent deployment—final report for the U.S. registry. *J Am Coll Cardiol* 1999;33:95A(abst).

D. AVE Stents

Navin Gupta, Alejandro N. Lopez, and Richard R. Heuser

Phoenix Heart, Phoenix, Arizona 83106

The introduction of coronary stenting promised to revolutionize interventional cardiology. Although the problems associated with percutaneous transluminal coronary angioplasty (PTCA), such as abrupt vessel closure and restenosis, could be attenuated with stenting (1,2,3), several years were required to appreciate and overcome the learning curves associated with optimal stent deployment, anticoagulation, and patient and lesion selection. (4–6) Currently accepted primary indications for coronary stenting include suboptimal angiographic result from balloon angioplasty and acute or threatened vessel closure due to dissection, as well as prevention of restenosis. The balance of apparent angiographic benefit must be weighed against the risks associated with stent usage, including thrombosis, restenosis, stent loss, and higher initial cost. Thus while great strides have been made in the development and utilization of stents, and hence, PTCA, the field remains dynamic. Whether newer stents with innovative technology, either alone or with adjunctive therapy, will improve clinical outcomes in coronary interventions remains to be seen. The need for novel devices and approaches to percutaneous interventions persists.

STENT DEVELOPMENT

Founded in 1991, Arterial Vascular Engineering (AVE) (Santa Rosa, CA) developed its first stent, the MicroStent PL in 1994. This stent was composed of 4-mm unconnected sinusoidal elements. These were laser-fused into 8-mm lengths, one or two of which were placed on a stent delivery system to form the company's first commercially available stent (outside the United States), the MicroStent. This was followed by the MicroStent II and the GFX stents, composed of 3-mm and 2-mm sinusoidal elements, respec-

tively. These third- and fourth-generation stents exhibit greater flexibility and trackability while retaining radial strength. The MicroStent II was introduced in the United States in November of 1995 by way of the Study of the MicroStent's Ability to Limit Restenosis Trial (SMART). The GFX stent was similarly introduced via registry within the SMART study. Both stents received FDA approval for distribution in the United States in December 1997. To date over 250,000 AVE stents have been implanted worldwide.

STENT CHARACTERISTICS

The MicroStent II is composed of sinusoidal elements formed from individual rings of 316L stainless steel. These elements are 3 mm in length and consist of eight struts with four crowns (Fig. 3.6). Elements are laser-fused to

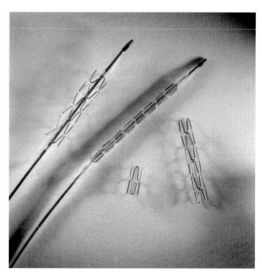

FIG. 3.6. The AVE Micro Stent II (Courtesy Arterial Vascular Engineering).

each other at a single point in a helical fashion along the length of the stent. This design avoids the creation of a rigid spine and provides greater flexibility and trackability to the stent than do the tubular slotted or wire coil designs. Maintaining the ring structure of the elements imparts significant radial strength to the stent, resulting in minimal stent recoil (<4%), while electropolishing creates smoother edges than laser-cut strut elements, providing smoother and more predictable handling characteristics. These characteristics allow for easier negotiation of tortuous vessels and greater approach to distal and side branch lesions. It may be surmised that the smoother finish of the stent as well as the parallel position of the struts to blood flow should provide less resistance to the flow of blood components and appear less thrombogenic (7).

The GFX stent (Fig. 3.7) represents the fourth-generation AVE stent and is composed of 2-mm sinusoidal elements. Each element consists of 12 struts arranged in an elliptorectangular shape to form six crowns (Figs. 3.8, 3.9). These elements are also laser-fused to each other at a single point in a helical fashion. This improvement in strut geometry gives the stent an exceptionally slim profile while increasing wall coverage by 30% over previous generations (Table 3.6). The moderate radiopacity of the MicroStent II and the GFX greatly improves stent visibility under fluoroscopy which, coupled with

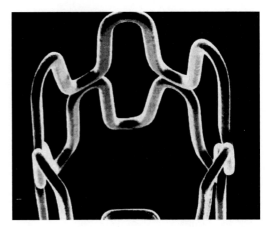

FIG. 3.8. GFX stent: Each element forms 12 struts arranged in an elliptorectangular design (Courtesy Arterial Vascular Engineering).

proximal and distal balloon markers, leads to greater accuracy of stent deployment and dilatation.

CLINICAL EXPERIENCE

Initial clinical experience with AVE stents was garnered by operators outside the United States. Ozaki and associates demonstrated a high level of procedural and angiographic success in the deployment of 28 MicroStents in 20 patients with acute or threatened closure after balloon

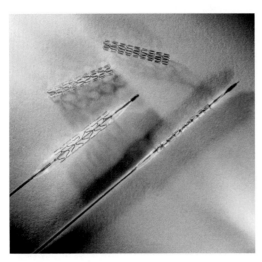

FIG. 3.7. The AVE GFX stent (Courtesy Arterial Vascular Engineering).

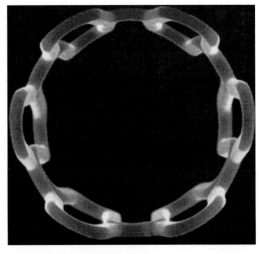

FIG. 3.9. GFX stent: Profile view (Courtesy Arterial Vascular Engineering).

TABLE 3.6. *Stent characteristics*

Diameter (mm)	Available lengths (mm)	Crossing profile	Wall coverage
MicroStent II:[a]			
3.0	6, 15, 20, 30	0.069"	17%
3.5	6, 15, 20, 30	0.069"	15%
4.0	6, 15, 20, 30	0.069"	13%
GFX:			
3.0	8, 12, 18, 24, 30	0.059"	23%
3.5	8, 12, 18, 24, 30	0.060"	20%
4.0	8, 12, 18, 24, 30	0.062"	17%

[a] For 30-mm. length crossing profile = 0.070"; Maximum guide wire = 0.014 in.

angioplasty, an experience corroborated by others (8,9). Colombo and associates found the MicroStent particularly well suited for tortuous vessels and to cross previously deployed stents (10). Short term results have also been favorable for deployment of the 30- and 39-mm-long MicroStent II in long lesions (average length 44 mm), which traditionally have high restenotic rates with balloon angioplasty alone (11).

Migration of segments of the MicroStent I was reported in three patients by Wong and associates from their experience of implantation in 30 patients (12). Failure to firmly embed the stent struts into the arterial wall, as well as the deployment of unconnected units across a bend point in the artery, appeared to contribute to these occurrences. Also, the MicroStent I is no longer used. The MicroStent II has all elements connected, making the migration problems unlikely to occur with the current design. A retrospective analysis by Agarwal and associates of 33 lesion-matched pairs of the MicroStent to the Palmaz-Schatz stent suggested a higher rate of binary restenosis in patients receiving MicroStents; however, the retrospective nature of the study, and the low number of patients presenting for angiographic follow-up, limit the power of the study to draw any conclusions (13). In this study, four MicroStents were deployed in lesions where the Palmaz-Schatz stent could not be placed, and an additional four MicroStents were passed through proximally deployed Palmaz-Schatz stents. These early experiences were the foundation for direct comparison of the MicroStent II to the Palmaz-Schatz stent.

THE SMART TRIAL

The SMART trial was a multi-center, randomized, prospective study comparing the AVE MicroStent II to the Palmaz-Schatz slotted tube stent. This trial was initiated to demonstrate clinical and angiographic equivalence of the MicroStent II to the Palmaz-Schatz stent in *de novo* and restenotic lesions up to 30 mm in length, as well as to obtain FDA approval for release in the United States.

Three-hundred-thirty patients were randomly assigned to receive treatment with the MicroStent II and 331 with the Palmaz-Schatz. Patients enrolled in the study were required to demonstrate objective evidence of ischemic heart disease requiring single lesion treatment in a native coronary artery. *De novo* as well as restenotic lesions in vessels ≥3.0 mm and ≤4.0 mm by visual inspection were included, provided the target lesion could be approached with one or two 15-mm Palmaz-Schatz stents or an appropriately sized MicroStent. The primary endpoint was the clinically driven need for target lesion revascularization at 9 months. Secondary endpoints included acute and late major adverse cardiac events.

Baseline characteristics reveal clinical and angiographic comparability between the two study groups (Tables 3.7, 3.8). While patients receiving the MicroStent II had a higher rate of restenotic lesions compared to patients receiving the Palmaz-Schatz stent, there was no difference in vessel diameter, percent diameter stenosis, or lesion length (SMART lesion morphology). Lesion success (99.1% for MicroStent II versus 96.8% for Palmaz-Schatz) as well as acute pro-

TABLE 3.7. *GFX registry: patient demographics*

Characteristic	GFX $n = 210$	Palmaz-Schatz $n = 331$
Age (years)	65 ± 10	64 ± 11
Male gender	69%	70%
Cigarette smoker	23%	26%
Diabetes mellitus	22%	17%
Hypertension (requiring treatment)	61%	58%
Hyperlipidemia (requiring treatment)	35%	31%
Prior CABG	10%	5%
Prior MI	35%	31%
CCS Class III & IV[a]	61%	69%
Number of diseased vessels		
Single	67%	73%
Double	21%	21%
Triple*	12%	6%

* Statistically Significant
[a] CCS, Canadian Cardiovascular Society.

cedural success (94.4% versus 95.7%) were high for both groups.

The most commonly used stent diameter was 3.0 mm, representing 48% of the MicroStents used versus 51% of the Palmaz-Schatz, with 15 mm being the most commonly used length, representing 80% of the MicroStents versus 99%

TABLE 3.8. *GFX registry: lesion morphology*

Characteristic	GFX $n = 210$	Palmaz-Schatz $n = 331$
Lesion length (mm)	13.7 ± 6.6	12.2 ± 6.2
Eccentric	43%	33%
Thrombus	2%	2%
Calcification (moderate–severe)	17%	13%
Lesion complexity[a]		
Type A	4%	10%
Type B1	23%	27%
Type B2	54%	52%
Type C	19%	11%

[a] Modified ACC/AHA.

TABLE 3.9. *GFX registry: 30-day adverse events*

Characteristic	GFX $n = 210$	Palmaz-Schatz $n = 331$
TLR	1.0%	2.1%
MACE[a]	3.8%	6.0%
Local vascular complications	0.5%	3.0%
Bleeding (requiring transfusion)	0.0%	0.5%
Stent thrombosis	1.0%	0.6%
Death	0.5%	0.3%
Myocardial infarction	2.9%	4.5%
Stroke	0.0%	0.0%

[a] In and out of hospital; TLR, target lesion revascularization (clinical restenosis); MACE, major adverse cardiac event (death, MI, TLR, stroke).

of the Palmaz-Schatz stents used. The average lesion length was 11.5 ± 6.4 mm in the Micro Stent II group versus 12.1 ± 6.2 mm in the Palmaz-Schatz group, with 63% of the stents deployed in vessels with type B2 or C lesions. This increase in lesion length and complexity compared to the STRESS and BENESTENT population indicates the growing experience and confidence of operators in deploying stents in highly complex lesions (1,2,14).

Target lesion revascularization at 9 months was 12.8% for the MicroStent compared to 12.1% for the Palmaz-Schatz (Table 3.9). Major adverse cardiac events were comparable between the two groups as well. An angiographic substudy was performed on 300 patients who underwent coronary angiography between 6 and 9 months (mean = 8.5 months). In-stent diameter stenosis was 38 ± 19% for the MicroStent group versus 33 ± 21% for the Palmaz-Schatz group while in-stent binary restenosis was 25.2% versus 22.1%. This data demonstrates clinical as well as angiographic equivalence between the MicroStent and the Palmaz-Schatz stent groups.

THE GFX REGISTRY

The GFX stent was evaluated within the SMART study in the form of a non-randomized

TABLE 3.10. *SMART: patient demographics*

Characteristic	MicroStent II n = 330	Palmaz-Schatz n = 331
Age (years)	63 ± 11	64 ± 11
Male gender	69%	70%
Cigarette smoker	23%	26%
Diabetes mellitus	19%	17%
Hypertension (requiring treatment)	58%	58%
Hyperlipidemia (requiring treatment)	34%	31%
Prior CABG[a]	10%	5%
Prior MI	27%	31%
CCS Class III & IV	65%	69%
Number of diseased vessels		
single	69%	73%
double	22%	21%
triple	9%	6%
Ejection fraction	57 ± 11%	57 ± 11%

[a] Statistically significant.

registry. Two-hundred-ten patients received the GFX stent and were compared to the 331 patients in the Palmaz-Schatz arm of the randomized trial. Baseline characteristics reveal a statistically significant trend toward more triple-vessel disease in the GFX population, while more patients in the Palmaz-Schatz group had CCS angina III or IV (Table 3.10). Lesion morphology and complexity were comparable, although a higher percentage (73% versus 63%) of GFX stents were deployed in vessels with type B2 or C lesions (Table 3.11). Despite the presence of more severe coronary artery disease in the GFX population, target lesion revascularization as well as major adverse cardiac events were comparable between the two groups at 30 days (Table 3.12).

INDICATIONS FOR STENTING

Suboptimal results achieved from balloon angioplasty due to elastic recoil remain the most

TABLE 3.11. *SMART: lesion morphology*

Characteristic	MicroStent II n = 330	Palmaz-Schatz n = 331
Reference vessel diameter (mm)	2.94 ± 0.54	2.94 ± 0.49
Percent stenosis	64 ± 13%	64 ± 13%
Target vessel:		
LAD	47%	42%
LCX	21%	22%
RCA	32%	36%
Restenotic lesion	6.4%	3.0%
Lesion length (mm.)	11.5 ± 6.4	12.1 ± 6.2
Eccentric	39%	33%
Thrombus	3%	2%
Calcification (moderate–severe)	16%	14%
Angulation >45 degrees	10%	9%
Lesion complexity[a]:		
type A	10%	10%
type B1	27%	26%
type B2	52%	52%
type C	11%	11%

[a] Modified ACC/AHA.

TABLE 3.12.   *SMART: endpoints*

Characteristic	MicroStent II n = 330	Palmaz-Schatz n = 331
Primary		
TLR at 9 months	12.8%	12.1%
CABG	5.5%	3.3%
PTCA	9.1%	10.6%
Secondary		
Acute success:		
Lesion success	99.1%	96.8%
Device success	97.8%	95.2%
Acute procedural success	94.4%	95.7%
MACE[a]	19.4%	16.3%
Death	2.1%	1.2%
Myocardial infarction	5.8%	3.9%
Emergent CABG	0.9%	1.2%
Stent thrombosis	0.0%	0.6%
Bleeding complications	1.8%	1.5%
Stroke	0.6%	0.0%
Surgical repair	1.2%	0.9%
Vascular complications	3.6%	3.3%

[a] In and out of hospital; TLR, target lesion revascularization (clinical restenosis); MACE, major adverse cardiac event (death, MI, TLR, stroke).

common indication for coronary stenting. Stenting also has demonstrated benefit in the treatment of acute or threatened vessel closure complicating balloon angioplasty (15). The AVE stents perform comparably to others in these situations. Their slim profile makes them particularly valuable in crossing coronary dissections, passing deployed stents to reach distal lesions, and to treat in-stent restenosis (16,17). There is growing evidence that using intracoronary stenting as an adjunct to or instead of balloon angioplasty in the treatment of acute myocardial infarction may be safe and highly effective (18,19,20). Reuben and associates achieved excellent clinical results in 11 patients receiving the MicroStent for severe dissection (8) and elastic recoil (5) following balloon angioplasty in the setting of acute myocardial infarction (21). Side branch occlusion occurred in 5% of 810 patients with bifurcation lesions

treated with Palmaz-Schatz stents in the Stent Antithrombotic Regimen Study (STARS) and was associated with an increased need for emergent bypass surgery and twice the rate of target lesion revascularization at 6 months (22). The unique design of AVE stents may be associated with less side branch occlusion, while increasing branch access. This may influence stent selection for lesions in close proximity to, or directly affecting, major branch vessels. In our experience, balloon dilatation may be safely performed through the AVE MicroStent II and the GFX stent.

FUTURE DEVELOPMENTS

Further advances in stent design and manufacturing, coupled with newer balloon technology, will define the next generation of AVE stents. Several AVE stents are currently in or entering clinical trials in Europe and the United States: the GFX 40-mm (length) stent, with significant trackability and a slim profile, should obviate the need for multiple stent deployment; the GFX 2.5-mm (diameter) stent will expand stenting options in patients with smaller coronary arteries as well as side branch and distal vessel lesions; while the GFX XP will utilize an extended pressure delivery system, allowing stent delivery, deployment, and postdilatation with a single balloon. An extended pressure balloon will also accompany the GFX II stents, which will have the added advantage of lower crossing profiles. This availability of a variety of sizes and lengths and concomitant balloon systems allows the interventionalist to optimize stent choice for a particular lesion and may decrease the use of equipment. The AVE stents exhibit exceptional handling characteristics, moderate radiopacity, and firm attachment to the delivery system, which combined with excellent clinical and angiographic outcomes make them an excellent choice for many coronary lesions.

REFERENCES

1. Fischman DL, Leon MB, Baim DS et al. A randomized comparison of coronary-stent placement and balloon angioplasty in the treatment of coronary artery disease. *N Eng J Med* 1194;331:496–501.

2. Serruys PW, De Jaegere P, Kiemeneij F et al. A comparison of balloon-expandable-stent implantation with balloon angioplasty in patients with coronary artery disease. *N Eng J Med* 1994;331:489–495.

3. Serruys PW, et.al. Randomized comparison of implantation of heparin coated stents with balloon angioplasty in selected patients with coronary artery disease (BENESTENT II). *Lancet* 1998;352:673–681.

4. Colombo A, Hall P, Nakamura S et al. Intracoronary stenting without anticoagulation accomplished with intravascular ultrasound guidance. *Circulation* 1995;91:1676–1688.

5. Schomig A, Neumann FJ, Kastrati A et al. A randomized comparison of antiplatelet and anticoagulation therapy after the placement of coronary-artery stents. *N Eng J Med* 1996;334:1084–1089.

6. Pomerantsev EV, Kim C, Kernoff RS et al. Coronary AVE MicroStent: serial quantitative angiography and histology in a canine model. *Cathet Cardiovasc Diagn* 1997;41:213–224.

7. Schatz RA. A view of vascular stents. *Circulation* 1989; 79: 445–457.

8. Ozaki Y, Keane D, Ruygrok P, de Feyter P, Stertzer S, Serruys PW. Acute clinical and angiographic results with the new AVE micro coronary stent in bailout management. *Am J Cardiol* 1995;76:112–116.

9. Antoniucci D, Valenti R, Santoro GM et al. Bailout coronary stenting without anticoagulation or intravascular ultrasound guidance: acute and six-month angiographic results in a series of 120 consecutive patients. *Cathet Cardiovasc Diagn* 1997;41:14–19.

10. Colombo A, Maiello L, Nakamura S et al. Preliminary experience of coronary stenting with the Micro Stent. *J Am Coll Cardiol* 1995(special issue)February:239A.

11. Rozenman Y, Mereuta A, Mosseri M, Lotan C, Nassar H, Hasin Y, Gotsman MS. Initial experience with long coronary stents: The changing practice of coronary angioplasty. *Am Heart J* 1997;134:335–361.

12. Wong P, Leung W, Wong C. Migration of the AVE micro coronary stent. *Cathet Cardiovasc Diagn* 1996; 38:267–273.

13. Agarwal R, Bhargava B, Kaul U et al. Long-term outcome of intracoronary Microstent implantation. *Cathet Cardiovasc Diagn* 1998;43:397–401.

14. Ellis SG, Vandormael MG, Cowley MJ, DiSciascia G, Deligonul U, Topol EJ. Coronary morphology and clinical determinants of procedural outcome with angioplasty for multivessel disease. *Circulation* 1990;82:1193–1202

15. George BS, Voorhees WO, Roubin GS et al. Multicenter investigation of coronary stenting to treat acute or threatened closure after percutaneous transluminal coronary angioplasty: clinical and angiographic outcomes. *J Am Coll Cardiol* 1993;22:135–143.

16. Hamon M, Monassier J-P. Stenting within a stent for treatment of residual dissection. *Cathet Cardiovasc Diagn* 1997;40:319–321.

17. Rozenman Y, Lotan C, Mosseri M, Nassar H, Hasin Y, Gotsman M. Experience with the AVE Micro Stent in native coronary arteries. *Am J Cardiol* 1996;78(Sep 15)(6):685–687.

18. Walton AS, Osterle SN, Yeung AC. Coronary artery stenting for acute closure complicating primary angioplasty for acute myocardial infarction. *Cathet Cardiovasc Diagn* 1995;34:142–146.

19. Ahmad T, Webb JG, Carere RR, Dodek A. Coronary stenting for acute myocardial infarction. *Am J Cardiol* 1995;76:77–80.

20. Stone GW, Brodie B, Griffin J, et. al. In-hospital and late outcomes following primary stenting in acute myocardial infarction—comparison with primary PTCA. *J Am Coll Cardiol* 1998;31(2)[Suppl A]:270A (1110–1149).

21. Reuben I, Weinstein JM, Abu-Ful A, Cafri C, Battler A. Coronary stenting with AVE microstents in acute myocardial infarction. *Int J Cardiol* 1997;59:247–250.

22. Abizaid AS, Popma JJ, Saucedo JF et al. Acute and late clinical outcome of bifurcation lesions treated with elective coronary stents: results from the STARS trial. *J Am Coll Cardiol* 1998;31(5)[Suppl C]:2553 (abst).

E. The Coronary NIR Stent

Roxana Mehran, Michael A. Peterson, and Martin B. Leon

The Cardiac Catheterization Laboratory, Washington Hospital Center and The Cardiovascular Research Foundation, Washington, DC 20010-2975

Coronary stenting has become an effective treatment for obstructive atherosclerotic coronary lesions. Randomized clinical trials and registry studies have shown a significant reduction in angiographic and clinical restenosis (reduced need for target lesion revascularization), and an improved rate of procedural success for stents compared to percutaneous transluminal coronary angioplasty (PTCA) in native coronary lesions (1–4) and in saphenous vein graft disease. (5–7) The first-generation "gold standard" Palmaz-Schatz (PS) coronary stent was granted approval by the Food and Drug Administration (FDA) in the U.S. in August 1994. Five years later, endovascular coronary metallic prostheses are being used in approximately 70% of all coronary interventions worldwide. The reasons for the current era of "stent frenzy" include: (a) simplified combination anti-platelet regimens that have dramatically reduced subacute stent closure without associated bleeding complications; (b) improved stent implantation techniques with post-stent high-pressure balloon inflations and guidance using intravascular ultrasound; (c) multiple clinical trials that have demonstrated efficacy and safety of stents in an expanding range of lesion subsets and patient cohorts; and (d) new "user-friendly" stents and delivery systems which have hastened acceptance in the catheterization laboratory milieu.

The first-generation stents clearly exhibited several limitations—reduced axial flexibility (tubular slotted designs), poor trackability through tortuous anatomy, inadequate scaffolding (coiled designs), very limited size ranges (lengths and diameters), and suboptimal radiopacity. These shortcomings were the impetus for the development of second- and third-generation intra-coronary stents. Newer designs exploit differences in material, geometry, and surface coverage to overcome the limitations of first-generation stents. Based upon randomized controlled trial data demonstrating equivalence compared with the Palmaz-Schatz stent, the ACS Multi-link stent (Guidant Corporation, Santa Clara, CA), the Medinol/Boston Scientific NIR stent (Jerusalem, Israel), and the AVE-gfx stent (Arterial Vascular Engineering, Santa Rosa, CA) are among these second-generation stents approved by the FDA for the prevention of restenosis in *de novo* or restenotic native coronary lesions.

This chapter is a detailed review of the coronary NIR stent (Medinol/Boston Scientific) including design specifications, early clinical investigations and pivotal randomized clinical trials.

DEVICE DESCRIPTION

The NIR stent (8) is made from 316 LVM surgical grade stainless steel sheets etched into a pre-specified geometric pattern. Automated rolling and laser welding forms these sheets into cylindrical stents containing either seven repeating cells (2.5, 3.0, and 3.5-mm diameters) or nine repeating cells (4.0, 4.5, and 5.0-mm diameters) spanning the tubular stent circumference (Tables 3.13 and 3.14).

Special Features: Transforming Geometry

The NIR stent geometry is a continuous uniform multicellular design with adaptive cells capable of differential lengthening, which confers flexibility in the unexpanded configuration, and

TABLE 3.13. *NIR stent technical specifications*

Material composition;	Stainless steel
Degree of radiopacity	Moderate
Ferromagnetism	None
Metallic area (expanded state)	11–18%
Metallic recoil	<1%
Strut design	Square, transform from flexible to rigid
Strut thickness	0.1 mm (0.004 inch)
Non-expanded profile	<1.0 mm (<0.04 inch)
Longitudinal flexibility	Excellent upon insertion, low after expansion
Percentage shortening on expansion	<3%
Available expanded diameters	2–5 mm
Lengths	9, 16, 25, and 32 mm
Other non-coronary types available	Peripheral stents for peripheral vessels, biliary, renal, and other uses: lengths: 14, 19, 39, and 59 mm. Expanded diameter range 5–12 mm.

(Adapted from Richter K, Almagor Y, Leon MB. The NIR stent, transforming geometry. In: Serruys PW, Kutryk MJ. *Handbook of coronary stents*. Second ed. London: Martin Dunitz, 1998:133.)

TABLE 3.14. *NIR stent delivery system*

Mechanism of deployment	Balloon expandable
Minimal internal diameter of guiding catheter	1.6 mm (0.064 inch)
Premounted on delivery catheter	Yes, available also as bare stent
Protective sheath/cover	No
Position radiopaque markers	On both ends of the stent
Further balloon expansion recommended	No
Recrossability of implanted stents	Excellent
Sizing diameter	Matching target vessel diameter

The stent delivery system specifications of the NIR stent. (Adapted from Richter K, Almagor Y, Leon MB. The NIR Stent, transforming geometry. In: Serruys PW, Kutryk MJ. *Handbook of coronary stents.* Second ed. London: Martin Dunitz, 1998:133.)

support with conformability to vessel curvature in the expanded configuration (Fig. 3.10). The "closed cell" design results in a much more flexible stent than previous slotted tube stents without straight bridge articulations. This design

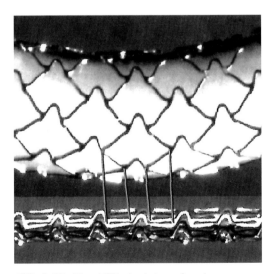

FIG. 3.10. The NIR stent, transforming geometry. Differential lengthening allows vertical struts to elongate as horizontal struts shorten, minimizing foreshortening.

also is a significant advance over connected ring stents in that excellent flexibility is achieved without sacrificing radial support and surface coverage—there are no large gaps that permit tissue prolapse.

Trackability and Flexibility Maximize Deliverability

The trackability of a stent in the naturally curved and tortuous anatomy of diseased coronary arteries is dependent upon profile, flexibility, and surface contour. The design of the NIR stent is based on uniform closed cells capable of elongating or foreshortening. The stent has no "free internal points." Loops or ends internal to the tubular structure are not connected longitudinally to their neighbors. This prevents the cells from flaring out and generating internal ridges that will create friction or adhere to the plaque surface upon insertion.

The Expanded Design Provides Rigidity and Radial Support

During expansion of the stent in the target lesion, the geometry of the basic uniform cell changes in a way that will cause the vertical loops of the cell to align with the horizontal loops and form a diamond-like cell. The "walls" of the cells align to form a long strut at about a 45-degree angle. This provides excellent hoop strength.

Continuous Closed Cells Confer Consistency

The uniform cellular design allows for a continuous support without gaps or increased distance between struts. The size of the individual cells decreases the chance for tissue prolapse into the lumen. By increasing the number of circumferential struts in the NIR stent (18 versus eight in the Palmaz Schatz stent), at an equal total radial force, the local force applied by each strut is significantly reduced.

Transforming Geometry Also Minimizes Foreshortening

The combination of vertical and horizontal loops in the NIR cell results in minimized foreshortening; upon expansion, the horizontal loops foreshorten while the vertical loops elongate. Therefore, the total length of the stent remains the same (See Fig 3.10).

NIR STENT DELIVERY SYSTEMS

The NIR stent delivery systems (NIR PRIMO and NIR-ON RANGER) are both over-the-wire and single operator exchange catheters with a balloon expandable NIR stent premounted over the semicompliant balloon. The system comes in nominal balloon diameters of 2.5, 3.0, 3.5, and 4.0 mm and lengths of 13, 20, 29, and 36 mm, corresponding to the NIR stent lengths of 9, 16, 25, and 32 mm, respectively. The stent is mounted on the balloon between two radiopaque markers, which, in conjunction with fluoroscopy, aid in the placement of the system's balloon segment and stent. Stent deployment is complete between 6 atm and 8 atm, but the balloons (with predictable growth) can be further inflated to 16 atm to facilitate complete stent expansion.

NIR-ON SOX

This is a unique delivery system with 2-mm-long restraining membranes on either end of the stent that release at 4 atm (Fig. 3.11). The "SOX" eliminate end-strut flaring, improve the crossing interface, and reduce likelihood of stent embolization without the increased rigidity and profile of a sheath system.

NIR STENT CLINICAL TRIALS

Milan Experience

Di Mario and associates reported the first "in-human" NIR stent coronary experience (9). This was a prospective single-center registry of 41 patients (mean age 59 yrs, 88% male), in whom 64 lesions were treated using 93 NIR stents. The inclusion criteria were broad and reflected "everyday experience." Ninety-eight percent of lesions were in native vessels, 50% left anterior descending (LAD) location, 48% ACC/AHA B2/C lesions, 31% of lesions were longer than 15mm in length, and 27% were in vessels smaller than 2.5 mm. All patients were treated with aspirin and ticlopidine for 1 month. Angiographic follow-up was available in 84% of the patients at 6 months. The in-hospital clinical outcomes were favorable: there were no deaths and no need for repeat revascularization, and one patient (2%) had a myocardial infarction. At 6-month follow-up, there was one death (2%), one non-Q wave MI (2%), and 17 (27%) target lesion revascularizations. By quantitative angiography, average reference vessel diameter was 2.86 mm. The minimum lumen diameter (MLD) at the lesion site increased from 1.01 mm preprocedure to 2.94 mm postprocedure, and decreased to 1.63 mm at 6-month follow-up. The diameter stenosis at 6 months was 43%, with a binary angiographic restenosis of 36%.

Singapore Experience

Lau and associates reported a similar registry experience (10). A series of 52 patients received 61 NIR stents in 55 vessels either electively, as "bailout" for threatened closure, or for failed PTCA. The acute success rate was 98% with no stent thrombosis, Q-wave MI, stroke or death. Long-term clinical follow-up (mean 9 ± 2.9 mo) showed no deaths or MI. Follow-up angiography in 43 patients (88%) at a mean of 4.8 ± 3.2 months demonstrated in-stent restenosis in 10 (23%), all of which were <3.0-mm vessels. Other registries confirmed these early favorable clinical results. (11)

Prospective Multicenter Trials

The First International Endovascular Stent Study (FINESS I) was a multi-center (11 sites), prospective registry of 255 patients (341 lesions) who underwent NIR stent placement (using 457 stents) for treatment of obstructive coronary dis-

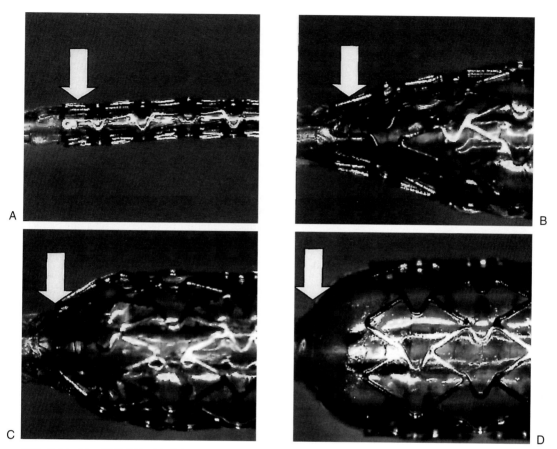

FIG. 3.11. The NIR ON with SOX. Note with expansion, the "SOX" membranes (*arrows*) retract off the stent to a low profile.

ease from December 1995 through March 1996 (12). The purpose of this study was to determine the feasibility, safety, and efficacy of elective and urgent deployment of the NIR stent in patients with simple and complex coronary lesions. Both native coronary and saphenous vein graft lesions were included for elective and 'bailout'' stenting indications. Only unprotected left main lesions, acute myocardial infarction, and bifurcation lesions were excluded. Nine-, 16-, and 32-mm-long NIR stents were manually crimped onto coronary balloons and deployed in native coronary (94%) and saphenous vein graft (6%) lesions. The mean age of the patients was 61 yrs. Eighty-four percent were male, 15% were diabetics, 48% had prior MI, and 45% had multivessel coronary disease. Seventy percent of the lesions were in LAD location, 6% had lesion

length >15 mm, and 31% had reference vessel diameter <2.5 mm, and 48% <2.75 mm. The early and late clinical outcomes are shown in Table 3.15. This study was limited because angiographic follow-up was not performed in these patients. Nevertheless, the mean lumen diameter increased by 1.51 ± 0.51 mm from pre- to post-procedure. A successful procedure with <50% diameter stenosis was accomplished in all lesions without any major adverse cardiac events (death, MI, or repeat revascularization) within 30 days in 95% of the patients. Event-free survival at 6 months was 82%. Despite the unfavorable clinical and angiographic characteristics of the patients enrolled in FINESS I, acute angiographic results and early clinical outcomes after NIR stent deployment were very promising.

FINESS II was designed as a multicenter (14

TABLE 3.15. *FINESS I, clinical outcomes*

	0–30 days (n = 255)	0–180 days (n = 255)
Any adverse event[a]	12 (4.7%)	47 (18.4%)
Death	3 (1.2%)	8 (3.1%)
MI: Q-wave	5 (2.0%)	7 (2.7%)
Non-Q MI	6 (2.4%)	8 (3.1%)
TLR (any)	4 (1.6%)	37 (14.5%)
Re-PTCA	0	24 (9.4%)
CABG	4 (1.6%)	13 (5.1%)

[a] Death or MI or TLR. MI, myocardial infarction; TLR, target lesion revascularization; PTCA, percutaneous transluminal coronary angioplasty; CABG, coronary artery bypass grafting.

sites) prospective international registry including 156 patients (mean age 60 yrs, 81% male) using 176 NIR stents (personal communication, PW Serruys). In this trial the inclusion criteria were more strict compared to those of FINESS I. Only single *de novo* native coronary lesions of ≤12mm length in vessels 3.0–5.0 mm in diameter were enrolled (similar to the STRESS/BENESTENT criteria). Angiographic and clinical follow-up was obtained in all patients at 12 months. The average reference vessel diameter by quantitative angiography was 2.94 ± 0.54 mm. At the lesion site, the acute gain (MLD post–MLD pre) was 1.60 mm (from 1.04 pre- to 2.64 postprocedure). At follow-up, late loss (MLD post–MLD follow-up) was 0.75 mm, with a loss index of 0.47. The six-month angiographic restenosis was 18% and TLR was 11.5% (Table 3.16). These improved late clinical out-

TABLE 3.16. *FINESS II, clinical outcomes*

	0–30 days (n = 156)	0–180 days (n = 156)
Any adverse event*	3 (1.9%)	21 (13.5%)
Death	0	0
MI: (total)	2 (1.3%)	3 (1.9%)
Q-wave	0	1 (0.6%)
Non-Q MI	2 (1.3%)	2 (1.3%)
TLR (any)	1 (0.6%)	18 (11.5%)
Re-PTCA	0	15 (9.6%)
CABG	1 (0.6%)	3 (1.9%)

*Death or MI or TLR; MI, myocardial infarction; TLR, Target lesion revascularization; PTCA, Percutaneous transluminal coronary angioplasty; CABG, Coronary artery bypass grafting.

comes clearly reflect the stricter inclusion criteria compared to FINESS I. These two early registry studies outside the U.S. prompted a prospective multi-center randomized trial comparing the NIR stent to other currently available stents.

The randomized NIR Vascular Advanced North American Trial (NIRVANA) randomized patients with single coronary lesions to treatment with the NIR stent or the Palmaz-Schatz stent (13). The study was designed to demonstrate equivalence (i.e., non-inferiority) of the NIR stent to the Palmaz-Schatz stent for the primary endpoint of target vessel failure (TVF defined as death, MI, or target vessel revascularization by 9 months). Secondary endpoints included acute procedure success, major adverse cardiac events, stent thrombosis, and measures of late angiographic results in a pre-specified subset undergoing routine angiographic follow-up. From January to April 1997, 849 patients with single *de novo* or restenotic native vessel lesions were randomized in 41 participating centers in the United States. The NIR stents used in this trial were seven-cell and nine-cell design in lengths of 9, 16, and 32 mm. The delivery system used was a single operator exchange Ranger platform (Scimed, Minneapolis, MN) and balloon diameters were 3.0, 3.5, and 4.0 mm. The baseline characteristics of the patients were similar between the two groups. The reference vessel sizes for both PS and NIR group were similar (3.0 mm). The post procedure in-stent diameter stenosis was lower for the NIR stent versus PS stent (7% versus 9%, $p = .04$). For the subset of patients with angiographic follow-up, the in-stent binary restenosis rate at six months was 20.0% for the NIR and 22.0% for the PS stent ($p = $ NS). The 9-month cumulative events are listed in Table 3.17. The rate of target lesion revascularization on all patients was 8.6% for the NIR stent versus 11.4% for PS stent ($p = $ NS). Multivariate logistic regression models showed that the independent predictors of restenosis were: post-in-stent MLD, longer lesion length, history of diabetes mellitus, and LAD target vessel. In summary, the randomized NIRVANA trial showed that the NIR stent is equivalent to the gold standard Palmaz-Schatz stent for

TABLE 3.17. *NIRVANA, clinical outcomes*

Cumulative events at 9 months	Palmaz-Schatz (n = 430)	NIR (n = 418)
Death	0.9%	1.0%
MI: (total)	4.2%	4.9%
Q-wave	0.9%	0.7%
Non-Q MI	3.3%	4.1%
TLR (any)	11.4%	8.6%
Re-PTCA	8.4%	6.5%
CABG	3.0%	2.1%
TVR	13.3%	11.5%
TVF[a]	14.4%	12.4%

[a] Death or MI or TVR. MI, myocardial infarction; TLR, target lesion revascularization; PTCA, percutaneous transluminal coronary angioplasty; CABG, coronary artery bypass grafting; TVR, target vessel revascularization; TVF, target vessel failure.

the treatment of focal *de novo* or restenotic lesions in native coronary arteries.

In addition, there were two NIR stent non-randomized registries including treatment of saphenous vein grafts and abrupt threatened closure lesions (14). The inclusion criteria were: (a) a single *de novo* or restenotic lesion (the prior restenosis must be >2 months from a previous non-stent procedure) with the target lesion <30 mm in length in a saphenous vein graft or (b) abrupt or threatened closure in a native coronary artery, with a reference vessel diameter (2.5 mm and ≤4.0 mm, due to treatment with a non-stent device. The SVG registry included 155 patients. The in-hospital major adverse cardiac event (MACE) rate was 3.2%, with a 6-month MACE rate of 16.1% and a TLR rate of 8.0%. The abrupt or threatened closure registry included 207 patients with in-hospital MACE of 6.8%, 6-month MACE rate of 23.2%, and TLR of 15.4% at 6 months.

In summary, completed clinical trials in the United States, Europe, and Asia support the safety and efficacy of the NIR stent. Compared to the Palmaz-Schatz stent, the NIR stent is equivalent (or better) for acute and long term results in the treatment of discrete coronary lesions. The NIR stent offers important advantages, especially improved flexibility without sacrificing radial support. The low profile delivery systems, including the SOX concept, insure stent securement which further facilitates stent deliverability and treatment of complex lesion morphologies. Clinical trials including more complex lesion subsets (both in Europe and in the United States) demonstrate excellent technical success, favorable procedural outcomes, and improved late clinical results.

THE NIR FUTURE

The NIR family of stents has grown to accommodate the wide range of challenging lesions that confront the practicing interventionalist. Stents have been developed for small vessels, lesions requiring exact positioning, bifurcation lesions, and extra-cardiac vessels.

Smaller Vessels

The NIR 5 Cell (Medinol/Boston Scientific) was designed especially for vessel diameters of 1.5–2.5 mm. The reduced number of cells maintains optimal surface coverage, radial support and trackability for smaller stent diameters. The crimped profile is 0.6 mm to help ensure deliverability. Fully expanded, the stent diameter is 2.5 mm and is available in lengths of 9, 16, 19 and 25 mm (Fig. 3.12).

Improved Radiopacity

The NIROYAL (Medinol/Boston Scientific) is a gold plated NIR stent which provides opti-

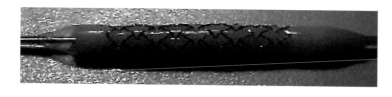

FIG. 3.12. The NIR 5 Cell stent expanded to 2.0 mm.

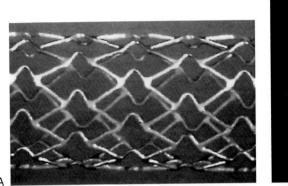
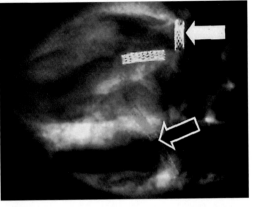

A

B

FIG. 3.13. The NIROYAL gold plated stent in detail **(A)**, and on X-ray **(B)**. Note the radiopacity of the NIROYAL (*solid arrow*) versus the NIR (*outlined arrow*).

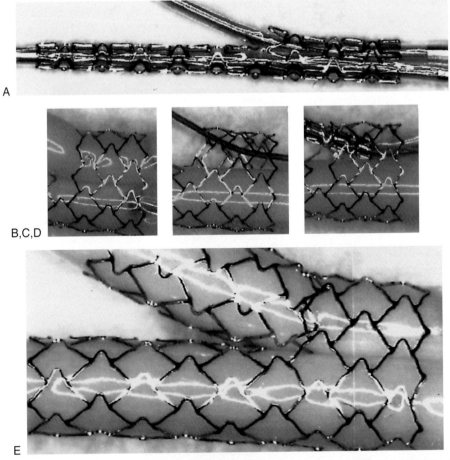

A

B,C,D

E

FIG. 3.14. The NIRSIDE crimped on two balloons with guidewires for each branch **(A)**. After inflation of both **(B)**, if the side branch result is not satisfactory a second stent may be deployed without difficulty or struts protruding into either vessel **(C–E)**.

mal radiopacity (Fig. 3.13). The stent is visible in both contracted and expanded states, but will not obscure angiographic details. NIROYAL struts are rounded, which may minimize vascular trauma. NIROYAL gold plating is available on all standard and peripheral NIR sizes and lengths.

Bifurcation Lesions

Interventional therapy of bifurcation lesions is associated with higher procedural complications (i.e., side branch occlusion) and higher restenosis rates, especially if both the parent and the daughter (side) branch vessels are treated (15).

The NIRSIDE (Medinol/Boston Scientific) stent was developed for "provisional" stenting of bifurcation lesions. The stent may be crimped on a dedicated balloon delivery system with guidewires for each of the branches (Fig. 3.14). Distally, the stent is a regular NIR; proximally, the stent is larger to better scaffold the parent vessel; and in between, there is an open cell. The daughter branch guidewire passes through the open cell. If the initial result is not optimal or threatens the daughter branch, a second stent may then be easily advanced through the side branch open cell. This system allows "cullote"

stenting without leaving stent struts protruding into parent or branch vessels, easier crossing of the parent stent, and reduced "jailing" of the branch vessels. In addition to superior results when both branches are stented, the NIRSIDE system allows the operator the discretion to choose facilitated stenting of the side branch only when absolutely necessary. All NIRSIDE stents feature NIROYAL gold plating for accurate deployment.

For Extra-Cardiac Applications

The NIR Peripheral (Medinol/Boston Scientific) stents maintain the transformable geometry features of coronary NIR stents for larger vessels (Fig. 3.15). By increasing the number of cells to seven, nine, or 11, the stents retain flexibility for insertion and provide excellent radial support after expansion. The seven- and nine-cell stents are 7 Fr-compatible, allowing use of traditional "coronary" equipment. The combination of low profiles and flexibility results in unprecedented trackability for a peripheral system (Fig. 3.16). The seven-and nine-cell stents are available in diameters from 5 to 9 mm and in lengths of 14, 19, and 39 mm. The 11-cell stent is available in 6–12-mm diameters with 19-, 39-, and 59-mm

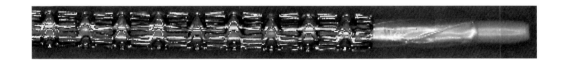

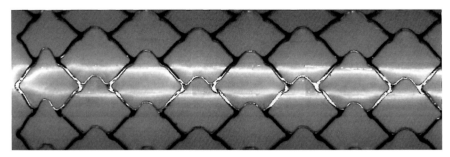

FIG. 3.15. The NIR Peripheral stent, crimped on an Ultrathin Diamond (*above*) and expanded to 10 mm (*below*).

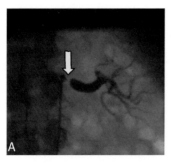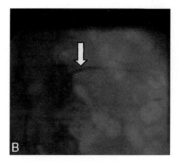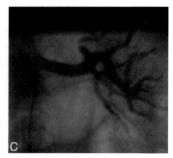

FIG. 3.16. A severe, ostial left renal artery stenosis **(A)**, is easily crossed with a NIR 9 cell via a 7 Fr system **(B)**, producing an excellent final result **(C)**.

lengths. All NIR Peripheral stents feature NIRO-YAL gold plating for positioning accuracy.

CONCLUSIONS AND SUMMARY

The NIR stent philosophy integrates advanced design concepts with practical technical requirements of the interventionalist to develop optimal clinical treatment strategies for patients with simple and complex ischemic vascular disease. Improved flexibility with maximal scaffolding and radial support is unique to the NIR closed cell stent design and remains a consistent theme throughout the full range of stent platforms available for coronary and peripheral vascular disease. Clinical trial data in patients with coronary artery disease substantiate the enhanced deliverability, improved peri-procedural results, and excellent long-term clinical and angiographic outcomes associated with the NIR coronary stent around the world. Further enhancements and additions to the NIR stent family to improve radiopacity, for the treatment of complex coronary lesion subsets, and in patients with peripheral vascular disease are already being subjected to early clinical trial evaluations.

REFERENCES

1. Fischman DL, Leon MB, Baim DS et al. A randomized comparison of coronary-stent placement and balloon angioplasty in the treatment of coronary artery disease. Stent restenosis study investigators. *N Engl J Med* 1994; 331:496–501.
2. George CJ, Baim DS, Brinker JA et al. One-year follow-up of the Stent Restenosis (STRESS I) Study. *Am J Cardiol* 1998;81:860–865.
3. Serruys PW, de Jaegere P, Kiemeneij F et al. A comparison of balloon-expandable-stent implantation with balloon angioplasty in patients with coronary artery disease. BENESTENT Study Group. *N Engl J Med* 1994; 331:489–495.
4. Macaya C, Serruys PW, Ruygrok P et al. Continued benefit of coronary stenting versus balloon angioplasty: One-year clinical follow-up of BENESTENT trial. BENESTENT Study Group. *J Am Coll Cardiol* 1996; 27:255–261.
5. Wong SC, Baim DS, Schatz RA et al. Immediate results and late outcomes after stent implantation in saphenous vein graft lesions: The multicenter U.S. Palmaz-Schatz stent experience. The Palmaz-Schatz Stent Study Group. *J Am Coll Cardiol* 1995;26:704–712.
6. Fenton SH, Fischman DL, Savage MP et al. Long-term angiographic and clinical outcome after implantation of balloon-expandable stents in aortocoronary saphenous vein grafts. *Am J Cardiol* 1994;74:1187–1191.
7. Piana RN, Moscucci M, Cohen DJ et al. Palmaz-Schatz stenting for treatment of focal vein graft stenosis: immediate results and long-term outcome. *J Am Coll Cardiol* 1994;23:1296–1304.
8. Richter K, Almagor Y, Leon MB. The NIR stent, transforming geometry. In: Serruys PW, Kutryk MJ, eds. *Handbook of coronary stents*. Second ed. London: Martin Dunitz, 1998:131–145.
9. Di Mario C, Reimers B, Almagor Y et al. Procedural and follow up results with a new balloon expandable stent in unselected lesions. *Heart* 1998;79:234–241.
10. Lau KW, He Q, Ding ZP, Quek S, Johan A. Early experience with the NIR intracoronary stent. *Am J Cardiol* 1998;81:927–929.
11. Zheng H, Corcos T, Favereau X et al. Preliminary experience with the NIR coronary stent. *Cathet Cardiovasc Diagn* 1998;43:153–158.
12. Almagor Y, Feld S, Kiemeneij F et al. First International New Intravascular Rigid-Flex Endovascular Stent Study (FINESS): Clinical and angiographic results after elective and urgent stent implantation. The FINESS trial investigators. *J Am Coll Cardiol* 1997; 30:847–854.
13. Baim DS, Cutlip DE, Sharma SK et al. The NIRVANA investigators. A randomized trial comparing the NIR stent to the Palmaz-Schatz stent in native coronary lesions. *J Am Coll Cardiol* in press.

14. Lansky AJ, Popma JJ, Mehran R et al. Late quantitative angiographic results after NIR stent use: results from the NIRVANA randomized trial and registries. *J Am Coll Cardiol* 1998;31:80A–81A(abst).

15. Lefevre T, Louvard Y, Morice MC et al. Stenting of bifurcation lesions. In: Marco J, Fajadet J, eds. *Ninth complex coronary angioplasty course book.* Paris: Europa Edition, 1998:311–318.

F. Self-Expanding Stents

David P. Foley and *Michael J.B. Kutryk

Thoraxcenter, University Hospital Rotterdam, 3015 GD Rotterdam, The Netherlands;
°Department of Cardiology, Saint Michael's Hospital, Toronto M5B1W8, Canada

There are currently three self-expanding stent designs available for clinical use.

1. The Schneider Wallstent (Schneider AG, Bülach, Switzerland), which was the pioneering endocoronary prosthesis;
2. the SCIMED Radius (Maple Grove, MN) stent, which was introduced in 1995 and has undergone clinical evaluation in registry as well as randomized trial; and
3. the recently introduced Medtronic Instent (Medtronic, Minneapolis, MN), which has yet to be clinically evaluated.

The evolution of the Wallstent is a chronicle of the development of coronary stent practice, particularly in Europe, in a treatise on self-expanding stents, deserves to be elaborately described. The completed trials of the Radius stent will also be detailed and the technical design of the Medtronic Instent will be described and illustrated.

THE CORONARY WALLSTENT

Historical Perspective

In 1985, the initial results of the percutaneous implantation of spring-loaded, self-expanding Z-type stents in dogs were described by Cesare Gianturco and colleagues (1). They appreciated the importance of oversizing the stent in relation to the size of the target vessel to prevent migration of the prostheses. However, the inflexibility of this early device, difficulties in its precise placement, and its apparent thrombogenicity in the canine coronary circulation led to the abandonment of its development and a reconsideration of a balloon-expandable stent which had been initially investigated by Gianturco and associates at MD Anderson Hospital in Houston, Texas, in 1981. In collaboration with Gary Roubin, the design of the original device was modified to an incomplete serpentine coil structure, and the first-generation stainless-steel Gianturco-Roubin Flex-Stent was released.

In Europe, the concept of a self-expanding coronary prosthesis was more successfully elaborated and in 1986, the self-expanding Wallstent became the first stent to undergo clinical evaluation in human coronary arteries, inaugurating a new era in interventional cardiology. The initial evaluation of what was eventually to become the coronary Wallstent began with Rousseau and coworkers (2), who tested a flexible, self-expanding, stainless-steel mesh stent that was restrained with a protective sheath. Despite partial or total thrombotic occlusions in 35% of the treated porcine arteries, this early experience provided the impetus for the implantation of a stent in an atheromatous human coronary artery. Clinical evaluation of the Wallstent began in 1986, with the first human implantations done by Jacques Puel (Toulouse, France)(3), followed shortly after by Ulrich Sigwart (Lausanne, Switzerland), and Patrick Serruys (Rotterdam, the Netherlands). The results of the implantation of 24 self-expanding mesh stents (Medinvent SA, Lausanne, Switzerland) in the coronary arteries of 19 patients were reported in 1987 (4). In that year, two additional centers in Lille (France) and London joined the collaboration, followed in 1989 by Geneva (Switzerland). The European Wallstent experience was an open-ended feasibility study for the possible uses of a coronary stent. At the outset, there was no study protocol to be followed, and each investigator selected the type of lesion to be stented and the anticoagulation regimen. As with all new procedures, operators had to struggle with the technical learning curve and develop clinical indications and contraindications from their experience. In May 1988, the five European centers testing the Wallstent agreed to set up a core laboratory in Rotterdam for quantitative angiographic analysis, to independently assess the results objectively (5,6). This decision was also an important milestone in establishing the standards for appropriate evaluation of all new intracoronary treatments.

Early Clinical Results

By January 1988, 117 Wallstents had been implanted (94 in native coronary arteries, 23 in aortocoronary-bypass grafts) in 105 patients (5), mainly electively for prevention of re-restenosis after prior balloon angioplasty in 71, to improve on unsatisfactory results of elective balloon angioplasty of primary lesions in 27, for acute vessel occlusion during balloon angioplasty in 14, and after recanalizing and dilating chronic total occlusion in five. A high rate of stent thrombosis emphasized the controversy that surrounded the choice of a suitable anticoagulation regimen that could minimize postprocedural complications without increasing the risk of excessive hemorrhagic side-effects. Adjunctive anticoagulation varied between centers and patients, ranging from sub-cutaneous heparin to routine intracoronary urokinase periprocedurally. Postprocedurally, many of the initial patients received no oral anticoagulation while others received some aspirin, Coumadin (Du Pont Pharmaceuticals), dipyridamole, and sulfinpyrazone, or combinations thereof.

The results of intermediate-term follow-up of this first series were sobering, with four patient deaths before repeat angiography and complete occlusion of 27 stents in 25 (24%) patients. However, a long-term restenosis rate of 14% in those that remained patent was extremely en-

couraging (5). The geometric aspects of Wallstent implantation were well studied in the early phase (7,8), but evaluation of the early implantation techniques with a critical eye today (10 years later) illustrates the naievete of the belief held by early investigators that merely releasing the stent in the coronary was sufficient and appropriate. As has been the trend in the rapidly evolving specialty of interventional cardiology, empirical remedies evolved rapidly and the early, and excessively high thrombosis rates were reduced to 10% by the combination of postdilating the Wallstent and improved anticoagulation regimes. (The postdilation technique was termed the ''Swiss Kiss'' by Patrick Serruys, referring to Ulrich Sigwart's idea to accelerate early expansion of the stent.) These parallel developments may be compared to more recent steps in reducing acute and sub-acute thrombosis by replacing anti-coagulant by anti-platelet therapy simultaneously with a strategy of optimal stent deployment, so that the independent contribution of each of the changes in the previous conventional approach cannot be easily quantified, but both steps were clearly appropriate. Despite the improvement in stent thrombosis achieved in 1990, the impending publication of the first major report in the New England Journal of Medicine in 1991 concerning the coronary Wallstent, incorporating the early learning curve experience as well as the more improved later results, led to the coronary Wallstent being withdrawn from the market in late 1990 because of the unacceptably high acute and sub-acute thrombosis rate. By March 1990, a total of 265 patients with 308 lesions had been included in the European multicenter Wallstent evaluation study. Significant differences were observed between the early (March 1986 to January 1988) and later (February 1988 to March 1990) experiences in terms of patient and lesion selection. In the later period, a greater percentage of bypass grafts and primary stenoses were treated and the early occlusion rate dropped from 24 to 10%. At the time it was not completely evident that the high early thrombosis rates in the early trials were not a result of properties intrinsic to the stent itself; since then, it has been pointed out that the problems could be attributed to the early learning curve of implantation techniques and errors in periprocedural management (9).

The small glimmer of hope in what has been called the "Pandora's box" of stenting (10) fortunately encouraged persistence by the pioneers. The observation of lower early occlusion rates in bypass grafts compared with native coronaries led in 1991 to recommencement of evaluation of the "less-shortening" Wallstent for venous bypass graft lesions. A total of 29 patients had successful implantation of 35 (out of 36 attempted) stents in 30 lesions between November 1991 and March 1993 at six centers in the Netherlands, Belgium, and Germany (11). All five cases of additional stent placement were required for proximal coverage. Thus, the need for additional stent placements was still a consequence of stent shortening from proximal to distal. This shortening may have been related to unawareness or misjudgment by the physician in choosing the appropriate length of stent to allow for the expected degree of shortening. (This in turn may have been due to lack of appropriate data from the manufacturer at that time.) No patient experienced a major adverse cardiac event (MACE) in-hospital. Sixteen percent had a hemorrhagic complication. By 6 month follow-up, one patient had experienced a non-Q-wave infarction (CPK 300 u/l) at 22 days with an angiographically patent stent, one patient underwent a repeat CABG due to progression of native coronary artery disease, and five patients had a reintervention (one for occlusion); thus the implantations resulted in a 76% event-free survival rate. These results were considered extremely favorable and indicated the need for more extensive clinical studies with this second-generation Wallstent.

Technical Design Evolution

After the stent was acquired from Medinvent SA (Lausanne, Switzerland), by Schneider (Bülach, Switzerland) in 1990, technical redevelopment was considered necessary. In particular, it had been observed that the use of multiple stents per lesion with stent overlap was a predictor of both early thrombosis and restenosis and that this was partly due to the unpredictable and excessive shortening on expansion of the stent. In addition, the stent was poorly visible on fluoroscopy. The original stainless steel mesh was replaced by a device made of strands of a non-ferromagnetic cobalt-based alloy with a platinum core. The wire was arranged into a self-expanding mesh that relies on the elastic range of metal deformation to expand (Fig. 3.17). The composition and design afforded the stent excellent longitudinal flexibility and good radiopacity. In the expanded state, the metallic surface area of the first-generation devices was roughly 20% of the stented surface, whereas with modification of the wire braid angle, the surface area of later devices was reduced to 14% and the device shortened less on expansion, allowing more precise placement (thus the term "the less-shortening Wallstent" [11]), which was first evaluated in the previously mentioned study in venous bypass grafts between 1991 and 1993. Thereafter, a diameter/length chart was provided to aid in tailoring stent selection to the target vessel. In the first and second generations, three radiopaque markers were present on the delivery catheter. Two markers were intended to indicate the distal and proximal extremities of the stent mounted on the delivery catheter, and the third marker was intended to give an approximate location of the proximal edge of the implanted stent in an appropriately expanded state.

In first-generation devices, the Wallstent was compressed and thus elongated on the delivery system, constrained by a doubled-over rolling membrane system. After positioning the stent was deployed by first re-inflating the indeflator to 4 atm–5 atm to facilitate rolling of the membrane. The rolling of the membrane was achieved by holding the steel rod and progressively retracting the catheter shaft onto the rod, thus releasing the stent from distal to proximal, thereby anchoring the stent against the arterial wall (See Fig. 3.17). As the stent began to deploy, there was a commitment to release, with the opportunity to drag the stent more proximally, if desired. On expansion, the stent shortened by about 15 to 20% of its constrained length. Its unconstrained length varied between 15 and 40 mm and its diameter in the fully expanded state ranged from 4.0 mm to 6.0 mm.

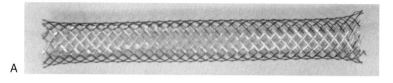

A

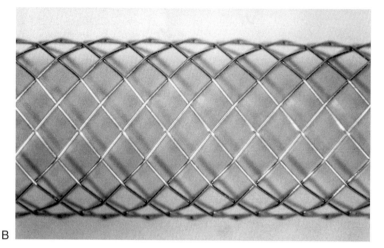

B

FIG. 3.17. A: The unconstrained Wallstent, first-generation. Flaring at the ends allows anchorage of the stent in the vessel wall, but with the potential to cause dissection, which partly explains the frequent need for additional stents as described in the early studies. **B:** The tight mesh structure is appreciated, rendering side branch access extremely difficult, although recent experience indicates that dilatation and even stenting with very low-profile stent is possible, although of dubious long term value.

With the introduction of the newer Magic Wallstent, a few of the disadvantages of the previous design were addressed. Principally, the Magic Wallstent uses a single-layer retractable sheath (instead of a rolling membrane system), so that no contrast injection is required to retract the membrane. In addition, the lower profile makes the device compatible with a 6 Fr guiding catheter. Furthermore, even more practically relevant, a partially deployed stent (officially up to 50%) may be retracted in the sheath and repositioned. This improved system allows more precise placement of the stent, especially with the more-difficult-to-place shorter units. A broader range of units has been introduced with this generation, ranging from "Mini," which is 3.5 mm in diameter and 11 mm long when fully unconstrained, to "Extra long," which is 48 mm long in its completely unconstrained state, ranging from 4.0 mm to 6.0 mm in diameter. This information is instantly readable from the Wallchart (Schneider) for convenient display in the catheterization laboratory, as well as on every stent package. Furthermore, the Magic Wallstent has recently been further modified to incorporate a monorail delivery.

Wallstent Implantation Recommendations

The inner and outer packaging for each Wallstent features bold-print recommendations specifying vessel diameter and the expected stent length at that diameter. Each package also provides a series of stent length-diameter relationships, starting with the unconstrained length and listing lengths expected at half-millimeter diameter increments. For example, a 5.0-mm "medium" stent would be 32 mm long in a 5-mm-diameter vessel, 35 mm at 4.5 mm (the recommended maximal vessel size for use of a 5-mm-diameter Wallstent), 38 mm at 4.0 mm, 41 mm at 3.5 mm, and 45 mm at 3.0 mm. It is recommended to select a Magic Wallstent using this information, based on the maximum target segment lumen diameter and the lesion length, so that the stent is at least 4 mm longer than the segment to be covered (to allow at least 2 mm of stent for anchorage proximal and distal to the lesion). These dimensions are ideally measured objectively, using the dilating balloon length or the opaque part of the guidewire, on-line quantitative coronary angiography (QCA) or intravascular ultrasound (IVUS). In early experience,

Schneider recommends adding at least 8 mm to the stent length selection to allow for possible underestimation of shortening after placement and postdilation.

The Magic Wallstent is generously 6 Fr- (0.064 inch lumen) compatible. An exchange-length guide wire (ideally with good support characteristics) was necessary until the monorail Magic Wallstent became available. Standard predilatation and optimizing postdilatation is generally recommended, although due to its self-expanding properties, the Wallstent can be implanted without predilatation in old, friable bypass grafts where instrumentation, especially by balloon angioplasty, provokes a high risk of embolization. Several centers have advocated the Wallstent as the device of choice for this indication (12,13). On the other hand, if an optimal predilatation has been achieved and in non-resistant lesions, after placement, postdilatation may not be necessary if good stent apposition is apparent after deployment with a satisfactory angiographic result (<20% diameter stenosis). There is compelling evidence of continuing stent expansion by serial IVUS studies even after an optimal initial placement (14,15).

The Wallstent's smooth exterior polyurethane restraining membrane and its longitudinal flexibility provide one of the most easily trackable and deliverable stents available, even in the longer units, with the capacity to successfully negotiate tortuous, stiff, and calcified vessels. This is sometimes only achievable by firm continuous forward pressure on the catheter, simultaneously with traction applied to the guidewire (which should have good support characteristics). It has been our experience over the years, especially with the first-generation rigid balloon-expandable stents, but even today (although less frequently), the Wallstent is an excellent trouble-shooting or bail-out stent. It will go where you need it to go and will almost always cover the entire segment that needs to be stented, using a single stent (with lengths up to 50 mm). The combination of the flexible-sheathed wall stent with 6 Fr guide catheters for safe and easy deep vessel intubation makes virtually every anatomical circumstance accessible to a Wallstent. The Wallstent is not, however, recommended for elective use in the region of important side-branches, because the mesh structure will imprison them. It is possible to pass through the mesh to dilate side branches with modern, low-profile balloons, and we have stented a side-branch using a NIR stent through a previously placed Wallstent, but the stent occluded after 3 months, partly due to recoil of the Wallstent mesh. Although anecdotes must not dictate policy, based on the cumulative experience over the years, we try to avoid jailing side-branches >2 mm in diameter with a Wallstent. Many of the trials described below have included a majority of target lesions in the right coronary artery. This may be because the absence of important left ventricular branches between the ostium and crux and the usually larger diameter (compared with the LAD) lend themselves better to optimal tailored Wallstent placement (Fig. 3.18B). Because of the available length as mentioned, complete ''reconstruction'' of chronically occluded or diffusely diseased right coronary arteries or venous grafts is particularly suited for the Wallstent, using 3 or less stents (11–13,16)(see Fig. 3.18B).

Recent Clinical Studies and Trials

A number of non-randomized studies using the second-generation, ''less-shortening'' Wallstent have reported excellent acute results with implantation success generally close to 100% and hospital event rates <5%, but with varying late clinical and angiographic results. Our group previously reported 30-day freedom from events in 97% of patients, 83% event-free survival after 6 months, and a luminal loss of 0.74 mm (16). However, that was a single-center study, in 36 patients treated by the same experienced team of operators, selecting larger vessels and using an aggressive post-dilatation strategy, as exemplified by the postprocedural minimum lumin diameter (MLD) of 3.06 mm. On the basis of what has become generally accepted as the ''bigger is better'' philosophy, the achievement of such a postprocedural MLD is entirely consistent with a clinical event rate of 15% (17).

The Wellstent Studies

The Wellstent multicenter European clinical evaluations of the less-shortening Wallstent

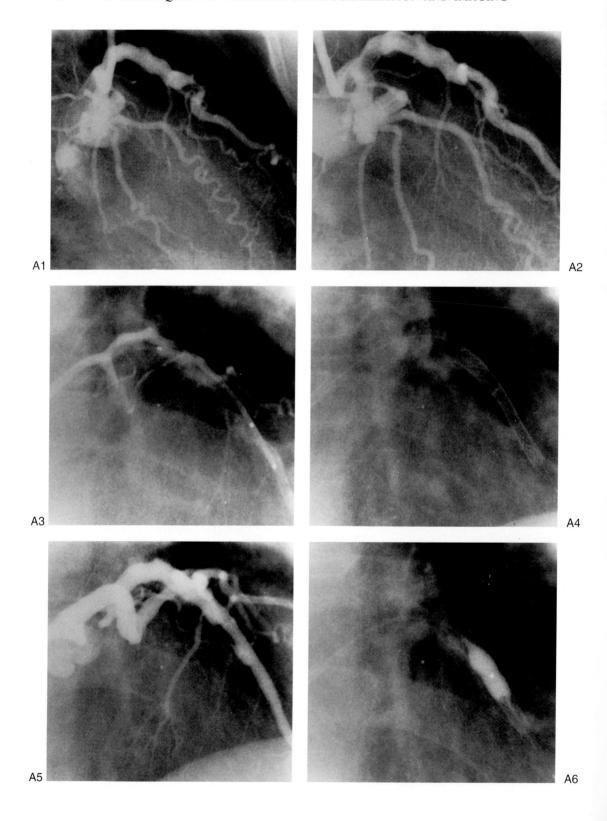

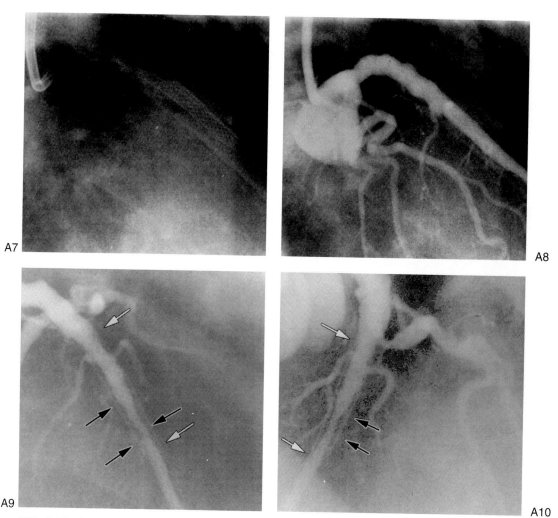

A7

A8

A9

A10

FIG. 3.18. Clinical examples. **A: Panel 1** shows an extremely eccentric and severe proximal LAD lesion with a double bend immediately distal in a 56-year-old female with Braunwald Class IIB angina pectoris. **Panel 2** is after predilatation. **Panel 3** shows positioning of a 4.5-mm-diameter, 27-mm-length (unconstrained) second-generation Wallstent. This length is chosen to adequately cover the lesion proximally and distally, encompassing the tortuous segment. Opacification of the vessel is achieved with difficulty, despite the use of an 8 Fr guiding catheter. **Panel 4** shows the radiopacity of the released stent and **panel 5** shows that postdilatation is required to reach an optimal result. **Panel 6** shows post-dilatation at the site of worst stenosis with a 4.0-mm "Chubby" balloon (Schneider, Switzerland). **Panel 7** shows the more expanded Wallstent, now perceptibly shortened compared to panel 4. **Panel 8** is the final result, with optimal tapering of the segment from the considerably larger proximal segment, measured at 4.53 mm by online QCA, to the smaller mid-LAD, with a diameter of 2.55 mm immediately distal to the stent and MLD of 2.92 mm within the stent. At routine 6-month follow-up, the patient was asymptomatic, with a negative maximal exercise test. **Panel 9** shows the non-opacified stent and **panel 10** shows the contrast-filled segment, showing marginally significant restenosis. The visibility of the stent appears to overemphasize the degree of stenosis, raising the dilemma of what to do, and stimulating the oculostenotic reflex . To help decision making, intravascular ultrasound examination was performed, revealing a minimal diameter in the treated segment of 1.88 mm. Based on all aspects, no intervention was carried out. One year later, the patient remains symptom free. *(Figure continues.)*

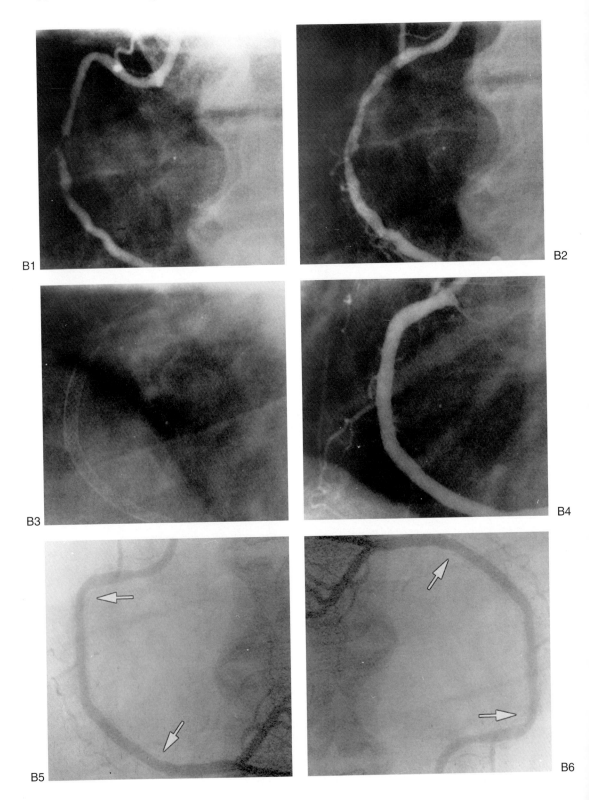

combined with aspirin and ticlopidine in native vessels (Wellstent Native Study [18]) and venous bypass grafts (Wellstent Bypass Study [19]) have been completed. In the native study in 105 patients, of whom 43% had unstable angina with 111 lesions (74% of which were type B2 or C) acute procedural success (successful stent implantation with residual stenosis <20%) was achieved in 99%. Mean reference vessel diameter was 3.18 ± 0.66 mm, MLD was 1.00 ± 0.50 mm pre- and 2.84 ± 0.47 mm poststent (diameter stenosis 16 ± 6%). Mean hospital stay was 2.2 days. At 30 days, 95% of patients were free of MACE. At 6-month and 1-year clinical follow-ups, 75% and 72% of patients, respectively, remained free of MACE. The majority of the MACE that did occur (63%) were re-interventions at follow-up re-angiography and most of these were not clinically driven. In 90% of eligible patients, MLD at follow-up was 1.65 ± 0.75 mm (late loss 1.20 ± 0.66 mm), late loss index was 0.65, diameter stenosis was 42 ± 15%, and the restenosis rate was 32%. Implantation of longer stents was associated with greater luminal loss ($p = .001$) and less favorable clinical outcome. It was concluded that the stent was safe and acutely effective, even in this high risk group, with excellent 30-day clinical results. Late restenosis was superficially greater than the rate reported in other studies (i.e., BENESTENT and STRESS), in more stable patients with shorter and less complex lesions. However, it must be noted that non-clinically driven repeat angioplasty (i.e., occu-

lostenotic reflex during routine follow-up angiography) represented more than 60% of late events, many of which might have never occurred had angiography only been performed where clinically indicated. This was strikingly demonstrated in the BENESTENT 2 trial, where routine follow-up angiography after stenting was associated with an artificial increase in "clinical events" (19). In the case of the Wallstent, the occulostenotic reflex may be even greater than that observed with other stents, being particularly eye-catching because of the excellent radiopacity of the Wallstent (Fig. 3.18). Not intervening in these cases without symptoms or demonstrable ischemia has been shown to be associated with an excellent 3-year outcome (20,21), and this principle needs to be more widely applied in the appropriate context. Use of additional rapidly performable and informative diagnostic tests, such as translesional pressure gradient and fractional flow reserve (21) measurement, or coronary flow reserve, may reassure the physician that the apparent in-stent restenosis is not physiologically important and need not be treated.

In the Wellstent Bypass trial conducted between October 1995 and July 1996, 109 patients were included by 15 European centers (19). A total of 122 lesions were treated with 164 stents, of which 16 were not Wallstents. Mean patient age was 66 ± 8 years, which is somewhat older than in most native vessel studies, and there was an expectedly high prevalence of adverse characteristics and risk factors. Thirty-six percent of

FIG. 3.18. *Continued.* **B:** Case to illustrate the potential use of the Wallstent for "reconstruction" of a diffusely diseased right coronary artery. **Panel 1** in the left inferior oblique projection shows the preintervention image, with a localized severe tandem stenosis in the mid-segment and diffuse narrowing throughout, which appears anything but enticing for percutaneous therapy. The patient had Braunwald Class IIIB angina and needed urgent intervention. **Panel 2** is after placement of a support guidewire and pre-dilatation with a 40-mm-long, 3-mm-diameter balloon at nominal pressure. **Panel 3** shows fluoroscopic image after placement of two 4.0-mm-diameter, 39-mm-long Wallstents and a 16-mm NIR stent to reach the ostium. **Panel 4** is the final optimal result, which is almost unimaginable beforehand. However, with almost 10 cm of implanted stent, the possibility of restenosis would appear to be high. Fortunately, on this occasion, nature was kind and at 6 months (**panel 5** showing the fluoroscopic image and **panel 6** showing the contrast opacified vessel) there was no significant renarrowing. Perhaps this case is illustrative of the need to achieve the most optimal acute results safely achievable at the time of coronary intervention and worry about the possibility of restenosis only if and when it happens.

patients had unstable angina, mainly Braunwald class IIB, and of the remainder, more than half had Canadian Cardiovascular Society Class 3 or 4 angina. Not unexpectedly, 95% of lesions were classified as ACC/AHA type C, a functional or total occlusion was present in 10.6%, and thrombus was present in 2.5%. Wallstents could be successfully deployed in all but one of the 122 target lesions. Postdilatation of the Wallstent was carried out in 87% of cases, with postdilation-related complications occurring in 2.5%. A single Wallstent was sufficient in 64.8% of patients. Two stents were needed in 25%, three stents in 5.6%, four stents in 2.8%, and five stents in 1.9%. The reference vessel diameter preintervention was 3.24 mm, with an MLD of 1.05 mm and diameter stenosis of 67%. Postprocedurally, the MLD increased to 2.93 mm with a diameter stenosis of 16%. Postprocedurally, patients were treated with aspirin and ticlopidine 500 mg daily for 1 month, in addition to whatever other medication was prescribed. The mean duration of hospital stay was 2.9 ± 3.8 days. At 30-day follow-up, the predetermined evaluation time for the primary endpoint of safety and efficacy, a total of 6.4% had experienced MACE, one of whom died from postdilatation-induced graft rupture. Five patients experienced periprocedural non-Q-wave myocardial infarction (three of which were diagnosed by asymptomatic enzyme increase) and one patient underwent a new PTCA procedure 12 days after a successful index procedure.

At 1 year, 42.2% of patients had experienced one or more events, ten patients (9%) had a fatal outcome, 11% had myocardial infarction (3.7% Q-wave and 7.3% non-Q-wave), 4.6% underwent repeat CABG, and 17.4% underwent repeat PTCA. The cause of death was cardiac in seven patients (one of whom was described above), two died within 2 days after the repeat CABG, two died suddenly out of hospital, and two died within 24 hours of hospital readmission with acute myocardial infarction in the months after successful graft stenting. Mean duration between stenting and death was 167 days.

Only 57.8% of the patients remained event-free at 1 year, which is significantly less than in the stented group of the SAVED trial and similar to the results achieved in the balloon angioplasty group in simple vein graft lesions (23). However, the population treated in this Wellstent study represents the more extreme end of the risk spectrum, as described. The results are in fact somewhat superior to those reported by Morrison and associates in similar types of patients (24) using an aggressive balloon angioplasty approach in the early 1990s. The mortality rate of 9% at 1 year is slightly higher than the 5% to 7% perioperative mortality for repeat CABG (25), but similar to or lower than that of "high-risk" repeat CABG (26,27). Both mortality and event rates were similar to those reported by Frimerman and associates in their high-risk patient cohort treated by Palmaz-Schatz stent implantation (28) and also similar to those in a previous Thoraxcenter study using the first-generation Wallstent (29).

Although only 50% of patients were symptom-free at clinical follow-up, a further 25% of patients had only mild angina (CCS Class 2 or less), whereas at baseline 71% of patients had CCS class 3 or worse angina (including 36% with unstable angina). Thus, despite the apparently high incidence of MACE during the follow-up period, there was on average a considerable improvement in patient symptomatic status as a consequence of Wallstent treatment. It was concluded that the Wallstent is acutely safe and effective for intervention in symptomatic venous bypass graft disease, represents an improvement over conventional balloon angioplasty, and offers an alternative palliative therapy to those at increased risk of operative mortality. The high event rate in the first year is indicative of the aggressive nature of venous graft and native coronary disease in patients a mean of 8.8 years post-CABG.

The WIN Trial

The effectiveness of the Wallstent in reducing the rate of restenosis compared with conventional balloon angioplasty was evaluated in the WIN (Wallstent In Native arteries) trial, in which 586 eligible patients were randomized to receive treatment either with implantation of a Wallstent (287) or with conventional balloon angioplasty (299) (30). Patients with both *de novo* and restenotic lesions in the native coronary circulation were included in this trial by 26 centers. The objectives were the assessment of clinical and angiographic restenosis as indicated by event-free survival and repeat angiography at 6 months after treatment. The first eight stented patients were treated with aspirin and Coumadin (Du Pont Pharmaceuticals), the remaining with aspirin and ticlopidine postimplantation, while patients in the PTCA-only group were treated with aspirin alone. The Wallstent was sized 0.5 mm to 1.0 mm greater than the online maximum reference diameter. Of the stented patients, 14.4% were treated for restenosis; of the balloon angioplasty patients, 12.2% were treated for restenosis. At 6-month follow-up, there was no difference in the clinical event rates (death, MI, target lesion revascularization, cerebrovascular accident) between the two groups (28.1% stent versus 26.8% balloon). Restenosis rates of the two treatment groups were identical (39% stent versus 39% balloon). Thus, in this selected native vessel population, elective stenting with the Wallstent offered no advantage when compared with balloon angioplasty.

The ITALICS Trial

Based on the *a priori* awareness of the somewhat increased tendency to luminal renarrowing associated with the Wallstent, a single-center trial at the Thoraxcenter examined the potential for locally delivered antisense oligonucleotides to prevent or reduce this intimal hyperplasia. The ITALICS (Investigation by the Thoraxcenter on Antisense DNA given by Local delivery and assessed by IVUS after Coronary Stenting) trial examined the effects on in-stent restenosis of a synthetic 15-mer antisense phosphorothioate oligodeoxynucleotide (LR-3280, Lynx Therapeutics, Haywood, CA) directed against the translation-initiation region of the c-myc nuclear proto-oncogene (31). Antisense to c-myc has been shown to inhibit smooth muscle cell migration, proliferation, and matrix protein synthesis *in vitro,* and to inhibit the restenosis process effectively in several animal models of vascular injury (32). In this trial, 84 patients were ran-

domized after successful placement of a Wallstent, to receive either a placebo or the antisense compound using a local drug-delivery catheter (Transport, SCIMED Life Systems) inside the stented segment. The primary endpoint for this trial was the in-stent neointimal volume at 6 month follow-up as assessed by intravascular ultrasound. Results of this trial showed that 10 mg LR-3280, given by the Transport catheter immediately after Wallstent implantation, did not reduce the clinical event rate or decrease the neointimal proliferative response as determined by IVUS and QCA.

Trials Using the New Magic Wallstent

The TRAPIST Trial

The beneficial effect of trapidil, an inhibitor of PDGF-activated protein kinase, to prevent neo-intimal hyperplasia was evaluated in the 21-center, double blind, placebo-controlled TRAPIST (TRAPidil In STent) trial, in patients undergoing implantation of a single Magic Wallstent for a native primary coronary lesion (33). The primary endpoint of this trial was the in-stent neointimal volume measured by IVUS at 6 month follow-up. A total of 353 patients were randomized to receive trapidil (200 mg three times a day) or placebo starting prior to the Wallstent implantation procedure. Final results showed no difference in neointimal volume as measured by IVUS between the two treatment groups (228 mm^3 trapidil versus 226 mm^3 placebo). No difference was seen in any of the angiographic parameters or in the incidence of MACE (death, myocardial infarction, need for bypass surgery, or target lesion revascularization). A significant difference was seen, however, in the incidence of unstable angina (6.1% versus 0.6%, $p = .009$) and silent ischemia (6.1% versus 1.2%, $p = .03$) between the two groups, with the placebo-treated group showing a better outcome.

The Magic 5 L Trial

This multicenter, non-randomized study was set up to comparatively evaluate five different lengths of Wallstent—namely, mini, extra short, short, medium, and long—with 50 patients in each group. Thus, it involved recruitment of 250 patients with native coronary lesions suitable for implantation of one of these lengths of stent, which were available in diameters from 3.5 mm to 6.0 mm. The purpose was to determine the applicability of the Wallstent across a wide range of lesion lengths in a variety of vessel diameters and to examine the influence of lesion length and stent length on clinical and angiographic outcome at 6 months. The inclusion period has been completed and the trial is now in the follow-up phase.

MEDTRONIC SELF-EXPANDING NITINOL STENT

The Medtronic Nitinol Stent (Medtronic Instent) is a self-expanding nitinol tubular device with a "Christmas tree" mesh design (Fig. 3.19). It is supplied on a single operator exchange (SOE) delivery catheter protected by an overtube which radially constrains the stent prior to deployment. Upon retraction of the overtube, the stent is self-expanded *in situ* to the required vessel diameter. The stent is available in diameters of 3.0 mm to 4.5 mm and in lengths of 8,

15, 25, and 36 mm. Registry studies are currently underway.

THE RADIUS STENT

The SCIMED Radius stent has a multiple zigzag segment design, and is cut from a single cylinder of nitinol metal (Fig. 3.20). The stent is delivered by wire pull-back of the restraining sheath, and does not shorten after full stent expansion. There is no mechanical recoil of this stent, but because the stent does not expand beyond its nominal size, proper sizing is very important. In clinical application, implantation of the Radius stent is associated with a low injury score (34) and, with modest oversizing, the stent continues to expand after implantation, which has been reported to exert a favorable influence on the luminal diameter measured at follow-up (35). With human implantations, it has also been shown that the nitinol Radius stent induces less platelet aggregation than the stainless steel Palmaz-Schatz and GR-II stents (36). This finding may be due to the type of metal used, the unique architecture of the Radius stent, or both. A disadvantage of the Radius stent design is the limitation to side branch access. Favorable results of animal testing (37) have led to the initiation of

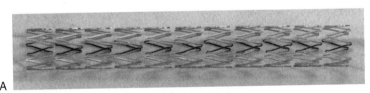

A

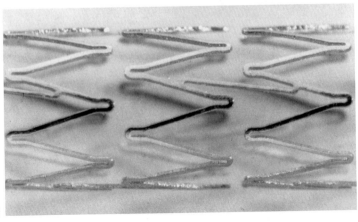

B

FIG. 3.19. Low- and high-power photographs of the Medtronic self-expanding stent, illustrating the "Christmas tree" design.

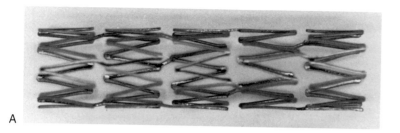

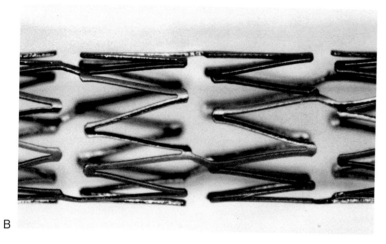

FIG. 3.20. The SCIMED Radius stent in low and high power.

a clinical registry series, the European ESSEX trial (38), and to an equivalency trial comparing the Radius with the Palmaz-Schatz stent available (SCORES; Stent COmparative REStenosis trial [39,40]), all of which have shown this stent to be safe and acutely effective and to be associated with 6-month clinical and angiographic outcomes comparable with best alternatives.

EPILOGUE

With the acquisition of Schneider by Boston Scientific/SCIMED, future plans for the self-expanding Radius stent and Magic Wallstent remain to be announced, particularly in view of the comparative success internationally of the balloon-expandable NIR stent, also approved in the United States. In the absence of any clinical data on the Medtronic self-expanding stent, it would appear that the future of the self-expanding stent is in doubt. It must be acknowledged that the potential benefit of the continuous expansion over time of self-expanding stents per se remains to be harnessed in a meaningful way,

possibly by avoiding excessive postdilatation after implantation to reduce unnecessary injury (41) and by using effective anti-proliferative therapy at the time of or prior to implantation (such as was attempted in the ITALICS and TRAPIST trials).

Technically, the availability of a sheathed (not to be compared with the rather cumbersome and stiff Stent Delivery System of some balloon-expandable stents) flexible stent in various lengths and diameters is particularly desirable for difficult anatomic circumstances and in complex lesions in venous bypass grafts, offering a definite advantage over even the most flexible and low profile balloon-expandable stents. The non-shortening Radius stent would appear to offer some practical advantages over the shortening Wallstent, in terms of predictability of behavior on implantation, precision of placement at the level of vessel ostia, avoiding unnecessary entrapment of side branches, and suitability for vessels smaller than 3 mm (as small as 2.5 mm). The Wallstent offers greater length-diameter combinations and has been successfully applied to wide variety of anatomical substrates since 1986, whereas the Radius stent has only been clinically evaluated by a limited number of centers in the two mentioned trials, mainly in 14 mm-length, so it has to stand the tests of applicability and time.

REFERENCES

1. Wright KC, Wallace S, Charnsangavej C, Carrasco CH, Gianturco C. Percutaneous endovascular stents: an experimental evaluation. *Radiology* 1985;156:69–72.
2. Rousseau H, Puel J, Joffre F et al. Self-expanding endovascular prosthesis: an experimental study. *Radiology* 1987;164:709–714.
3. Puel J, Joffre F, Rousseau H, Guermonprez B, Lancelin B, Morice MC. Endo-prothèses coronariennes auto-expansives dans le prévention des resténoses après angioplastie transluminale. *Arch Mal Coeur* 1987;8: 1311–1312.
4. Sigwart U, Puel J, Mirkovitch V, Joffre F, Kappenberger L. Intravascular stents to prevent occlusion and restenosis after transluminal angioplasty. *N Engl J Med* 1987; 316:702–706.
5. Serruys PW, Strauss BH, Beatt KJ et al. Angiographic follow-up after placement of a self-expanding coronary artery stent. *N Engl J Med* 1991;324:13–17.
6. Strauss BH, Serruys PW, Bertrand ME et al. Quantitative angiographic follow-up of the coronary Wallstent in native vessel and bypass grafts (European experience: March 1986–March 1990). *Am J Cardiol* 1992;69: 475–481.
7. Serruys PW, Juilliere Y, Bertrand ME, Puel J, Rickards AF, Sigwart U. Additional improvement of stenosis geometry in human coronary arteries by stenting after balloon dilatation. *Am J Cardiol* 1988;61:71G–76G.
8. Puel J, Juilliere Y, Bertrand ME, Rickards AF, Sigwart U, Serruys PW. Early and late assessment of stenosis geometry after coronary arterial stenting. *Am J Cardiol* 1988;61:546–553.
9. Serruys PW, Di Mario C. Who was thrombogenic: the stent or the doctor? [editorial; comment]. *Circulation* 1995;91:1891–1893.
10. Serruys PW, Strauss BH, van Beusekom HM, van der Giessen WJ. Stenting of coronary arteries: has a modern Pandora's box been opened? [see comments]. *J Am Coll Cardiol* 1991;17:143B–154B.
11. Keane D, de Jaegere P, Serruys PW. Structural design, clinical experience, and current indications of the coronary Wallstent. *Cardiol Clin* 1994;12:689–697.
12. Kelly P.A., Kurbaan AS, Clague JR, Sigwart U. Total endovascular reconstruction of occluded saphenous vein grafts using coronary or peripheral Wallstents. *J Invas Cardiol* 1997;9:513–517.
13. Joseph T, Fajadet J, Jordan C et al. Reconstruction of old diffusely degenerated saphenous vein grafts with less-shortening Wallstents. *Circulation* 1997;96 [Suppl]:I-275(abst).
14. Von Birgelen C, Airiian SG, de Feyter PJ, Foley DP, van der Giessen WJ, Serruys PW. Coronary Wallstents show significant late, postprocedural expansion despite

15. König A, Regar E, Henneke K-H et al. Interaction of the Wallstent with the coronary artery during a longterm follow-up: morphological assessment by serial intravascular ultrasound with a motorized pullback system. *J Am Coll Cardiol* 1998;31[Suppl]:494A(abst).
16. Ozaki Y, Keane D, Ruygrok P, van der Giessen WJ, de Feyter P, Serruys PW. Six-month clinical and angiographic outcome of the new, less-shortening Wallstent in native coronary arteries. *Circulation* 1996;93: 2114–2120.
17. Kuntz RE, Safian RD, Carrozza JP, Fishman RF, Mansour M, Baim DS. The importance of acute luminal diameter in determining restenosis after coronary atherectomy or stenting. *Circulation* 1992;86:1827–1835.
18. Foley DP, Heyndrickx G, Macaya C et al, on behalf of the Wellstent Native Investigators. Implantation of the self-expanding less-shortening Wallstent for primary, coronary artery lesions: final results of the Wellstent Native study. *Eur Heart J* 1997;18[Suppl]:156(abst).
19. Serruys PW, van Hout B, Bonnier H, al e. Effectiveness, costs and cost-effectiveness of a strategy of elective heparin-coated stenting compared to balloon angioplasty in selected patients with coronary artery disease: The BENESTENT II Study. *Lancet* 1998 (*in press*).
20. Foley DP, Wijns W, Suryapranata H et al. Bypass graft angioplasty using the self-expanding less-shortening Wallstent—results of the Wallstent CABG study. *Eur Heart J* 1997;18[Suppl]:157(abst).
21. Kimura T, Yokoi H, Nakagawa Y et al. Three-year follow-up after implantation of metallic coronary-artery stents. *N Engl J Med* 1996;334:561–566.
22. Pijls NH, De Bruyne B, Peels K et al. Measurement of fractional flow reserve to assess the functional severity of coronary-artery stenoses. *N Engl J Med* 1996;334: 1703–1708.
23. Savage MP, Douglas JS, Jr., Fischman DL et al. Stent placement compared with balloon angioplasty for obstructed coronary bypass grafts. Saphenous Vein *De Novo* Trial Investigators. *N Engl J Med* 1997;337: 740–747.
24. Morrison DA, Crowley ST, Veerakul G, Barbiere CC, Grover F, Sacks J. Percutaneous transluminal angioplasty of saphenous vein grafts for medically refractory unstable angina. *J Am Coll Cardiol* 1994;23: 1066–1070.
25. Rogers WJ, Alderman EL, Chaitman BR et al. Bypass Angioplasty Revascularization Investigation (BARI): baseline clinical and angiographic data. *Am J Cardiol* 1995;75:9C–17C.
26. Rosengart TK, Krieger K, Lang SJ et al. Reoperative coronary artery bypass surgery. Improved preservation of myocardial function with retrograde cardioplegia. *Circulation* 1993;88:II330–II335.
27. Lemmer JH, Jr., Ferguson DW, Rakel BA, Rossi NP. Clinical outcome of emergency repeat coronary artery bypass surgery. *J Cardiovasc Surg* 1990;31:492–497.
28. Frimerman A, Rechavia E, Eigler N, Payton MR, Makkar R, Litvack F. Long-term follow-up of a high risk cohort after stent implantation in saphenous vein grafts. *J Am Coll Cardiol* 1997;30:1277–1283.
29. de Jaegere PP, van Domburg RT, Feyter PJ et al. Long-term clinical outcome after stent implantation in saphenous vein grafts. *J Am Coll Cardiol* 1996;28:89–96.

30. Bilodeau L, Schreiber T, Hilton JD et al. The Wallstent In Native coronary arteries (WIN) multicenter randomized trial: in-hospital acute results. *J Am Coll Cardiol* 1998;31[Suppl]:80A(abst).

31. Kutryk MJB, Serruys PW, Bruining N et al. Randomized trial of antisense oligonucleotide against c-myc for the prevention of restenosis after stenting: results of the Thoraxcenter "ITALICS" trial. *Eur Heart J* 1998; 19[Suppl]1:569(abst).

32. Bennet MR, Schwartz SM. Antisense therapy for angioplasty restenosis: some critical considerations. *Circulation* 1995;92:1981–1993.

33. Serruys PW, Pieper M, Foley DP et al. TRAPIST study: a randomised double-blind study to evaluate the efficacy of Trapidil on restenosis after successful elective coronary stenting. *Circulation* 1998(abst).

34. Kobayashi Y, Mukai S, Brown CL III et al. Geometric expansion in a self-expandable stent and a balloon-expandable stent: interim results from the IVUS substudy of the SCORES trial. *Circulation* 1998;96[Suppl]:I-584(abst).

35. Kobayashi Y, Teirstein PS, Bailey SR et al. Self-expandable stent versus balloon-expandable stent: a serial volumetric analysis by intravascular ultrasound [abstract]. *J Am Coll Cardiol* 1998;31[suppl]:396A.

36. Isshiki T, Eto K, Ochiai M et al. Nitinol Radius stent induces less platelet aggregation than stainless steel Palmaz-Schatz/Gianturco-Rubin II stents. *J Am Coll Cardiol* 1998;31[Suppl]:312A(abst).

37. Carter AJ, Scott D, Laird JR et al. Progressive vascular remodeling and reduced neointimal formation after placement of a thermoelastic self-expanding nitinol stent in an experimental model. *Cathet Cardiovasc Diagn* 1998;44:19–201.

38. van der Giessen WJ, Grollier G, Hoorntje JC, Heyndrickx G, Morel MM, Serruys PW. The ESSEX Study: first clinical experience with the self-expanding, nitinol Radius stent. *Eur Heart J* 1997;18[Suppl]:158(abst).

39. Goldberg S, Schwartz RS, Mann TJ, III et al. Comparison of a novel self-expanding Nitinol stent (RADIUS™) with a balloon expandable (Palmaz-Schatz™) stent: initial results of a randomized trial (SCORES). *Circulation* 1997;96[Suppl]:I-654(abst).

40. Han RO, Schwartz RS, Mann JT et al. Comparative efficacy of self expanding and balloon expandable stents for the reduction of restenosis. *J Am Coll Cardiol* 1998; 31[Suppl]:314A(abst).

41. Wilson S, Han RO, Schwartz RS, Goldberg S. Angiographic outcomes in self-expanding and balloon-expandable stents: importance of procedural technique in determining late patency. *Circulation* 1998;98[Suppl]: I–160(abst).

G. Impact of the Stented Segment Length on Clinical Outcome—Observations from the beStent Registry

Ariel Roguin and Rafael Beyar

Technicon-Israel Institute of Technology, Heart System Research Center, Department of Biomedical Engineering, The Julius Silver Institute, Technicon City, Haifa, 32000 Israel

Percutaneous transluminal coronary angioplasty is an effective treatment for selected patients with symptomatic coronary artery disease. Yet, in spite of great improvement in angioplasty and related technology, long-term success is compromised by the occurrence of restenosis, ranging between 15 and 50% of patients within the first 6 months (1–9).

Long lesions have been known for their negative impact on the acute success and long-term outcome of various catheter based coronary interventions (10). Longer lesions have a higher risk of dissection, vessel occlusion and restenosis. Angiographic restenosis rates of up to 58% have been reported for balloon angioplasty of long lesions (11,12). The development of devices such as excimer laser and rotational atherectomy have increased procedural success, but restenosis remained a major problem (6). In contrast, longer lesions could be successfully and safely treated with stents as the acute complications were reportedly reduced (9–11). Yet, in spite of adequate acute results, long-term results with stents for long lesions have been discouraging, with angiographic restenosis rates of 48% for lesions greater than 20 mm (13).

Recent observations suggest an increasing association with lesion length or stent multiplicity and angiographic restenosis rates, yet these studies are limited by multiple stent designs and incomplete angiographic follow-up. It has been recently demonstrated that mandatory angiographic follow-up interferes with the natural history of the procedure related course (14). Therefore, we reasoned that a clinical rather than angiographic follow-up study, with uniform stent design may have additional important information on the clinical effectiveness of stented angioplasty in long lesions.

We performed an analysis of the first 185 patients treated with the serpentine design stent in phase 1A of the beStent multicenter study and compared the early and 6-month clinical events with respect to the length of the stented segment.

METHODS

Patients

Between March and October 1996, 266 stents were deployed in 185 patients, undergoing elective angioplasty in eight Medical Centers worldwide. The patients signed informed consent for the procedure. The inclusion criteria included: 3 mm–5 mm native vessels, *de novo* and restenotic lesions, and no myocardial infarction within 8 days prior to implantation. The indication for stenting in this cohort of patients were treatment of suboptimal results, bailout conditions, and prevention of restenosis.

All patients were clinically monitored with regular visits at 1, 3, and 6 months after implantation. All main adverse coronary events (MACE), including death, myocardial infarction, CABG, and TLR, were recorded and reported to the clinical control committee.

Stent Design

The stent is made of 316 L stainless steel tube cut into a unique serpentine design. Upon expansion the stent utilizes the principles of rotational non-stress junctions and orthogonal locking. The stent has no shortening and two radiopaque end-markers for adequate visibility allowing precise positioning. The rotational low-stress junctions dissipate stress concentration upon expansion and lead to orthogonal locking, maximizing radial strength. The stent lengths used in this study were 15, 25, and 35 mm, available in both a small-diameter (BES series; 2.5 mm–3.0 mm) and large-diameter ranges (BEL series; 3.0 mm–5.5 mm).

Stent Implantation Procedure

The implantation of the beStent is similar in principles to implantation of other unmounted balloon-expandable stents. The stent was mounted on the appropriate balloon for delivery (a 15-mm stent is mounted on a 20-mm balloon, a 25-mm stent on a 30-mm balloon, and a 35-mm stent is mounted on a 40-mm balloon). If possible, a semicompliant or a noncompliant balloon was generally used so that the same balloon can be used for the high (14 atm or higher) pressure inflation, thus optimizing balloon usage. The selection of the guiding catheter ranged between 6 Fr and 8 Fr. The stent was sledded on the balloon using the special tube and stylet system for mounting. It was then gently crimped on the balloon, which was mounted over the angioplasty wire, and then firmly crimped on the balloon, verifying a smooth stent surface with no protruding struts and no stent slippage over the balloon. In general, a floppy 0.014-inch wire was selected for stent implantation; however, if excessive tortuosity was suspected, an extra-support wire and a low-profile balloon were used.

Once the lesion was crossed, the stent was positioned using its gold end-markers. Since there is no shortening of the stent, the markers precisely define the stent's final deployment position. Initial deployment was done at a pressure of 8 atm. After complete balloon expansion, 10 to 30 seconds were allowed for equilibration before the balloon was deflated. The balloon was then repositioned so that it did not protrude distal to the stent, and reinflated to a pressure of 14 atm or higher. If the delivery balloon could not be used at high pressure, further dilatation with a high pressure balloon was employed.

Anticoagulation Protocol

All patients received aspirin before stent deployment. A bolus of 10,000 units of heparin was given after sheath insertion, with a repeat bolus of 5,000 units given as needed to maintain the activated clotting time >300 seconds. Heparin was discontinued after the procedure and the sheath removed 4 hours later. Most patients received aspirin 100 mg daily indefinitely unless contraindicated. Ticlopidine 500 mg daily was started on the day of the procedure and continued for 1 month.

Definitions

The patients were categorized according to their stented lesion length. Lesions were characterized as short (<15 mm in length), medium (16 mm–25 mm in length), or long (>26 mm in length). All events were classified according to the stented lesion length involved. There were several cases where a single event was counted for more than one lesion length. The arterial-lumen dimensions were obtained using selected end-diastolic cine frames demonstrating the stenosis in its most severe and non-foreshortened projection. The same projection was used to measure the final results. Angiographic success was defined as an ability to deploy the stent without acute complications, leading to angiographic result of <50% residual stenosis. Clinical in-hospital, 30-day and 6-month successes were defined as angiographic success without major adverse events during hospitalization or the follow-up terms, respectively.

Follow Up

All treated patients were seen routinely at 1, 3, and 6 months after the procedure. All patients were interviewed and a treadmill exercise test was done if not contraindicated. The patients reported any complaint and were treated promptly as needed.

RESULTS

Patient, Angiographic, and Procedural Characteristics

The patients' ages ranged 32 to 78 years (mean 60 ± years). The majority of the patients were males (84%). Angiographic baseline characteristics were similar for the 3 lesion length groups (Table 3.18). A total of 254 lesions were treated with 266 stents in 185 patients. The majority of the lesions were complex: A 36, 13%, B1 57, 22%, B2 75, 28%, and C 98, 37%. The distribution among the different lesion lengths was similar. Multiple stents required to treat tandem lesions or long lesions that could not be treated with a single stent were implanted in 58 of 185 patients (32%). The stents were 15 ($n = 125$, 48%), 25 ($n = 98$, 37%), or 35 ($n = 39$, 15%) mm long and 2.5–3.0 ($n = 123$, 52%) or 3.0–5.5 ($n = 112$, 48%) mm in diameter.

Technical Consideration and Procedural Success

Full lesion coverage was attempted in all cases. Failure to deploy the stent occurred in five patients and retrieved successfully in four. No adverse events were reported in these cases. Stent loss in the peripheral circulation occurred in one patient. Patients with unsuccessful deployment were not included for the follow-up aimed to specifically test the effect of lesion coverage.

TABLE 3.18. *Angiographic baseline characteristics, divided according to stented lesion lengths*

Stented lesion length	<15mm	16–25mm	>26mm
Number of patients	84	66	35
Reference arterial diameter			
Pre	3.30 ± 0.52	3.23 ± 0.35	3.23 ± 0.54
Post	3.10 ± 0.57	2.97 ± 0.47	2.96 ± 0.58
Stenosis (%)			
Pre	85 ± 13	80 ± 17	77 ± 15
Post	3 ± 1	3 ± 1	3 ± 1

TABLE 3.19. *In hospital, 30-day, and 6-month clinical success, divided according to stented lesion lengths*

Stented Lesion length	<15mm	16–25mm	>26mm
Number of patients	84	66	35
Event-free survival			
Hospitalization	98.8%	100%	90%
At 30 days	96.4%	100%	90%
At 6 months	89.2%	89.5%	83%

In-Hospital and Short-Term (30 day) Clinical Success and Complications

The acute and in-hospital results are detailed in Table 3.19. In all stented lesion length groups the in-hospital and short-term complication rates were low, without statistical difference between the groups. Therefore, the acute and short-term safety of long lesion stent treatment is demonstrated.

Six-Month Follow-Up

All the patients were under close clinical follow-up and were seen routinely at 1, 3, and 6 months after the procedure, or as needed. The overall (in-hospital, 30-day, and 6-month) event-free survival was 85.2% for this group of patients with simple and complex lesions. The majority of events occurred in patients with lesions longer than 26 mm (Figs. 3.21 and 3.22). Therefore, it seems that some of the events are related to the length of the treated lesions, although not reaching statistically significance. Event-free survival was 83% for lesions >26 mm versus 89% for lesions <25 mm ($p = .32$). It is noteworthy that lesions covered with one 25-mm stent had excellent long-term results comparable to the short (15 mm) stented lesions.

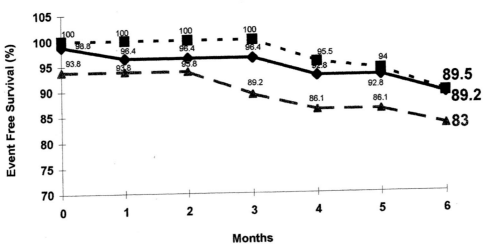

FIG. 3.21. Event-free survival curve of death, MI, CABG, and TLR, according to stented lesion length. (*lines: continuous*,15 mm; *small dotted*, 16 mm–25 mm; *big dotted* >26 mm).

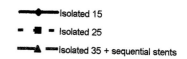

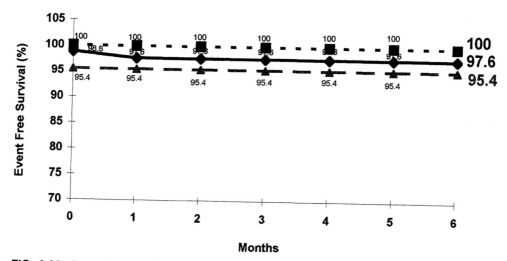

FIG. 3.22. Event-free survival curve of death and MI, according to stented lesion length. (*lines*: *continuous*,15 mm; *small dotted*, 16 mm–25 mm; *big dotted* >26 mm).

DISCUSSION

In the current study we have demonstrated the short-term safety of treatment of long lesions with stents. Yet, a trend for higher 6-month clinical event rates was noted for stented lesion lengths higher than 25 mm. Moreover, the event rates in long lesions in this study (17% in the >26 mm group) are relatively lower than earlier studies of roughly 50% restenosis rates. This highlights the difference between angiographic restenosis rates and clinically based need for repeat angiography and revascularization. In addition, it should be stressed that long-term events after stent implantation go beyond 6 months and a longer-term follow-up may be required for more accurate description of long-term stent results.

Itoh and associates (13) report, on 120 lesions (stent length >20 mm) using several stent types, a restenosis rate of 35% to 48% with no difference among the different stents used. Another report by the same group (15) of the use of the Wallstent in diffuse disease in native and saphenous vein grafts showed a restenosis rate of 33%. The influence of lesion length on restenosis is controversial (16). Savage and associates (17), in a prospective evaluation of 826 patients in the Multi-Hospital Eastern Atlantic Restenosis Trial (M-HEART), did not find a correlation between primary coronary angioplasty success and the stenosis length. Hirshfeld and associates (12), using a subset of the same study population, demonstrated a direct relationship between lesion length and restenosis (17). Some reports confirmed that observation (17) but others have failed to demonstrate such an association (18). In the present study a trend toward more events in the longer stented segments was noted, but this trend did not reach statistical significance.

Theoretically, treatment of long lesions could be improved by the use of longer stents. The advantage of long stents may be not only economical, but also in eliminating stent gaps or unnecessary stent overlaps that may contribute to restenosis (19). Despite this hypothesis and despite the findings with IVUS that documented the lower gain obtained at the articulation site of the Palmaz-Schatz, experience with the use of longer stents has not so far been rewarded for a low restenosis rate (20). In addition, long stents have a higher delivery failure rate as noted by Kobayashi and associates (21) that may in itself complicate the clinical outcome. In this observational study, 2,853 stented lesions were divided into three groups according to stented segment length of <20 mm, from 20 mm to 35 mm and >35 mm. Restenosis rates (with 69% angiographic follow-up) were 19%, 31%, and 39%, respectively.

Another predictor of restenosis is vessel size (22–24). Vessel size and lesion length add to each other when associated in the same lesion (25). Due to natural vessel tapering it is likely that in a discrete number of cases at least the distal portion of long stents is located in a vessel segment with less than 3.0 mm lumen diameter. Thus, both stenting and balloon angioplasty are associated with a high risk of restenosis.

To date, in long diffuse coronary narrowings, the superiority of one treatment over the other is not yet established. A study comparing percutaneous transluminal coronary angioplasty with and without additional stenting is warranted. The presence of stents as ''backup'' allows a more aggressive angioplasty with ''oversizing balloons'' achieving ''stent-like'' results. This permits us to reassess the long-term outcome of balloon angioplasty of long lesions by increasing the safety of the procedure as dissections and even occlusions can be well managed. This approach of optimal-result percutaneous transluminal coronary balloon angioplasty gave promising procedural results and may ameliorate long-term results of long lesion treatment (26).

In summary, the most appropriate and suitable treatment for the long coronary lesion is presently under evaluation. The initial experience with the beStent demonstrates its safety and efficiency for treating simple as well as complex coronary disease. Tubular stents can be safely used to treat long lesions with expected low clinical event rates for lesions covered with <25-mm stents. For longer stented lesions a trend for a higher event rates observed here probably reflects the higher restenosis rates that are known for long lesions.

REFERENCES

1. Serruys PW, de Jagere P, Kiemeneij F et al. A comparison of balloon expandable stent implantation with balloon angioplasty in patients with coronary artery disease. *N Engl J Med* 1994;331:489–495.
2. Fischman DL, Leon MB, Baim DS et al. A randomized comparison of coronary stent placement and balloon angioplasty in the treatment of coronary artery disease. *N Engl J Med* 1994;331:496–501.
3. Colombo A, Hall P, Nakamura S et al. Intracoronary stenting without anticoagulation accomplished with intravascular ultrasound guidance. *Circulation* 1995;91:1676–1688.
4. Kimura T, Yokoi H, Nakagawa Y et al. Three-year follow-up after implantation of metallic coronary artery stents. *N Engl J Med* 1996;334:561–566.
5. Savage M, Fischman D, Schatz RA et al. Long term angiographic and clinical outcome after implantation of balloon-expandable stents in the native coronary *circulation. J Am Coll Cardiol* 1994;24:1207–1212.
6. Leon MB, Wong SC. Intracoronary stents; a breakthrough or just another small step. *Circulation* 1994;89:1323–1327.
7. Rodriguez AE, Santaera O, Larribau M et al. Coronary stenting decreases restenosis in lesions with early loss in luminal diameter 24 hours after successful PTCA. *Circulation* 1995;91:1397–1402.
8. Macaya C, Serruys PW, Ruygrok P et al. Continued benefit of coronary stenting versus balloon angioplasty: one year clinical follow up of BENESTENT trial. *J Am Coll Cardiol* 1996;27:255–261.
9. Versaci F, Gaspardone A, Tomai F, Crea F, Chiariello L, Gioffre PA. A comparison of coronary-artery stenting with angioplasty for isolated stenosis of the proximal left anterior descending coronary artery. *N Engl J Med* 1997;336:817–822.
10. Meier B, Gruentzig AR, Hollman J, Ischinger T, Bradford JM. Does length or eccentricity of coronary stenoses influence the outcome of transluminal dilatation. *Circulation* 1983;67:497–499.
11. Cannon AD, Roubin GS, Hearn JA, Iyer SS, Baxley WA, Dean LS. Acute angiographic and clinical results of long balloon percutaneous transluminal coronary angioplasty and adjuvant stenting for long narrowings. *Am J Cardiol* 1994;73:635–641.
12. Hirshfeld JW Jr, Schwartz JS, Jugo R et al. Restenosis after coronary angioplasty: a multivariate statistical model to relate lesion and procedure variables to restenosis. *J Am Coll Cardiol* 1991;18:647–656.
13. Itoh A, Hall P, Maiello L, Blengino S, Finci L, Ferraro M, Martini G, Colombo A. Coronary stenting of long lesions (greater than 20 mm)—a matched comparison of different stents. *Circulation* 1995;92[Suppl II]:I-688.
14. Legrand V, Serruys PW, Emanuelsson H et al. BENESTENT II—final results of visit I: a 15 day follow up. *J Am Coll Cardiol* 1997;29:170A(abst).
15. Colombo A, Itoh A, Hall P et al. Implantation of the Wallstent in native coronary arteries and venous bypass

grafts without subsequent anticoagulation. *J Am Coll Cardiol* 1996;27A A

16. Savage MyP, Goldberg S, Hirshfeld JW and the M-HEART investigators, Clinical and angiographic determinants of primary coronary angioplasty success. *J Am Coll Cardiol* 1991;17:22–28.

17. Ellis SG, Roubin GS, King SB III et al. Importance of stenosis morphology in the estimation of restenosis risk after elective percutaneous transluminal coronary angioplasty. *Am J Cardiol* 1989;63:30–34.

18. Leimgruber PP, Roubin GS, Hollman J et al. Restenosis after successful coronary angioplasty in patients with single vessel disease. *Circulation* 1986;73:710–717.

19. Elderman ER, Rogers C. Hoop dreams: stents without restenosis. *Circulation* 1996;94:1199–1202.

20. Hoffmann R, Mintz G, Dussaillat G et al. Patterns and mechanisms of in-stent restenosis: a serial intravascular ultrasound studies. *Circulation* 1996;94:1247–1254

21. Kobayashi Y, Di Mario C. Immediate and follow up results following single long coronary stent implantation. *Circulation* 1997;96[Suppl]:I-472.

22. Dussaillant GR, Mintz GS, Pichard AD et al. Small stent size and intimal hyperplasia contribute to restenosis; a volumetric intravascular ultrasound analysis. *J Am Coll Cardiol* 1995;26:720–724.

23. Perursson MK, Jonmundsson EH, Brekkan A, Hardarson T. Angiographic predictors of new coronary occlusions. *Am Heart J* 1995;129:515–520.

24. Kaul U, Upasani PT, Agarwal R, Bahl VK, Wasir HS. In-hospital outcome of percutaneous transluminal coronary angioplasty for long lesions and diffuse coronary artery disease. *Cathet Cardiovasc Diagn* 1995;35:294–300.

25. Ellis SG, Savage M, Fischman D et al. Restenosis after placement of Palmaz-Schatz stents in native coronary arteries: initial results of a multicenter experience. *Circulation* 1992;86:1836–1844.

26. Stone GW, Hodgson JM, Frederick G et al. Improved procedural results of coronary angioplasty with intravascular ultrasound-guided balloon sizing. the CLOUT pilot trial. *Circulation* 1997;95:2044–2052.

4

Intravascular Ultrasound: Practical Use in the Cardiac Catheterization Laboratory

Hiroyuki Okura, Heidi N. Benneau, Paul G. Yock, and *Peter J. Fitzgerald

*Division of Cardiovascular Medicine, *Department of Medicine (Cardiology), Stanford University School of Medicine, Stanford, California 94305*

Intravascular ultrasound (IVUS) has become an important tool in today's cardiac catheterization laboratory for serial assessment of the coronary arteries before and after interventions. IVUS allows two-dimensional, cross-sectional vessel visualization that augments information provided by the "silhouette" technique of coronary angiography. In addition, ten years of clinical experience with IVUS in the cardiac catheterization laboratory has provided useful information regarding device selection and endpoint assessment of various interventional strategies. In this chapter, the practical uses of intravascular ultrasound in today's cardiac catheterization laboratory will be reviewed, including case scenarios as well as highlights from recent clinical trials.

CATHETER TECHNOLOGY

Two configurations of IVUS catheter systems have evolved for routine use in the cardiac catheterization laboratory (Fig. 4.1). One is a mechanical implementation (1) and the other, a solid state design strategy (2). In the mechanical design, a flexible cable traveling the length of the catheter is used to rotate a single transducer, which is mounted at the distal tip. Solid state design catheters have multiple imaging elements (up to 64) fixed to the surface of the distal tip and obtain real-time cross sectional images perpendicular to the catheter axis. Both design strategies feature flexible assemblies, providing

similar high quality images in tortuous coronary arteries, permitting accurate sizing of vessels and detailing plaque architecture.

The size of the catheter has continually decreased to diameters of less than 1 mm, allowing compatibility with 6 Fr guiding catheter platforms. Imaging frequencies have also increased, now in the range of 40 to 50 MHz, and provide substantially higher resolution for delineating subtle plaque variations in the vessel wall (Fig. 4.2).

TARGET LESION ASSESSMENT

Preintervention

The development of lower profile IVUS catheters allows routine and safe assessment of criti-

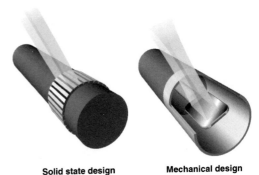

Solid state design　　　　**Mechanical design**

FIG. 4.1. Diagram of the two basic IVUS imaging catheter configurations. A solid state and a mechanical design.

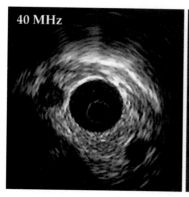
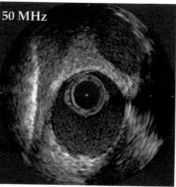

FIG. 4.2. Ultrasound images obtained by high frequency catheters, 40 MHz (*left*) and 50 MHz (*right*), which provide higher resolution at the expense of increased signal strength in blood and decreased signal penetration in tissue.

cal lesion subsets prior to intervention (3). This is particularly helpful during diagnostic cardiac catheterization for delineating complex coronary anatomy such as ostial lesions that may be elusive or ambiguous by angiography. For example, detection of "occult" left main disease by IVUS can dramatically alter the overall patient triage and therapeutic strategy. Recent studies have supported IVUS criteria for the confirmation of critical left main disease, defined as lumen area stenosis greater than 80%, minimum lumen diameter (MLD) less than 2.0 mm, and/or minimal lumen area less than 4.0 mm^2 (4,5). Figure 4.3 demonstrates a coronary angiogram

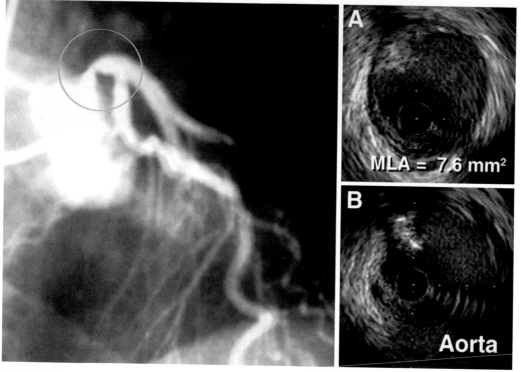

FIG. 4.3. The appearance of possible proximal left main narrowing by angiography with little evidence for disease based on IVUS in this 51-year-old man. **Panel A** represents the cross-sectional image in the left main just beyond the ostium (MLA = 7.6 mm^2). **Panel B** represents the left main at the ostium, showing the oblique view of the aorta. MLA, minimum lumen area.

and IVUS image sequence of a 51-year-old man with vague symptoms of exertional angina. The angiogram suggests severe narrowing at the left main ostium. Ultrasound images, however, demonstrate a large luminal area (7.6 mm^2) at the ostium with a mild amount of fibrocalcific plaque. Thus, despite compelling angiographic images, the more definitive IVUS assessment of "true" cross-sectional anatomy revealed that this patient did not require surgical intervention. In comparison, Figure 4.4 shows an angiogram of a 72-year-old woman that suggests only mild stenosis of the left main despite a large anterior wall defect documented by Thallium stress test. IVUS examination of the left main showed significant superficial calcium with a luminal area less than 2.0 mm^2 and a lumen area stenosis of

80% compared to the proximal reference segment. This patient, in contrast to the first one, was triaged from the cardiac catheterization laboratory directly to bypass surgery.

Beyond defining left main anatomy, the most critical information derived from preintervention ultrasound scanning in the coronary tree is an accurate assessment of both vessel size and plaque composition. These features often impact on the size and type of an interventional device. Figure 4.5 illustrates the marked discrepancy between the angiogram and IVUS with respect to vessel size. The size of the right coronary artery in this patient appears no larger than 3.0 mm (guiding catheter is 6 Fr). Prior treatment for this patient, without the use of IVUS, had been limited to balloon angioplasty, to a maximum of

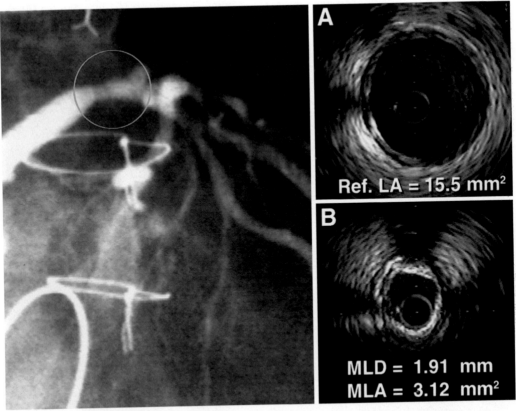

FIG. 4.4. The appearance of mild distal left main narrowing by the angiogram but significant disease on IVUS in this 72-year-old woman. **Panel A** represents the proximal reference with minimum disease (LA = 15.5 mm^2). **Panel B** represents a significant lesion in the distal left main with extensive superficial calcification (MLD = 1.91 mm, MLA = 3.12 mm^2). LA, reference lumen area; MLD; minimum lumen diameter; MLA, minimum lumen area.

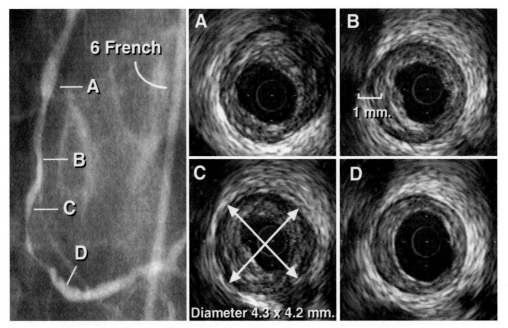

FIG. 4.5. Marked discrepancy with respect to the vessel size between the angiogram and ultrasound images. On the left panel, angiography shows that the size of the right coronary artery is no greater than 3.0 mm, compared to the 6 Fr guiding catheter. On the right panel, IVUS images positioned at **A**, **B**, **C**, and **D** demonstrate a vessel size to exceed 4.0 mm in diameter throughout the lesion.

3.0 mm in size, resulting in two separate episodes of restenosis over the course of seven months. On the third visit to the cardiac catheterization laboratory, IVUS was used to evaluate the vessel size. Ultrasound scanning of the artery revealed vessel size to be in excess of 4.5 mm, providing a broader choice of therapeutic options for the patient. Treatment with two 4.0-mm stents within the target lesion resulted in excellent short-term results. Follow-up at nine months for this patient revealed no effort angina and full angiographic patency within the stented vessel segment.

In a recent study, the discrepancy of vessel size between the angiographic and ultrasound images was investigated to elucidate practical guidelines for routine use in the cardiac catheterization laboratory (6). In the CLOUT (Clinical Outcomes With Ultrasound Trial) study, balloon size was determined as the midpoint between the medial-adventitial border and the true lumen diameter by IVUS in the reference segment (6). This IVUS-guided strategy increased acute luminal gain during PTCA, using balloons tradi-

tionally considered as oversized based upon the angiogram. This aggressive approach resulted in significantly improved target lesion dimension without increased rates of dissection or in-hospital ischemia. These guidelines may be particularly important as provisional stenting with "aggressive" balloon sizing has now become an option for first line therapy in *de novo* lesions (7,8). Further support for aggressive PTCA comes from subgroup analysis from the BENESTENT-1 trial, which revealed excellent long-term results of standalone balloon angioplasty when "stentlike" results (residual diameter stenosis $\leq$30%) were obtained—especially in non-LAD lesion subsets (7). Recent results from OCBAS (Optimal Coronary Balloon Angioplasty with Provisional Stenting versus Primary Stent) support the concept of provisional stenting with regard to similar restenosis rates (19.2% vs. 16.4%; p = NS) and target vessel revascularization rates (17.5% vs. 13.5%; p = NS) between the two strategies. In addition, aggressive "stentlike" angioplasty showed a small but significant cost benefit with this provisional approach (8).

Another key preinterventional IVUS feature impacting device selection is the detection and quantification of calcific patterns in the vessel wall. Several studies have clearly demonstrated that ultrasound is more sensitive than fluoroscopy in the catheterization laboratory for detecting the extent of calcium (9,10). Greater than 180° arc of calcium seen on the cross-sectional ultrasound image is needed before the fluoroscopic image begins to exhibit calcification. In addition, IVUS can determine the location and extent of calcification; deep at the medial border, at the luminal surface, and/or within the plaque substance itself. The presence of large amounts of luminal calcification in the target lesion (generally greater than 180° arc occupying at least 50% of the lesion length) may influence the operator to choose high-speed rotational atherectomy to debulk and enhance lesion compliance for stand alone therapy and/or to facilitate definitive stent expansion (11).

Recently, a nonrandomized, single-center analysis of 306 patients, comparing stenting with or without rotational atherectomy and balloon angioplasty with rotational atherectomy for calcified lesions, showed beneficial acute and long-term effects by partial decalcification by high-speed rotational atherectomy prior to stenting (12). In this study, significantly larger ($p <$ .0001) final MLDs were achieved by rotational atherectomy plus Palmaz-Schatz stenting (3.21 ± 0.49 mm) compared to stent alone (2.88 ± 0.51 mm) or rotational atherectomy plus balloon angioplasty (2.29 ± 0.55 mm) (Fig. 4.6A). Additionally, nine months follow-up revealed a higher event-free survival for patients treated by "rotastenting" versus either stent alone or rotational atherectomy plus balloon angioplasty (85%, 77%, and 67%, respectively, log-rank p = .0633) (Fig. 4.6B).

In the setting of extensive superficial calcification, the neolumen created by rotational atherectomy appears round and regular, with a final lumen diameter approximately equal to the definitive burr size. Conversely, in soft plaque which is more likely to undergo spasm, the postprocedural lumen is typically less round and tends to be smaller than the final burr size. Although adjunct balloon angioplasty can augment the final luminal area, it is important to use low pressure (< 1.5 atm) so as to minimize extensive vessel barotrauma and dissection at calcified edges (13).

POSTINTERVENTION FINDINGS

Nonstent Vessels

Recently, postprocedural plaque burden has been reported to have significant impact on late

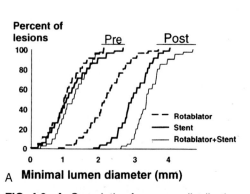
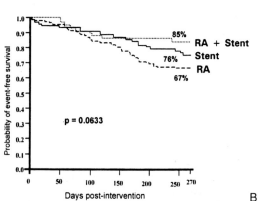

FIG. 4.6. A. Cumulative frequency distribution curves for minimal lumen diameters before and after interventions. A larger minimum lumen diameter was achieved with a combination of rotational atherectomy and stent. **B.** Event-free survival-curves for each treatment strategy during 9-month follow up. (Reprinted from ref. 22, with permission from Excerpta Media Inc.)

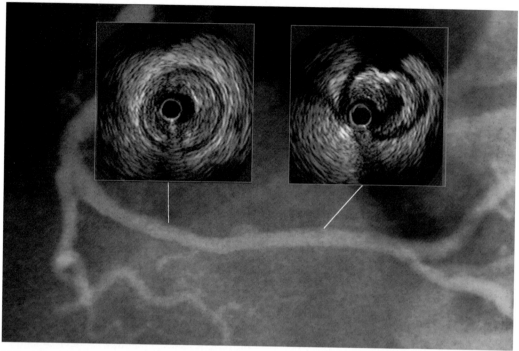

FIG. 4.7. An angiogram and IVUS scan of distal right coronary artery lesion following directional atherectomy. The IVUS images show a large residual plaque accumulation (*left*) and a large plaque burden with dissection (*right*) despite a reasonable angiographic appearance.

outcome following balloon angioplasty and directional atherectomy (Fig. 4.7). Two single-center studies have shown that residual plaque burden as assessed by IVUS is a strong independent predictor of late outcome despite a "good" angiographic result in the target segment (14,15). Mintz et al. showed that the IVUS post-intervention cross-sectional narrowing (plaque plus media cross-sectional area divided by external elastic membrane cross-sectional area) was the most consistent predictor of restenosis (14). Similarly, Görge et al. demonstrated that percent area stenosis and a MLD measured by IVUS were strong correlates of angiographic restenosis (15).

More recently, two multicenter trials have addressed IVUS predictors of outcome following balloon angioplasty. The PICTURE (Post-Intra-Coronary Treatment Ultrasound Result Evaluation) study investigated 200 patients to identify whether morphological features of the dilated segment, as assessed by IVUS after successful

PTCA, were predictive of restenosis. Results of this trial showed that a larger lumen, vessel area, and smaller plaque area as evidenced by IVUS were related to a larger angiographic MLD at follow-up, though these parameters were not significantly related to the categorical restenosis rate (16). Phase II of the GUIDE (Guidance by Ultrasound for Decision Endpoints) Trial, which was a multicenter prospective trial involving over 500 patients, investigated the relationship between IVUS lesion characteristics after a successful angiographic result and late patient outcome. Multivariate analysis at follow-up demonstrated that the ultrasound measurement of residual plaque was the single most powerful predictor for both angiographic and clinical outcomes among all the angiographic and ultrasound variables tested (17).

The concept of residual plaque evident by IVUS stimulated several directional coronary atherectomy (DCA) studies targeted toward aggressive plaque removal during the primary in-

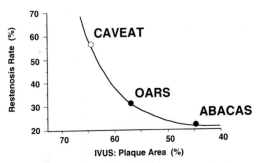

FIG. 4.8. Relationship of residual percent plaque area (percent plaque area = plaque area / vessel area) and restenosis. For comparison, the mean data for plaque residuals and restenosis rates from three atherectomy trials are superimposed. Both OARS (Optimal Atherectomy Restenosis Study) and ABACAS (Adjunctive Balloon Angioplasty following Coronary Atherectomy Study) used IVUS to guide debulking strategy, whereas CAVEAT (Coronary Angioplasty Versus Excisional Atherectomy Trial) used only the angiogram to guide debulking.

tervention. In the OARS (Optimal Atherectomy Restenosis Study) trial, aggressive or "optimizing" of the atherectomy procedure using IVUS guidance and additional balloon angioplasty resulted in a low residual percent diameter stenosis of 7% as assessed by quantitative coronary angiography and an acceptable angiographic restenosis rate of 28.9% at 6 months (18). In this trial, despite angiographic success, IVUS still revealed (although less than historical experience) a significant amount of residual plaque area of 58% immediately after DCA (19). In a

similar trial led by experienced interventionalists in Japan, the ABACAS (Adjunctive Balloon Angioplasty following Coronary Atherectomy Study) trial showed that even more aggressive debulking, guided by IVUS, resulted in lower residual plaque (43%), which ultimately led to an incremental lowering of the angiographic restenosis rate to 21% (Figs. 4.8, 4.9) (20,21).

Recently, serial IVUS observations have addressed new insights regarding the mechanisms of restenosis in nonstented lesions. Several studies have shown that the predominant mechanism responsible for late lumen loss after angioplasty is pathological remodeling (i.e., vessel shrinkage) rather than tissue growth (22–24). In addition, Kimura et al. demonstrated that the remodeling process following interventions was characterized by an early adaptive enlargement and late constriction of the vessel (25). Taken together, these IVUS studies, tracking the vessel size and plaque burden over time, have modified the restenosis concept following device manipulation in the coronary arteries. Both postprocedural residual plaque and vessel remodeling play key roles in the prediction and mechanism of restenosis, respectively.

Stented Vessels

Intracoronary stenting has emerged as the generally preferred definitive therapy for coronary artery disease because it completely blunts subsequent vessel contraction. Thus, in accordance with this mechanical scaffold in the coro-

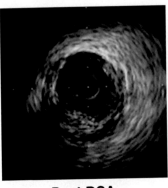

Post DCA

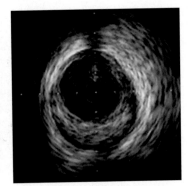

6M Follow up

FIG. 4.9. Tracking vessel morphology over time following directional atherectomy. IVUS shows reduced plaque by IVUS-guided "aggressive" debulking at baseline procedure (*left panel*). Repeat IVUS at 6 months reveals vessel expansion (positive remodeling) with mild increase in plaque burden (*right panel*). DCA, directional coronary atherectomy; 6M, six months.

nary artery, stents have provided a favorable impact on the restenosis rate in a wide spectrum of both *de novo* and restenotic lesion subsets. This is especially true in vessels ≥3.0 mm in size, and in particular, the LAD location (26–28). Early in the learning phase of stent therapy, IVUS was used to guide stent deployment procedures and directed the use of adjunct high-pressure balloon dilatation (mean pressure exceeding 15 atm) as well as determining the need for larger-diameter balloons to achieve "optimal" geometric stent expansion. IVUS-guided stent therapy, combined with a specific regimen of antiplatelet management, reduced subacute thrombosis to acceptable, safe, and predictable levels (29). In several landmark studies, IVUS showed that 80% of stents implanted using conventional angiographic deployment strategies with inflation pressures of 6 to 8 atm had one or more of the following problems: (a) incomplete expansion (MLD not achieving the desired size), (b) incomplete apposition (struts not touching the vessel wall), and (c) edge dissections (29–31). Figure 4.10 highlights these common scenarios tracked well by IVUS, which are often silent by angiography.

In the era of "high pressure" stenting, the role or influence of IVUS on long-term outcomes (angiographic restenosis rate or clinical surrogates such as myocardial infarction and/or repeat revascularization) is perhaps a more rele-

vant issue. The final MLD by angiography immediately after coronary stenting has been suggested as essential to minimize the likelihood of restenosis (32). Recently, IVUS findings have yielded additional geometric information for predicting restenosis and target vessel revascularization (TVR) rate following stent deployment. Single-center studies have demonstrated that the minimal stent area (MSA) is a powerful predictor of both independent adjudicated TVR or angiographic core laboratory binary restenosis (33–36).

In the recent multicenter study, CRUISE (*Can Routine Ultrasound Improve Stent Expansion*), the value of IVUS guidance was tested to determine the clinical impact on stent deployment in the high-pressure era (37). This study directly compared adjunctive IVUS guidance to angiography guidance alone for stent implantation. In the IVUS-guidance group, 38% of patients required additional therapy due to incomplete apposition, edge dissection and most commonly, suboptimal MSA. As a result, the MSA in this IVUS subgroup increased from a mean of 6.25 mm² to 7.14 mm², shifting the MSA cumulative distribution curve rightward (Fig. 4.11). Follow-up at 9 months demonstrated that the IVUS-guidance group experienced a 44% relative reduction in TVR (8.5% vs. 15.2%, $p < .05$), with no difference in death or myocardial infarction. Similarly, the RESIST (*REStenosis after Ivus*

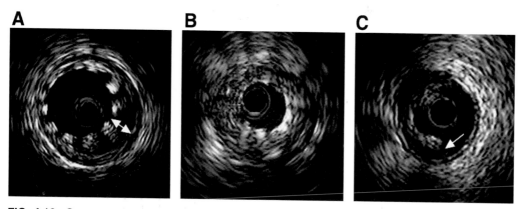

FIG. 4.10. Common ultrasound findings after stenting—incomplete apposition (**A**), incomplete expansion (**B**), and edge tear (**C**). **Panel A** shows a gap between a portion of stent and the vessel wall (*arrow*). **Panel B** shows incomplete expansion of the stent relative to the vessel size. In panel **C**, an edge tear or "pocket flap" is shown at the stent margin (*arrow*).

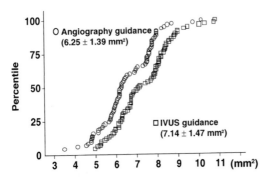

FIG. 4.11. Cumulative frequency distribution curve of minimal stent area illustrating the impact (rightward shift) of IVUS-guided stenting in the CRUISE trial.

Guide *ST*enting) study showed a 6.3% absolute reduction in the angiographic restenosis rate (22.5% vs. 28.8%) and a 20% increase in late lumen cross sectional area in the IVUS-guidance group compared to angiography guidance alone

(38). Other ongoing randomized trials using IVUS combined with stents, where overall cost is an additional endpoint, will be completed in the very near future.

Even with IVUS guidance, 20% to 30% of cases do not achieve the IVUS criteria for "optimal" stent deployment. Suboptimal results may be partially related to large plaque burdens limiting vessel compliance and inhibiting complete stent expansion as well as promoting longitudinal plaque redistribution (39). Debulking prior to stent placement to achieve favorable compliance characteristics of a given lesion segment may lead to further improved long-term results. The SOLD registry, which tested plaque removal using DCA prior to stent placement, showed a remarkably low angiographic restenosis rate of 11% at 6 months follow-up (40). In addition, for lesions with large amounts of preintervention superficial calcium, "rotastenting" may be a preferable approach. In Figure 4.12,

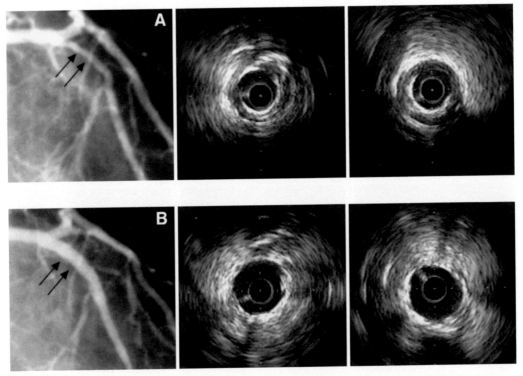

FIG. 4.12. Debulking by rotational atherectomy prior to stenting. Effective luminal patency was achieved following 2.0-mm burr (**Panel A**). **Panel B** shows facilitated expansion of the lumen by the stent after rotational atherectomy.

preintervention IVUS images show superficial calcium at the target lesion (left panel). After rotational atherectomy with use of 2.0-mm burr, stenting resulted in a significantly larger lumen than standalone rotational atherectomy. Debulking by rotational atherectomy prior to stent placement, in these lesion subsets, allows for safe delivery of "sheathless" stent designs and provides the potential for optimizing geometric expansion.

INTRACORONARY PRESSURE AND FRACTIONAL FLOW RESERVE

As intravascular ultrasound has matured as a technique for precise *anatomic* characterization of lesions, a new technique has emerged for *physiologic* assessment—the pressure-derived fractional flow reserve (FFR). Here again a combination of technical and scientific advances has made the new approach possible.

On the technical side, the main advance has been the development of high-fidelity pressure monitoring guidewires. There are two basic designs: solid state and fluid-filled. The solid state designs have micromanometers incorporated into the guidewire just proximal to the flexible distal segment (3 cm from the tip). The wire is connected by a cable to a small signal conditioning box, which in turn routes to the standard catheterization laboratory hemodynamic equipment and monitor displays. Two companies currently have FDA-approved solid state wires: the WaveWire (Endosonics, Rancho Cordova, CA) and the PressureWire (Radi, Uppsala, Sweden). Both of these wires are 0.014 inches in caliber and can be used as an interventional wire, although the guidewire delivery and performance characteristics are not quite as good as those of current, front-line guidewires. The second main design is a fluid-filled guidewire (a hypo tube construction) with pressure monitoring ports just proximal to the flexible wire tip. This wire requires a special transducer which attaches to the proximal end of the guidewire; a cable then goes from this adapter into the standard hemodynamic monitoring equipment. At the time of writing this chapter, there is no FDA-approved wire of this design, though at least two companies have advanced prototypes in testing.

Although measuring pressure gradients has been possible using catheters since the beginning of coronary angioplasty, the development of the pressure guidewires is critically important for two reasons. First, even the smallest catheters create an artifactual increase in pressure when delivered across a stenosis. With the guidewires there is only a minimal increase in pressure due to the wire except in the most severe stenoses—where the gradients are obviously high in any event. Second, the guidewire platform is much more practical than catheter-based pressure measurements. Pressure gradient determinations can be made in the diagnostic setting using wires delivered through small caliber catheters (5 Fr) with minimal chance of disrupting the vessel. In the interventional setting, the pressure wire can be used as the working wire, left in place to provide monitoring as different therapeutic catheters are exchanged.

The scientific development that has enabled the practical use of coronary pressure measurements is the concept of FFR. Based on the early work of Gould (41), Piljs and DeBruyne conceived and validated a new index of coronary flow reserve that is more robust than the coronary velocity reserve measured by Doppler methods (42–45). The key to the FFR concept is the fact that the flow in a coronary bed is directly proportional to the driving pressure. The driving pressure in a nonobstructed coronary artery is the difference between the ostial pressure (which is the same as the aortic pressure) and the coronary venous pressure (which is negligible in almost all cases). In an artery with a lesion, the driving pressure that the myocardium "sees" is the pressure distal to the stenosis. The fractional flow reserve is simply a ratio between these two driving pressures: the actual driving pressure distal the lesion (P_d, measured by the guidewire across the lesion) and the pressure in the aorta (P_a, measured by the guiding catheter). The pressures are determined at maximal hyperemia, for example, with adenosine administration (Fig. 4.13). This ratio can be thought of as the ratio of the actual maximal flow in the artery—which is proportional to the real myocardial driving pressure—to the flow that would be present if there was no obstruction, which is proportional

RESTING GRADIENT

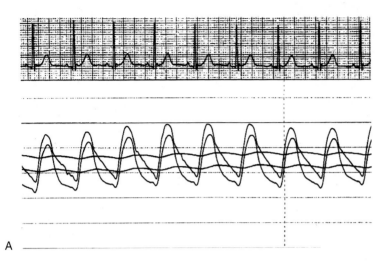

A

FFR: 55/74 = 0.74

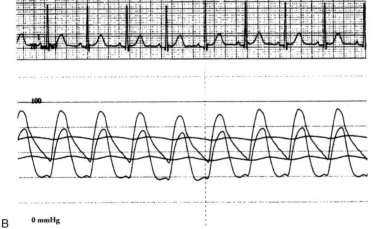

B   0 mmHg

FIG. 4.13. A: Mean and phasic recordings from pressure wire (*lower tracings*) and guiding catheter (*upper tracings*) under resting conditions. **B:** With adenosine-induced hyperemia, the gradient increases. The FFR is calculated from the ratio of the mean pressures.

to the aortic pressure. Although the FFR is calculated as a ratio of pressures, it in fact reflects the ratio of actual to ideal flow (hence the name fractional *flow* reserve).

There are several attractive features to the FFR as a measurement of functional flow impairment. First, there is an unambiguously normal value, which is 1.0. An FFR of 1.0 means the myocardial driving pressure is the same as the aortic pressure, since there is no obstruction in the vessel. As the lesion worsens, the FFR decreases. A number of studies comparing FFR

to noninvasive perfusion studies have suggested that an FFR of 0.75 is the most discriminating threshold for ischemia (if the FFR is below 0.75, the myocardium will be ischemic under conditions of stress) (42,44,46). Interestingly, since flow correlates directly with cross-sectional area, this means that the clinical FFR studies corroborate the early experimental observations that reductions in cross-sectional area to 75% or less create ischemia in the provoked state (47).

Two other advantages of FFR over the coronary flow reserve are worth mentioning. First, the FFR measures obstruction in the epicardial vessels, but is independent of the resistance in the myocardial bed. This is generally an advantage from the interventional standpoint, where the practical clinical questions are (a) whether a stenosis needs to be treated and (b) whether it has been treated optimally. On the other hand, the FFR technique does not provide a measure of small vessel disease in those clinical conditions where this issue is important, such as diabetes or syndrome x. Another favorable aspect of the FFR measurement is that it is relatively independent of the hemodynamic condition of the patient (48). By virtue of the aortic pressure measurement, the FFR is internally calibrated to the instantaneous hemodynamic status of the patient. The Doppler-derived coronary velocity reserve, on the other hand, can vary more widely during hemodynamic swings.

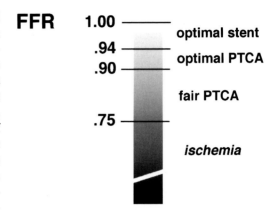

FIG. 4.14. The gradient of FFR results in diagnostic and interventional settings. Below 0.75, the territory served by the vessel will be ischemic, at least during exercise. Following balloon angioplasty, an FFR of 0.84 to 0.90 is acceptable, but is associated with higher recurrence rates than is seen with an FFR greater than 0.90. With a fully deployed stent (and no significant disease elsewhere in the vessel) an FFR of 0.94 can be achieved.

Clinical Applications

There are two major areas of clinical use for the FFR: assessment of the intermediate lesion and optimization of procedure outcomes. As mentioned above, there are several studies corroborating an FFR 0.75 as the threshold of ischemia. A patient coming to the catheterization laboratory with an angiographically intermediate or obscure narrowing who has an FFR above 0.75 is unlikely to benefit symptomatically from treating that narrowing (49). A prospective, multicenter trial (the DEFER trial) is underway to evaluate the clinical outcome of not treating lesions with an FFR over 0.75.

In the area of procedural optimization, there is a gradient of FFR findings depending on the particular technique (Fig. 4.14). Because stenting is the most effective technique for acutely improving flow, the FFR results are generally higher than for balloon angioplasty. An FFR of 0.94 or greater means that the stent is fully expanded and there are no significant inflow or outflow problems (50). With balloon angioplasty, an optimal result correlates with an FFR of 0.90 or greater; moderately good results yield FFRs in the 0.84 to 0.90 range. A recent single-center study suggests that in patients undergoing angioplasty where the FFR is greater than 0.90 the clinical outcomes are comparable to those achieved with stenting (51). A practical implication of this finding is that FFR can provide a guide for provisional stenting: if an FFR greater than 0.90 can be achieved using a balloon, it is not necessary to stent; for an FFR less than 0.90, the clinical outcome can probably be improved by stenting.

Limitations and Subtleties

The FFR is a robust, reproducible, and fairly simple measurement, but there are certain pitfalls. From a practical standpoint, one important issue is the need to achieve maximal hyperemia. The most convenient agent and route for administration is intracoronary adenosine. Unfortunately, in about 10% of patients maximal hyperemia will not be achieved with this approach. Intravenous adenosine is a more reliable stimulus, but is considerably more expensive (because of the larger dose of adenosine required), involves more time and the infusion equipment and causes angina-like chest discomfort in the large majority of patients. Even intravenous adenosine may provide suboptimal hyperemia in some cases so that operator judgment is mandatory in interpreting the results of a particular FFR value.

A second important consideration is that the FFR provides a cumulative assessment of the pressure drop across the entire vessel length between the ostium and the position of the guidewire sensor. In many cases there will be obstruction to flow elsewhere in the vessel in addition to the lesion that appears important by angiography. If this is the situation, it will obviously not be possible to optimize the FFR by treating the target segment alone. The location of the residual stenosis can be identified by performing a pullback of the guidewire while administering a constant infusion of intravenous adenosine.

THE FUTURE OF CATHETER-BASED ULTRASOUND

Both the IVUS catheter and ultrasound system are now in a rapid technical development phase. Ultrasound catheters are now in sizes less than 1 mm and thus are deliverable to the majority of anatomical configurations in the coronary tree. The transducer frequencies are approaching 50 MHz and the ultrasound systems are being developed to be smaller, compact units with an "all digital" front and back end. This digital solution will add significantly to both pre and postprocessing techniques allowing for refine-

ments in tissue characterization by Radio Frequency (RF) signal analysis, three-dimensional display in real time, and automatic border detection.

As the frequency increases, the echo pattern for blood becomes significantly enhanced and may obscure the luminal border using control display algorithms. However, postprocessing techniques in real-time permit digital filters to distinguish blood variation signals (uncorrelated process) compared to tissue signals (correlated process). Ultimately, postprocessing techniques to reduce blood speckle and, hence, detect lumen borders, will be possible in real time. Figure 4.15 shows blood noise reduction for a 45-MHz transducer system with automatic border detection of the luminal border. Being able to track luminal dimensions (i.e., vessel and/or stent geometry) instantaneously in the catheterization laboratory will facilitate the integration of IVUS catheters into a busy catheterization schedule.

Digital archiving of 30 frames per second for several minutes directly into computer memory will allow real-time three-dimensional reconstruction. This feature would enable the interventionalists to reconstruct the spatial configurations of target vessels by looking "inside" the vessel. For example, rather than interpret hundreds of frames, one can immediately determine the extent of the disease and the relationship to branch vessels (Fig. 4.16A) as well as determine incomplete stent geometry by these composite presentations (Fig. 4.16B).

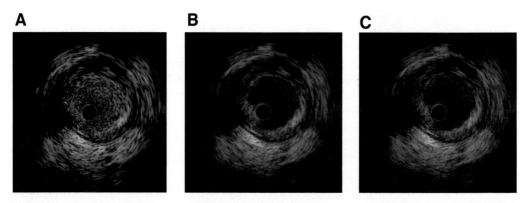

FIG. 4.15. Blood noise reduction and automatic border detection. IVUS image of a 45-MHz transducer demonstrates remarkable blood signal noise (**A**). Blood signal was suppressed by using a specialized digital filter (**B**), allowing automatic luminal border detection (**C**).

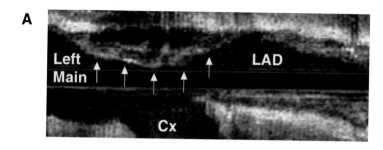

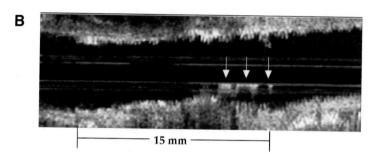

15 mm

FIG. 4.16. Longitudinal reconstructed images of the proximal left anterior descending artery. **Panel A** shows a discrete amount of plaque (*arrows*) in the left main extending into the proximal left anterior descending artery. **Panel B** demonstrates incomplete apposition of the stent at the distal edge (*arrows*). LAD, left anterior descending; Cx, Circumflex.

Finally, the ultimate goal of coronary plaque visualization is to identify the vulnerable plaque, thought to be the ultracellular plaque substructure responsible for acute coronary syndromes. Having a digital system with upfront RF signal processing, including the features of both amplitude and phase variations, would permit the detection of subtle tissue signal interactions. Recently the ability to analyze the "raw" signals has shown promise for characterizing different tissue types *in vivo* (52). The ability to provide this service on-line in the cardiac catheterization laboratory would lend insight not only for tracking the natural history of plaque but also potentially recognizing plaques that may require alternative therapies for stabilization.

REFERENCES

1. Yock PG, Fitzgerald PJ, Sudhir K, Linker DT, White W, Ports A. Intravascular ultrasound imaging for guidance of atherectomy and other plaque removal techniques. *Int J Card Imaging* 1991;6:1791–1789.
2. Nissen SE, Gurley JC, Grines CL et al. Intravascular ultrasound assessment of lumen size and wall morphology in normal subjects and patients with coronary artery disease. *Circulation* 1991;84:1087–1099.
3. Pichard AD, Mintz GS, Satler LF, Kent KM, Popma JJ, Kovach JA, Leon MA. The influence of preintervention intravascular ultrasound imaging on subsequent trans-

catheter treatment strategies. *J Am Coll Cardiol* 1993; 21:133A.
4. Burns W, Hermiller J, Kisslo K, Culp S, Davidson C. Prognostic significance of left main coronary artery disease detected by intravascular ultrasound. *J Invasive Cardiol* 1995;7:119–121.
5. Higano ST, Yeo TC, Lerman A, Nishimura RA, Holmes DR. Intracoronary ultrasound guided clinical decision making in indeterminate left main disease: 18 Month follow-up study. *J Am Coll Cardiol* 1998;31:224 A.
6. Stone GW, Hodgson JM, St Goar FG et al. Improved procedural results of coronary angioplasty with intravascular ultrasound-guided balloon sizing: the CLOUT Pilot Trial. Clinical Outcomes With Ultrasound Trial (CLOUT) Investigators. *Circulation* 1997;95: 2044–2052.
7. Serruys P, Azar A, Sigwart U et al. Long-term follow-up of "stent-like" (≤30% diameter stenosis post) angioplasty: a case for provisional stenting. *J Am Coll Cardiol* 1996;27:15A.
8. Rodriguez A, Ayala F, Bernardi V et al. Optimal coronary balloon angioplasty with provisional stenting versus primary stent (OCBAS): immediate and long-term follow-up results. *J Am Coll Cardiol* 1998;32: 1351–1357.
9. Mintz GS, Douek P, Pichard AD et al. Target lesion calcification in coronary artery disease: an intravascular ultrasound study. *J Am Coll Cardiol* 1992;20: 1149–1155.
10. Honye J, Mahon DJ, Jain A et al. Morphological effects of coronary balloon angioplasty *in vivo* assessed by intravascular ultrasound imaging. *Circulation* 1992;85: 1012–1025.
11. Mintz GS, Potkin BN, Keren G, Satler LF, Pichard AD, Kent KM, Popma JJ, Leon MB. Intravascular ultrasound evaluation of the effect of rotational atherectomy in ob-

structive atherosclerotic coronary artery disease. *Circulation* 1992;86:1383–1393.

12. Hoffmann R; Mintz GS; Kent KM; Pichard AD; Satler LF; Popma JJ; Hong MK; Laird JR; Leon MB. Comparative early and nine-month results of rotational atherectomy, stents, and the combination of both for calcified lesions in large coronary arteries. *Am J Cardiol* 1998; 81:552–557.

13. Kovach JA, Mintz GS, Pichard AD, Kent KM, Popma JJ, Satler LF, Leon MB. Sequential intravascular ultrasound characterization of the mechanisms of rotational atherectomy and adjunct balloon angioplasty. *J Am Coll Cardiol* 1993;22:1024–1032.

14. Mintz GS, Popma JJ, Pichard AD et al. Intravascular ultrasound predictors of restenosis after percutaneous transcatheter coronary revascularization. *J Am Coll Cardiol* 1996;27:1678–1687.

15. Görge G, Liu E, Ge J, Haude M, Baumgart D, Caspary G. Intravascular ultrasound variables predict restenosis after PTCA. *Circulation* 1995;92:I-148.

16. Peters RJG, Kok WE, Di Mario C et al. Prediction of restenosis after coronary balloon angioplasty. Results of PICTURE (Post—IntraCoronary Treatment Ultrasound Result Evaluation), a prospective multicenter intracoronary ultrasound imaging study. *Circulation* 1997;95: 2254–2261.

17. The GUIDE trial investigators. IVUS-determined predictors of restenosis in PTCA and DCA: final report from the GUIDE trial, phase II. *J Am Coll Cardiol* 1996; 27:156A.

18. Simonton CA, Leon MB, Baim DS et al. ''Optimal'' directional coronary atherectomy: final results of the Optimal Atherectomy Restenosis Study (OARS). *Circulation* 1998;97:332–339.

19. Baim DS, Simonton CA, Popma JJ et al. Mechanism of luminal enlargement by optimal atherectomy—IVUS insights from the OARS study. *J Am Coll Cardiol* 1996; 27:291A.

20. Hosokawa H, Suzuki T, Ueno K, Aizawa T, Fujita T, Takase S, Oda H. Clinical and angiographic follow-up of adjunctive balloon angioplasty following coronary atherectomy study (ABACAS). *Circulation* 1996;94:I-318

21. Suzuki T, Kato O, Ueno K et al. Initial and long-term results of the adjunctive ballon angioplasty following coronary atherectomy study (ABACAS). *J Am Coll Cardiol* 1997;29:68A.

22. Post MJ, Borst C, Kuntz RE. The relative importance of arterial remodeling compared with intimal hyperplasia in lumen renarrowing after balloon angioplasty. A study in the normal rabbit and the hypercholesterolemic Yucatan micropig. *Circulation* 1994;89:2816–2821.

23. Kakuta T, Currier JW, Haudenschild CC, Ryan TJ, Faxon DP. Differences in compensatory vessel enlargement, not intimal formation, account for restenosis after angioplasty in the hypercholesterolemic rabbit model. *Circulation* 1994;89:2809–2815.

24. Mintz GS, Popma JJ, Pichard AD, Kent KM, Satler LF, Wong C, Hong MK, Kovach JA, Leon MB. Arterial remodeling after coronary angioplasty: a serial intravascular ultrasound study. *Circulation* 1996;94:35–43.

25. Kimura T, Kaburagi S, Tamura T et al. Remodeling of human coronary arteries undergoing coronary angioplasty or atherectomy. *Circulation* 1997;96:4754–4783.

26. Serruys PW, de Jaegere P, Kiemeneij F et al. A compari-

son of balloon-expandable-stent implantation with balloon angioplasty in patients with coronary artery disease. Benestent Study Group. *N Engl J Med* 1994;331: 4894–4895.

27. Fischman DL, Leon MB, Baim DS et al. A randomized comparison of coronary-stent placement and balloon angioplasty in the treatment of coronary artery disease. Stent Restenosis Study Investigators. *N Engl J Med* 1994;331:496–501.

28. Erbel R, Haude M, Hopp HW et al. Coronary-Artery Stenting Compared with Balloon Angioplasty for Restenosis after Initial Balloon Angioplasty. *N Engl J Med* 1998;339:1672–1678.

29. Colombo A, Hall P, Nakamura S et al. Intracoronary stenting without anticoagulation accomplished with intravascular ultrasound guidance. *Circulation* 1995;91: 1676–1688.

30. Goldberg SL, Colombo A, Nakamura S, Almagor Y, Maiello L, Tobis JM. Benefit of intracoronary ultrasound in the deployment of Palmaz-Schatz stents. *J Am Coll Cardiol* 1994;24:996–1003.

31. Schwarzacher SP, Metz JA, Yock PG, Fitzgerald PJ. Vessel tearing at the edge of intracoronary stents detected with intravascular ultrasound imaging. *Cathet Cardiovasc Diagn* 1997;40:152–155.

32. Kuntz RE, Safian RD, Carrozza JP, Fishman RF, Mansour M, Baim DS. The importance of acute luminal diameter in determining restenosis after coronary atherectomy or stenting. *Circulation* 1992;86:1827–1835.

33. Ziada KM, Tuzcu EM, De Franco AC et al. Absolute, not relative, poststent lumen area is better predictor of clinical outcome. *Circulation* 1996;94:I-453.

34. Moussa I, Di Mario C, Moses J, Reimers B, Blengino S, Colombo A. The predictive value of different intravascular ultrasound criteria for restenosis after coronary stenting. *J Am Coll Cardiol* 1997;29:60A.

35. Hoffmann R, Mintz GS, Mehran R et al. Intravascular ultrasound predictors of angiographic restenosis in lesions treated with Palmaz-Schatz stents. *J Am Coll Cardiol* 1998;31:43–49.

36. Kasaoka S, Tobis JM, Akiyama T et al. Angiographic and intravascular ultrasound predictors of in-stent restenosis. *J Am Coll Cardiol* 1998;32:1630–1635.

37. Fitzgerald PJ, Hayase M, Mintz GS et al. CRUISE: Can routine intravascular ultrasound influence stent expansion? Analysis of outcomes. *J Am Coll Cardiol* 1998; 31:396A.

38. Schiele F, Meneveau N, Vuillemenot A et al. Impact of intravascular ultrasound guidance in stent deployment on 6-month restenosis rate: a multicenter, randomized study comparing two strategies—with and without intravascular ultrasound guidance. RESIST Study Group. REStenosis after Ivus guided STenting. *J Am Coll Cardiol* 1998;32:320–328.

39. Honda Y, Yock C, Hermiller JB, Fitzgerald PJ, Yock PG. Longitudinal redistribution of plaque is an important mechanism for lumen expansion in stenting. *J Am Coll Cardiol* 1997;29:281A.

40. Moussa I, Moses J, Di Mario C et al. Stenting after optimal lesion debulking (SOLD) registry. Angiographic and clinical outcome. *Circulation* 1998;98: 1604–1609.

41. Gould KL, Kirkeeide RL, Buchi M. Coronary flow reserve as a physiologic measure of stenosis severity. *J Am Coll Cardiol* 1990;15:459–474.

42. De Bruyne B, Bartunek J, Sys SU, Heyndrickx GR. Relation between myocardial fractional flow reserve calculated from coronary pressure measurements and exercise-induced myocardial ischemia. *Circulation* 1995;92:39–46.

43. De Bruyne B, Baudhuin T, Melin JA et al. Coronary flow reserve calculated from pressure measurements in humans. Validation with positron emission tomography. *Circulation* 1994;89:1013–1022.

44. Pijls NH, De Bruyne B, Peels K et al. Measurement of fractional flow reserve to assess the functional severity of coronary-artery stenoses [see comments]. *N Engl J Med* 1996;334:1703–1708.

45. Pijls NH, van Son JA, Kirkeeide RL, De Bruyne B, Gould KL. Experimental basis of determining maximum coronary, myocardial, and collateral blood flow by pressure measurements for assessing functional stenosis severity before and after percutaneous transluminal coronary angioplasty. *Circulation* 1993;87:1354–1367.

46. Pijls NH, Van Gelder B, Van der Voort P et al. Fractional flow reserve. A useful index to evaluate the influence of an epicardial coronary stenosis on myocardial blood flow [see comments]. *Circulation* 1995;92: 3183–3193.

47. Gould KL, Lipscomb K. Effects of coronary stenoses on coronary flow reserve and resistance. *Am J Cardiol* 1974;34:48–55.

48. De Bruyne B, Bartunek J, Sys SU, Pijls NH, Heyndrickx GR, Wijns W. Simultaneous coronary pressure and flow velocity measurements in humans. Feasibility, reproducibility, and hemodynamic dependence of coronary flow velocity reserve, hyperemic flow versus pressure slope index, and fractional flow reserve [see comments]. *Circulation* 1996;94:1842–1849.

49. Bech GJ, De Bruyne B, Bonnier HJ et al. Long-term follow-up after deferral of percutaneous transluminal coronary angioplasty of intermediate stenosis on the basis of coronary pressure measurement. *J Am Coll Cardiol* 1998;31:841–847.

50. Hanekamp C KJ Pijls N, Michels H, Bonnier H. Comparison of quantitative coronary angiography, intravascular ultrasound and coronary pressure measurement to assess optimum stent deployment. *Circulation* 1999;99: 1015–1021.

51. Bech G, DeBruyne B, Peels K, Michels R, Bonnier H, Koolen J. Usefulness of fractional flow reserve to predict clinical outcome after balloon angioplasty. *Circulation* 1999;99:883–888.

52. Jeremias A, Kolz ML, Oshima A. *In vivo* intravascular ultrasound tissue characterization for the early detection of allograft rejection. *Circulation* 1998;17:I-691.

5

Developing or Niche Techniques

A. Angiogenesis and Myogenesis

Stephen G. Ellis

*Sones Cardiac Catheterization Laboratories, Department of Cardiology, The Cleveland Clinic
Foundation, Cleveland, Ohio 44195-5066 and Department of Medicine, Ohio State University,
Columbus, Ohio 43210*

Despite dramatic advances in revascularization options developed over the last two decades, many patients with advanced coronary disease are left with little hope for relief of angina or for long-term survival. This is especially true for the estimated 150,000 patients with severe angina undergoing cardiac catheterization annually in the United States who are no longer candidates for bypass surgery or standard percutaneous coronary intervention, and for the over 200,000 patients diagnosed annually with congestive heart failure related to advanced coronary artery disease. While neither angiogenesis nor myogenesis will be approved therapies at the time this textbook goes to press, they offer molecular biology–based interventions that, with refinement, will likely offer hope to the previously untreatable patient.

ANGIOGENESIS

Physiology

Angiographically apparent collateral blood vessels often develop to compensate for and partially ameliorate ischemia consequent to slowly developing severe epicardial stenoses. These collaterals are sometimes sufficient to minimize ischemia and angina, and also to limit significant myocardial damage in the event the collateralized artery occludes.

Billinger and colleagues (1) studied 201 patients undergoing percutaneous coronary inter-vention to assess parameters that discriminated between patients with and without ischemia (ST segment elevation or depression ≥ 1 mm) during transient coronary artery occlusion. Seventy-five percent of patients demonstrated an ischemic response. As noted in Table 5.1 and Fig. 5.1, these investigators found that both the Rentrop collateral score (0 = no evident collaterals, 1 = contrast opacification of the collateral vessels only, 2 = partial opacification of the recipient epicardial vessel, 3 = complete opacification of the recipient vessel) and collateral flow index $[(p_{occlusion\text{-}CVP}) \div (p_{AO\text{-}CVP})]$ to be strongly protective against ischemia.

Factors involved in the degree of collateralization relative to ischemia are incompletely understood. Animal studies suggest that aging and hyperlipidemia may impair collateral formation. The normal physiologic response of viable myocardium to sustained or intermittent severe ischemia is complex, and some patients develop decreased contractility or myocardial "hibernation," possibly in response to calcium overload or oxidant stress. In addition, a cascade of intracellular signaling events is set into play, culminating in (a) increasing sensitivity (upregulation) of receptors of growth factors that stimulate angiogenesis and (b) increased production of vascular endothelial growth factor (VEGF) and other growth factors that directly stimulate angiogenesis by augmenting the migration and proliferation of endothelial and smooth muscle

TABLE 5.1. *Relationship between baseline clinical and angiographic factors and collaterization*

	Sufficient collaterals	Insufficient collaterals	*p*
n	50	151	
Age	59 ± 10	58 ± 10	NS
CFI	0.48 ± 0.18	0.17 ± 0.09	<0.0001
Rentrop (0–3)	2.0 ± 0.7	0.8 ± 0.8	<0.0001
AP	9%	91%	<0.0001

AP, angina pectoris during PTCA; CFI, collateral flow index.
From ref. 1, with permission.

cells in the adjacent vascular structures, as well as progenitor stem cells in the bone marrow and blood, which are capable of becoming transformed into vascular elements. A very large number of growth factors and cytokines are involved in this complicated process, often with important interplay between elements (Fig. 5.2).

Proof of Principle

It is premature to speculate which combination of growth factors and delivery mechanisms

Collateral Flow Index, CFI
0.8
0.6
0.4
0.2
0
p < 0.0001
Sufficient collaterals
Insufficient collaterals

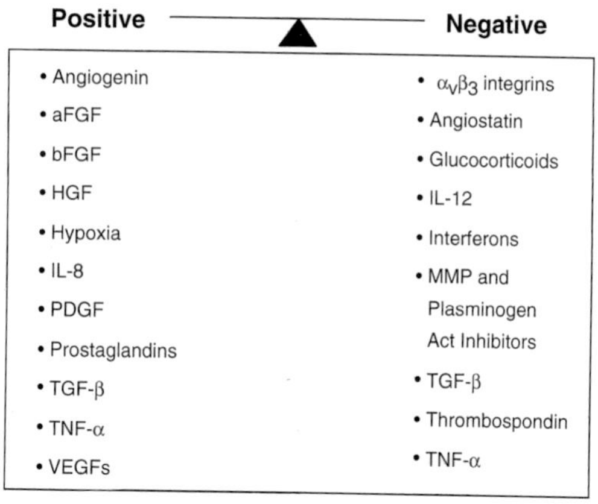

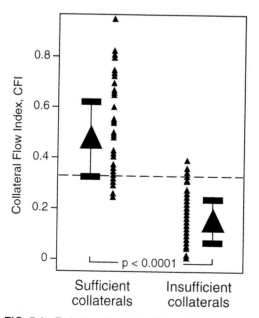

FIG. 5.1. Relation of collateral flow index to presence (insufficient collaterals) or absence (sufficient collaterals) of ECG changes during balloon occlusion of the collateralized vessel. (From ref. 1, with permission.)

Positive
Negative
• Angiogenin
• aFGF
• bFGF
• HGF
• Hypoxia
• IL-8
• PDGF
• Prostaglandins
• TGF-β
• TNF-α
• VEGFs
• $\alpha_v\beta_3$ integrins
• Angiostatin
• Glucocorticoids
• IL-12
• Interferons
• MMP and Plasminogen Act Inhibitors
• TGF-β
• Thrombospondin
• TNF-α

FIG. 5.2. Growth factors and cytokines modulating angiogenesis.

will ultimately become most clinically useful. It is not too soon, however, to acknowledge the tremendous potential of the general approach of therapeutic angiogenesis.

The finding that VEGF could be used to achieve angiogenesis that was therapeutic was first demonstrated by Takeshita et al. (2), who administered recombinant VEGF as a single intraarterial bolus to rabbits with unilateral hindlimb ischemia and demonstrated increased blood flow. Similar findings with recombinant VEGF administration in canine and porcine models of myocardial ischemia were published shortly thereafter.

Building on this preclinical work from Takeshita's and other laboratories, Baumgartner and colleagues (3) moved to perform the initial human experiments in patients with limb-threatening ischemia. The capacity to transfer genetic information into a human cell with "naked" plasmid DNA is quite limited, often necessitating the use of viruses (stripped of their cellular mechanisms to replicate) that provide cellular machinery to enter the target cell and to generate the desired protein product—a controversial approach. Fortunately, ischemic skeletal myocytes are fairly receptive to the uptake and utilization of naked DNA. Aided by the fact that VEGF is a protein secreted by transformed cells, Baumgartner and colleagues were able to overcome the modest transfection rates, allowing demonstration of "proof of principle" of therapeutic angiogenesis for human limb ischemia (3).

Isner (4) has studied direct skeletal injection of cDNA for phVEGF$_{165}$, using tuberculin syringes in over 70 carefully selected patients. More than 95% of patients with rest pain without ulcers or gangrene have demonstrated improvement in symptoms and objective measures of perfusion, such as ankle brachial index. Preliminary data suggest that the clinical benefit extends for at least 2 years. Patients with gangrene or ulcers have had a more varied response, with only 55% to 77% of patients improving. Preliminary analysis suggests that younger patients and those with a patent dorsalis pedis (recipient) artery are most likely to respond. In patients with disease so advanced that significant tissue regrowth is necessary for recovery, coadministration of blood or bone marrow–derived progenitor stem cells may be required for clinical benefit. Similar, but less well developed, results have also been reported using basic fibroblast growth factor (FGF).

Isner subsequently extended his work to patients with myocardial ischemia, using direct myocardial injection of naked plasmid cDNA encoding VEGF$_{165}$ via a minithoracotomy. Sixteen patients have been treated to date. Others, such as Rosengart and Schumacher, have reported similar results with a similar approach in fewer patients. Perhaps as is true with patients with rest pain of the extremities but without ulcers or gangrene, patients with severe myocardial ischemia may respond. Myocardial scar and necrosis might be considered the equivalent of gangrene and ulceration, and patients with no evidence of reversible perfusion defects prior to treatment have been avoided in these series. Angina commonly begins to diminish by 2 weeks and reaches a maximum improvement by 2 to 3 months. Reduction in angina class is often dramatic (although a placebo effect could account for some of the benefit). All patients recruited to date have had Class IV angina prior to treatment, yet by 6 weeks the mean angina class has been 0.7 (Fig. 5.3). Interestingly, improvement in both transient and fixed sestamibi defects has been noted (recall that reperfusion of "fixed de-

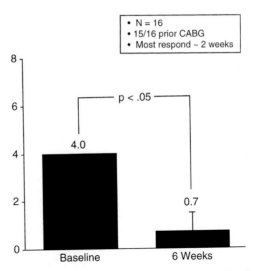

FIG. 5.3. Improvement in angina class with direct myocardial injection of phVEGF$_{165}$.

fects" will, in 50% to 70%, lead to improvement in regional ventricular function) (Fig. 5.4).

Growth Factors

Although there are many potential therapeutic growth factors, those from the VEGF and FGF families have been studied most closely. VEGF, in its various forms, is a potent mitogen for endothelial cells, and also induces the expression of urokinase-type and tissue-type plasminogen activators that facilitate sprouting of endothelial cells. It is also known as vascular permeability factor. VEGF may exist in one of four molecular forms, denoted VEGF$_{121}$, VEGF$_{165}$, VEGF$_{189}$, and VEGF$_{206}$, formed by alternate splicing of a single VEGF gene. The higher molecular weight isoforms bind heparin avidly, accounting for their longer plasma half-life. The Flt-1 and KDR/Flk-1 VEGF receptors are upregulated by tissue ischemia. The FGF family is comprised of at least nine polypeptides, among which acidic FGF (or FGF-1) and basic FGF (FGF-2) are the most carefully characterized. At least four high-affinity receptors have been identified, stimulation of which is mitogenic for smooth muscle cells, fibroblasts, and endothelial cells. Additional low-affinity, high-capacity receptors provide an extracellular storage site for the FGFs

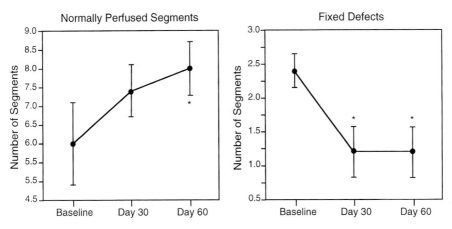

FIG. 5.4. SPECT-sestamibi perfusion imaging: summary of findings in five patients. Short-axis views were divided into a total of 13 segments and graded as normal (no perfusion defect), reversible (perfusion defect during stress that partially or completely reversed at rest), or fixed (perfusion defect during stress that persists at rest). Values represent mean ± SEM for all five patients at baseline, 30 days, and 60 days post–gene therapy. *p* < .05 compared with baseline. (From ref. 4, with permission.)

from which the growth factors may be released upon the addition of exogenous heparin. Heparan sulfate binding appears to facilitate FGF dimerization and enhanced receptor binding. Basic FGF has been shown to directly upregulate VEGF transcription.

Vehicles and Delivery Devices

The concepts and observations that (a) receptors for VEGF and other growth factors are considerably upregulated in the presence of ischemia; (b) the initial human ischemic limb data suggest benefit from a methodology known to have limited capacity to transfect smooth muscle cells; and (c) other studies showing a limited dose-response relationship between growth factor and increase in blood flow have led to the hope that the direct surgical approach to transfer gene therapy to ischemic myocardial cells might be avoided. Response in experimental models of ischemia to intravenous and intraarterial application of growth factors has been mixed. The best test of the concept that nondirect intravenous administration of growth factors might be clinically effective to date has been the Phase II Genentech study of protein VEGF$_{165}$. Building on initial Phase I nonplacebo-controlled studies of intraarterial and intravenous injection of this

form of VEGF, wherein some apparent clinical response was noted, investigators randomized 178 patients with Class II or III angina, demonstrated ischemia to involve at least 20% of the left ventricular myocardium and well-preserved left ventricular function, to a high-dose infusion of VEGF, low-dose administration of VEGF, or matching placebo. VEGF and placebo were administered with a single intracoronary injection followed by three intravenous infusions. The doses utilized had been based on the maximum doses tolerated in earlier studies (flushing and hypotension are common side effects). Initial 60-day results have, unfortunately, suggested no benefit in terms of relief of angina or improvement in exercise time, compared with placebo-treated patients who, interestingly, did demonstrate considerable clinical improvement. These results serve to cast doubt on the utility of unaided intravenous application of growth factors in this manner. Initial work from Mukherjee and colleagues (7) at the Cleveland Clinic suggest that the myocardial uptake of intravenously administered VEGF may be augmented tenfold by the coapplication of ultrasound energy to the myocardium. The potential utility of this and other ways to augment intravenous uptake remain to be tested.

Given the initial response to direct myocardial

injection and intravenous application of these agents, it would seem possible that successful percutaneous application of growth factors will also require direct myocardial injection. Several catheters have been developed for just this purpose—modifying catheters already in use for transmyocardial application of laser energy for PMR. Preliminary studies indicate that application of 0.2 to 0.3 mL of methylene blue, or adenoviruses modified to express β-galactosidase, which stains blue with the application of X-gal, in a similar volume of fluid suggests that injected material "spreads" approximately 0.5 to 0.7 mm in all directions. Whether this can be safely applied using biplane fluoroscopy or will require more sophisticated guidance systems, such as the Biosense Noga electromagnetic orientation and guidance system, has yet to be determined. Thus far, application of VEGF during

surgery has been via multiple injections spanning the ischemic region, and it is not certain whether uniform application will be required.

The success of the application of naked plasmid DNA has dampened enthusiasm for the utilization of virus transfection as a means to increase cellular transfection of these growth factors. Clearly, viruses are taken up 10- to 20-fold more readily than naked DNA, but given the possible complications associated with viruses, they may not be needed. Adenovirus and retrovirus vector systems have been best studied to date. The DNA encoding for the desired structural proteins, as well as their promoter and other regulatory elements, are identified and inserted into a cloning vector, using restriction endonucleases and standard molecular biology techniques (Fig. 5.5). Retrovirus-mediated gene transfer has the advantage of yielding prolonged

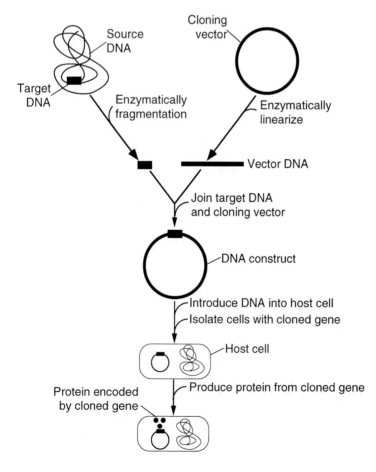

FIG. 5.5. Shown is the recombinant DNA cloning procedure. DNA from a source organism is cleaved with a restriction endonuclease and inserted into a cloning vector. Then the cloning vector–insert DNA construct is introduced into a target host cell, and those cells that carry the construct are identified and grown. If required, the cloned gene can be expressed in the host cell, and its protein can be produced and harvested.

treatment effect due to the insertion of the retrovirus into the cells' own DNA, but initial retrovirus vector systems were limited in that they could transfect only dividing cells and by the concern about insertional mutagenesis—the inadvertent ''turning on'' of proto-oncogenes, leading to cancer by insertion of the virus genetic material into the host genome. Early experience with replication-deficient retrovirus systems in over 200 patients has shown apparent safety, but clearly more patients will need to be treated to have a better understanding of the safety profile. More recently, retroviral vectors have been modified to enhance the efficiency of their transduction, engineering them to infect nondividing cells and specifying the cell types that can be infected. Adenovirus-mediated gene transfer is attractive in some ways: The vector systems are well characterized and reasonably easy to build, and adenovirus vectors do not require cell division for their transfection efficacy, but they appear limited greatly by the immune response that they provoke. Consequently, protein product yields diminish considerably after 10 to 14 days following transfection. Adeno-associated virus and herpes simplex virus vector systems have also been studied.

The so-called naked DNA approach uses plasmid DNA. Plasmids are self-replicating, double-stranded, circular DNA molecules that are maintained in bacteria and other eukaryotic cells as independent, extrachromosomal entities. Virtually all bacteria have plasmids. Some plasmids carry information for their own transfer from one cell to another (F plasmids), others encode resistance to antibiotics (R plasmids), and others carry specific sets of genes for the utilization of unusual metabolites or appear to have no useful function. These plasmids typically range in size from 1 to 500 kb. Each plasmid has a sequence that functions as an origin of DNA replication to enable it to replicate separately in a host cell.

Safety Concerns

The principal safety concern regarding the utilization of growth factors to stimulate angiogenesis in areas of myocardial ischemia is that these growth factors have been observed to augment tumor growth and metastases. In fact, antiangiogenesis agents are being studied as chemotherapeutic agents. It is hoped that the relatively brief exposure apparently required to stimulate therapeutic angiogenesis will be inadequate to stimulate growth and/or metastases of nascent or quiescent tumors in humans. Concern has also been raised that the application of growth factors may lead to stimulation and/or rupture of atherosclerotic plaques. To date, only long-term exposure ($\geq$16 weeks) antiangiogenesis drugs has been shown to diminish plaque formation in animal models (5). Other concerns are that growth factors may stimulate neovascularization in ischemic retina (e.g., from diabetes or macular degeneration), hence possibly leading to retinal hemorrhage and blindness, as well as other growth factor–specific complications (e.g., protein-losing nephropathy with repeated administration of basic FGF). Clearly, the application of growth factors needs to be studied in very large numbers of patients over a protracted period to examine the incidence of these potential unwanted, yet serious, side effects. While it might seem that the direct myocardial injection of genetic or protein material would eliminate the possibility of such untoward side effects, initial data suggest some spread to adjacent vascular tissues, such as the lung, thymus, and, potentially, the liver (6). Obviously, the intravenous application of such agents would also be cause for concern, but perhaps the brevity of their exposure to potential unwanted targets might minimize unwanted side effects.

The Future

There seems little reason to believe that direct myocardial injection using percutaneous catheters will not replicate the initial results seen with the surgical application of such growth factors. Both methods would likely be clinically useful, as many patients requiring such treatment might also benefit from concomitant bypass surgery or percutaneous intervention. Rather widespread clinical investigation of both approaches will likely take place in calendar year 1999, with the surgical trials moving somewhat ahead of the percutaneous application trials. Whether such treatments may soon become available for patients is uncertain. The Food and Drug Administration has yet to deal with attempts to balance the potential clinical usefulness against the potential long-term clinical risk of such a "drug class." Initially, however, it would seem prudent to treat only patients with severe and debilitating angina until the long-term safety profile of these agents can be determined. At the same time, further safety information will need to be developed in patients with a propensity toward other complications, such as retinal hemorrhage. Early retinopathy may not be an absolute contraindication. This has major implications, as 28% of patients otherwise eligible for angiogenesis trials (symptomatic and not well suited for CABG or PCI) are diabetics (7). A tremendous amount of clinical data is yet needed before we can place these potentially active therapeutic agents in their proper perspective.

MYOGENESIS

With the aging of the U.S. population, as well as the salvage with reperfusion therapy of many patients who might otherwise have died of myocardial infarction, the incidence of severe congestive heart failure is increasing rapidly. Despite the well-demonstrated survival benefits associated with application of angiotensin-converting enzymes and β-blockers in this population, and our ability to partially ameliorate symptoms with utilization of diuretics and digitalis preparations, the outlook for many patients with advanced congestive heart failure is bleak. This is fundamentally due to our inability to effect an adequate repair of the infarcted myocardium, short of heart transplantation.

As a terminally differentiated cell type, a cardiac myocyte cannot replicate in response to adjacent injury and its hypertrophic response is severely limited. Nonetheless, it is apparent that *in situ* cellular transplantation (myogenesis) may be possible by using a wide variety of cell sources. If such cells could be transplanted en masse and their function coordinated, one might

actually be able to repair infarcted myocardium. A number of investigators, including our own group, have begun to study just these processes. The primary limitation at present is the absence of cardiomyocytes to transplant. Adult sources are limited and would require immunosuppression therapy similar to that required by total heart transplant patients, and the utilization of fetal myocardial cardiomyocytes is problematic on ethical bases. Further, the genetic machinery required to transform a related cell into a cardiomyocyte (similar to myo-D with skeletal myocytes) is as yet unknown. Some investigators have reported apparent milieu-based transformation of injected skeletal myoblasts into cells with markers and function consistent with cardiomyoblasts (8), but the degree to which this may be accomplished remains greatly uncertain. Nonetheless, Taylor et al. (9) and Li et al. (10) have demonstrated some improvement in ventricular function after intramyocardial injection of skeletal myocytes or myoblasts in animal models. Certainly, long-term engraftment of such cells is feasible. It may well be that uptake of skeletal myocytes into an area of infarction might be able to limit infarct expansion without actually augmenting myocardial contractility. Another interesting and provocative approach makes use of the fact that a small number of bone marrow progenitor stem cells can be induced to transform into phenotypic cardiac myocytes. In fact, Li and colleagues have reported an improvement in rat myocardial function after direct injection of marrow-derived stem cells.

Given the pace of molecular biology, it would seem likely that the genetic information necessary to transform fibroblasts or cellular myoblasts into cardiac myoblasts will soon be characterized. While it will also be necessary to assure electromechanical coupling of transplanted cells to the adjacent viable myocardium, it seems very likely that such approaches will move into clinical testing very early in the next decade. Clearly, a variety of risks and unknowns, such as the potential for stimulating clinical, important ectopic arrhythmias must be overcome, but barring induction of serious complications, it seems quite likely that *in situ* cell transplantation to enhance ventricular function and treat congestive heart failure may well be a clinical reality in the next or following decades.

REFERENCES

1. Billinger M, Fleisch M, Garachemani A, Eberli F, Meier B, Seiler C. How much coronary collateral flow protects against myocardial ischemia? *J Am Coll Cardiol* 1999; 33:90A.
2. Takeshita S, Zheng LP, Brogi E, et al. Therapeutic angiogenesis: a single intra-arterial bolus of vascular endothelial growth factor augments revascularization in a rabbit ischemic hindlimb model. *J Clin Invest* 1994;93: 662–670.
3. Baumgartner I, Pieczek A, Manor O, et al. Constitutive expression of phVEGF$_{165}$ after intramuscular gene transfer promotes collateral vessel development in patients with critical limb ischemia. *Circulation* 1998;97: 1114–1123.
4. Isner J, as presented at Myocardial Reperfusion XII, New Orleans, LA, March 6, 1999.
5. Moulton KS, Heller E, Konerding MA, Palinski W, Folkman J. Angiogenesis inhibitors reduce plaque growth. 1998;98:I–454.
6. Magovern CJ, Mack CA, Zhang J, et al. Direct in vivo gene transfer to canine myocardium using a replication-deficient adenovirus vector. *Ann Thorac Surg* 1996;62: 425–434.
7. Mukherjee D, Bhatt DL, Roe MT, Patel V, Ellis SG. Direct myocardial revascularization and angiogenesis—how many patients might be eligible? *Am J Cardiol* 1999 (accepted).
8. Chiu R C-J, Zibaitis A, Kao RL. Cellular cardiomyoplasty: myocardial regeneration with satellite cell implantation. *Ann Thorac Surg* 1995;60:12–18.
9. Taylor DA, Atkins BZ, Hungspreugs P, et al. Regenerating functional myocardium: improved performance after skeletal myoblast transplantation. *Nat Med* 1998;4: 929–933.
10. Li R-K, Jia Z-Q, Weisel RD, et al. Cardiomyocyte transplantation improves heart function. *Ann Thorac Surg* 1996;62:654–661.

B. Directional Coronary Atherectomy Prior to Stent Implantation: Rationale, Technique, and Long-term Outcome

Issam Moussa, Jeffery Moses, and *Antonio Colombo

*Department of Clinical Research, Interventional Cardiology, Lenox Hill Hospital, New York, New York 10021; *Cardiac Catheterization Laboratory, Centro Cuore Columbus, 20145 Milan, Italy*

Prospective, randomized, clinical trials have demonstrated the superiority of coronary stents in reducing angiographic restenosis and clinical events compared with PTCA in focal *de novo* lesions in native coronary arteries (1–3). However, restenosis remains a problem when stents are implanted in ''complex lesion subsets,'' such as: long lesions (4), ostial lesions (5–7), chronic total occlusions (8–10), and bifurcational lesions (11). Restenosis after implantation of slotted tube stents is mainly due to neointimal proliferation (12). It has been postulated that the degree of neointimal hyperplasia after stenting is proportional to the degree of vessel wall stretch (13). The stretching force needed to expand the vessel is proportionate to the vessel wall resistance manifested by the absolute amount and consistency of the plaque. Therefore, it is logical that the maximal stretching force will need to be applied where the plaque is most severe to achieve an adequate lumen gain. Theoretically, this stretching effect would lead to more propensity for neointimal hyperplasia at the original plaque site. In fact, preliminary experimental data in animal models (14) support this concept. In humans, observational intravascular ultrasound data (15,16) indicate that a larger preintervention plaque burden leads to a higher rate of late lumen loss after stenting. In addition, observational angiographic data (17) indicate that in patients who had stent implantation, restenosis tends to occur at the original lesion site (where the plaque burden is largest). Based on these observations, it may be postulated that the removal of atherosclerotic plaque prior to stenting may lead to a reduction in neointimal hyperplasia, therefore reducing the incidence of restenosis.

The efficacy of interventional devices in excising the atherosclerotic plaque depends primarily on plaque composition (i.e., noncalcified vs. calcified). Directional coronary atherectomy (Devices for Vascular Interventions, Temecula, CA) has been shown to be the most effective device in removing fibrotic noncalcified plaque (18), thus transforming the rigid atherosclerotic arterial wall to a more elastic structure that is amenable for dilatation (19). However, despite the reduction in restenosis with "optimal" directional atherectomy, compared with PTCA, restenosis remains about 30%, with no difference in the need for repeat revascularization at 1-year follow-up (20).

Therefore, the failure of *stand-alone* debulking or *stand-alone* stenting in significantly reducing restenosis in complex lesion subsets and the mechanisms underlying this process, namely pathologic arterial remodeling after debulking (21,22), highlight the need to explore the possible synergistic role of combining both techniques in an attempt to reduce restenosis in these lesion subsets.

THE STENTING AFTER OPTIMAL LESION DEBULKING "SOLD" REGISTRY

To examine the safety and efficacy of directional atherectomy prior to coronary stent implantation, we conducted a prospective registry between February 1996 and January 1998. A total of 128 patients with 168 lesions were enrolled. Patients were enrolled in this registry if they had all of the following: (a) clinical or functional evidence of ischemia; (b) no myocardial infarction within 48 hours; and (c) the culprit lesion was ≥15 mm in length and located in a vessel with a reference diameter ≥2.75 mm by visual estimate. Ostial and bifurcational lesions were considered for enrollment regardless of vessel size and lesion length. Restenotic lesions

and chronic total occlusions were also included. Directional atherectomy was performed using methods previously described (23). The endpoint of the atherectomy procedure was to achieve a <20% residual diameter stenosis by visual estimate. A 7 Fr GTO cutter was used in 96% of lesions, with an average of 14 ± 7 cuts per lesion. Coronary stenting was performed with the goal of achieving a near zero angiographic residual stenosis. Only slotted tube stents were used: The Multilink stent (15 and 25 mm) (Advanced Cardiovascular Systems, Inc., Temecula, CA) was used in 51 lesions (30%); the Palmaz-Schatz stent (Johnson & Johnson Interventional systems, Warren, NJ) in 45 lesions (27%); the NIR stent (16, 19, 25, and 32 mm) (SciMed, Inc., Minneapolis, MN) in 26 lesions (15%); and other slotted tube stents in 46 lesions (28%). The AVE Microstent (18, 24, and 39 mm) (Arterial Vascular Engineering, Santa Rosa, CA) was used in situations in which other stents could not be delivered. Intravascular ultrasound guidance was used in a subset of patients preintervention, after DCA and after stenting. All patients were discharged on aspirin 325 mg once a day and ticlopidine 250 mg twice a day for 2 weeks. Clinical follow-up was obtained in all patients at 1 month and 1 year postprocedure.

Patients' clinical profiles and baseline angiographic characteristics are shown in Table 5.2. Intravascular ultrasound-guided stent implantation was used in 95% of lesions. Stents were expanded using a balloon-to-artery ratio of 1,19 ± 0.16 and an inflation pressure of 16 ± 4 atm. The quantitative angiographic and intravascular ultrasound measurements are shown in Table 5.3. Mean residual percentage plaque area after DCA was 54% ± 14%, but as illustrated in (Fig. 5.6), about 40% of lesions had a residual percentage plaque area greater than 0.60. Clinical success was achieved in 96% of patients. Major procedural and in-hospital complications occurred in four patients (3.2%): emergency bypass surgery in two patients (1.6%), both of whom died during hospitalization; and two other patients (1.6%) had nonfatal Q-wave myocardial infarction. Non–Q-wave myocardial infarction occurred in 17 patients (13.3%). No other events occurred at 1-month follow-up. Angiographic

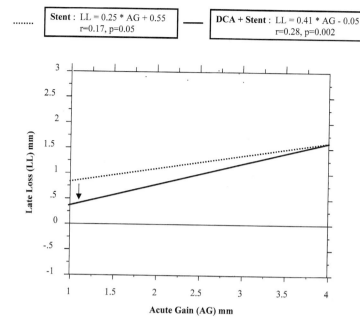

Stent : LL = 0.25 * AG + 0.55 r=0.17, p=0.05

DCA + Stent : LL = 0.41 * AG - 0.05 r=0.28, p=0.002

FIG. 5.9. Shown are simple linear regression lines of late loss (*LL*) against acute gain (*AG*) for the atherectomy stent group (*dotted line*) and the stent alone group (*solid line*). Note the downward shift in the regression line.

tersect when large acute lumen gain is achieved. This may suggest that in vessels where large acute lumen gain can be achieved with stenting alone, such as in large vessels, the addition of DCA might be of less benefit. Alternatively, perhaps more plaque removal in these lesions might have maintained the favorable balance between acute gain and late loss.

The results of this registry are in concordance with several other reports utilizing DCA before stenting in different lesion subsets. Keitz et al. (31) reported on 44 patients treated with directional atherectomy prior to stenting, using the Palmaz-Schatz stent. A total of 51 stents were deployed in 47 vessels. Aortoostial lesions were present in 14 patients (32%). The diameter stenosis increased from 73.6% ± 9.6% at baseline to 30.7% ± 13.6% after DCA, and to −8.2% ± 12.6% after stenting. Bramucci et al. (32) reported on 68 patients (71 lesions) who underwent directional atherectomy prior to elective Palmaz-Schatz stent implantation. This cohort included focal lesions that required a single Palmaz-Schatz stent. At 6-month follow-up, target lesion revascularization was needed in 7% of patients.

WHY DOES PLAQUE REMOVAL PRIOR TO STENT IMPLANTATION REDUCE RESTENOSIS?

It has been demonstrated previously that restenosis after coronary stent implantation is a multifactorial process in which patient, lesion and postprocedural factors (33,34) interact to produce a given outcome. To understand the role of plaque removal in this complex process, we matched for all the clinical, angiographic and procedural factors between the DCA plus stent group and the stent alone group. Despite matching, the postprocedure lumen dimensions were significantly larger in the DCA plus stent group. This is theoretically expected because plaque removal facilitates stent expansion that in turn would translate into larger lumen gain. Restenosis was significantly lower in the DCA plus stent group. The important question that arises concerns whether the lower restenosis rate in the DCA plus stent group is entirely due to the acute lumen gain achieved or whether it is also due to the attenuation of late lumen loss. To answer this, we performed multivariate logistic regression analysis in the group of lesions that had

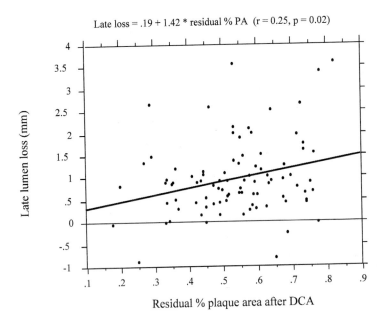

Late loss = .19 + 1.42 * residual % PA (r = 0.25, p = 0.02)

FIG. 5.10. Simple linear regression of late lumen loss after stent placement against residual percentage plaque area after atherectomy. Note that the larger the residual plaque burden before stent implantation, the higher the late lumen loss at follow-up.

IVUS interrogation post-DCA and poststenting and returned for angiographic follow-up (see Table 5.5). In this model, only a lower residual plaque burden after DCA and a larger lumen area after stenting predicted a lower probability of restenosis. Interestingly, the influence of residual plaque burden after DCA (before stent implantation) on the probability of restenosis was more prominent than that of postprocedure lumen CSA. Figure 5.10 further illustrates the linear positive relationship between residual plaque burden after DCA and late lumen loss after stenting. Figure 5.10 illustrates that the larger the residual plaque burden before stent implantation, the higher the degree of late lumen loss, but the degree of this correlation, albeit statistically significant, is weak ($r = .25$). This may be due to two factors: (a) This correlation equation does not account for the other important variables that are known to influence the process of restenosis, such as vessel size, lesion length, stent length, and other patient related factors; and (b) there may be a threshold phenomenon by which plaque removal beyond a certain level ceases to impact late lumen loss in the same magnitude. These findings add further support to the concept that the residual plaque burden

after catheter-based coronary interventions (15,16,35,36) is a risk factor for restenosis. Furthermore, it seems that plaque removal prior to stent implantation does reduce restenosis to a magnitude that is partially dependent on the amount of the plaque removed.

CASE STUDIES

Case 1

A 57-year-old man with a history of HTN was admitted with unstable angina pectoris. Coronary angiography showed a distal left main artery stenosis (Fig. 5.11A). Intravascular ultrasound interrogation showed a fibrotic noncalcified plaque at the lesion site. An intraaortic balloon pump (IABP) was inserted and directional atherectomy performed using a 7 Fr GTO cutter (12 cuts were performed). One 15-mm ACS Multilink stent was implanted, protruding into the LAD artery. A kissing balloon technique was used for final stent expansion: a 4.0-mm balloon inflated to 20 atm in the LM artery and a 3.5-mm balloon inflated to 10 atm toward the LCX artery. The postprocedure angiogram is shown in Fig. 5.11B. The patient received ticlop-

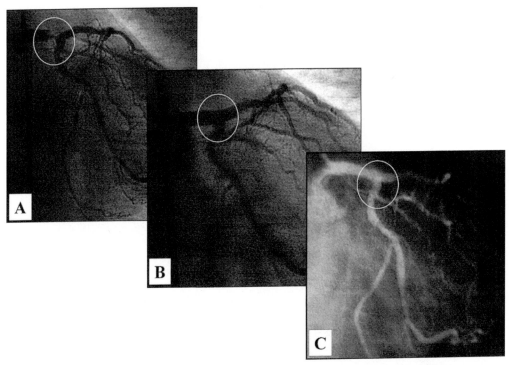

FIG. 5.11. A: Coronary angiogram of the left coronary artery system in the RAO projection shows an unprotected distal left main coronary artery stenosis (*white circle*); reference vessel diameter measured 3.53 mm. **B:** Postprocedure angiogram after directional atherectomy (12 cuts) and implantation of 1 ACS Multilink stent toward the LAD (*white circle*). **C:** Coronary angiogram 5 months postintervention; note the minimal late lumen loss (*white circle*).

idine and aspirin and was discharged after 48 hours, with no in-hospital events. Follow-up angiography was performed at 5 months, demonstrating the absence of restenosis (Fig. 5.11C). Late clinical follow-up was performed at 11 months, and the patient remained free of angina and other cardiac events.

Case 2

A 63-year-old man with a history of HTN, hyperlipidemia admitted with progressive exertional angina. Coronary angiography showed a total occlusion in the proximal segment of the RCA (Fig. 5.12A). After recanalization, severe atherosclerosis appeared to involve a very long segment of the artery (Fig. 5.12B). Directional atherectomy was performed using a 7 Fr GTO cutter (40 cuts were performed); an angiogram after DCA is shown in Fig. 5.12C. Three AVE II 39-mm stents were implanted and expanded, using a 4.0-mm balloon inflated to 20 atm (Fig. 5.12D). The patient was discharged after 24 hours on aspirin and ticlopidine, with no in-hospital events. Follow-up angiography was performed at 5 months (Fig. 5.12E), demonstrating the absence of restenosis. The patient remained free of angina and other cardiac events 10 months postprocedure.

CLINICAL IMPLICATIONS

Directional atherectomy prior to stent implantation is an approach that is based on sound theoretical, experimental, and clinical observations. Preliminary nonrandomized experience has shown the feasibility and favorable long-term outcome of selected patients undergoing this ap-

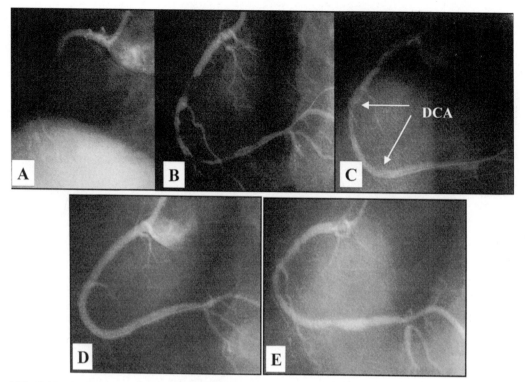

FIG. 5.12. A: Baseline coronary angiography showed a total occlusion in the proximal segment of the RCA. **B:** A coronary angiogram after vessel recanalization. **C:** A coronary angiogram after DCA (40 cuts). **D:** A coronary angiogram after implantation of three AVE II 39-mm stents expanded with a 4.0-mm balloon inflated to 20 atm. **E:** Coronary angiogram at 5-month follow-up.

proach. However, several important issues remain to be addressed: (a) The incidence of non–Q-wave myocardial infarction is increased with directional atherectomy compared with PTCA or stent alone. Despite the controversy concerning the impact of this event on long-term clinical outcome, this remains a limitation that has to be addressed by the utilization of potent antiplatelet agents and/or by the development of new atherectomy devices that produce a lower rate of embolization. (b) Considering the increased procedural time and cost, this approach has to be applied in selected patient subsets in which debulking or stenting as a stand-alone strategy is associated with a high restenosis rate. Randomized clinical trials testing this approach, using the various debulking devices, are in progress. However, until the results of such randomized trials are available, this approach may

serve an important clinical purpose when applied in the following lesion subsets: (a) noncalcified lesions located in vessels >2.75 mm in diameter that require two or more stents, (b) aortoostial lesions, (c) bifurcational lesions, (d) restenotic lesions, and (e) chronic total occlusions that are successfully recanalized through the true lumen.

REFERENCES

1. Serruys P, Jaegere P, Kiemeneij F, et al. A comparison of balloon expandable stent implantation with balloon angioplasty in patients with coronary artery disease. *N Engl J Med* 1994;331:489–495.
2. Fischman DL, Leon MB, Baim D, et al. A randomized comparison of coronary stent placement and balloon angioplasty in the treatment of coronary artery disease. *N Engl J Med* 1994;331:496–501.
3. Macaya C, Serruys PW, Ruygrok P, et al, for the Benestent Study Group. Continued benefit of coronary stent-

ing compared to balloon angioplasty: one year clinical follow-up of the Benestent trial. *J Am Coll Cardiol* 1996; 27:255–261.

4. Itoh A, Hall P, Maiello L, et al. Coronary stenting of long lesions (greater than 20 mm): a matched comparison of different stents. *Circulation* 1995;92[Suppl I]:I-688(abst).

5. Zampieri P, Colombo A, Almagor Y, et al. Results of coronary stenting of ostial lesions. *Am J Cardiol* 1994; 73:901–903.

6. Rocha-Singh K, Morris N, Wong SC, et al. Coronary stenting for treatment of ostial stenoses of native coronary arteries or aorto-coronary saphenous vein grafts. *Am J Cardiol* 1995;75:26–29.

7. Mehran R, Mintz GS, Bucher TA, et al. Aorto-ostial instent restenosis: mechanisms, treatment, and results. A serial quantitative angiographic and intravascular ultrasound study. *Circulation* 1996;94[Suppl I]:I-200.

8. Goldberg SL, Colombo A, Maiello L, et al. Intracoronary stent insertion after balloon angioplasty of chronic total occlusions. *J Am Coll Cardiol* 1995;26:713–719.

9. Sirnes P, Golf S, Myreng Y, et al. Stenting in chronic coronary occlusion (SICCO): a randomized, controlled trial of adding stent implantation after successful angioplasty. *J Am Coll Cardiol* 1996;28:1444–1451.

10. Moussa I, Di Mario C, Moses J, et al. Comparison of angiographic and clinical outcome of coronary stenting of chronic total occlusions versus subtotal occlusions. *Am J Cardiol* 1998;81:1–6.

11. Colombo A, Maiello L, Itoh A, et al. Coronary stenting of bifurcational lesions: immediate and follow-up results. 1996;27[Suppl A]:277A(abst).

12. Hoffmann R, Mintz G, Dussaillant G, et al. Patterns and mechanisms of in-stent restenosis: a serial intravascular ultrasound study. *Circulation* 1996;94:1247–1254.

13. Rogers C, Edelman E. Endovascular stent design dictates experimental restenosis and thrombosis. *Circulation* 1995;91:2195–3001.

14. Carter AJ, Farb A, Laird J, et al. Neointimal formation is dependent on the underlying arterial substrate after coronary stent placement. *J Am Coll Cardiol* 1996; 27(February special issue):320A(abst).

15. Moussa I, Di Mario C, Moses J, et al. The impact of preintervention plaque area as determined by intravascular ultrasound on luminal renarrowing following coronary stenting. *Circulation* 1996;94:1528(abst).

16. Hoffman R, Mintz GS, Mehran R, et al. Intravascular ultrasound predictors of angiographic restenosis in lesions treated with Palmaz-Schatz stents. *J Am Coll Cardiol* 1998;31:43–49.

17. Corvaja N, Moses J, Moussa I, et al. Stent restenosis: where does it occur? An angiographic analysis. *Eur Heart J* 1997;18:P2193.

18. Holmes D, Topol E, Adelman A, Cohen E, Califf R. Randomized trials of directional coronary atherectomy: implications for clinical practice and future investigation. *J Am Coll Cardiol* 1994;24:431–439.

19. Ibrahim A, Kronenberg M, Boor P, et al. Atherectomy and angioplasty improve compliance and reduce thickness of iliac arteries—an in vitro ultrasound study. *Circulation* 1994;90:I-534(abst).

20. Baim DS, Cutlip D, Sharmin SK, et al., for the BOAT investigators. Final results of the Balloon versus Optimal Atherectomy Trial (BOAT). *Circulation* 1998;97: 322–331.

21. Mintz GS, Popma JJ, Hong MK, et al. Intravascular ultrasound to discern device-specific effects and mechanisms of restenosis. *Am J Cardiol* 1996;78[sSuppl 3]: 18–22.

22. de Vrey E, Mintz GS, Kimura T, et al. Arterial remodeling after directional coronary atherectomy: a volumetric analysis from the Serial Ultrasound Restenosis (SURE) Trial. *J Am Coll Cardiol* 1997; (February special issue): 280A(abst).

23. Simonton CA, Leon MB, Baim DS, et al. "Optimal" directional coronary atherectomy: final results of the Optimal Atherectomy Restenosis Study (OARS). *Circulation* 1998;97:332–339.

24. Cutlip DE, Chauhan M, Senerchia C, et al. Influence of myocardial infarction following otherwise successful coronary intervention on late mortality. *Circulation* 1997;96:162(abst).

25. Simoons ML, Harrington R, Anderson KM, et al. Small, non-Q-wave myocardial infarctions during PTCA, are associated with increased 6 months mortality. *Circulation* 1997;96:163(abst).

26. Lefkovits J, Blankenship JC, Anderson KM, et al. Increased risk of non-Q-wave myocardial infarction after directional atherectomy is paletelet dependent: evidence from the EPIC trial. *J Am Coll Cardiol* 1996;28: 849–855.

27. Reimers B, Moussa I, Akiyama T, et al. Long-term clinical follow-up after successful repeat percutaneous intervention for stent restenosis. *J Am Coll Cardiol* 1997; 30:186–192.

28. Christophe B, Banos J, Belle EV, et al. Six-month angiographic outcome after successful repeat percutaneous intervention for in-stent restenosis. *Circulation* 1998; 97:318–321.

29. Mehran R, Hong M, Lansky A, et al. Vessel size and lesion length influence late clinical outcomes after native coronary artery stent placement. *Circulation* 1997; 96:1520(abst).

30. Kornowsky R, Mehran R, Hong M, et al. Procedural results and late clinical outcomes after placement of three or more stents in single coronary lesions. *Circulation* 1998;97:1355–1361.

31. Kiesz R, Rozek MM, Mego DM, et al. Device synergy: directional atherectomy and stenting significantly reduces residual stenosis. *Eur Heart J* 1996;17: P974(abst).

32. Bramucci I, Angoli L, Merlini PA, et al. Acute results of adjunct stents following directional coronary atherectomy. *J Am Coll Cardiol* 1997;29(February): 415A(abst).

33. Kastrati A, Schomig A, Elezi S, et al. Predictive factors of restenosis after coronary stent placement. *J Am Coll Cardiol* 1997;30:1428–1436.

34. Kuntz RE, Safian RD, Joseph P, et al. The importance of acute luminal diameter in determining restenosis after coronary atherectomy or stenting. *Circulation* 1992;86: 1827–1835.

35. Mintz GS, Popma JJ, Pichard AD, et al. Intravascular ultrasound predictors of restenosis after percutaneous transcatheter coronary revascularization. *J Am Coll Cardiol* 1996;27:1678–1687.

36. The GUIDE trial investigator. IVUS-determined predictors of restenosis in PTCA and DCA: final report from the GUIDE trial, phase II. *J Am Coll Cardiol* 1996;29: 156A.

C. Transluminal Extraction Coronary Atherectomy

Mauricio G. Cohen, *Brian H. Annex, and †Michael H. Sketch, Jr.

*Cardiac Catheterization Laboratory, *Department of Medicine, Division of Cardiology, and
†Diagnostic and Interventional Cardiac Catheterization Laboratories, Department of Medicine,
Division of Cardiology, Duke University Medical Center, Durham, North Carolina 27710*

Since the introduction of balloon angioplasty, it has become the preferred strategy for coronary revascularization in certain subsets of patients. Improvements in angioplasty equipment and technique have allowed the operator to approach increasingly complex coronary lesions. Despite these improvements, a 2% to 12% incidence of abrupt closure, a 4% to 10% incidence of myocardial infarction, and a 30% to 45% incidence of restenosis remain the main limitations of this modality of treatment (1–6). Complex lesion morphology and unstable coronary syndromes have been associated with lower procedural success and poorer clinical outcomes (7–10). To improve the safety and efficacy of interventional therapies for the approach of unfavorable coronary anatomy, several alternative devices have been and are being developed. This chapter addresses the current applications and limitations of one of these devices, the transluminal extraction-atherectomy catheter (TEC).

DEVELOPMENT AND MECHANISM OF ACTION

The TEC was developed by the Duke Interventional Cardiac Catheterization Program in conjunction with Interventional Technologies, Inc. (San Diego, CA). The mechanism of this device is a combination of excision and aspiration of atherosclerotic plaque and intraluminal detritus, especially thrombus. In early *in vivo* canine experiments, the catheter showed good trackability through tortuous coronary arteries. None of the treated vessel showed evidence of dissection or perforation. Histologic examination revealed that the excision under the plaque was superficial, with occasional extension into the innermost 25% of the media (11).

In further assessment of the aspiration component of this device, angioscopic studies revealed complete or partial thrombus removal in 75% to 100% of vein graft lesions. In these studies, the TEC was shown to be effective in removing globular thrombus, which is more loosely attached to the wall and protruding into the lumen than is laminar thrombus (12). Despite the reduction in thrombus burden at the treatment site, intraluminal defects and haziness were visualized with coronary angiography in up to 26% of lesions after TEC (13). Angioscopy and intravascular ultrasound revealed that these findings might have corresponded to intimal dissection rather than to intraluminal detritus (12,14,15).

However, the mechanism of TEC remains controversial. Pizzulli et al. (16) examined aspirated blood following a TEC procedure. There was a scarcity of intimal cells and fibrous tissue found in the aspirated blood, leading the authors to interpret that mechanical dilatation (Dotter effect) may be implicated in the mechanism of action of extraction-atherectomy.

DESCRIPTION OF THE DEVICE

The TEC device is a percutaneous over-the-wire, motor-driven system. The components include a catheter, a drive unit, and a battery pack (Fig. 5.13). The shaft of the catheter is a hollow torque tube with a conical tip that has two stainless steel blades with adjacent windows (Fig. 5.14). The drive unit consists of a motor that rotates the catheter at 750 rpm when activated by a trigger. A thumb lever on the top of the unit is used to control the advancement of the cutter over the target lesion. A glass vacuum

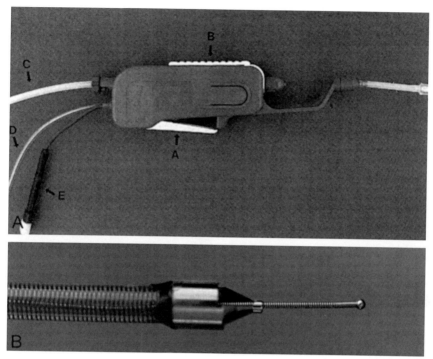

FIG. 5.13. A: The transluminal extraction-endarterectomy catheter (TEC) drive unit. *A*, trigger; *B*, advancement control lever; *C*, rear extension tubing; *D*, suction tubing; *E*, power connector. **B:** A close-up of the cutter head and torque tube of the TEC catheter over a 0.014-in. TEC guidewire. (From Sketch MH, Phillips HP, Lee M, Stack RS. Coronary transluminal extraction-endarterectomy. *J Invest Cardiol* 1991;3:23–28, with permission.)

bottle attaches to the drive unit and provides 1 atm of negative pressure for aspiration of the excised material. The battery pack, composed of eight energy cells, is plugged into the drive unit.

The system is advanced over a special 0.014-in. guidewire made of stainless steel. The stiffness of the shaft of the wire provides support for the rotation of the catheter and straightens

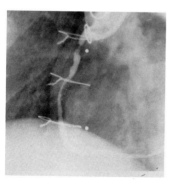
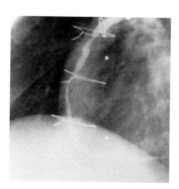
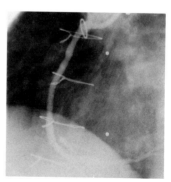

A,B

C

FIG. 5.14. A: Angiogram demonstrating a 95% diffuse stenosis in the proximal body of a saphenous vein graft to the distal portion of the right coronary artery. **B:** Repeat angiogram showing the interval result after three passes with a 7 Fr TEC cutter. **C:** Final result obtained after adjunctive stenting with three 15-mm Palmaz biliary stents deployed with a 4.0-mm balloon.

the artery for coaxial cutting in order to avoid vessel perforation. It has a floppy tip and a terminal 0.020-in. ball to prevent advancement of the cutter beyond the tip of the wire. When the cutter is advanced over the wire, the trigger at the drive unit activates the motor and the suction simultaneously. The blades excise the plaque and the debris is aspirated through the catheter to the vacuum bottle.

TEC PROCEDURE

During the 24 to 48 hours prior to the procedure, all patients should be treated with a 325 mg dose of aspirin and 250 mg of ticlopidine twice daily or clopidigrel in anticipation of possible stent deployment (17). After femoral access is obtained, a bolus of 100 U per kilogram of body weight of intravenous heparin is administered, with additional boluses as needed, to achieve and maintain an activated clotting time (ACT) between 300 and 350 seconds. If the patient receives abciximab, the dose of heparin should be lowered to 70 U per kilogram of body weight to obtain an ACT greater than 200 seconds (18).

The procedure is performed via a percutaneous transfemoral technique, as with conventional angioplasty. A 10 Fr arterial sheath is placed to allow the insertion of a 10 Fr guide catheter, preferably with side-holes. Several configurations of guide catheters are available: JL, JR, multipurpose, modified Amplatz, left Amplatz, right bypass graft, and hockey stick. To avoid traumatizing the wall of the aorta and to reduce blood loss, either this large guiding catheter is advanced over a 0.063-in. J-wire, or a 6 Fr multipurpose catheter is advanced over a 0.035-in. J-tipped guidewire. Because these guiding catheters are stiffer, deep seating and overrotation must be avoided to reduce the risk of vessel injury. A special rotating, dual hemostatic valve is attached to the back of the catheter. Once the ostium is engaged, intracoronary nitroglycerin (100 to 200 g) is administered to minimize coronary spasm.

The lesion can be crossed directly with the TEC wire. In the presence of tortuous anatomy, any 300-cm angioplasty guidewire can be used, and once across the lesion, it can be exchanged for the TEC wire by using an end-hole catheter. The tip of the wire should be placed as far distal as possible to ensure cutting over the stiff radiolucent portion.

The cutter size is selected according to the reference diameter of the target vessel. Several sizes, from 5.5 to 7.5 Fr (1.8 to 2.50 mm), are available. In general, a cutter diameter undersized at least 1 mm in relation to the reference vessel diameter is preferred. Smaller cutters should be employed in tortuous vessels to prevent perforation. In thrombus-laden lesions, a larger cutter (i.e., 7.0 or 7.5 Fr) is initially selected to facilitate clot aspiration. In severely stenotic lesions, a smaller cutter is initially utilized, with progression to larger cutters, as necessary, to maximize resection of the lesion.

The TEC device is assembled and the motor drive tested on the table. Care must be taken to introduce the back end of the wire through the central bushing of the cutter and not through the adjacent windows. The cutter is then advanced under fluoroscopic guidance and positioned 1 to 2 cm proximal to the target lesion. A lactated Ringer's solution is infused under pressure through the guide catheter during periods of cutter activation to create a particulate slurry, facilitating aspiration of the excised material. The cutter is activated to a platform speed and then advanced very slowly across the lesion. Activation of the cutter in the lesion must be avoided, as it may increase the risk of dissection and embolization. The blood flow into the vacuum bottle must be monitored before and during advancement of the cutter. Usually, three to five passes with the device across the lesion are necessary to achieve the desired result. After use of the TEC, adjunctive therapies can include balloon angioplasty and/or stenting.

PATIENT SELECTION AND CONTRAINDICATIONS

A unique feature of this device is aspiration of intraluminal debris. The main niche application for TEC appears to be the treatment of diffusely diseased, degenerated saphenous vein by-

TABLE 5.6. *Contraindications for TEC*

Total occlusions unable to be crossed with a wire
Heavily calcified lesions
Severe coronary ectasia
Severe eccentricity or angulation of the target lesion
Tortuous anatomy proximal to the target lesion
Evidence of dissection
Severe peripheral vascular disease

pass grafts and lesions in native coronary vessels with angiographic or clinically suspected thrombus. As new technology evolves and clinical randomized data become available, the indications and contraindications for TEC must be reassessed.

The general contraindications are depicted in Table 5.6. Proximal tortuosity can impede the advancement of the cutter. Severely calcified lesions are resistant to excision and can restrict the progression of the catheter. Angulated, eccentric, and dissected lesions are at a higher risk of perforation. Because larger sheath and guide catheter sizes are required for extraction-atherectomy, peripheral artery disease may imply an increased risk for the patient. These criteria are in constant evolution as experience with this device grows.

CLINICAL EXPERIENCE

The US TEC Registry, the NACI Registry, and the William Beaumont Hospital study report the initial clinical experience with TEC and represent the largest series of extraction-atherectomy for coronary artery disease (19–22). These three studies completed enrollment before coronary stents and glycoprotein IIb/IIIa inhibitors became widely available. The data from these studies are presented in Tables 5.7 through 5.10. In addition, several smaller studies have been reported (15,23–26). The high proportion (45% to 73%) of vein graft interventions in these studies reflects a physician preference to treat vein graft lesions with this device. In contrast, the National Heart, Lung and Blood Multicenter PTCA Registry had only 4% saphenous vein graft interventions (27). Results in native coronaries and vein grafts were analyzed separately in the three studies.

Vein Graft Cohorts: Acute Outcome

The baseline characteristics for the vein graft cohorts in all three studies were similar (see Table 5.7). The majority of patients were men, with a mean age of 65 to 67 years. As expected, multivessel disease was present in 87% to 92%. The mean ejection fraction was 47%, and a myocardial infarction was the admission diagnosis in 14% of the cases. The mean graft age was 8.3 years. Thrombus, at the treatment site, was present in 28% to 43%.

Procedural success was achieved in 89% to 93% of the patients (see Table 5.8) with a high rate of adjunctive angioplasty (74% to 91%). Major in-hospital complications included death in 2% to 5.3%, emergency bypass surgery in 0.4% to 0.7%, and periprocedural myocardial

TABLE 5.7. *Baseline characteristics of vein graft cohorts*

	US TEC Registry (n = 538)	NACI Registry (n = 243)	Beaumont Study (n = 146)
Age (mean yrs)	65	66.6	65
Male gender	81.8%	77.8%	78.0%
Diabetes	N/A	29.6%	N/A
Multivessel disease	89.4%	92.2%	86.8%
Prior myocardial infarction	49.8%	65%	N/A
Prior PTCA	30.5%	30.5%	22%
Unstable angina	43.5%	66.3%	45%
Congestive heart failure	13.2%	17.4%	N/A
Myocardial infarction on admission	13.8%	14.4%	N/A
Ejection fraction	47%	47.7%	47%
Graft age (mean yrs)	8.3	8.3	8.3

PTCA, percutaneous transluminal angioplasty; CABG, coronary artery bypass surgery; N/A, not applicable.

TABLE 5.8. *Procedural outcomes and in-hospital complications of the vein graft cohorts*

	US TEC Registry (n = 538)	NACI Registry (n = 243)	Beaumont Study (n = 146)
Procedural success	89%	85.5%	93%
TEC alone success	75%	50.2%	39.2%
Adjunctive PTCA	74%	87%	91.2%
Distal embolization persisting after PTCA	8%	3.7%	3.2%
Complications			
• Death	3.2%	5.3%	2.0%
• Emergency CABG	0.4%	0.4%	0.7%
• Periprocedural MI	0.7%	1.6%	4.7%
• Combined MACE	4.3%	6.2%	N/A

TEC, transluminal extraction-atherectomy catheter; PTCA, percutaneous transluminal angioplasty; CABG, coronary artery bypass surgery; MI, myocardial infarction; MACE, major adverse cardiac events; N/A, not applicable.

infarction in 0.7% to 4.7% (see Table 5.8). Distal embolization was apparent after TEC in 6.8% to 11.3% of procedures, and persisted at the completion of the case in 3.2% to 8.0%.

Predictors of adverse outcome were examined in all three series. In the NACI Registry, vein graft cohort, thrombus, calcium, and baseline minimal luminal diameter were angiographic predictors of in-hospital complications (20). Coronary embolization resulting in myocardial infarction occurred more frequently when thrombus was present at the site of the treated lesion (28). In the Beaumont study, univariate analysis showed that midbody location, *de novo* lesion, and the presence of thrombus were associated with higher angiographic complications, but none of these variables were significant in the multivariate analysis. The occurrence of no-reflow, distal embolization, and abrupt closure immediately after TEC, were the strongest independent predictors for clinical complications (22). Extraction-atherectomy as a stand-alone treatment for vein graft lesions correlated with a higher rate of complications in the US TEC registry (OR = 2.5, 95% CI = 1.8 to 3.1), highlighting the need for adjunctive therapy (29).

In addition to these large studies, two small retrospective studies showed increased complications associated with the presence of thrombus at the target lesion. In one of these studies that analyzed the outcome of 65 consecutive patients treated with TEC, distal embolization occurred in 12.8% of patients and resulted in a higher incidence of postprocedural adverse events.

Thrombus at the target lesion was more frequent in those patients with distal emboli (82% vs. 40%, $p = .02$) (24). Dooris et al. (13) reported the results of extraction-atherectomy in lesions with and without thrombus. A total of 183 lesions were treated in 175 consecutive patients. Angiographic evidence of thrombus was present at the treatment site in 32% of lesions. After TEC followed by adjunctive angioplasty, thrombus was removed in 74% of these lesions. Clinical success rates were higher among patients without thrombus (88% vs. 69%, $p < .01$). Unlike other studies, distal embolization and abrupt closure occurred equally often in lesions with and without thrombus; however, combined adverse events (death, coronary bypass surgery, and Q-wave myocardial infarction) were more frequent in the group of patients with thrombus (13.3% vs. 2.4%, $p < .01$) (13).

Native Cohorts: Acute Outcome

In contrast to the vein graft cohorts, patients in the native cohorts were younger and had a lower percentage of men. As expected, fewer patients had multivessel disease. Myocardial infarction precipitated the hospitalization in 18% of the cases. The mean ejection fraction was slightly higher, and only 12% to 24% had a prior bypass surgery (ee Table 5.9). Thrombus at the target lesion was identified in 5% to 24% (20,21,30).

Despite a more favorable risk factor profile, procedural results and clinical outcomes were

TABLE 5.9. *Baseline characteristics of the native cohorts*

	US TEC Registry (n = 609)	NACI Registry (n = 93)	Beaumont Study (n = 175)
Age (mean yrs)	60	61.7	61
Male gender	76%	64.8%	69.7%
Diabetes	N/A	22.7%	N/A
Multivessel disease	46%	55.7%	28%
Prior myocardial infarction	18%	58%	N/A
Prior PTCA	N/A	38.6%	44%
Prior CABG	12%	12.5%	24%
Unstable angina	41%	44.3%	30%
Congestive heart failure	7%	9.1%	N/A
Myocardial infarction on admission	18%	18.2%	N/A
Ejection fraction	N/A	54.2%	52%

PTCA, percutaneous transluminal angioplasty; CABG, coronary artery bypass surgery; N/A, not applicable.

somewhat worse in the native cohort. Procedural success was accomplished in 79% to 89% with a 79% to 92% use of adjunctive angioplasty. Overall, a trend toward increased major complications was observed in the native cohorts. In-hospital mortality was 2.0% to 5.3%. Myocardial infarction occurred in 1.1% to 3.4%, and emergency bypass surgery was performed in 2.8% to 3.6% (see Table 5.10). Distal embolization after TEC occurred in very few cases (0.0% to 0.5%) and persisted at the termination of the procedure in 0.0% to 2.6%.

In the Beaumont study, advanced age, treatment of an ulcerated lesion, and abrupt closure after TEC were independent correlates of major in-hospital complications (21). An analysis of the US TEC registry showed that atherectomy of a native vessel was an independent predictor of complications (29).

Randomized Studies

The TOPIT study (TEC or PTCA in Thrombus) is the only randomized study that compared balloon angioplasty versus extraction-atherectomy in native coronary vessels (31,32). A total of 250 patients were enrolled, and 115 patients were randomized to TEC. The principal clinical indications for enrollment included primary reperfusion for myocardial infarction, unstable angina, postinfarction angina, and failed thrombolytic therapy. Baseline and angiographic characteristics were similar in both groups. Thrombus was present at the target lesion in 52% of cases. Procedural success rates were 98% and 97%, respectively, for TEC and angioplasty. Adjuvant therapies included stenting (26% for TEC; 25.2% for PTCA) and abciximab (1.8% for TEC; 6% for PTCA). There was a

TABLE 5.10. *Procedural outcomes and in-hospital complications of the native cohorts*

	US TEC Registry (n = 609)	NACI Registry (n = 93)	Beaumont Study (n = 175)
Procedural success	89%	78.60%	84%
TEC alone success	N/A	40.50%	29%
Adjunctive PTCA	78.48%	92%	84%
Distal embolization persisting after PTCA	1.20%	2.60%	0%
Complications			
• Death	1.60%	1.10%	2.30%
• Emergency CABG	3.60%	0%	2.80%
• Periprocedural MI	1.10%	1.10%	3.40%
• Combined MACE	N/A	2.30%	6.40%

TEC, transluminal extraction-atherectomy catheter; PTCA, percutaneous transluminal angioplasty; CABG, coronary artery bypass surgery; MI, myocardial infarction; MACE, major adverse cardiac events; N/A, not applicable.

TABLE 5.11. *In-hospital events in the TOPIT study*

	TEC (n = 115)	PTCA (n = 135)	p Value
Death	1 (0.87%)	0	NS
CABG	1 (0.87%)	1 (0.87%)	NS
PTCA	5 (4.35%)	5 (3.70%)	NS
Threefold CPK elevation	1.63%	5.69%	.082

PTCA, percutaneous transluminal angioplasty; CABG, coronary artery bypass surgery; CPK, creatine-phosphokinase; NS, not significant.

trend toward a higher number of patients with a threefold increase in postprocedural cardiac enzymes in the PTCA group (5.7% vs.1.6%, p = .08). There were no statistically significant differences in the occurrence of major in-hospital cardiac adverse events between treatment groups (Table 5.11).

Angiographic Follow-Up

For patients undergoing extraction-atherectomy in native vessels, the US TEC registry and the Beaumont study obtained 6-month angiographic follow-up in 73% and 83%, respectively (Table 5.12). Angiographic restenosis, defined as diameter narrowing >50%, was found in 51% and 61% of patients, respectively. For the vein graft cohorts, follow-up catheterization was available in 65% of patients in the US TEC registry and 80% of patients in Beaumont study. Restenosis occurred in 60% and 69% of patients, respectively (19,21,22). A multivariate analysis of the US TEC registry identified that increased lesion complexity, with calcification or ulceration, independently correlated with a higher rate of restenosis after extraction-atherectomy (33).

TABLE 5.12. *Angiographic follow-up*

	US TEC Registry (%)	Beaumont Study (%)
Native Cohort		
Angiographic 6-mo follow-up	73	83
Restenosis	51	61
Vein Graft Cohort		
Angiographic 6-mo follow-up	65	80
Restenosis	60	69

The Duke Multicenter Coronary TEC registry provided additional information on restenosis. The study enrolled 313 patients between July 1988 and April 1991 in five centers. Angiographic follow-up at 6 months was achieved for 84% of all eligible patients. Using the same definition as other studies, the restenosis rate was 45%, and this frequency was similar for native vessels and saphenous vein grafts. A subgroup analysis revealed a restenosis rate of only 18% in native vessels when TEC alone was performed and the postprocedural narrowing was less than 25% (34). These findings are in accordance with the concept that the incidence of restenosis is inversely proportional to the acute luminal gain at the time of the procedure.

Ishizaka et al. (26) examined the angiographic evolution of 25 patients undergoing extraction-atherectomy with adjunctive balloon angioplasty. Follow-up coronary angiograms at 1 day and 3 months were obtained. Those patients without evidence of early restenosis at 3 months underwent a 6-month catheterization. Early and late restenosis occurred in 35% and 19%, respectively. Lesions that had increased the percentage diameter stenosis on day 1 were more likely to develop early restenosis. These results suggest that elastic recoil contributes significantly to restenosis after TEC. Tissue proliferation may contribute to a lesser degree and may be responsible for late restenosis. A lower reference diameter of the intervened vessel was identified as another predictor of restenosis (26).

Clinical Follow-Up

For the native cohorts, the Beaumont study obtained 6-month clinical follow-up in 92% patients. Adverse events included death in 1.9%, myocardial infarction in 1.3%, repeat percutaneous target lesion intervention in 13.5%, and bypass surgery in 11.8%. Combined major adverse cardiac events at 6 months occurred in 28.5% patients (21). The NACI registry followed 97% of the patients for 1 year. At the end of this period, death occurred in 4.5%, myocardial infarction in 9.1%, and percutaneous target lesion revascularization in 10.2%. Death, Q-wave

TABLE 5.13. *Clinical follow-up of the native cohorts at 6 months*

	NACI Registry (n = 87)	Beaumont Study (n = 153)
% Follow-up	98.9%	92%
Death	4.5%	1.9%
Q-wave myocardial infarction	2.3%	1.3%
Target lesion revascularization	8%	13.5%
Coronary bypass surgery	21.6%	11.8%

myocardial infarction, or revascularization occurred in 41% of patients (Table 5.13) (20).

In the vein graft cohort, 6-month clinical follow-up was complete in 92% of patients in the Beaumont study. Major adverse events included death in 7%, Q-wave myocardial infarction in 4%, repeat percutaneous intervention in 26%, and bypass surgery in 5%. The rate of combined events was 42% (22). In the NACI registry, adverse events at 1 year (92.2% complete follow-up) included death in 15.6%, myocardial infarction in 11.9%, percutaneous target vessel revascularization in 37.9%, and bypass surgery in 10.3%. One of these cardiac adverse events occurred in 51% patients (20) (Table 5.14).

Extraction-Atherectomy and Stenting

Coronary stenting has become a mainstay in the management of acute angioplasty complications and the prevention of elastic recoil with a consequent reduction of restenosis (35,36). In a randomized trial, stent placement for selected patients with vein graft disease had a higher success rate and showed a trend toward fewer post-

TABLE 5.14. *Clinical follow-up of the vein graft cohorts at 6 months*

	NACI Registry (n = 238)	Beaumont Study (n = 118)
% Follow-up	97.9%	92%
Death	10.3%	7%
Q-wave myocardial infarction	3.3%	4%
Target lesion revascularization	7%	26%
Coronary bypass surgery	8.2%	5%

procedural myocardial infarctions; however, the restenosis rate did not differ between groups (37). A combined strategy of thrombus removal with extraction-atherectomy followed by immediate stenting represents an attractive approach for atherosclerotic lesions in degenerated saphenous vein grafts.

Braden et al. (38) reported the experience of extraction-atherectomy in vein grafts followed by deployment of Palmaz-Schatz stents in 49 consecutive patients. The combined TEC–stent approach was successful in 52 (98%) of 53 saphenous vein grafts, with evidence of distal embolization in one case. Average cutter size was 2.2 mm, and 1.7 stents were deployed per lesion. In-hospital major events reported were death in 6% and non–Q-wave myocardial infarction in 4%. At a mean follow-up of 13 months, death occurred in 11% of patients, target vessel revascularization rate in 11%, and nonfatal myocardial infarction in 9%. The combined event rate was 28%, which appears favorable in this complex patient cohort (38).

Another study reported the use of the TEC–stent approach for the treatment of vein graft lesions in 36 patients with a high rate of procedural success (100%) in high-risk lesions. An increased rate (15.6%) of subsequent non–Q-wave myocardial infarction was reported (39).

TEC-BEST II is an ongoing multicenter randomized study comparing the effectiveness of extraction-atherectomy followed by stenting versus the more common approach of balloon angioplasty and stenting for vein graft lesions with length equal to or less than 30 mm without thrombus. Another arm of the trial is also evaluating the performance of TEC–stent with and without adjunctive abciximab for vein graft lesions more than 30mm long with visible thrombus. It is expected that this trial will provide definitive answers for the role of extraction-atherectomy in the management of high-risk vein graft anatomy.

Transluminal Extraction Catheter in Acute Myocardial Infarction

The role of percutaneous interventions in the acute management of myocardial infarction is well established. Several randomized studies have shown that balloon angioplasty is an effective and safe strategy for acute coronary flow restoration. Compared with thrombolytics, primary angioplasty was associated with better clinical outcomes at 30 days (40). Recently published data suggest that primary stenting constitutes another safe and effective percutaneous approach for acute myocardial infarction (41). In selected patients, the use of primary stenting resulted in a lower incidence of recurrent infarction and reduced need for repeat revascularization compared with balloon angioplasty (42).

Kaplan et al. (43) reported the application of TEC in 100 patients with acute coronary syndromes, including primary reperfusion for acute myocardial infarction in 32% of cases, postinfarct angina in 28% of cases, thrombolytic failure in 40% of cases, and cardiogenic shock in 11% of cases (43). Thrombus at the target lesion was visualized in 66%, and in 65% the flow in the culprit vessel was TIMI 0 or 1. The target lesion was located in a vein graft in 29% cases. Overall procedural success was achieved in 94% of patients. Distal embolization, no reflow, or both occurred in 6% of patients. The use of adjunctive angioplasty substantially improved the residual stenosis after TEC from 56% to 28% ($p < .001$), and the TIMI 2 or 3 flow after TEC from 89% to 96%. The in-hospital mortality was 5%, with three of the five deaths occurring in patients who initially presented with cardiogenic shock. A repeat percutaneous intervention was needed in 2% of cases. A predischarge catheterization, performed in 78% of patients, showed a 95% patency rate in the infarct vessel, with a 93% rate of TIMI 3 flow. The results of this nonrandomized study suggest that atherectomy may have a role in a high-risk population with acute coronary syndromes.

POTENTIAL CLINICAL APPLICATIONS

Saphenous Vein Bypass Grafts

Coronary artery bypass surgery is one of the most important advances in the treatment of coronary artery disease. Despite the long-term survival benefit provided by surgical revasculariza-

tion, the accelerated atherosclerosis that develops in vein grafts leads to symptom recurrence and the need for repeat revascularization in a significant proportion of patients. As compared with the initial surgery, reoperation entails increased mortality, a higher incidence of perioperative myocardial infarction, and reduced relief of angina. The rate of vein graft attrition has been reported to be 15% to 20% during the first year after surgery, 1% to 2% per year between 1 and 6 years after surgery, and 4% per year between 6 and 10 years after surgery. Therefore, graft patency is only 60% after 10 years of surgery (44).

Even though percutaneous revascularization procedures constitute an appealing alternative to repeat surgery, a greater incidence of thrombotic complications and embolization may occur, with a consequent effect on procedural outcomes. In a review of balloon angioplasty for vein grafts, de Feyter et al. (44) reported a combined overall success rate of 88% and a 6-month restenosis rate of 42% for selected patients in which high-risk lesions were likely to be excluded. Factors associated with unfavorable results included age of the graft (older than 4 to 6 years), total occlusion, diffuse disease, and the presence of thrombus. In the CAVEAT II trial (45), which compared balloon angioplasty with directional atherectomy for vein grafts, distal embolization occurred in approximately 10% of patients and strongly correlated with increased rates of death and myocardial infarction. The multivariate analysis showed that the presence of thrombus was an independent predictor of distal embolization (45).

The relationship between cardiac enzyme elevation and procedural complications has been described. The variables associated with CK and CK-MB enzyme release after an intervention included coronary embolism, a history of recent myocardial infarction, hemodynamic instability, transient abrupt closure, side-branch occlusion, vein graft procedures, complex lesions, higher residual stenoses, large dissections, and more severe preprocedural stenoses. These investigators found a relationship between a twofold to fivefold increase in CK-MB and the risk of death over a period of 36 months (46). The rates of

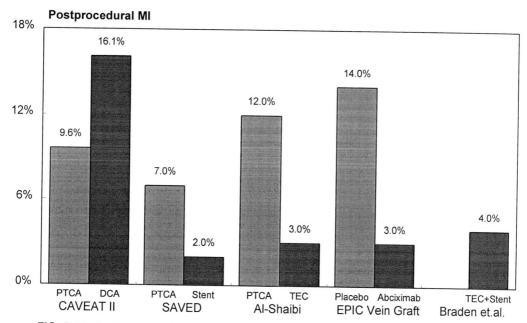

FIG. 5.15. Postprocedural non–Q-wave myocardial infarction in vein graft interventions.

non–Q-wave myocardial infarction in several vein graft intervention trials are outlined in Fig. 5.15.

Because of the potential of preventing distal embolization through aspiration of intraluminal thrombus, extraction-atherectomy constitutes an attractive method for the treatment of high-risk lesions in vein grafts. A retrospective study (25) showed a decrease in distal embolization with extraction-atherectomy compared with balloon angioplasty for vein grafts. This study compared the outcomes in 103 patients who underwent TEC with those of 60 patients who underwent balloon angioplasty. Treatment was assigned at the discretion of the operator. The characteristics of the lesions were similar in both groups, except for thrombus, which was more frequently visualized in lesions treated with atherectomy (52% vs. 36%, $p = .05$). Adjunctive angioplasty was used in 78% of TEC procedures. An overall lower incidence of distal embolization was reported in patients treated with extraction-atherectomy (3.9% vs. 16.7%, $p = .005$). When thrombus was present at the lesion, this difference was even greater (5.6% vs. 31.8%, $p = .002$) (25).

Al-Shaibi et al. (47) compared the postprocedural release of cardiac enzymes between TEC and balloon angioplasty in 124 consecutive patients. The results favored TEC, showing a reduction in total CK elevation of more than twice the normal value (3% vs. 12%, $p < .02$) and CK-MB (7% vs. 22%, $p < .02$) after the procedure.

Several studies have shown a substantial benefit of antiplatelet agents for those patients undergoing interventions in native vessels. It seems that this benefit has not been fully established for vein graft interventions. A subanalysis of 101 vein graft interventions from the EPIC study showed a reduced occurrence of distal embolization in patients treated with abciximab compared with those receiving placebo (3% vs. 21%, $p = .037$) (48). However, the lower rate of distal embolization did not translate into significant differences in the incidence of death, nonfatal myocardial infarction, and repeat urgent revascularization at 30 days and 6 months. A pooled analysis of vein graft interventions from the EPIC and EPILOG trials showed a combined adverse event rate of 11.9% in 59 patients that received placebo and 10.4% in 87 patients treated with a bolus plus infusion of abciximab. This difference was not statistically significant (49).

In most of the registries and retrospective studies, extraction-atherectomy was performed in high-risk patient cohorts based on the expected benefit of thrombus aspiration. This selection bias may account for the high rate of procedural complications and restenosis reported in these studies. The lower success rate after TEC as a sole therapy emphasizes the need for adjunctive balloon angioplasty. Additional therapies, such as stenting and glycoprotein IIb/IIIa inhibitors, constitute appealing strategies that may further reduce the incidence of restenosis and distal embolization when treating this problematic subset of patients. Unfortunately, due to the lack of prospectively randomized studies, the definitive role of TEC in vein graft lesions has not been completely assessed, and the results of an ongoing randomized trial are awaited. Based on operator experience, the main niche for this device appears to be the treatment of diffusely diseased, degenerated vein grafts containing thrombus. A combined approach of atherectomy immediately followed by stenting may reduce the incidence of distal embolization and achieve a larger residual diameter.

Native Coronaries

Even though the majority of interventionalists use TEC to extract thrombus from complex lesions in degenerated vein grafts, the only randomized study available has been performed in native vessels with complex lesion morphology. As previously discussed, the major finding of this study was a trend toward lower cardiac enzyme release after extraction-atherectomy (31). Whether this difference translates into a better long-term outcome is unknown. In previous nonrandomized studies, TEC in native vessels correlated with a higher incidence of major complications (29). The exact role of TEC in native arteries is unknown but appears to be limited primarily to thrombus extraction.

REFERENCES

1. Cowley M, Dorros G, Kelsey S, Raden KV, Detre K. Nonoperative dilatation of coronary artery stenosis: per-cutaneous transluminal coronary angioplasty. *Am J Cardiol* 1984;53:12C–16C.
2. Simpferdorfer C, Belardi J, Bellamy G, Galen K, Franco I, Hollman J. Frequency, management and follow-up of patients with acute coronary occlusion after percutaneous transluminal angioplasty. *Am J Cardiol* 1987;59:267–269.
3. McBride W, Lange R, Hillis D. Restenosis after successful coronary angioplasty: pathology and prevention. *N Engl J Med* 1988;318:1734–1737.
4. Roubin G, King S, Douglas JD Jr. Restenosis after percutaneous transluminal coronary angioplasty: the Emory University Hospital experience. *Am J Cardiol* 1987;60:39B–43B.
5. Tcheng JE, Fortin D, Frid D, et al. Conditional probabilities of restenosis following coronary angioplasty. *Circulation* 1990;82:III-1.
6. Blackshear J, O'Callaghan W, Califf R. Medical approaches to prevention of restenosis after coronary angioplasty. *J Am Coll Cardiol* 1987;59:267–269.
7. Breadlau C, Roubin G, Leimgruber P, et al. In-hospital morbidity and mortality in patients undergoing elective coronary angioplasty. *Circulation* 1985;72:1044–1052.
8. Ellis S, Roubin G, King SI, et al. Angiographic and clinical predictors of acute closure after native vessel angioplasty. *Circulation* 1988;77:372–379.
9. Ellis S, Vandermael M, Cowley M, et al. Coronary morphologic and clinical determinants of procedural outcome with angioplasty for multivessel coronary disease: implications for patient selection. Multivessel Angioplasty Prognosis Study Group. *Circulation* 1990;82:1193–1202.
10. Savage M, Goldberg S, Hirshfeld J, et al. Clinical and angiographic determinants of primary coronary angioplasty success: M-HEART Investigators. *J Am Coll Cardiol* 1991;17:22–28.
11. Stack R, Califf R, Phillips HR, et al. Advances in cardiovascular technologies: interventional cardiac catheterization at Duke Medical Center. *Am J Cardiol* 1988;62:1F–44F.
12. Annex BH, Larkin TJ, O'Neill WW, Safian RD. Evaluation of thrombus removal by transluminal extraction coronary atherectomy by percutaneous coronary angioscopy. *Am J Cardiol* 1994;74:606–609.
13. Dooris M, Hoffmann M, Glazier S, et al. Comparative results of transluminal extraction coronary atherectomy in saphenous vein graft lesions with and without thrombus. *J Am Coll Cardiol* 1995;25:1700–1705.
14. Kaplan BM, Safian RD, Grines CL, et al. Usefulness of adjunctive angioscopy and extraction atherectomy before stent implantation in high-risk aortocoronary saphenous vein grafts. *Am J Cardiol* 1995;76:822–824.
15. Popma JJ, Leon MB, Mintz GS, et al. Results of coronary angioplasty using the transluminal extraction catheter. *Am J Cardiol* 1992;70:1526–1532.
16. Pizzulli L, Manz M, Lüderitz B. Dotter effect rather than tissue removal as major dilatation mechanism of transluminal extraction atherectomy (TEC). *Circulation* 1992;86:I-780(abst).
17. Leon MB, Baim DS, Popma JJ, et al. A clinical trial comparing three antithrombotic-drug regimens after coronary-artery stenting. *N Engl J Med* 1998;339:1665–1671.
18. The EPILOG Investigators. Platelet glycoprotein IIb/IIIa receptor blockade and low-dose heparin during per-

cutaneous coronary revascularization. *N Engl J Med* 1997;336:1689–1696.

19. Meany TB, Leon MB, Kramer BL, et al. Transluminal extraction catheter for the treatment of diseased saphenous vein grafts: a multicenter experience. *Cathet Cardiovasc Diagn* 1995;34:112–120.

20. Sketch MH Jr, Davidson CJ, Yeh W, et al. Predictors of acute and long-term outcome with transluminal extraction atherectomy: the New Approaches to Coronary Intervention (NACI) Registry. *Am J Cardiol* 1997;80: 68K–77K.

21. Safian RD, May MA, Lichtenberg A, et al. Detailed clinical and angiographic analysis of transluminal extraction coronary atherectomy for complex lesions in native coronary arteries. *J Am Coll Cardiol* 1995;25: 848–854.

22. Safian RD, Grines CL, May MA, et al. Clinical and angiographic results of transluminal extraction coronary atherectomy in saphenous vein bypass grafts. *Circulation* 1994;89:302–312.

23. Twidale N, Barth CWD, Kipperman RM, Bowles MH, Galichia JP. Acute results and long-term outcome of transluminal extraction catheter atherectomy for saphenous vein graft stenoses. *Cathet Cardiovasc Diagn* 1994;31:187–191.

24. Hong MK, Popma JJ, Pichard AD, et al. Clinical significance of distal embolization after transluminal extraction atherectomy in diffusely diseased saphenous vein grafts. *Am Heart J* 1994;127:1496–1503.

25. Misumi K, Matthews RV, Sun GW, Mayeda G, Burstein S, Shook TL. Reduced distal embolization with transluminal extraction atherectomy compared to balloon angioplasty for saphenous vein graft disease. *Cathet Cardiovasc Diagn* 1996;39:246–251.

26. Ishizaka N, Ikari Y, Hara K, et al. Angiographic follow-up of patients after transluminal coronary extraction atherectomy. *Am Heart J* 1994;128:691–696.

27. Holmes DR Jr, Holubkov R, Vlietstra RE, et al. Comparison of complications during percutaneous transluminal coronary angioplasty from 1977 to 1981 and from 1985 to 1986: the National Heart, Lung, and Blood Institute Percutaneous Transluminal Coronary Angioplasty Registry. *J Am Coll Cardiol* 1988;12:1149–1155.

28. Moses J, Tierstein P, Sketch M, et al. Angiographic determinants of risk and outcome of coronary embolus and myocardial infarction with the transluminal extraction catheter: a report from the new New Approaches to Coronary Intervention (NACI) Registry. *J Am Coll Cardiol* 1994;23:220A(abst).

29. Gitlin J, Sutton J, Casale P, Whitlow P, Ellis S, et al. Transluminal extraction catheter atherectomy in bypass grafts vs. native vessels: are there significant differences? *J Am Coll Cardiol* 1994;23:220A(abst).

30. Annex BH, Sketch MH Jr, Stack RS, Phillips HR III. Transluminal extraction coronary atherectomy. *Cardiol Clin* 1994;12:611–622.

31. Schreiber T, Kaplan B, Gregory M, et al. Transluminal extraction atherectomy vs. balloon angioplasty in acute isquemic syndromes (TOPIT): hospital outcome and six-month status. *J Am Coll Cardiol* 1997; 29: 132A(abst).

32. Kaplan B, Gregory M, Schreiber T, et al. Transluminal extraction atherectomy versus balloon angioplasty in acute ischemic syndromes: an interim analysis of the TOPIT trial. *Circulation* 1996;94:I-317.

33. Sutton J, Gitlin J, Casale P, Whitlow P, Topol E, Ellis S. Complex lesion with ulceration or calcification are predictors of restenosis after transluminal extraction atherectomy. *J Am Coll Cardiol* 1993;21:442A(abst).

34. Sketch M Jr, O'Neill W, Galichia J, et al. Restenosis following coronary transluminal extraction-endarterectomy: the final analysis of a multicenter registry. *J Am Coll Cardiol* 1992;19:227A(abst).

35. Serruys PW, de Jaegere P, Kiemeneij F, et al. A comparison of balloon-expandable-stent implantation with balloon angioplasty in patients with coronary artery disease. Benestent Study Group. *N Engl J Med* 1994;331: 489–495.

36. Fischman DL, Leon MB, Baim DS, et al. A randomized comparison of coronary-stent placement and balloon angioplasty in the treatment of coronary artery disease. Stent Restenosis Study Investigators. *N Engl J Med* 1994;331:496–501.

37. Savage MP, Douglas JS Jr, Fischman DL, et al. Stent placement compared with balloon angioplasty for obstructed coronary bypass grafts. Saphenous Vein De Novo Trial Investigators. *N Engl J Med* 1997;337: 740–747.

38. Braden GA, Xenopoulos NP, Young T, Utley L, Kutcher MA, Applegate RJ. Transluminal extraction catheter atherectomy followed by immediate stenting in treatment of saphenous vein grafts. *J Am Coll Cardiol* 1997; 30:657–663.

39. Hong MK, Wong SC, Popma JJ, et al. Favorable results of debulking followed by immediate adjunct stent therapy for high risk saphenous vein graft lesions. *J Am Coll Cardiol* 1996;27:179A(abst).

40. Weaver WD, Simes RJ, Betriu A, et al. Comparison of primary coronary angioplasty and intravenous thrombolytic therapy for acute myocardial infarction: a quantitative review. *JAMA* 1997;278:2093–2098.

41. Stone GW, Brodie BR, Griffin JJ, et al. Prospective, multicenter study of the safety and feasibility of primary stenting in acute myocardial infarction: in-hospital and 30-day results of the PAMI stent pilot trial. Primary Angioplasty in Myocardial Infarction Stent Pilot Trial Investigators. *J Am Coll Cardiol* 1998;31:23–30.

42. Suryapranata H, van't Hof A, Hoorntje J, de Boer M, Zijlstra F. Randomized comparison of coronary stenting with balloon angioplasty in selected patients with acute myocardial infarction. *Circulation* 1998;97:2502–2505.

43. Kaplan BM, Larkin T, Safian RD, et al. Prospective study of extraction atherectomy in patients with acute myocardial infarction. *Am J Cardiol* 1996;78:383–388.

44. de Feyter PJ, van Suylen RJ, de Jaegere PP, Topol EJ, Serruys PW. Balloon angioplasty for the treatment of lesions in saphenous vein bypass grafts. *J Am Coll Cardiol* 1993;21:1539–1549.

45. Lefkovits J, Holmes DR, Califf RM, et al. Predictors and sequelae of distal embolization during saphenous vein graft intervention from the CAVEAT-II trial. Coronary Angioplasty Versus Excisional Atherectomy Trial. *Circulation* 1995;92:734–740.

46. Abdelmeguid AE, Ellis SG, Sapp SK, Whitlow PL, Topol EJ. Defining the appropriate threshold of creatine kinase elevation after percutaneous coronary interventions. *Am Heart J* 1996;131:1097–1105.

47. Al-Shaibi KF, Goods CM, Jain SP, et al. Does transluminal extraction atherectomy reduce distal embolization in saphenous vein grafts? *Circulation* 1995;92:I-329(abst).

48. Mak KH, Challapalli R, Eisenberg MJ, Anderson KM, Califf RM, Topol EJ. Effect of platelet glycoprotein IIb/IIIa receptor inhibition on distal embolization during percutaneous revascularization of aortocoronary saphenous vein grafts. EPIC Investigators. Evaluation of IIb/IIIa platelet receptor antagonist 7E3 in preventing is-chemic complications. *Am J Cardiol* 1997;80:985–988.

49. Tcheng J, Anderson K, Tardiff B, et al. Reducing the risk of percutaneous intervention after coronary bypass surgery: beneficial effects of abciximab treatment. *J Am Coll Cardiol* 1997;29:187A(abst).

D. Intracoronary Doppler Flow Velocity: Using Measurements of Coronary Blood Flow in Interventional Cardiology

Morton J. Kern and *Richard G. Bach

*Catheterization Laboratory, St. Louis University Medical Center, St. Louis, Missouri 63110; *Department of Internal Medicine, Division of Cardiology, St. Louis University Health Sciences Center, St. Louis, Missouri 63110*

Coronary physiologic data can be used to facilitate clinical decisions in the catheterization laboratory. Because angiography cannot determine the clinical or physiologic importance of coronary stenoses narrowed between 40% and 70% diameter (1), physiologic testing is often performed before proceeding with coronary interventions. Coronary blood flow, coronary vasodilatory reserve (CVR), and regional myocardial perfusion have demonstrated predictable relationships between the anatomic and physiologic parameters in experimental studies (2–4). Similar clinically reliable physiologic relationships in patients are now applicable to the catheterization laboratory because of recent conceptual and technical advances. Intracoronary Doppler flow velocity can be measured distal to a target stenosis. Employing individual reference flow data obtained from an adjacent angiographically nonobstructed artery, the presence of a lesion-specific abnormality of CVR can be established. Prior to angioplasty or during diagnostic angiography, poststenotic CVR can replace out-of-laboratory nuclear stress testing for target lesion assessment (5,6). Intracoronary velocity data can be obtained continuously for monitoring lesion stability and assessing outcome following

angioplasty. During multivessel angioplasty, secondary lesions can be physiologically assessed before undergoing additional interventions (Table 5.15).

FUNDAMENTAL DOPPLER VELOCITY PRINCIPLES

A shift in signal frequency occurs as the transmitter moves to or away from a target. The

TABLE 5.15. *Clinical uses of intravascular Doppler coronary flow velocity*

1. Intermediate (40%–70%) lesion assessment
2. Angioplasty
   Endpoint
   Monitoring complications
   Assessing additional lesions
   Collateral flow
   Stent
   Atherectomy
3. Coronary vasodilatory reserve
   Syndrome X
   Transplant coronary arteriopathy
   Saphenous vein graft, internal mammary artery
4. Coronary research
   Pharmacologic studies
   Intraaortic balloon pumping
   Coronary physiology of vascular disease
   Myocardial perfusion imaging correlations

change in the signal frequency is proportional to the speed of the target (or transmitter), a phenomenon called the Doppler effect. Using a piezoelectric crystal which both emits and receives high-frequency sound, mounted on the tip of an intravascular device, the velocity of red blood cells flowing through an artery can be determined.

$$\text{Velocity} = \frac{(F_1 - F_0) \times (C)}{(2F_0)(\cos \varnothing)}$$

where

V = velocity of blood flow
F_0 = transmitting (transducer) frequency
F_1 = returning frequency
C = constant: speed of sound in blood
$\varnothing$ = angle of incidence

Volumetric flow can be determined from a velocity value as the product of vessel area (cm^2) and flow velocity (centimeters per second) yielding a value in cubic centimeters per second. Volumetric flow rate can also be computed by multiplying vessel cross-sectional area × mean flow velocity (estimated at 0.5 × average peak velocity) (7,8). Changes in absolute Doppler flow velocities are equal to changes in volumetric coronary flow when the vessel cross-sectional area remains constant. Assuming a constant vessel diameter, a parabolic flow profile and an interrogating Doppler angle of <20%,

the volumetric flow rate can be calculated from the velocity measurements within 5% of absolute values in 3- to 5-mm vessels. The velocity signals, processed on-line by fast Fourier transform, correlated with absolute coronary flow measurements in *in vitro* and *in vivo* validation studies (8, 9).

For very severe lesions, the cross-sectional area of the Doppler guidewire (0.164 mm^2 or 21% of the cross-sectional area of a 1-mm diameter lumen) will impair blood flow. Flow will therefore not be impacted for intermediate lesions in the typical coronary artery (Fig. 5.16).

APPROACHES TO THE PATIENT WITH CORONARY STENOSES

After diagnostic angiography or during angioplasty, the Doppler guidewire is passed through an angioplasty Y-connector attached to a diagnostic or guiding catheter. Intravenous heparin (5,- to 10,0000-U bolus) is required. Intracoronary nitroglycerin (100 to 200 μg) is given to minimize flow-mediated vasodilation, which would result in an underestimation of coronary flow reserve. The guidewire is advanced into the artery. The guidewire is then advanced at least 5 to 10 artery-diameter lengths (>2 cm) beyond the stenosis to permit signals to be acquired under conditions of reestablished laminar flow. After obtaining baseline velocity, maximal coro-

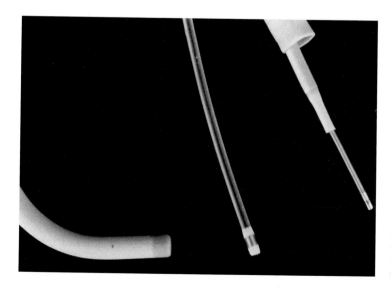

FIG. 5.16. From left to right: 6 Fr angiographic catheter, 2.2 Fr Tracker catheter (Target Therapeutics) for pressure gradient measurements; 0.014-in. Doppler FloWire (Cardiometrics, Inc. Mountain View, CA) residing within a 2.9 Fr IVUS catheter (CVIS, Palo Alto, CA) with an 8 Fr guide catheter. Scale is 1mm.

nary hyperemia is induced by intracoronary adenosine (8 to 12 μg in the right coronary artery and 18 to 24 μg in the left coronary artery) (10). Alternatively, intravenous adenosine or dipyridamole may be used. CVR is computed as the quotient of hyperemic and basal mean flow velocity. After obtaining CVR in the target vessel, CVR is then measured in an adjacent reference vessel. Relative CVR (rCVR) is computed as $CVR_{target}/CVR_{reference}$.

Normal Phasic Flow Velocity Patterns

The normal phasic coronary artery flow pattern in humans is diastolic predominant (11). With increasing severity of epicardial artery stenoses, diastolic flow is blunted. Systolic flow provides a small contribution to mean normal flow that may relatively increase with stenosis severity. The normal diastolic-to-systolic flow velocity ratio (DSVR) is >1.8 and is maintained in both the proximal and distal segments (>2.0-mm diameter) of the left coronary and distal branches of the right coronary artery in patients with normal left ventricles (Fig. 5.17).

The phasic coronary artery blood flow velocity pattern is altered distal to significant coronary stenoses. Segal et al. (12) examined flow velocity in 38 patients undergoing angioplasty and in 12 patients having flow measured in normal vessels as controls. Before angioplasty, the mean DSVR distal to a significant stenosis was decreased compared with that of normal vessels (1.3 ± 0.5 vs. 1.8 ± 0.5, $p < .01$). After angioplasty, the abnormal phasic velocity pattern generally returned toward normal, increasing from 1.3 ± 0.5 vs. 1.9 ± 0.6 ($p < .01$). The flow velocity measurements corresponded to angiographic increases in lumen area, despite the fact that coronary reserve did not improve in most patients. As was later learned (13), CVR likely remained impaired in this study due to incomplete lumen enlargement despite what appeared to be a satisfactory angiographic appearance.

Ofili et al. (11) also examined coronary flow dynamics before and after angioplasty in patients compared with flow in angiographically normal arteries. In 29 patients after angioplasty, the distal average peak hyperemic velocity was

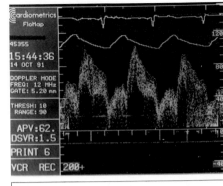

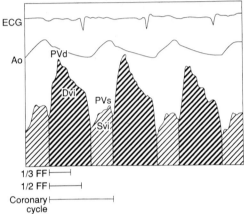

FIG. 5.17. Top: Normal coronary Doppler velocity spectral flow pattern. Velocity scale is 0 to 200 cm per second. Electrocardiogram and aortic pressure readings are shown above the spectral velocity signal. **Bottom:** Diagram showing measurements obtained from spectral signals. Dvi, diastolic velocity integral; FF, flow fraction; Pvd, peak diastolic velocity; Pvs, peak systolic velocity; Svi, systolic velocity integral. (From ref.11, with permission.)

significantly increased after balloon dilation. Distal mean velocity increased more than proximal velocity, decreasing the proximal-to-distal velocity ratio, another marker of lesion severity (Table 5.16).

NORMAL CORONARY VASODILATORY RESERVE

The most sensitive and specific physiologic correlate of coronary stenosis severity in experimental and clinical studies is the poststenotic CVR. The question of what is normal CVR as-

TABLE 5.16. *Baseline and hyperemia velocity parameters in individual coronary arteries*

	Baseline			Hyperemia[a]		
	LAD (n = 24)	LCX (n = 19)	RCA (n = 12)	LAD	LCX	RCA
Proximal						
Peak D Vel	49 ± 20	40 ± 15	37 ± 12	104 ± 28[b]	79 ± 20	72 ± 13
Mean Vel	31 ± 15	25 ± 8	26 ± 7	66 ± 18[b]	50 ± 14	48 ± 13
D Vel Int	18 ± 11[c]	13 ± 5	11 ± 4	37 ± 55[b]	27 ±	22 ± 9
1/3 FF (%)	45 ± 4[c]	44 ± 5	40 ± 5	44 ± 5	43 ± 6	41 ± 4
D/S	2.0 ± 0.5[c]	1.8 ± 0.7	1.5 ± 0.5	2.0 ± 0.5	1.9 ± 0.6	1.9 ± 0.8
Distal						
Peak D Vel	35 ± 16	35 ± 8	28 ± 8	70 ± 17	71 ± 22	67 ± 16
Mean Vel	23 ± 11	21 ± 6	21 ± 9	45 ± 12	45 ± 12	42 ± 9
D Vel Int	13 ± 9	10 ± 3	8 ± 5	9 ± 6	11 ± 8	9 ± 2
1/3 FF (%)	46 ± 2	45 ± 9	39 ± 6	45 ± 3	42 ± 7	40 ± 9
D/S	2.4 ± 0.8[c]	2.1 ± 0.8	1.4 ± 0.3	2.2 ± 1.0	1.9 ± 0.8	1.6 ± 0.3

Anova: Scheffe F test $p < .05$

D, diastolic; D/S, peak diastolic/systolic velocity; D Vel Int, diastolic flow velocity integral (units); Vel, velocity (cm/sec); 1/3 FF, one-third flow fraction.

[a] All three coronary arteries had significantly higher absolute velocity parameters during hyperemia ($p < .001$).
[b] LAD vs. LCX and RCA.
[c] LAD vs. RCA.
Modified from ref. 11.

sessed using the Doppler guidewire and bolus intracoronary adenosine in patients in the cardiac catheterization laboratory was addressed in a study of 416 coronary arteries in 214 patients with atypical chest pain syndromes and angiographically normal coronary arteries, coronary artery disease and angiographically normal vessels, and angiographically normal transplant recipients (14). CVR responses were compared by vessel, gender, status post–heart transplant, and the presence of remote coronary artery disease in another artery. In normal patients with chest pain syndromes, CVR was 2.7 ± 0.6, lower than in transplant recipients (3.0 ± 0.6, $p < .05$) and higher than in poststenotic diseased vessel coronary flow reserve (1.8 ± 0.6). CVR tended to be higher in men than in women ($p < .07$). CVR was similar among left anterior descending, circumflex, and right coronary arteries in normal patients (2.8 ± 0.6, 2.7 ± 0.05, and 2.9 ± 0.6, respectively). Regional differences were also not present in the transplant population.

Di Mario et al. (15) evaluated the long-term reproducibility of Doppler coronary flow velocity in patients with coronary artery disease. Coronary flow velocity was recorded twice in the mid-vessel location in 31 patients over a 6-month follow-up period. Baseline velocity was

similar (23 ± 8 cm per second) to values at follow-up (22 ± 5 cm per second), but the correlation was weak (slope = 0.3, r = .46). Initial coronary flow reserve was 2.9 ± 0.8 and 3.0 ± 0.8 at follow-up, with a larger scatter over the line of identity (slope = 0.22, r = .22). The standard deviation of the difference between initial and follow-up measurements was higher in baseline conditions (±31%) than during hyperemia (±23%). The largest variation was for coronary flow reserve (SD ± 36%). Long-term reproducibility improved when flow velocity was normalized for the cross-sectional area at the site of measurement.

TRANSLESIONAL HEMODYNAMICS AND ISCHEMIC STRESS TESTING

Excellent correlations with myocardial perfusion imaging and poststenotic coronary flow velocity reserve have been reported by several single-center studies (5,6,16) and one multicenter trial (17). An abnormal distal CVR (<2.0) corresponded to reversible myocardial perfusion imaging defects with high sensitivity (86% to 92%), specificity (89% to 100%), predictive accuracy (89% to 96%), and positive and negative predictive values (94% to 100% and 77% to

95%), respectively. A guidewire pressure technique to determine coronary flow, the fractional flow reserve of the myocardium (FFRmyo; discussion follows), has also been validated against myocardial perfusion using positron emission tomography (18–20), and normal range values (>0.75) can easily discriminate among stenoses responsible for positive exercise stress testing (20) with excellent (>90%) specificity and sensitivity and high diagnostic accuracy (93% when compared with all noninvasive ischemic stress studies).

HEMODYNAMIC CRITERIA OF A SIGNIFICANT CORONARY LESION

The use of flow velocity to assess hemodynamics of a coronary stenosis is based on the concept that the coronary circulation is comprised of two major components: a conduit (epicardial arteries) and a microcirculation (capillary and myocardial vascular bed). If poststenotic CVR is normal, then both components are assumed to be normal. If CVR is abnormal, then examination of lesion-specific indices will separate conduit obstruction, which can be treated mechanically (angioplasty) from microcirculatory disturbances, which are theoretically unlikely to benefit from such intervention and which may be more appropriately treated medically.

For a borderline CVR value or where the operator has low confidence in an accurate signal, a lesion-specific index should be acquired. Two lesion-specific measurements, thus far validated, are (a) relative coronary vasodilatory reserve ratio ($CVR_{target}/CVR_{normal}$) and (b) a translesional pressure gradient at hyperemia (FFR [fraction flow reserve]). The accuracy of translesional gradients for FFR calculation may be affected (overestimated) when a small plastic catheter instead of an angioplasty sensor guidewire is used (see Coronary Pressure Measurements).

CORONARY PRESSURE MEASUREMENTS FOR DETERMINATION OF CORONARY BLOOD FLOW

Translesional pressure measurements using sensor guidewires have reemerged as another

TABLE 5.17. *Equations from Pijls et al. (17) for calculation of myocardial, coronary, and collateral fraction flow reserve from pressure measurements during maximal hyperemia*

Myocardial fraction flow reserve (FFR):	
FFR	$= 1 - \Delta P/(P_a - P_v)$
	$= (P_c - P_v)/(P_a - P_v)$
	$= P_c/P_a$
Coronary fractional flow reserve (FFR_{cor}):	
FFR_{cor}	$= 1 - \Delta P(P_a - P_w)$
Collateral fractional flow reserve (FFR_{coll}):	
FFR_{coll}	$= FFR - FFR$

P_a, mean aortic pressure; P_c, distal coronary pressure; P, mean translesional pressure gradient; P_v, mean right atrial pressure; P_w, mean coronary wedge pressure or distal coronary pressure during balloon inflation.

significant adjunctive physiologic technique for lesion assessment before and after angioplasty, especially when questionable angiographic or coronary flow data are obtained.

The determination of coronary blood flow from guidewire pressure measurements, the FFR, has been validated (7–12,14–20). The FFR is defined as the ratio of maximal hyperemic flow in the stenotic artery to the theoretic maximal hyperemic flow in the same artery without a stenosis. FFR is computed as the ratio of mean distal coronary pressure and mean aortic pressure during maximal hyperemia and is a specific index to describe the influence of the coronary stenosis on maximal perfusion of the subtended myocardium. FFR is normally 1.0 for all vessels and independent of changes in hemodynamics and microcirculatory status (Table 5.17). It is important to note that there is good agreement between FFR and rCVR by Doppler (20).

PRESSURE MEASURING TECHNIQUE

Using standard angioplasty technique, the pressure wire is positioned in the proximal coronary artery segment and the pressure signal is matched to the aortic (guide catheter) pressure. The guidewire is advanced into the artery beyond the target stenosis. The two pressures are simultaneously recorded at baseline and during hyperemia induced by intracoronary or intravenous adenosine. FFR is computed as $Pressure_{distal}/Pressure_{aorta}$ during maximal hyperemia. The pressure wire can then be pulled back proximal to the stenosis to recheck signal drift (Fig. 5.18).

Pijls et al. (21) correlated FFR in 45 patients with moderate coronary stenosis and chest pain of uncertain origin with bicycle exercise testing, thallium scintigraphy, and stress dobutamine echocardiography. In all 21 patients with fractional flow reserve < 0.75, reversible myocar-

dial ischemia was demonstrated unequivocally on at least one noninvasive test. After coronary revascularization, all positive results reverted to normal. In 21 of 24 patients with fractional flow reserve of ≥ 0.75, tests were negative for reversible myocardial ischemia on all tests. No revascularization procedures were performed, and all patients were stable and did not require further intervention over 14 months of follow-up. The sensitivity of fractional flow reserve for reversible ischemia was 88%, specificity 100%, positive and negative predictive value 100% and

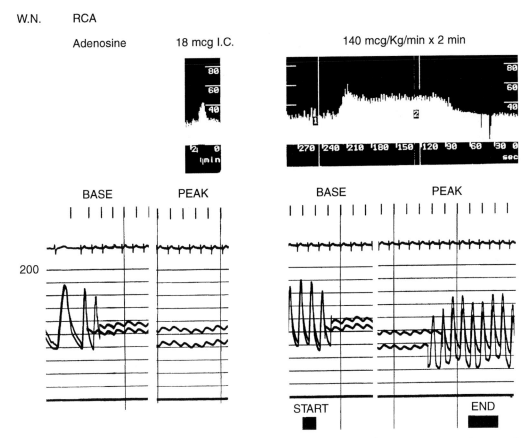

FIG. 5.18. Coronary pressure and flow measured at rest (base) and during maximal hyperemia (peak) across an intermediately severe right coronary artery lesion, demonstrating an increase from the resting gradient of 16 mm Hg to 30 mm Hg. **Top panel:** The flow velocity response of intracoronary and intravenous adenosine showing a CVR of 2.0. **Lower panels:** The aortic distal coronary pressures. Fractional flow reserve is computed from the maximal hyperemic distal pressure and aortic pressure. Aortic pressure equals 106 mm Hg, distal coronary pressure equals 80 mm Hg, fractional flow reserve is 80/106 = 0.75, a normal value corresponding to a negative stress thallium study in this individual. Intravenous adenosine reduced systemic pressure more than intracoronary, but did not change the FFR (76/98 = 0.78).

88%, respectively, with a predictive accuracy of 93%.

In patients with an impaired microvascular circulation, the absence of a significant hyperemic transstenotic gradient may theoretically be related to either the absence of a flow-limiting stenosis or to low flow due to either an impaired distal vasodilation or a well-developed collateral circulation. This situation is under study.

CLINICAL USE OF TRANSLESIONAL PHYSIOLOGIC MEASUREMENTS

For interventional cardiology, there are several major indications for coronary Doppler flow measurements: (a) assessment of the angiographically intermediate lesion, (b) decision for angioplasty of secondary lesions in multivessel angioplasty, (c) endpoint determination after angioplasty, and (d) coronary physiology research.

INTERMEDIATELY SEVERE STENOSIS

An intermediate stenosis (40% to 70% diameter narrowing) is encountered in nearly 50% of all patients with coronary arter disease. As noted earlier, intracoronary flow velocity measurements parallel stress testing results and can therefore identify clinically important lesions, assisting in immediate decision making. When intermediate coronary lesions are not associated with abnormal physiology, angioplasty can be safely deferred (21,22).

A prospective study of deferring angioplasty based on normal translesional flow reported outcome results in 88 patients with 100 lesions (26 single-vessel, 74 multivessel coronary artery stenoses) (22). The percent lumen area reduction, percent diameter stenosis, and obstruction diameter in the deferred group were 77% $\pm$ 8%, 54% $\pm$ 7%, and 1.32 $\pm$ 0.33 mm, respectively. Translesional pressure gradients were lower for the deferred compared with a reference angioplasty group (10 $\pm$ 9 mm Hg vs. 46 $\pm$ 22 mm Hg, $p < .01$). Proximal-to-distal velocity ratios demonstrated similar values for both the normal and deferred groups, with significant differences compared with the angioplasty group (1.1 $\pm$ 0.35 for the normal, 1.3 $\pm$ 0.55 for the deferred,

and 2.3 $\pm$ 1.2 for the angioplasty group; $p < .05$ vs. both normal and deferred groups).

Clinical follow-up data were available in 84 of 88 (95%), with a mean follow-up of 10 $\pm$ 8 months and a minimum follow-up period of 6 months (range 6 to 30 months). In the deferred group, rehospitalization due to both noncardiac and angina-like symptoms occurred in 18 patients, 12 of whom had cardiac events. No patient had a myocardial infarction. One patient died due to postangioplasty complications of a nontarget artery. One patient with multivessel coronary artery disease and decreased left ventricular function had sudden death due to ventricular fibrillation 12 months after lesion assessment. Ten patients required either coronary artery bypass grafting ($n = 6$) or coronary angioplasty ($n = 4$), only six of which involved target arteries. Of the six patients who required bypass surgery, only three involved a target artery with previously normal translesional flow velocity. There were no complications related to translesional pressure or flow velocity measurements in any patient studied.

This study demonstrated that in patients with angiographically intermediately severe lesions, normal translesional hemodynamic data can be acquired safely and that angioplasty can be deferred, with approximately 92% of target arteries evaluated remaining stable without the need for intervention. Similar data have been obtained for patients with intermediate coronary stenoses assessed by intracoronary pressure measurements (FFR) (21). Translesional flow velocity-pressure measurements can thus provide objective functional evidence of lesion significance to assist in selecting patients for appropriate coronary interventions.

OUTCOME OF ANGIOPLASTY AND CORONARY FLOW VELOCITY

The predictive value of coronary flow velocity measurements after angioplasty was reported in the results of a European multicenter prospective study DEBATE, Doppler Endpoint Balloon Angioplasty Trial Europe (13). In 224 patients after single-vessel angioplasty, poststenotic coronary vasodilatory reserve, proximal-to-distal flow ratio, and DSVR were compared with early and late clinical events.

After angioplasty, there was no difference in the angiographic minimal lumen diameter between patients with early ischemic events ($n = 35$) and asymptomatic patients ($n = 189$, 1.81 ± 0.38 mm vs. 1.79 ± 0.29 mm, respectively). However, the CVR (2.73 ± 0.93 vs. 2.22 ± 0.65; $p < .05$) was higher in asymptomatic patients compared with those experiencing early events. These data indicated that, on average, the symptomatic group could be differentiated but, because of the spread of data points, an isolated CVR value would not be prognostic except in the extremes. An analysis combining the postprocedural coronary flow reserve (>2.5) with satisfactory anatomic results (quantitative angiographic percent diameter stenosis $<35\%$) identified 44 of 224 patients with a 16% rate of repeat angioplasty and angiographic restenosis at 6 months, values similar to restenosis rates in the major stent trials.

Notably, the combined anatomic and functional postangioplasty data were a better prognostic index than either parameter alone and were strongly predictive of early and late clinical events. Prospective trials using physiologically guided decisions to assess the need for stenting will further define clinical scenarios for selective rather than universal stenting in angioplasty patients.

STENTING AND CORONARY FLOW VELOCITY

From ultrasound imaging and Doppler flow data, traditional balloon angioplasty may not achieve an optimal result for luminal enlargement, despite a satisfactory angiographic appearance. After coronary angioplasty, CVR often remains impaired. If this result is due to unappreciated luminal narrowing, then coronary stenting may normalize CVR. Decisions for stenting or larger balloon catheters after coronary angioplasty may therefore be facilitated using coronary physiologic data.

To demonstrate the relationship between anat-

omy and physiology after angioplasty and stenting, 42 patients undergoing elective angioplasty and stent placement had measurements of coronary flow velocity reserve (0.014-in. Doppler FloWire; Cardiometrics, Inc., Mountain View, CA) and intravascular ultrasound (IVUS) imaging (2.9F CVIS) before and after balloon angioplasty and again after stent placement (23).

The percent diameter stenosis decreased from 84% $\pm$ 13% to 37% $\pm$ 18% after angioplasty to 8% $\pm$ 8% after stent placement. CVR increased from 1.7 ± 0.79 to 1.89 ± 0.6 after angioplasty to 2.49 ± 0.68 after stent placement (Figs. 5.19 and 5.20). The poststent CVR was similar to that found in normal adjacent reference vessels (2.61 ± 0.46). There was no relationship between CVR and angiographic percent diameter stenosis or absolute QCA dimensions. IVUS vessel cross-sectional area was significantly larger after stenting (5.1 ± 2.0 mm^2 after angioplasty vs. 8.4 ± 2.1 mm^2 after stent; $p < .01$) (Fig. 5.21).

The increase in CVR after stenting, incrementally more than balloon angioplasty, suggests that the postlesional CVR after angioplasty is related to the degree of lumen expansion or, conversely, the degree of residual lesion encroachment, which is not always appreciated by angiography. A physiologically guided intervention to achieve an optimal lumen for flow may lead to improved angioplasty techniques and improved outcomes, and may potentially limit unnecessary stent placement.

CORONARY BLOOD FLOW MONITORING AFTER CORONARY INTERVENTIONS

Monitoring flow for variations due to slowly progressive dissection, thrombus formation, or vasospasm is easily performed using the velocity trend plot. The flow velocity trend changes often precede angiographic signs of vessel occlusion (24) (Fig. 5.22). Monitoring flow can also reduce total contrast volume when assessing stability of angioplasty results and can identify potential unstable flow associated with vessel closure, a benefit that has obvious clinical ad-

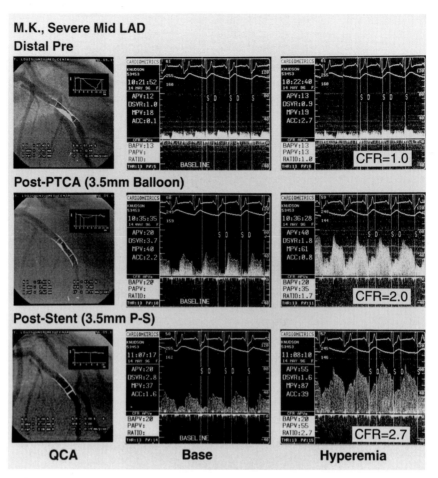

FIG. 5.19. Example of angiographic and coronary flow velocity data before and after coronary angioplasty and again after stent placement. **Left panel:** Cineangiographic frames and **(middle and right panels)** coronary basal and hyperemic flow velocity are shown for each study period. Coronary flow reserve (CFR) is 1.0 before angioplasty, 2.0 after angioplasty, and 2.7 after stenting. Velocity scale is 0 to 160 cm per second. Each velocity panel displays ECG, aortic pressure, and spectral flow velocity with phasic markers of systole (*S*) and diastole (*D*). (From ref. 23, with permission.)

vantages. In the DEBATE study (13), the observation of unstable flow velocity (cyclic flow variations) immediately following balloon dilation, although infrequent, was highly predictive of abrupt vessel closure (four of five patients) (13). Interruption of unstable flow with conversion to a stable postprocedure flow pattern reduces morbidity related to an out-of-laboratory acute vessel closure and reduces the need for a repeat procedure, angioplasty catheters, and/or stent placement. Early warning signs of an adverse outcome derived from flow trend monitoring can potentially save the cost of the repeat angioplasty and/or bypass surgery.

CORONARY BLOOD FLOW VELOCITY DURING INTERVENTION FOR ACUTE MYOCARDIAL INFARCTION

The semiquantitative but clinically predictive TIMI angiographic grade flow is an established standard of reperfusion therapies. Angiographic TIMI flow grade in the infarct-related artery is a strong correlate of subsequent mortality. To

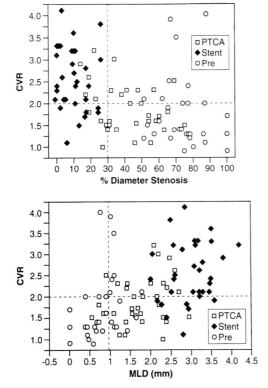

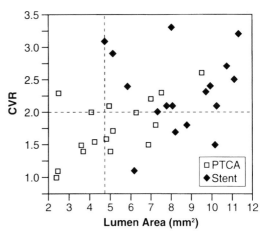

FIG. 5.20. Relationship between percent diameter stenosis by quantitative coronary angiography (QCA, **top panel**), minimal lumen diameter (MLD, **bottom panel**), and coronary vasodilatory reserve (CVR). o, preangioplasty; □, postangioplasty; ◆, poststent. (From ref. 23, with permission.)

FIG. 5.21. Relationship between coronary vaso-dilatory reserve (CVR) and intravascular ultrasound lumen area. □, postangioplasty; ◆, poststent. (From ref. 23, with permission.)

assess the quantitative aspect of TIMI flow grade, primary or rescue angioplasty was performed using a 0.014 to 0.018-in. Doppler-tipped angioplasty guidewire in 41 acute myocardial infarct patients (25). TIMI angiographic flow grade, assessed by two independent observers and quantitated by the frames-to-opacification method from cinefilm, was compared with measured flow velocity. Of 41 patients, 33 had primary and 8 had rescue angioplasty, 34 within 24 hours of acute myocardial infarction. Before angioplasty, 34 patients had TIMI grade 0 or 1, 5 patients had TIMI grade 2, and 3 patients had TIMI grade 3 flow in the infarct artery. Following angioplasty, diameter stenosis improved from 95% ± 7% to 22% ± 10%. One patient had TIMI grade 1, 5 patients had TIMI grade 2,

and 35 patients had TIMI grade 3 flow. Poststen-otic flow velocity increased from 6.6 ± 6.1 to 20.0 ± 11.1 cm per second ($p < .01$) following angioplasty. Before angioplasty, there were no statistical differences between poststenotic flow velocity values among infarct vessels with TIMI grade 0, 1, or 2, however, TIMI grade 3 had higher flow velocity (9.4 ± 5cm/sec vs 16 ± 5.4; $p < 0.05$). Following angioplasty, TIMI grade 3 flow increased to 21.8 ± 10.9 cm per second ($p < .05$ vs. preangioplasty distal TIMI grade 3 flow). Postangioplasty flow velocity correlated with angiographic frame count ($r = .45$; $p < .02$). However, for TIMI grade 3, there was a large overlap with low TIMI ≤2 flow velocity (<20 cm per second), despite frames-to-opacification of <60. Nine of 11 clinical events (i.e., death, recurrent myocardial infarction, or need for repeat coronary revascularization) occurred in the TIMI 3 group with flow velocity <20cm per second.

These results indicate that semiquantitative TIMI perfusion grades are distinguished by differences in coronary flow velocity, with TIMI grade ≤2 consistently associated with low-flow values. On average, TIMI grade 3 flow velocity is higher than TIMI grades ≤2 flow, but there is a substantial overlap with low-flow values of TIMI ≤2 flow. Quantitative assessment of flow

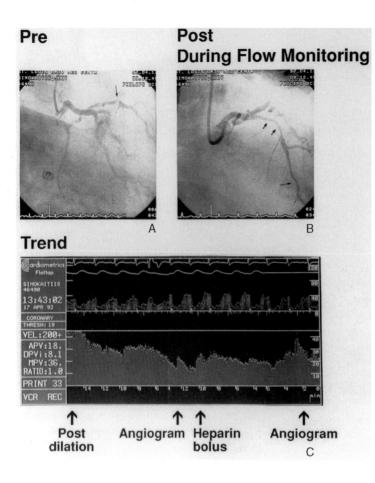

FIG. 5.22. Shown are cineangiographic frames of lesion in left anterior descending (LAD) artery stent/ stenosis **(A)** (*arrow*) before angioplasty. **B:** After angioplasty **(top right panel)** during velocity monitoring, angiographic haziness and mottling (*two arrows*) at angioplasty site was associated with cyclical flow variations measured at tip of Doppler guidewire (*distal arrow*), as shown on flow velocity trend plot. **C:** Trend plot displays the following signals (from top to bottom): ECG, aortic pressure, phasic velocity (0- to 200-cm per second scale) and continuous plot of average peak velocity (APV, 0- to 50-cm per second scale). Events at *arrows* are described in text. (Reproduced with permission from Kern MJ, Donohue T, Bach R, et al. Monitoring cyclical coronary blood flow alterations following coronary angioplasty for stent restenosis using a Doppler guidewire. *Am Heart J* 1993;125: 1159–1160.)

velocity after reperfusion could potentially establish important physiologic correlations among clinical outcomes for prognosticating after various reperfusion therapies.

USE OF CORONARY FLOW VELOCITY FOR STENTING

Case Example

The following case illustrates a practical application of intracoronary Doppler for additional stenting.

A 58-year-old man with unstable angina underwent coronary arteriography, which demonstrated minimal luminal irregularities in the left coronary artery system, normal left ventricular function, and significant, highly eccentric, and irregular stenoses in ectatic proximal and mid portions of the right coronary artery (Fig. 5.23).

Quantitative coronary angiography of the proximal stenosis demonstrated that its most severe percent diameter narrowing was 82%. Coronary angioplasty was undertaken with coronary flow guidewire, which demonstrated a poststenotic distal coronary reserve ratio of 1.1 (Fig. 5.24).

Balloon angioplasty was undertaken with a 3.5-mm balloon. The result was a hazy, irregular angiographic result, considerably improved compared with the initial presentation but still irregular with evidence of dissection. The flow velocity after initial angioplasty demonstrated an improvement with a poststenotic CVR of 1.8 (Fig. 5.25).

A 3.5-mm Palmaz-Schatz stent was then de-

LAO

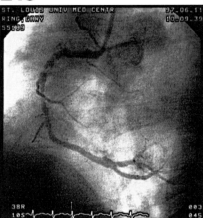

RAO

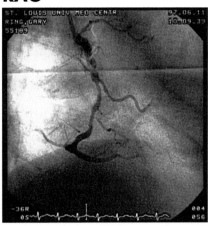

FIG. 5.23. Cineangiogram of a 58-year-old man with unstable angina. **Left panel:** The left anterior oblique (*LAO*) projection. **Right panel:** The right anterior oblique (*RAO*) projection shows eccentric irregular stenosis in the proximal portion of the right coronary artery, with luminal irregularities throughout the distal coronary artery.

RCA: QCA 82%

Distal RCA, CFR=1.1

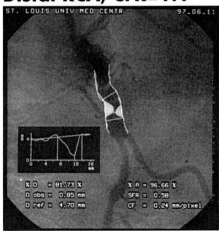

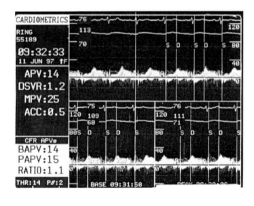

FIG. 5.24. **Left panel:** Quantitative coronary angiographic frame of the right coronary artery in the left anterior oblique (LAO) projection, showing the most severe stenosis at 81.7% diameter stenosis. The reference vessel segment diameter was 4.7 mm. Coronary flow reserve measured distal to the stenosis (**right panel**) demonstrated a basal average peak velocity (*BAPV*) of 14, peak average peak velocity (*PAPV*) of 15, and a coronary reserve (*ratio*) of 1.1. The coronary flow velocity panel is split into top and bottom. Top portion shows the continuous flow velocity signal. The scale on the right side shows velocity range from 0 to 120 cm per second. The electrocardiographic signal is shown at the top, with the aortic pressure underneath. Systole and diastole are demarcated by *S* and *D*, respectively. The numbers in the upper left corner demonstrate the heart rate (76 bpm) and blood pressure (113/70 mm Hg). The lower portion is split into the left and right side. The basal flow velocity is on the left side. The peak hyperemic flow velocity is on the right side. The scale is the same as the top portion of the flow screen.

Distal RCA, CFR=1.8

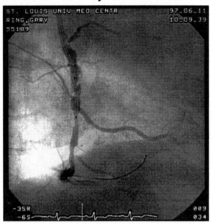

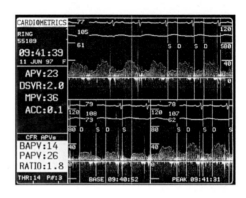

FIG. 5.25. Left panel: Angiogram in the right anterior oblique (*RAO*) projection, showing improvement in the proximal right coronary stenosis but a hazy and dissected portion at the site of balloon angioplasty. **Right panel:** The flow velocity data demonstrating basal average peak velocity (*BAPV*) increasing from 14 to 26 cm per second during maximal hyperemia, for a CVR of 1.8. Format as in Fig. 5.24.

ployed in the proximal right coronary artery, with dramatic improvement in the angiographic appearance. There remained a distal approximately 50% narrowing beyond the stent in the mid and distal portions of the right coronary artery. Given the angiographic appearance of the distal right coronary artery and the positioning

of the proximal stent, is a second or third stent required?

Based on the subsequent physiologic measurements, a decision can be made whether the remaining coronary artery disease results in residual flow limitation, with consideration that a purely angiographic approach using multiple

LAO

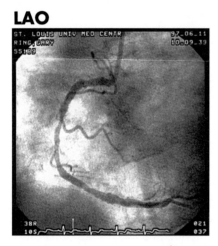

RAO

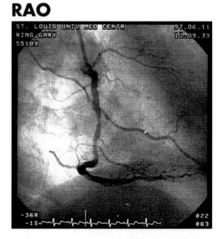

FIG. 5.26. Left anterior oblique (*LAO*) and right anterior oblique (*RAO*) views of the right coronary artery after a 3.5-mm Palmaz-Schatz stent and high-pressure balloon inflations. Is subsequent stenting of the right coronary artery necessary? Following stenting, CVR was measured again in the distal portion of the right coronary artery.

Post-Stent

Distal RCA, CFR=2.9

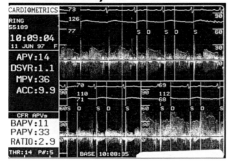

Circumflex, CFR=2.9

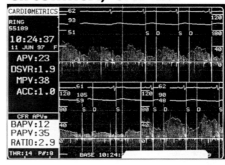

FIG. 5.27. CVR in the distal right coronary artery and in the normal reference circumflex artery after stenting. CVR was 2.9 in the right coronary artery and 2.9 in the circumflex artery, for a relative coronary flow reserve ratio of 1.0. This is a normal value, and no further stenting was performed on the basis of this data.

stents may prove both technically complicated and costly without clear superiority with respect to outcome. Figure 5.26 shows the angiographic result after Palmaz-Schatz placement. Coronary flow reserve was then measured.

CVR in the distal right coronary artery after proximal stenting was 2.9, with basal flow increasing from 11 to 33 cm per second (Fig. 5.27). To assess whether this was in the normal range for the myocardium under study for the existing hemodynamic conditions, CVR was also measured in the angiographically normal circumflex artery segment as a reference measurement. Coronary flow reserve was also 2.9. The flow reserve was normal for the poststented artery, and further stenting was successfully deferred at this point.

SUMMARY

From the foregoing discussion and case illustrations, considerable experience has established that incorporation of translesional flow velocity into clinical practice can assist in identification of appropriate angioplasty candidates, improve the technical approach to complex intervention, and potentially improve the outcome of interventional procedures. Additional vascular information using coronary Doppler flow or pressure

provides important adjunctive data on which to base decisions, rather than accept subjective impressions as to the requirements for different intervention approaches.

ACKNOWLEDGMENT

The authors wish to thank the J.G. Mudd Cardiac Catheterization Laboratory team and Donna Sander for manuscript preparation.

REFERENCES

1. White CW, Wright CB, Doty DB, et al. Does visual interpretation of the coronary arteriogram predict the physiologic importance of a coronary stenosis? *N Engl J Med* 1984;310:819–824.
2. de Feyter PJ, Serruys PW, Davies MJ, Richardson P, Lubsen J, Oliver MF. Quantitative coronary angiography to measure progression and regression of coronary atherosclerosis: value, limitations, and implications for clinical trials. *Circulation* 1991;84:412–423.
3. Harrison DG, White CW, Hiratzka LF, et al. The value of lesion cross-sectional area determined by quantitative coronary angiography in assessing the physiologic significance of proximal left anterior descending coronary arteries stenosis. *Circulation* 1984;69:1111–1119.
4. Gould KL, Lipscomb K, Hamilton GW. Physiologic basis for assessing critical coronary stenosis. *Am J Cardiol* 1974;33:87–94.
5. Miller DD, Donohue TJ, Younis LT, et al. Correlation of pharmacologic 99mTc-sestamibi myocardial perfusion imaging with poststenotic coronary flow reserve in patients with angiographically intermediate coronary artery stenoses. *Circulation* 1994;89:2150–2160.

6. Joye JD, Schulman DS, Lasorda D, Farah T, Donohue BC, Reichek N. Intracoronary Doppler guide wire versus stress single-photon emission computed tomographic thallium-201 imaging in assessment of intermediate coronary stenoses. *J Am Coll Cardiol* 1994;24: 940–947.

7. Hatle L, Angelsen B. Physics of blood flow. In: Hatle L, Angelsen B, eds. *Doppler ultrasound in cardiology*. Philadelphia: Lea & Febiger, 1982:8–31.

8. Doucette JW, Corl PD, Payne HM, et al. Validation of a Doppler guide wire for intravascular measurement of coronary artery flow velocity. *Circulation* 1992;85: 1899–1911.

9. Labovitz AJ, Anthonis DJ, Craven TL, Kern MJ. Validation of volumetric flow measurements by means of a Doppler-tipped coronary angioplasty guide wire. *Am Heart J* 1993;126:1456–1461.

10. Wilson RF, Wyche K, Christensen BV, Zimmer S, Laxson DD. Effects of adenosine on human coronary arterial circulation. *Circulation* 1990;82:1595–1606.

11. Ofili EO, Kern MJ, Labovitz AJ, et al. Analysis of coronary blood flow velocity dynamics in angiographically normal and stenosed arteries before and after endoluminal enlargement by angioplasty. *J Am Coll Cardiol* 1993;21:308–316.

12. Segal J, Kern MJ, Scott NA, et al. Alterations of phasic coronary artery flow velocity in man during percutaneous coronary angioplasty. *J Am Coll Cardiol* 1992;20: 276–286.

13. Serruys PW, Di Mario C. Prognostic value of coronary flow velocity and diameter stenosis in assessing the short and long term outcome of balloon angioplasty: the DEBATE study (Doppler endpoints balloon angioplasty trial Europe). *Circulation* 1996;94:I-317(abst).

14. Kern MJ, Bach RG, Mechem C, et al. Variations in normal coronary vasodilatory reserve stratified by artery, gender, heart transplantation and coronary artery disease. *J Am Coll Cardiol* 1996;28:1154–1160.

15. Di Mario C, Gil R, Serruys PW. Long-term reproducibility of coronary flow velocity measurements in patients with coronary artery disease. *Am J Cardiol* 1995; 75:1177–1180.

16. Deychak YA, Segal J, Reiner JS, et al. Doppler guide wire flow-velocity indexes measured distal to coronary stenoses associated with reversible thallium perfusion defects. *Am Heart J* 1995; 129:219–227.

17. Heller LI, Popma J, Cates C, et al. Functional assessment of stenosis severity in the cath lab: a comparison of Doppler and tl-201 imaging. *J Interven Cardiol* 1995; 7:23A.

18. Pijls NHJ, van Son AM, Kirkeeide RL, De Bruyne B, Gould KL. Experimental basis of determining maximum coronary, myocardial, and collateral blood flow by pressure measurements for assessing functional stenosis severity before and after percutaneous transluminal coronary angioplasty. *Circulation* 1993;87:1354–1367.

19. de Bruyne B, Baudhuin T, Melin JA, et al. Coronary flow reserve calculated from pressure measurements in humans: validation with positron emission tomography. *Circulation* 1994;89:1013–1022.

20. Baumgart D, Haude M, Goerge G, et al. Improved assessment of coronary stenosis severity using the relative flow velocity reserve. *Circulation* 1998;98:40–46.

21. Pijls NHJ, de Bruyne B, Peels K, et al. Measurement of myocardial fractional flow reserve to assess the functional severity of coronary artery stenosis. *N Engl J Med* 1996;334:1703–1708.

22. Kern MJ, Donohue TJ, Aguirre FV, et al. Clinical outcome of deferring angioplasty in patients with normal translesional pressure-flow velocity measurements. *J Am Coll Cardiol* 1995;25:178–187.

23. Kern MJ, Dupouy P, Drury JH, et al. Role of coronary artery lumen enlargement in improving coronary blood flow after balloon angioplasty and stenting: a combined intravascular ultrasound Doppler flow and imaging study. *J Am Coll Cardiol* 1997;29:1520–1527.

24. Kern MJ, Aguirre FV, Donohue TJ, et al. Coronary flow velocity monitoring after angioplasty associated with abrupt reocclusion. *Am Heart J* 1994;127:436–438.

25. Kern MJ, Moore JA, Aguirre FV, et al. Determination of angiographic (TIMI grade) blood flow by intracoronary Doppler flow velocity during acute myocardial infarction. *Circulation* 1996;94:1545–1552.

E. Percutaneous Myocardial Revascularization

Sidney T.H. Lo, David P. Lee, and *Stephen N. Oesterle

*Division of Cardiovascular Medicine, Stanford University Medical Center, Stanford, California 94305-5246; *Department of Medicine, Harvard Medical School, Department of Cardiology, Massachusetts General Hospital, Boston, Massachusetts 02114*

For many years, aortocoronary bypass graft surgery and percutaneous coronary intervention have been the mainstays of coronary revascularization therapy. There began to be recognized an increasing number of patients with refractory symptoms which were unsuitable for further conventional therapies due to poor surgical risks, repeated surgical bypass failures, diffuse or small-vessel coronary disease and chronic coronary artery occlusions. These patients with ''end-stage'' coronary disease have limited therapeutic options available. Experimental techniques such as laser revascularization and delivery of angiogenic growth factors have recently become available in a clinical trial setting. Transmyocardial revascularization (TMR) utilizes laser energy to create a multitude of transmural myocardial channels in the hope of improving myocardial perfusion. Initially performed via a surgical approach, this has recently evolved into a feasible percutaneous procedure. Percutaneous transmyocardial laser revascularization (PMR , PTMR, or PMLR) has now emerged as a promising technique of reperfusing ischemic myocardium in end-stage coronary artery disease (CAD) patients.

BACKGROUND

Transmyocardial revascularization was inspired by the reptilian circulation. In reptiles, blood is supplied directly to the myocardium from the ventricular cavity via a network of branching channels without the need for epicardial vessels. In addition, contrary to mammals, filling occurs during systole rather than diastole. In the 1930s, direct vascular communications between the left ventricular cavity and coronary arteries in humans was described as ''myocardial sinusoids'' by Wearn et al. (1). In the 1960s, Sen et al. (2) created left ventriculomyocardial channels in dogs, using needle acupuncture which reduced infarct size and improved survival postepicardial artery ligation. In the 1980s, Mirhoseini et al. (3,4) created transmyocardial channels in a canine infarct model, using a CO_2 laser, which proved to be protective from ischemia. This was the setting that led to laser TMR trials in humans.

TMR (TMLR)

Mirhoseini et al. (5) reported the results of the first human TMR series in 1988. He utilized CO_2 laser TMR in 12 patients as an adjunct to coronary bypass surgery to treat areas not suitable for grafting. Unfortunately, the TMR results could not be separated from those of bypass revascularization in these patients, but improvement in perfusion in the TMR-treated segments was seen on follow-up stress thallium imaging, and the patency of channels was documented on follow-up left ventriculography. Cooley et al. (6) reported significant reduction in angina class 12 months after TMR sole therapy for refractory angina in 21 patients (average angina class of 3.7 ± 0.4 before vs. 1.8 ± 0.6 after; $p < .01$). A multicenter study of TMR sole treatment for 200 patients with refractory angina, who were considered not amenable to coronary angioplasty or bypass grafting, demonstrated efficacy in angina relief, decreased hospital admissions (2.5 vs. 0.5 admissions per patient year), and improved perfusion in myocardial segments with a perioperative mortality of 9% (7). A prospective, multicenter randomized trial of TMR versus maximum medical management in 162 patients with class IV angina demonstrated significantly reduced hospitalization at 3 months (20% vs. 43%) and improved angina class without significant increase in mortality (8). TMR appears to be an effective method of angina relief for end-stage CAD patients, with an almost immediate benefit postprocedure persisting to at least 1 year but which has a significant perioperative mortality risk.

MECHANISMS OF ACTION

The exact mechanism of action of TMR and PMR is much debated and remains poorly understood. There is conflicting evidence as to the long-term patency of the channels created. Channels patent as long as 3 years postprocedure have been reported (9–12). In human postmortem studies, the majority of these channels were found to be closed as early as 1 day postprocedure (13–15). Angiogenesis (14,16,17) and denervation (18,19) are postulated to be more likely mechanisms of action.

PMR (PMLR)

The disadvantage of CO_2 laser TMR is the need for general anesthesia and thoracotomy, with their associated risks. Thoracotomy is required because CO_2 laser energy is not transmissible via a flexible fiberoptic system, unlike a holmium:yttrium-aluminium-garnet (Ho:YAG) laser. Using Ho:YAG lasers and optical fibers, Jeevanandam et al. (20) and Yano et al. (21) created nontransmural channels from the endocardium via a left atrial approach in canines. They postulated that the procedure could be performed percutaneously and channels created from the endocardial surface. Kim and colleagues (22) demonstrated the feasibility of the percutaneous approach using a novel endovascular system in a canine model. This led to PMR use in clinical trials in humans. Currently, there are three PMR systems under study:

1. CardioGenesis PMR (CardioGenesis Corporation, Sunnyvale, CA) (Fig. 5.28): A 9 Fr braid-reinforced aligning or guiding catheter with a soft tip, which allows the passage of a 6 Fr braid-reinforced laser delivery catheter into the left ventricle. The laser delivery catheter has a central 400-μm optical fiber with a 1.75-mm lens mounted at the distal tip. The Ho:YAG laser has an output wavelength of 2.1 μm and produces 2-J pulses with a peak power of 5.7 kW and a fluence of 83 J per centimeter. Pulses are delivered in groups of two at a frequency of 17 Hz (''burst'').

2. Eclipse PTMR (Eclipse Surgical Technologies Inc., Sunnyvale, CA): Very similar to the previous system. There is no lens attached to

the optical fiber tip. This system also utilizes a Ho:YAG laser and has a wavelength of 2.1 μm and a 5- or 15-Hz pulse frequency.

3. NaviStar (Biosense Inc., Division of Johnson and Johnson, Cordis, Miami,FL) This is a 7 Fr system that incorporates an *in vivo* navigation technology using a magnetic sensor on the distal catheter tip. A three-dimensional roadmap is produced to allow accurate channel location. The Ho:YAG laser energy is delivered via a 300 μm optical fiber. Electrical and mechanical tip sensors offer the potential advantage of detecting viable myocardium for channel creation. This procedure has been named *direct myocardial revascularization* (DMR).

PROCEDURE

A 9 Fr femoral arterial sheath and a 7 or 8 Fr femoral venous sheath is introduced in the usual manner. Systemic anticoagulation is achieved with heparin bolus doses aiming for an activated clotting time (ACT) of 250 to 300 seconds. Occasionally, it may be necessary to use an esmolol infusion to reduce movement of the guiding catheter (which sits in the left ventricle) if a highly contractile ventricle confounds the operator's ability to torque and position the laser delivery catheter. Biplane coronary and/or bypass angiography and left venticulography are performed to aid delineation of the target treatment area. This is done using a transparent film that is

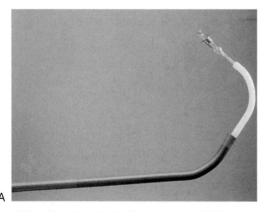
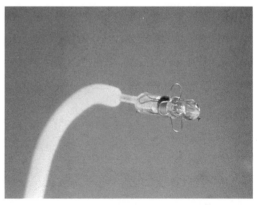

A   B

FIG. 5.28. The CardioGenesis Axcis PMR coaxial catheter system. **A:** 9 Fr aligning catheter delivers 6 Fr laser delivery catheter, a 400-μm optical fiber capped by a 1.75-mm lens. **B:** Close-up of the lens cap with extended nitinol "stops."

taped onto the two video monitors, which permit tracings of the coronary tree and left ventricular outline to be marked. This roadmap is used to help guide the laser catheter. The laser catheter is calibrated and checked before use. The CardioGenesis PMR guiding catheter is loaded onto a 6 Fr diagnostic catheter and introduced into the left ventricle. After the removal of the pigtail catheter, the laser catheter is advanced through the Tuohy-Borst valve, and once it exits the guiding catheter, the extendible optical fiber is positioned onto the endocardium. The coaxial catheter system permits multiple degrees of rotational and longitudinal movement so that the laser can reach all endocardial sites (Fig. 5.29). The tip is capped by a lens that has a series of petal-like structures made of nitinol (see Fig. 5.28). These stops retard full transmural advancement of the fiber–lens assembly during laser activation. Mild pressure is applied, and when firm contact between the laser fiber and the endocardium is achieved, the laser is fired (using the foot control). Contact should be confirmed fluoroscopically in orthogonal views by observing the laser catheter tip. Typically, a change of the tip motion from a slight reciprocating motion to a rhythmic beating constitutes adequate contact. This may be associated with the presence of ventricular extrasystoles. Typically, two "bursts" of two pulses (2 J per pulse) are delivered to create a channel. The laser delivers bursts approximately 100 to 150 ms after the QRS complex on the electrocardiogram (late systole). The channel site is marked on the roadmap in both planes. The laser catheter tip is retracted and repositioned under fluoroscopy for the next channel site. Using the roadmap, care is taken to avoid channel overlapping, which increases the possibility of ventricular perforation. Ten to 20 channels are created, depending on the area treated, with a suggested spacing of one channel per square centimeter. On completion, a postprocedure left ventriculogram is performed to assess myocardial function, channels (rarely seen), and undetected perforation (or ventricular septal defect if septum was treated). Sheaths may be removed once the ACT is < 180 seconds, or immediately if an arterial closure device is used. Patients are usually discharged the following day if the postprocedure echocardiogram excludes the presence of a pericardial effusion.

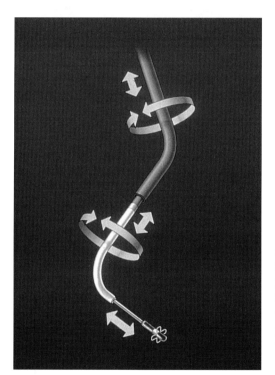

FIG. 5.29. Schematic representation of the CardioGenesis catheter system, demonstrating the multiple longitudinal and rotational aspects of movement.

ADVERSE EVENTS

In addition to the risks normally associated with a cardiac catheterization procedure, PMR increases the likelihood of left ventricular perforation, pericardial effusion, and potential tamponade. Immediate pericardiocentesis may be required. Channels created are approximately 6 mm in depth. PMR should be avoided if the preprocedural echocardiogram demonstrates the wall thickness of the target treatment area to be <8 mm. A ventricular septal defect may be formed if perforation of the septum occurs. Significant aortic stenosis is a contraindication to PMR, because the guiding catheter may critically impede flow. Arrhythmias and new bundle branch block may be alleviated with catheter repositioning in the majority of cases.

EFFICACY

Little has been published on the effectiveness of PMR. Initial experience in pilot studies suggests that PMR is technically feasible and safe (23). There was no procedural or immediate postprocedure mortality in 30 treated patients, but one ventricular perforation necessitated pericardiocentesis (23). Lauer et al. (24) reported 16 PMR-treated patients, six of which had improved angina class with a nonsignificant trend toward improved exercise capacity and improved myocardial perfusion at 3 months. Large-scale PMR efficacy studies are ongoing:

THE PACIFIC STUDY

Potential Angina Class Improvement from Intramyocardial Channels

This is a large randomized multicenter trial in the United States and the United Kingdom comparing CardioGenesis PMR (system) and maximal convention medical therapy in 200 patients with Canadian angina class III or IV symptoms. These patients have advanced coronary disease that is not amenable to coronary angioplasty or bypass grafting. Additionally, presence of reversible ischemia on dipyridamole thallium scanning and an LVEF >30% is required for inclusion in the study. Angina class, exercise tolerance (treadmill test), myocardial perfusion (dipyridamole thallium scan), and quality of life (Seattle angina questionnaire) are assessed at 3, 6, and 12 months postprocedure. The trial completed recruitment as of July 1998.

The six-month clinical results were presented at the American College of Cardiology in March of 1999. The data suggested that 70% of the patients treated with PMR had their angina reduced to Class I or II after six months, as compared to less than 10% with medical therapy (25).

CURRENT STATUS

PMR is emerging as a feasible alternative myocardial revascularization technique for the end-stage CAD patient. Current studies seek to confirm its safety and efficacy in this setting.

Despite reports of lowered TMR perioperative mortality rates (26), the lower procedural risks of PMR make it more appealing and may lead to its use in a broader range of patients. PMR as an adjunct to coronary intervention is currently under study. TMR has also been used with some success in allograft CAD (27), suggesting another possible role for PMR.

REFERENCES

1. Wearn JT, Mettier SR, Klempp TG, Zschiesche LJ. The nature of the vascular communications between the coronary arteries and the chambers of the heart. *Am Heart J* 1933;9:143–164.
2. Sen PK, Udwadia TE, Kinare SG, Parulkar GB. Transmyocardial acupuncture: a new approach to myocardial revascularization. *J Thorac Cardiovasc Surg* 1965;50:181–189.
3. Mirhoseini M, Cayton MM. Revascularization of the heart by laser. *J Microsurg* 1981;2:253–260.
4. Mirhoseini M, Muckerheide M, Cayton MM. Transventricular revascularization by laser. *Lasers Surg Med* 1982;2:187–198.
5. Mirhoseini M, Shelgikar S, Cayton MM. New concepts in revascularization of the myocardium. *Ann Thorac Surg* 1988;45:415–420.
6. Cooley DA, Frazier OH, Kadipasaoglu KA, et al. Transmyocardial laser revascularization: clinical experience with twelve month follow-up. *J Thorac Cardiovasc Surg* 1996;111:791–799.
7. Horvath KA, Cohn LH, Cooley DA, et al. Transmyocardial laser revascularization: results of a multicenter trial with transmyocardial laser revascularization used as sole therapy for end-stage coronary artery disease. *J Thorac Cardiovasc Surg* 1997;113:645–654.
8. Allen KB, Fudge TL, Selinger SL, Dowling RD. Prospective randomized multicenter trial of transmyocardial revascularization versus maximal medical management in patients with class IV angina. *Circulation* 1997;96(Suppl I):I-564.
9. Horvath KA, Smith WJ, Laurence RG, Schoen FJ, Appleyard RF, Cohn LH. Recovery and viability of an acute myocardial infarct after transmyocardial laser revascularization. *J Am Coll Cardiol* 1995;25:258–263.
10. Cooley DA, Frazier OH, Kadipasaoglu KA, Pehlivanoglu S, Shannon RL, Angelini P. Transmyocardial laser revascularization: anatomic evidence of long-term channel patency. *Tex Heart Inst J* 1994;21:220–224.
11. Okada M, Shimizu K, Ikuta H, Horii H, Nakamura K. A new method of myocardial revascularization by laser. *Thorac Cardiovasc Surg* 1991;39:1–4.
12. Whittaker P, Rakusan K, Kloner RA. Transmural channels can protect ischemic tissue: assessment of long-term myocardial response to laser- and needle-made channels. *Circulation* 1996;93:143–152.
13. Krabatsch T, Schaper F, Leder C, Tulsner J, Thalmann U, Hetzer R. Histological findings after transmyocardial laser revascularization. *J Cardiovasc Surg* 1996;11:326–331.
14. Gassler N, Wintzer HO, Stubbe HM, Wullbrand A, Helmchen U. Transmyocardial laser revascularization:

histological features in human nonresponder myocardium. *Circulation* 1997;95:371–375.

15. Burkhoff D, Fisher PE, Apfelbaum M, Kohmoto T, DeRosa CM, Smith CR. Histological appearance of transmyocardial laser channels after 4 1/2 weeks. *Ann Thorac Surg* 1996;61:1532–1535.

16. Kohmoto T, Fisher PE, DeRosa C, Smith CR, Burkhoff D. Evidence of angiogenesis in regions treated with transmyocardial laser revascularization. *Circulation* 1996;94(Suppl II):294

17. Kohmoto T, DeRosa CM, Yamamoto N, et al. Evidence of vascular growth associated with laser treatment of normal canine myocardium. *Ann Thorac Surg* 1998;65:1360–1367.

18. Whittaker P, Kloner R, Przyklenk K.Laser-mediated transmural myocardial channels do not salvage acutely ischemic myocardium. *J Am Coll Cardiol* 1993;22:302–309.

19. Kwong KF, Kanellopoulos GK, Nickols JC, et al. Transmyocardial laser treatment denervates canine myocardium. *J Thorac Cardiovasc Surg* 1997;114:883–889.

20. Jeevanandam V, Auteri JS, Oz MC, Watkins J, Rose EA, Smith CR. Myocardial revascularization by laser induced channels. *Surg Forum* 1990;41:225–227.

21. Yano OJ, Bielefeld MR, Jeevanandam V, et al. Prevention of acute regional ischemia with endocardial laser channels. *Ann Thorac Surg* 1993;56:46–53.

22. Kim CB, Kesten R, Javier M, et al. Percutaneous method of laser transmyocardial revascularization. *Cathet Cardiovasc Diagn* 1997;40:223–228.

23. Oesterle SN, Reifart N, Meier B, Lauer B, Schuler G. Laser-based percutaneous myocardial revascularization (PMR): initial human experience. *Am J Cardiol* 1998;82:659–662.

24. Lauer B, Junghans U, Stahl F, Brennan E, Oesterle S, Schuler G. Percutaneous myocardial revascularization, a new approach to patients with intractable angina *pectoris.J Am Coll Cardiol* 1998;31(Suppl A):214A.

25. Oesterle SN, Yeung A, Ali N, et al. The CardioGenesis Percutaneous Myocardial Revascularization (PMR) Randomized Trial: Initial clinical results. *J Am Coll Cardiol* 1999;33:380A(abstr).

26. Krabatsch T, Tambeur L, Lieback E, Shaper F, Hetzer R. Transmyocardial laser revascularization in the treatment of end stage coronary artery disease. *Ann Thorac Cardiovasc Surg* 1998;4:64–71.

27. Frazier OH, Kadipasaoglu KA, Radovancevic B, et al. Transmyocardial laser revascularization in allograft coronary artery disease. *Ann Thorac Surg* 1998;65:1138–1141.

F. Catheter-Based Radiation Therapy for Restenosis

Ron Waksman

Experimental Angioplasty and Vascular Brachytherapy, Cardiology Research Foundation, Washington Hospital Center, Washington, DC 20010

Restenosis following coronary intervention remains a significant clinical concern (1,2). It has proven refractory to numerous pharmacologic interventions in clinical trials using several different classes of compounds, including growth inhibitors, anticoagulants, calcium channel blockers, fish oils, lipid-lowering drugs, and others (3–5).

The major components of restenosis are felt to be due to elastic recoil that occurs immediately after all interventions except stenting. Second is an exuberant cellular proliferation and matrix synthesis, and third is vascular constriction that occurs late in the healing process (6,7).

Since the discovery of x-rays by Roentgen 100 years ago, ionizing radiation has been recognized to interact biologically. The earliest applications for brachytherapy were to treat surface lesions. Brachytherapy was later developed for intracavity treatment of cervical and uterine tumors. Later, ionizing radiation demonstrated effectiveness in the treatment of benign diseases, such as prevention of keloid formation, pterigium of the eye, and osteotrophic bone formation after hip replacement, and so on (8–12). In 1965, before the angioplasty and the restenosis eras, Friedman et al. (13) reported the use of iridium 192 (14 Gy) delivered intraluminally to injured aorta of cholesterol-fed rabbits, and demonstrated inhibition of smooth muscle cell proliferation and intimal hyperplasia in the irradiated atherosclerotic arteries.

The effect of radiation therapy for the prevention of restenosis was tested initially by using external beam radiation. Sporadic early reports suggested the effectiveness of this treatment in reducing neointimal formation after vascular injury in rat carotid. External radiation following stent implantation in porcine coronaries was reported to give unfavorable results (14).

In the last decade of this century, a new initiative to deliver the radiation intraluminally was examined in preclinical models and in a few clinical trials, with encouraging results. Those facilitated the creation of a new field in interventional cardiology and radiation oncology: vascular brachytherapy.

This chapter discusses basic radiation biology and radiation physics, and reviews the status of preclinical and clinical studies in the field.

RADIATION PHYSICS

Isotope selection and dosimetry for intracoronary brachytherapy are derived from the anatomy of the vessel and the treated lesion and by knowing the target tissue for this therapy. Other important parameters are the diameter and the curvature of the vessel, the eccentricity of the plaque, the lesion length, the composition of the plaque, the amount of calcium, and the presence or absence of stent in the treated segment. Gamma- and beta-emitting radionuclides are currently being investigated and are in use in the clinical trials for vascular brachytherapy. A selected list of radioisotopes tested and used in clinical trials is presented in Table 5.18. The requirements for ideal radioisotopes for vascular brachytherapy should include the following: dose distribution of a few millimeters from the source with minimal dose gradient, low dose levels to the surrounding tissues and minimal exposure to the patient and the personnel, treatment time less than 10 minutes, and sufficient half-life for multiple applications when used for catheter-based systems. Other considerations of source selection are the source energy, availability in the right activity, and low cost.

Dosimetry is the determination of the dose at different distances from the source. Among the methods of dosimetry is theoretical modeling, such as the Monte Carlo calculations using standard algorithms. The use of point sources for vascular brachytherapy requires determination of the dose distribution of point sources, called point kernels or point dose functions, which can also be reconstructed from results of serial of measurements. There are various methods of actual measurements and detection of the dose. The most common are the use of films and scanners at various distances from the source and the use of thermoluminescent dosimeters (TLDs) made from lithium fluoride. Other methods are use of ion chambers, calorimeters, and liquid scintillation counters and semiconductor spectrometers to determine the energy of the emission.

The American Association of Physicists in Medicine established Task Group 60 and published their recommendations of dose prescription points at a depth of 2 mm from the source for the intracoronary application, and at 1 mm larger than the average lumen radius for peripheral application (15).

The dosimetry of radioactive stents is even more complicated and dependent on the stent geometry, which varies across stent designs. The currently tested radioactive stents lack dose

TABLE 5.18. *Radionucleides for vascular brachytherapy*

Isotope	Emission	Half-life	Energy maximum (MeV)	Energy average (MeV)	Activity required
^{192}Ir	γ	74 d	0.67	0.18	500 mCi
^{125}I	x-ray	60 d	0.035	0.028	3 Ci
^{103}Pd	x-ray	17 d	0.021	0.021	4 Ci
^{90}Sr/Y	β	29 yr	2.28	0.93	50 mCi
^{90}Y	β	64 h	2.28	0.93	50 mCi
^{32}P	β	14 d	1.71	0.69	40 mCi
^{188}W/Re	β, γ	69 d	2.12^a	0.77^a	50 mCi
^{133}Xe	β, γ	5.2 d	0.35^a	0.10^a	300 mCi
^{186}Re	β	90 h	1.08	0.38	300 mCi
^{188}Re	β, γ	17 h	2.12^a	0.77^a	100 mCi
^{106}Rh	β, γ	130 d	3.54^a	1.42^a	30 mCi

^{a} Beta energy only.

homogeneity across their entire lengths (16). This could affect the biologic response to radiation, especially at the stent edges. In addition, low-activity radioactive stents may be associated with ineffective low-dose rate, while radioactive stents with high activity may deliver toxic doses to the stented area, may delay the reendothelialization, and will promote stent thrombosis and necrosis in tissue surrounding the stent.

UNDERSTANDING GAMMA RADIATION

Gamma rays are photons originating from the center of the nucleus, as opposed to x-rays, which originate from the orbital outside of the nucleus. Gamma rays have energies between 20 keV and 2 MeV, and they are deeply penetrating, which requires an excess of shielding in comparison with the use of beta and x-ray emitters. The only gamma ray isotope currently in use is iridium 192 (^{192}Ir). Other isotopes that emit both gamma and x rays are iodine 125 (^{125}I) and palladium 103 (^{103}Pd), which have lower energies and require high activities for the dose prescribed for this application within an acceptable dwell time (<20 minutes). The latter either are not available in such activities or are too expensive for this application. Iridium 192 is available in activities up to 10 Ci, but due to its high penetration, an average shielding of a catheterization laboratory will not be sufficient to handle activity above 0.5 Ci. This limitation is associated with a prolonged dwell time of more than 12 minutes for doses above 15 GY when prescribed at a 2-mm radial distance from the source; in addition, personnel are required to leave the room during treatment.

UNDERSTANDING BETA RADIATION

Beta rays are high-energy electrons emitted by nuclei and contain too many or too few neutrons. These negatively charged particles have a wide variety of energies. Several of these have transition energy, especially in the parent–daughter pair. An example of such a pair is the strontium/yttrium 90 (^{90}Sr/Y) pair of pure beta emitters, which have transition energies of 0.54 and 2.27 MeV, respectively.

Beta emitters have a wide range of half-lives, from several minutes (^{62}Cu) to almost 30 years (^{90}Sr/Y). Beta emitters rapidly lose their energy to the surrounding tissue, and their range is within 1 cm of tissue. Therefore, they are associated with a higher gradient to the near wall. The use of beta sources for vascular application is attractive from the radiation exposure and the safety points of view. Shielding requirements are minimal due to lower levels of radiation exposure, personnel are allowed to stay in proximity to the source, and the dwell time is shorter compared with the use of gamma radiation. However, the electrons, by interacting with the electric field of the atomic nucleus, can create a photon; this mechanism creates the bremsstrahlung phenomenon, which is associated with additional exposure. The short range of penetration of the beta sources can limit their use in larger vessels and requires precise positioning of the source, with wide margins to cover the treated lesions and to prevent the edge effect. When beta emitters are selected for vascular brachytherapy, shielding of previous stents and calcified plaque may require an increase in the prescribed dose of up to 20%. Dose distribution measurements of beta emitters are often more complicated than with gamma emitters. Another limitation of beta sources is the requirements of the use of sealed sources, which may affect their size and flexibility for use in coronary arteries. Finally, beta sources require more centered delivery systems to secure homogeneity of the dose to the surrounding tissue.

RADIATION BIOLOGY AND MECHANISM

The principal mechanism of radiation biology for prevention of restenosis is one that causes death to radiosensitive cells, especially those that are undergoing mitosis following vascular injury. Cell death results from chromosomal damage and is dependent on the cumulative dose, the dose rate, and the cell cycle.

An understanding of the action of radiation is gained by performing survival cell curves for different doses of radiation. A linear curve represents a direct relation between the prescribed dose and the number of killed cells. A nonlinear curve is seen more frequently with a single high dose of radiation, and cell kill increases disproportionately. The result is variability of responses among different types of cells. The damage of radiation is done at the molecular level within nanoseconds after irradiation, but the cells do not die immediately; the damage continues for years.

Repair occurs immediately after the induction of the radiation, and with low doses may be associated with complete repair. Potentially, therefore, recurrence of restenosis may be delayed if the dose of radiation is not sufficient to inhibit complete repair.

For some cells, radiation-induced apoptosis (programmed cell death) may occur, although this may not be the main mechanism for the effect of radiation on myofibroblasts (17). Hall et al. (18) have shown that human endothelial and smooth muscle cells have similar survival curves and suggested that inhibition of smooth muscle cells will result in inhibition of endothelial cells. Cells can repair radiation damage; therefore, a subtherapeutic dose may only delay the restenosis, because the surviving cells will continue to divide and eventually occupy the lumen wall.

Lower dose rates are less effective and require higher cumulative doses to reach the therapeutic window. Thus, there is a minimum dose rate that would be effective for intervening in the cell cycle to stop cell division (15).

Late effects of vascular brachytherapy may be seen 5 to 10 years following the treatment. Among potential late effects are late thrombosis, fibrosis, thinning of the media, and aneurysm formation (19).

Some of the potential mechanisms by which radiation may reduce restenosis were examined in a series of studies performed on pig coronary arteries by Waksman et al. (17).

Following balloon overstretch injury, the arteries were treated with ^{90}Sr/Y (14 or 28 Gy prescribed to a depth of 2 mm), and animals were killed 3, 7, and 14 days later. 5-Bromo-2-deoxyuridine (BrdU) was administered 24 hours before sacrifice to label proliferating cells. By 3 days postinjury, cell proliferation, assessed by BrdU immunostaining, was significantly reduced in the media and the adventitia of irradiated vessels as compared with control arteries.

However, there were no significant differences in the adventitia and the media by 7 days in the irradiated arteries when compared with controls. Alpha-actin staining for smooth muscle cells and myofibroblasts, which was used as an index for remodeling, was lower in the adventitia of the irradiated vessels by 2 weeks after the injury. A larger vessel perimeter was found in irradiated vessels in a dose-dependent fashion, suggestive of favorable remodeling. Additionally, TUNEL (terminal deoxyribonucleotidyl transferase end labeling) detected apoptosis at 3 and 7 days in injured arteries and irradiated injured segments, with no significant difference in the degree of apoptosis between these two groups (17). The degree of apoptosis at earlier or later time points has not been analyzed; it is possible that earlier (at day 1) or later (at day 14), there would be a significant difference between irradiated and nonirradiated vessels. However, it is not expected that substantial apoptosis will be detected in long-term (>6-month) follow-up.

These studies suggest that endovascular radiation reduces restenosis by inhibiting the first wave of cell proliferation in the adventitia and the media, and by inducing favorable remodeling. Long-term studies are necessary to determine whether this effect is long lasting or merely delays intimal proliferation and negative remodeling. Additional studies are also necessary to determine whether proinflammatory cytokines such as interferon-γ (IFN-γ), tumor necrosis factor-α (TNF-α), and interleukin-1 (IL-1), as well as antiinflammatory cytokines such as transforming growth factor-β1 (TGF-β1), known to be induced by radiation, are involved in the antirestenotic effect of endovascular radiation (20–22).

DEVICES AND TECHNOLOGY

The platforms for delivery of radionuclides into the coronary arteries are via either catheter-based systems (high dose rate) or radioactive stents (low dose rate). Among the catheter-based systems used in clinical trials are fixed radioactive wire lengths of 26 to 30 mm (Angiorad, Louisiana), radioactive seeds embedded in a nylon ribbon (Best International, Springfield, VA), and radioactive seeds delivered hydrauli-

TABLE 5.20. *Summary of completed beta and gamma clinical trials*

Study Investigator Sponsor	Study design	Radiation system	Dose (Gy)	Results and status
Venezuela Condado et al.(40) Angiorad	Open-label, radiation post balloon angioplasty in 21 pts (22 native coronary arteries)	Hand delivered 0.014-in. or 0.018-in., 30-mm iridium wire into a noncentered 4 Fr closed-end lumen catheter. (Angiorad)	20 and 25 actual doses 19–55	Completed. Clinical and angiographic follow-up at 8 and 36 mo demonstrated safety and low late loss
SCRIPPS Teirstein et al. (42) Best Medical	Single-center, double-blind, randomized in 55 pts with restenosis and stenting	Hand-delivered 0.030-in. ribbon with ^{192}Ir seeds (Best Medical) into a closed-end lumen, noncentered 4.5 Fr catheter (Navius)	≥8 to <30 to media by IVUS	Showed reduction of restenosis in irradiated group by clinical, IVUS, and angiogram at 6 mo
WRIST Waksman et al. (43) CRF, WHC	Single-center, double-blind, randomized in 130 pts with in-stent restenosis (100 native; 30 SVG)	Hand-delivered 0.030-in. nylon ribbon with seeds (Best Medical) into a noncentered, closed-end lumen, 5 Fr catheter (Medtronic)	15 Gy at 2.0 mm from source in vessels 3–4 mm	Significant reduction in restenosis rate (67%) and need for revascularization (63%)
GAMMA 1 Leon et al. (44) Cordis	Multicenter, double-blind, randomized in 250 pts with in-stent restenosis	Hand-delivered 0.030-in. ribbon with seeds into a noncentered, closed-end lumen 4 Fr catheter	≥8 to <30 to media (IVUS)	Significant reduction in restenosis rate and need for revascularization
ARTISTIC Waksman et al. (45) Vascular Therapies	Multicenter, double-blind, randomized in 290 pts with in-stent restenosis	Mechanical delivery of 0.014-in., fixed-wire, 30-mm (Angiorad) into a monorail closed-end lumen balloon centering	12, 15, 18 to 2-mm distance	Feasibility phase in 25 pts completed, with low restenosis rate multicenter initiated in the summer of 1998
ARREST Faxon et al. (46) Vascular Therapies	Double-blind, randomized in 700 pts post PTCA and provisional stenting	Mechanical delivery of 0.014-in., fixed-wire, 30-mm (Angiorad system) centering balloon, 3.2 Fr catheter	>8 to <35 to media by IVUS	Feasibility phase completed, 25 pts, multicenter will start in 1999
Geneva Verin et al. (47) Schneider	Open-label in 15 pts after PTCA In *de-novo* lesions	Mechanical loading of 0.014-in., 29-mm, fixed-wire via a segmented, centered, 30-mm balloon (2.5–4.0 mm)	18 to vessel wall	Demonstrated feasibility, safety, restenosis rate (40%)
BERT King et al. (48) Novoste	Open-label in 84 pts post PTCA in *de novo* lesions	Hydraulic hand delivery of a train of 12 radioactive seeds (30 mm) in a noncentered 5 Fr catheter	[90]Sr/Y 12, 14, 16 at 2 mm	Demonstrated safety, restenosis rate of 17% with late loss of 0.05 at 6 mo
PREVENT Raizner (28) Guidant	Multinational, open-label feasibility study in 80 pts after PTCA or stenting. (Phase I)	Automatic afterloader (Nucletron), 0.018-in., 27-mm, fixed-wire ^{32}P via a helical centering balloon (2.5–4.0 mm)	[32]P 16, 20, 24 at 1 mm	Demonstrated safety, lower late loss, TLR in irradiated group vs. control

pts, patients.

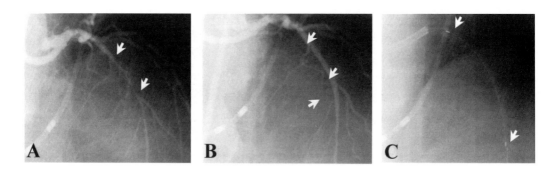

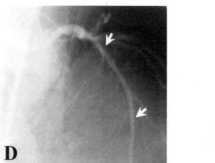
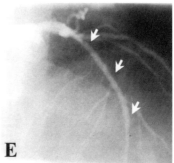

FIG. 5.31. A series of angiograms of a patient treated with gamma radiation from the Gamma radiation trial for in-stent restenosis. **A:** Preintervention. **B:** After rotational atherectomy and restenting. **C:** Radiation therapy. **D:** Final result after radiation therapy. **E:** Six-month follow-up angiogram.

There was a 79% decrease in the need for revascularization and a 63% decrease in major cardiac events (death, Q-wave myocardial infarction, and any revascularization) in the irradiated group compared with control. Intravascular ultrasound subanalysis demonstrated regression of tissue in 53% at follow-up of the irradiated arteries. The WRIST study is considered to be a landmark in the establishment of gamma radiation for the treatment of in-stent restenosis. Other studies in this series include LONG WRIST, which examined the effectiveness of the same system in long lesions (36 to 80 mm) in 120 patients. LONG WRIST HIGH DOSE is a registry of 60 patients, with the same inclusion exclusion criteria as the LONG WRIST study for vessels up to 4 mm in diameter. The prescribed dose is 15 Gy at 2.4 mm from the source. SVG WRIST is a multicenter study using the same system and protocol for 120 patients with in-stent restenosis in a vein graft.

GAMMA 1 is a multicenter, randomized, double-blind trial in which 250 patients were being enrolled for treatment for in-stent restenosis with a hand-delivered ^{192}Ir ribbon source, while the dosimetry is guided by intravascular ultrasound (doses between 8 and 30 Gy). Recently, the 6-month angiographic results showed a significant reduction in the in-stent angiographic restenosis rate in the radiation arm (21.6%) compared with control (52%). Subanalysis for lesion length demonstrated a 70% reduction in the angiographic restenosis rate for lesions <30 mm in length versus only a 48% reduction for lesion lengths between 30 and 45 mm (44). In addition, an edge effect was noted in patients who did not have enough coverage of the lesion by the radioactive seeds.

ARTISTIC (Angiorad Radiation Technology for In-Stent restenosis Trial in native Coronaries) is a study in which a 0.014-in., fixed, 30-mm ^{192}Ir wire is being used in a blinded, randomized manner in 300 patients with in-stent restenosis in native coronary arteries. The pilot phase of the study in 26 patients has been completed, and 6-month angiographic follow-up was reported: low binary restenosis rates (10%), lower late loss index (0.12), and lower major cardiac adverse events (15%) (45).

ARREST (Angiorad Radiation for Restenosis Trial) is a multicenter pilot study in 25 patients and was recently completed. Patients enrolled with *de novo* or restenotic lesions and were treated with balloon angioplasty alone and then with open-label radiation therapy using the Angiorad radiation system with a fixed ^{192}Ir wire source and dosimetry based on IVUS findings. The pilot study demonstrated feasibility and safety. However, the angiographic restenosis rate in this feasibility cohort was 45% and was explained by the underdosing of the target area (< 8 Gy to the adventitia) (46).

SMARTS (SMall Artery Radiation Therapy Study) is a randomized trial in 180 patients with small-vessel disease (2.0 to 2.75 mm) treated with gamma radiation (^{192}Ir).

Beta Clinical Trials

The clinical trials using beta emitters were initially designed to examine the effectiveness of beta radiation therapy for prevention of restenosis for *de novo* lesions in native coronaries. More recent studies have been initiated to test the effectiveness of beta radiation for in-stent restenosis.

The Geneva Experience examined the ^{90}Y source following PTCA in a small cohort of 15 patients. Although the investigators were able to demonstrate the feasibility of the radiation system, the outcome of this study was disappointing, because five of 15 patients in this trial experienced angiographic and clinical restenosis (47). The investigators related their results to insufficient dose to the adventitia (<5 Gy) and have since initiated a dose-finding multicenter study of 160 patients in Europe, utilizing doses of 9 to 18 Gy prescribed to 1 mm from the surface of the balloon with the use of an automatic afterloader.

BERT (Beta Energy Restenosis Trial) was a feasibility study approved by the Food and Drug Administration and was limited to 23 patients in two centers (Emory University and Brown University). The study was designed to test the ^{90}Sr/Y source delivered by a hydraulic system (Novoste Corp., Norcross, GA). The prescribed doses in this study were 12, 14, or 16 Gy, and the treatment time was not to exceed 3.5 minutes. The radiation was successfully delivered to 21 of 23 patients following conventional PTCA without any complications or adverse events at 30 days. At follow-up, two patients (at 6 months) and one patient (at 9 months) underwent repeat revascularization to the target lesion (48). The Canadian arm of this study included 30 patients from the Montreal Heart Institute (49,50), and the European arm, BERT 1.5, was conducted in an additional 30 patients at the Thoraxcenter in Rotterdam, utilizing the same system under the same protocol. At 6-month follow-up, the angiographic restenosis rate for the entire cohort of 84 patients was 17%, with a lower late loss of 9%. However six more patients required revascularization due to an edge effect near the treated lesion. A case profile using the system is presented in Fig. 5.32.

The BETACATH trial was initiated in July 1997 as a prospective, randomized, placebo-controlled trial to evaluate the safety and effectiveness of the ^{90}Sr/Y BetaCath System versus placebo in *de novo* or restenotic lesions of native coronary arteries. A total of 1,100 patients who underwent elective PTCA or provisional stent placement were enrolled in 27 centers, and the angiographic follow-up at 8 months will be available by the beginning of the year 2000. The results of this study will determine the future of this technology for clinical use for prevention of restenosis.

BRIE (Beta Radiation in Europe) is a registry of 150 patients that will allow treatment of multivessels with the BetaCath system, using ^{90}Sr/Y source doses of 14 and 16 Gy.

PREVENT (Proliferation Reduction with Vascular Energy Trial) is a prospective, randomized, blinded, multinational, multicenter study, the objective of which is to demonstrate the safety of the Guidant (Santa Clara, CA) beta radiation system in human coronaries immediately

Pre-Treatment   **Post-Treatment**   **6-Month FU**

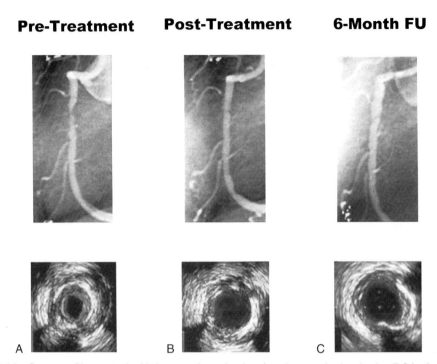

A   B   C

FIG. 5.32. Case profile treated with beta catheterization for *de novo* lesion in the RCA. **A:** Prior to the procedure. **B:** Following balloon angioplasty and radiation. **C:** Six-month angiographic follow-up.

following PTCA or stent placement. The system consists of a ^{32}P isotope, 27 mm in length, delivered into a centering helical balloon delivery catheter via an automatic afterloader apparatus. The doses used in this open-label phase are 16, 20, and 24 Gy prescribed to 1 mm from the source. The feasibility phase of the study was completed in May 1998, and the preliminary results suggest low rates of late loss in the irradiated group (4.8%) compared with control (51.3%), with a significant reduction in the need for target lesion revascularization (4% vs. 18%). However, due to an increase in the edge effect, the target lesion revascularization rates were similar in the treated vessels (24%) versus control (29%). Subanalysis of patients with in-stent restenosis treated with ^{32}P demonstrated lower rates of recurrence compared with a matched control group from the WRIST study.

CURE (Columbia University Radiation Energy) is the first use of a liquid-filled balloon system in a feasibility clinical trial. It was used in 30 patients after balloon angioplasty or in 30 patients who are underwent intracoronary stenting (51,52). The study was initiated at Columbia University (New York, NY) under an institutional IDE (Institutional Device Exemption). The isotope in the liquid form is ^{188}Re, retrieved from a tungsten 188 generator and injected via syringe into a perfusion balloon (Lifestream, Guidant, Santa Clara, CA) to allow a dwell time of up to 10 minutes. The restenosis rate in this cohort was 24%. The system demonstrated feasibility and safety.

MARS (Mallinckrodt Angioplasty Radiation Study) is a multicenter feasibility study utilizing a liquid ^{186}Re beta emitter source for prevention of restenosis in *de novo* and restenotic lesions. The study was initiated in the Netherlands and is about to expand to Canada.

Studies to examine the effectiveness of beta radiation systems in preventing recurrence of in-stent restenosis have been launched; among them are BETA WRIST (^{90}Y), INHIBIT (^{32}P), and START 90 (^{90}Sr/Y). These studies are similar in design and aim to address the efficacy of beta emitters for the treatment of restenosis, in order to get an expedited approval for marketing in the United States.

BETA WRIST is the first study to report about the efficacy of beta radiation for prevention of in-stent restenosis. This is a registry of 50 patients that underwent treatment for in-stent restenosis in native coronaries and were treated with a beta radiation system using the ^{90}Y source, a centering catheter, and an afterloader system. The clinical outcome of these patients underwent comparison with the control group of the original cohort of WRIST, which demonstrated a reduction of >50% for the need of target lesion or vessel revascularization. Comparison of the outcome of the irradiated beta group with the gamma group did not detect major differences between them (53).

The BETA WRIST study suggested that in-stent restenosis treatment with beta emitters may produce an outcome similar to that shown with gamma emitters.

So far, the lessons from the beta feasibility studies were that the radiation effect is confined to the length of the source, and longer beta sources are required to cover the entire segment undergoing intervention to eliminate the edge effect phenomenon.

CONCLUSIONS AND FUTURE PERSPECTIVES

Initial data from the preclinical work and the clinical experience from the feasibility clinical trials lead to the conclusion that vascular brachytherapy is a breakthrough adjunct therapy to vascular intervention. So far, gamma radiation using ^{192}Ir was proved in three randomized clinical trials to have a robust effect on prevention of recurrences for patients with in-stent restenosis following intervention. Based on the SCRIPPS, WRIST, and Gamma 1 trials, this therapy should be standard for patients who present with in-stent restenosis.

Another observation from all clinical trials is the effect on reduction of angiographic late loss with radiation therapy. BETA WRIST provides insights that beta emitters will be effective as well for the treatment of in-stent restenosis if

the right dose is provided to the right target. Dosimetry still seems to play a major role in the success of the technology, and although not proved by a head-to-head study, delivery systems with centering capability should provide a more homogenous dose to the target area.

The latest data from the clinical trials identified two major complications that require a solution. The edge effect phenomenon, which is seen primarily with the radioactive stent, is also reported to occur with a catheter-based system, both with beta and gamma emitters, especially when the treated area is not covered with wide margins. Late thrombosis after vascular brachytherapy is a serious complication reported in every clinical trial. This phenomenon of late thrombosis was associated more frequently with additional stent implantation, probably due to the delayed healing associated with radiation. A potential solution to the occurrence of late thrombosis is to prolong treatment with the use of antiplatelet therapy, which is currently being done in a few protocols prescribed to 3 months.

With continuing positive results from the ongoing clinical trials, it is likely that catheter-based radiation therapy will play a permanent role in the field of interventional cardiology and radiology for the prevention of restenosis. Currently, we are in the midst of investigation and exploration of the mechanisms by which radiation prevents restenosis. Furthermore, numerous studies looking at new isotopes and delivery systems should enable interventionists to use this technology more comfortably in the cardiac catheterization laboratory. In Europe, several systems have already received the CE market. In the United States, however, the first indication for marketing approval will probably be for in-stent restenosis, and the first approval is estimated to occur in the year 2000.

REFERENCES

1. Holmes DR Jr, Vlietstra RE, Smith HC, et al. Restenosis after percutaneous transluminal coronary angioplasty (PTCA): a report from the PTCA registry of the National Heart, Lung and Blood Institute. *Am J Cardiol* 1984; 53:77C–81C.
2. Pickering JG, Weir L, Janowski J, Kearney MA, Isner JM. Proliferative activity in peripheral and coronary ath-

erosclerotic plaque among patients undergoing percutaneous revascularization. *J Clin Invest* 1993;91:1469–1480.

3. Thornton MA, Gruentzig AR, Hollman J, King SB III, Douglas JS. Coumadin and aspirin in prevention of recurrence after transluminal coronary angioplasty: a randomized study. *Circulation* 1984;4:721–727.

4. Ellis SG, Roubin GS, Wilentz J, Douglas JS Jr, King SB III. Effect of 18- to 24-hour heparin administration for prevention of restenosis after uncomplicated coronary angioplasty. *Am Heart J* 1989;41(17):777–782.

5. Pepine CJ, Hirshfield JW, Macdonald RG, et al. A controlled trial of corticosteroids to prevent restenosis after coronary angioplasty. *Circulation* 1990;81:1753–1761.

6. Post MJ, Borst C, Kuntz RE, et al. The relative importance of arterial remodeling compared with intimal hyperplasia in lumen renarrowing after balloon angioplasty. A study in the normal rabbit and the hypercholesterolemic Yucatan micropig. *Circulation* 1994;89:2816–2821.

7. O'Brien ER, Alpers CE, Stewart DK, et al. Proliferation in primary and restenotic coronary atherectomy tissue: implications for antiproliferative therapy. *Circ Res* 1993 :223–231.

8. Puck TT, Morkovin D, Marcus PI, et al. Action of x-rays on mammalian cells: II. Survival curves of cells from normal human tissues. *J Exp Med* 1957;106:485–500.

9. Sinclair WK. Cyclic x-ray response in mammalian cells *in vitro*. *Radiat Res* 1968;63:620–643.

10. Fischer-Dzoga K, Dimitrievich GS, Griem ML. Differential radiosensitivity of aortic cells *in vitro*. *Radiat Res* 1984;99:536–546.

11. Fischer-Dzoga K, Dimitrievich GS, Schaffner T. Effect of hyperlipemic serum and irradiation on wound healing in primary quiescent cultures of vascular cells. *Exp Mol Pathol* 1989;52:1–12.

12. Nickson JJ, Lawrence W Jr, Rachwalsky I, et al. Roentgen rays and wound healing: II. Fractionated irradiation: experimental study. *Surgery* 1953;34:859–862.

13. Friedman M, Byers SO. Effects of iridium 192 radiation on thromboatherosclerotic plaque in the rabbit aorta. Arch Pathol 19XX':285–291.

14. Schwartz R, Huber K, Murphy J, Edwards W, Vilestra R, Holmes DR Jr. Restenosis and the proportional neointima response to coronary artery injury results in the porcine model. *J Am Coll Cardiol* 1992;19:267–274.

15. Nath R, Amols H, Coffey C, et al. Intravascular brachytherapy physics: report of the AAPM Radiation Task Group No. 60. *Med Phys* 1998.

16. Janicki C, Duggan DM, Coffey CW, Fischell DR, Fischell TA. Radiation dose from a phosphorous-32 impregnated wire mesh vascular stent. *Med Phys* 1995;24(3):437–445.

17. Waksman R, Rodriquez JC, Robinson KA, et al. Effect of intravascular irradiation on cell proliferation, apoptosis and vascular remodeling after balloon overstretch injury of porcine coronary arteries. *Circulation* 1997;96:1944–1952.

18. Hall EJ, Miller RC, Brenner DJ. The basic radiobiology of intravascular irradiation. In: Waksman R, ed. *Vascular brachytherapy,* 2nd ed. Futura Publishing, 1999:63–72.

19. Gillette EL, Powers BE, McChensey SM, Park RD, Withlow SJ. Response of aorta and branch arteries to experimental intraoperative irradiation. *Int J Radiat Oncol Biol Phys* 1989;17:1247–1255.

20. Pickering JG, Weir L, Janowski J, Kearney MA, Isner JM. Proliferative activity in peripheral and coronary atherosclerotic plaque among patients undergoing percutaneous revascularization. *J Clin Invest* 1993;91:1469–1480.

21. Weichselbaum RR, Hallahan DE, Sukhatme V, Dritschillo A, Sherman ML, Kufe DW. Biological consequences of gene regulation after ionizing radiation exposure. *J Natl Cancer Inst* 1991;83:480–484.

22. Wiedermann JG, Marboe C, Amols H, Schwartz A, Weinberger J. Intracoronary irradiation markedly reduces neointimal proliferation after balloon angioplasty in the swine: persistent benefit at 6-month follow-up. *J Am Coll Cardiol* 1995;25:1451–1456.

23. Waksman R, Robinson KA, Crocker IR, Gravanis MB, Cipolla GD, King SB III. Endovascular low dose irradiation inhibits neointima formation after coronary artery balloon injury in swine: a possible role for radiation therapy in restenosis prevention. *Circulation* 1995;91:1533–1539.

24. Wiedermann JG, Marboe C, Amols H, Schwartz A, Weinberger J. Intracoronary irradiation markedly reduces neointimal proliferation after balloon angioplasty in swine: persistent benefit at 6-month follow-up. *J Am Coll Cardiol* 1995;25:1451–1456.

25. Mazur W, Ali MN, Dabaghi SF, et al. High dose rate intracoronary radiation suppresses neointimal proliferation in the stented and ballooned model of porcine restenosis. *Int J Radiat Oncol Biol Phys* 1996;36:777–788.

26. Verin V, Popowski Y, Urban P, et al. Intra-arterial beta irradiation prevents neointimal hyperplasia in a hypercholesterolemic rabbit restenosis model *Circulation* 1995;92:2284–2290.

27. Waksman R, Robinson KA, Crocker IR, et al. Intracoronary low dose beta irradiation inhibits neointima formation after coronary artery balloon injury in the swine restenosis model. *Circulation* 1995;92:3025–3031.

28. Raizner A. Endovascular radiation: the Baylor Experience. Highlights in intracoronary radiation therapy. *Thoraxcenter* 1996;(December):10–11.

29. Waksman R, Chan RC, Kim WH, Vodovotz Y, Lavie E. Intracoronary delivery of rhenium-186 radioactive coil after balloon injury inhibits neointima formation in swine coronary arteries. *Circulation* 1998;98:17, I-557:2933.

30. Waksman R, Robinson K, Crocker I, et al. Intracoronary radiation prior to stent implantation inhibits neointima formation in stented porcine coronary arteries. *Circulation* 1995;92:1383–1386.

31. Waksman R, Robinson KA, Crocker IR, Gravanis MB, Palmer SJ, Cipolla GD. Intracoronary beta radiation before versus after stent implantation for inhibition of neointima formation in the porcine model. *Circulation* 1996;94:I-147(abst).

32. Weiderman JG, Marobe C, Amols H, Schwartz A, Weinberger J. Intracoronary irradiation fails to reduce neointimal proliferation after oversized stenting in a porcine model. *Circulation* 1995;92:I-146(abst).

33. Waksman R, Bhargava B, Saucedo JF, et al. Yttrium-90 delivered via a centering catheter and afterloader, given both before and after stent implantation, completely inhibits neointima formation in swine coronary arteries. *Am Coll Cardiol* 1999;33:2:20A.

34. Amols HI, Trichter F, Weinberger J. Intracoronary radiation for prevention of restenosis: dose perturbations caused by stents. *Circulation* 1998;98(19):2024–2029.

35. Liermann DD, Boettcher HD, Kollatch J, et al. Prophylactic endovascular radiotherapy to prevent intimal hyperplasia after stent implantation in femoro-popliteal arteries. *Cardiovasc Intervent Radiol* 1994;17:12–16.

36. Schoppel D, Liermann LJ, Pohlit R, et al. 192-Ir endovascular brachytherapy for avoidance of intimal hyperplasia after percutaneous transluminal angioplasty and stent implantation in peripheral vessels: years of experience. *Int J Radiat Oncol Biol Phys* 1996;36:835–840.

37. Waksman R, Laird JR, Benenati J, et al. Intravascular radiation for prevention of restenosis after angioplasty of narrowed femoral-popliteal arteries: preliminary six month results of a feasibility study. *Circulation* 1998; 98:I-66.

38. Nori K. External radiation for AV-dialysis fistulas: results from pilot studies (abst). Presented at Advances in Cardiovascular Radiation Therapy III, Washington DC, February 17–19, 1999.

39. Condado JA, Waksman R, Gurdiel O, et al. Long-term angiographic and clinical outcome after percutaneous transluminal coronary angioplasty and intracoronary radiation therapy in humans. *Circulation* 1997;96(3): 727–732.

40. Condado JA, Saucedo JF, Caldera C, et al. Two year angiographic evaluation after intracoronary 192 iridium in humans. *Circulation* 1997;96:I-220.

41. Teirstein PS, Massullo V, Jani S, et al. Catheter-based radiotherapy to inhibit restenosis after coronary stenting. *N Engl J Med* 1997;336(24):1697–1703.

42. Teirstein PS, Massullo V, Jani S, et al. Two-year follow-up after catheter-based radiotherapy to inhibit coronary restenosis. *Circulation* 1999;99:243–247.

43. Waksman R, White RL, Chan RC, et al. Intracoronary radiation therapy for patients with in-stent restenosis: 6-month follow-up of a randomized clinical study. *Circulation* 1998;98:I-651.

44. Leon MB, Teirstein PS, Lansky AJ, et al. Intracoronary gamma radiation to reduce in-stent restenosis: the Multicenter Gamma 1 Randomized Clinical Trial. *J Am Coll Cardiol* 1999;33:56A(abst).

45. Waksman R, Porrazzo MS, Chan RC, et al. Results from the ARTISTIC feasibility study of 192-iridium gamma radiation to prevent recurrence of in-stent restenosis. *Circulation* 1998;98:I-442.

46. Faxon DP, Buchbinder M, Cleman MW, et al. Intracoronary radiation to prevent restenosis in native coronary lesions: the results of the Pilot Phase of the ARREST Trial. *J Am Coll Cardiol* 1999;33:19A(abst).

47. Verin V, Urban P, Popowski Y, et al. Feasibility of intracoronary beta-irradiation to reduce restenosis after balloon angioplasty. A clinical pilot study. *Circulation* 1997;95(5):1138–1144.48. King SB, Williams DO, Chougule P, et al. Endovascular beta-radiation to reduce restenosis after coronary balloon angioplasty. Results of the beta energy restenosis trial (BERT). *Circulation* 1998;97:2025–2030.

49. Meerkin D, Bonan R, Tardif JC, et al. Reduction of the hyperplastic response following balloon angioplasty by beta-radiation. *J Am Coll Cardiol* 1998;31(2):222A.

50. Bonan R, Arsenault A, Tardif JC, et al. Beta energy restenosis trial, Canadian arm. *Circulation* 1997;96:I-219.

51. Amols HI, Reinstein LE, Weinberger J. Dosimetry of a radioactive coronary balloon dilatation catheter for treatment of neointimal hyperplasia. *Med Phys* 1996; 23:1783–1788.

52. Weinberger J. Clinical experience with the liquid-filled balloon: the CURE study (abst). Presented at Advances in Cardiovascular Radiation Therapy III, Washington DC, February 17–19, 1999.

53. Waksman R, White RL, Chan RC, et al. Intracoronary beta radiation therapy for in-stent restenosis: preliminary report from a single center clinical study. *J Am Coll Cardiol* 1999;33:19A(abst).

54. Makkar R, Whiting J, Li A, et al. A beta-emitting liquid isotope filled balloon markedly inhibits restenosis in stented porcine coronary arteries. *J Am Coll Cardiol* 1998;31(2):350A.

55. Robinson KA, Pipes DW, Bibber RV, et al. Dose response evaluation in balloon injured pig coronary arteries of a beta emitting ^{186}Re liquid filled balloon catheter system for endovascular brachytherapy *Advances in Cardiovascular Radiation Therapy II*, Washington DC, 1998, March 8–10.

56. Waksman R, Chan RC, Vodovotz Y, et al. Radioactive 133-Xenon Gas-filled Angioplasty Balloon: A novel intracoronary radiation system to prevent restenosis. *J Am Coll Cardiol* 1998;31(2):346A.

G. Radioisotope Stents: Evolution and Current Status

Tim A. Fischell

Heart Institute at Borgess Medical Center, Michigan State University, Kalamazoo, Michigan 49001

BACKGROUND

Restenosis remains a significant problem after PTCA and stenting, particularly in long lesions, in smaller diameter vessels, and in diabetics (1,2). Experimental and clinical data have demonstrated that in-stent restenosis is principally caused by neointimal formation (3–6). Endovascular radiation has been proposed as a method to reduce neointimal formation and, thus, prevent restenosis (7–17).

Teirstein et al. (12) reported a significant reduction in late lumen loss and restenosis in a randomized, placebo-controlled clinical trial utilizing 8- to 25-Gy irradiation delivered via an endovascular iridium 192 (^{192}Ir) source, combined with stenting, in patients with restenosis lesions (12). An alternative approach using a beta-emitting source has proved feasible and possibly effective (17). Another alternative, and simpler, approach to intravascular brachytherapy is the use of a stent as the platform for local radiation delivery.

RATIONALE FOR RADIOISOTOPE STENT

Coronary stenting has rapidly evolved to become the most popular primary treatment of obstructive coronary artery disease. It is estimated that approximately 60% to 80% of all coronary interventions are now performed with a strategy of primary stenting. Table 5.21 lists the proposed reasons for the popularity of stents as a primary treatment. Interventional cardiologists cite the ease and time efficiency, predictability of hemodynamic and angiographic results, and lack of early vessel closure as the primary factors motivating their increased use of primary stenting as

TABLE 5.21. *Rationale for primary stenting*

- Stent placement can be performed quickly
- Predictably excellent angiographic results
- Predictable hemodynamic and clinical results
- Patients' demand/expectation for stent treatment
- Predictable in-hospital course with very low subacute closure rate
- Improved long-term angiographic and clinical outcome

opposed to plain old balloon angioplasty (POBA). Interestingly, the modest improvements in late clinical and angiographic results with stents, as compared with balloon angioplasty, are likely to play a lesser role in the interventionalist's decision making. If this analysis is correct, it becomes clear that as stents improve, primary stenting will likely be performed in the large majority of cases independently of the decision whether or not to use radiation therapy to try to improve long-term outcomes. It follows that the radiation delivery strategy that provides the quickest, simplest, and most cost-effective primary stent–compatible approach will be used most often. Assuming that radioisotope stents are proved as safe and effective as catheter-based radiation, it is likely that this will be a preferred method for intravascular brachytherapy. Other potential advantages of the radioisotope stent over catheter-based systems include (a) the ability to deliver therapeutic treatment using pure beta emitters with approximately 1/100,000 of the radioactivity of the catheter-based source (e.g., 0.005 mCi of ^{32}P for stent vs. up to 500 mCi of gamma emitter ^{192}Ir for catheter-based system), (b) lack of requirements for in-laboratory dosimetry calculations, and (c) time efficiency (eliminates the entire procedure of catheter-based irradiation).

EVOLUTION OF RADIOISOTOPE STENT

Initial *in vitro* feasibility studies to examine the possible efficacy of continuous low-dose-rate radiation from a stent source were performed in 1992. In these experiments, it was demonstrated that low-dose beta-particle irradiation inhibited smooth muscle proliferation and possibly migration *in vitro* (13). Experimental studies have demonstrated that stents ion implanted with ^{32}P reduce neointimal formation at activities as low as 0.14 μCi (7,8,10,14). However, as with catheter-based irradiation, the clinical results with stent-based brachytherapy are likely to be complex and highly dose dependent.

The dose-response data using radioisotope stents in animal models of restenosis have been variable and somewhat inconsistent. In a porcine single-injury model, activities of 0.5 μCi in a 15-mm-long stent appears to be reasonably effective in reducing neointimal hyperplasia, particularly at 1 month. At activities of 1.0 μCi, there appears to be increased neointima in a juvenile swine model. At activities of 3 to 23 μCi, there is substantial inhibition of neointima at 1 month but with evidence of incomplete vessel healing. At these higher activities in a double-injury porcine model, there appears to be more neointima than in controls at a 6-month follow-up. This appears similar to recently presented data using beta catheters, which also showed increased neointima at 6 months in a single-injury porcine model at doses that appeared to inhibit neointima at 1 month.

Hehrlein et al. (10) reported a series of experiments using varying activities of ^{32}P stents in rabbit iliac arteries. In contrast to results from the porcine experiments, these authors reported a substantial, dose-dependent reduction in neointimal formation with the maximal effect evident at 3 months after placement of a 13.0 μCi, 7-mm-length stent (equivalent to a 26 μCi, 15-mm-long coronary stent). The contrasting results with the doses of continuous beta-particle irradiation used in these experimental studies suggest a species- or model-dependent response to endovascular irradiation delivered via a stent. As will be discussed later, recent human data suggest that the rabbit model rather than the porcine model may be more predictive of results seen in diseased human coronary arteries.

DOSIMETRY

Determinants of Vessel Dosing with Radioisotope Stents

There are a number of important determinants of vessel wall dosing with a beta-particle–emitting radioisotope stent. Table 5.22 lists a number of the variables that may determine dosing to target tissue with a radioisotope stent.

The dosimetry of a ^{32}P stent have previously been described in detail. Janicki et al. (18) characterized the near-field dose of a 1.0 μCi, 15-mm-length Palmaz-Schatz (Cordis, a Johnson and Johnson Co., Warren, NJ) using a modification of the dose-point-kernel method. Modification of the dose distribution around a uniform cylinder of ^{32}P to account for the geometry of a tubular, slotted Palmaz-Schatz stent with mathematic modeling allowed construction of three-dimensional dose maps. For a 1.0 μCi, 15-mm-length ^{32}P stent at a distance of 0.1-mm, dose values of approximately 2,500 cGy are delivered at the strut wires (peaks) and approximately 800 cGy between the wires (valleys) over one half-life (14.3 days). The nonuniformity of dosing reflective of the stent geometry decreases at distances of 1 to 2 mm from the surface. While these data provide an *in vitro* analysis of dosing from a radioactive stent, the actual dose distribution will be affected by variations in atherosclerotic plaque morphology and the symmetry of stent expansion.

Dr. Jerry Williams et al., from Johns Hopkins University, has presented some intriguing data regarding inhibition of smooth muscle cell pro-

TABLE 5.22. *Variables affecting dose to target tissue with radioisotope stent*

- Activity of stent (microcuries)
- Half-life of radioisotope
- Beta-particle energy
- Vessel geometry and size
- Stent geometry/design
- Plaque morphology

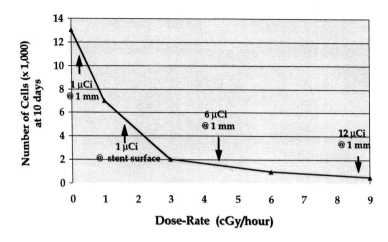

FIG. 5.33. Inhibition of proliferating human smooth muscle cells *in vitro* as a function of dose rate with continuous low-dose-rate beta-particle irradiation. These data suggest that stents of 4 to 20 μCi (15 mm long) may be needed to achieve therapeutic dose rates. *Arrows* denote the dose rate at 14 days after implant with varying ^{32}P stent activities and at various depths.

liferation using continuous low-dose-rate beta-particle irradiation (Fig. 5.33, Washington Hospital Center Radiation Symposium, 1998). These data demonstrate that continuously delivered dose rates of 6 to 10 cGy per hour from a beta source are highly effective in stopping proliferation of human vascular smooth muscle cells. Although one must be careful in extrapolating these types of *in vitro* dose-response data to the clinic, they may shed some light on a range of dose rates that one may need to achieve to inhibit smooth muscle cell proliferation with an implanted, continuous, low-dose-rate beta emitter such as a ^{32}P stent. Based on these human smooth muscle cell experiments, we currently estimate the effective stent activity for *de novo* lesions to be in the 4.0- to 20.0-μCi range (initial clinical trial used mean activity was 0.7 μCi). It should be noted that in the rabbit model, the most effective activity was approximately 26 μCi.

The data from these experiments also have interesting implications regarding where the dose and dose rates are delivered to achieve inhibition of smooth muscle cell growth. The dose and dose rates are greater at the plane of the stent at 14 to 28 days than they are at a depth of 1 mm at the time of implant. This may suggest that the critical treatment zone (target tissue) for a radioisotope stent is at the plane of the stent (electron fence theory) rather than at 1 to 2 mm deep to the luminal surface, as has been proposed for catheter-based intravascular brachytherapy.

Comparison of Dosing from Radioisotope Stent and Catheter-Based Systems

It should be noted that in both animal trials and clinical experience, the effects of intravascular brachytherapy, particularly with beta emitters, is highly dose dependent. In the porcine coronary artery injury model, rapidly delivered doses (beta or gamma) of < 800 cGy are ineffective in preventing neointimal hyperplasia. In the Geneva trial, low doses of beta-particle irradiation appeared to be ineffective in reducing neointimal hyperplasia.

Other clinical results with catheter-based brachytherapy techniques for the prevention of restenosis have been encouraging. In the SCRIPPS trial, there was a substantial reduction in late lumen loss and angiographic restenosis in a randomized, placebo-controlled clinical trial with 8- to 25-Gy irradiation delivered via an endovascular ^{192}Ir source in patients with refractory restenosis (12). Similar 6-month results were reported with the beta emitter ^{90}Y/Sr in the Beta Particle Radiation Restenosis Trial (17). These investigators prescribed a dose of radiation that was similar to the cumulative dose provided by a 1.0-μCi ^{32}P radioactive at a distance of 0.1 mm from the stent surface, but less than 20% of the catheter delivered dose in the deeper vessel wall. It is important to appreciate that the catheter-based approach gives the radiation at a much greater dose rate, which may be as important as the cumulative dose in preventing neointimal formation. With the ^{32}P catheter-based system from Neocardia, dose rates at a depth of 1 mm from the luminal surface may be in the range of 25,000 cGy per hour, with a cumulative dose of approximately 2,500 cGy. In contrast, the initial Isostent for Restenosis Intervention Study (IRIS) 1A trial with the ^{32}P radioisotope stent delivered a dose rate of only 1 cGy per hour and 500 cGy during the first 2 weeks to the same target tissue. This dose rate and total dose are not likely to have therapeutic effects in restenosis prevention, particularly in *de novo* lesions.

CLINICAL STUDIES USING ^{32}P RADIOISOTOPE STENT

The first radioisotope stent was implanted in a patient on October 7, 1996, at Borgess Medical Center in Kalamazoo, Michigan. The stent is easily shielded within a lucite shield, which contains the distal end of the stent (Fig. 5.34). In the Phase 1 IRIS, very low activity (0.5 to 1.0 μCi) ^{32}P 15-mm-length Palmaz-Schatz coronary stents were used in patients with symptomatic *de novo* or restenosis native coronary lesions. The enrollment for this trial was completed on January 14, 1997, with 32 patients receiving a beta-particle–emitting stent. Stent placement was successful in all patients. There were no cases of subacute stent thrombosis, target lesion revascularization, death, or other major cardiac events within the first 30 days (primary safety endpoint), thus demonstrating acceptable early event-free survival. At 6-month follow-up, there was a binary restenosis rate of 31% (10 of 32) and a clinically driven target vessel revascularization (TVR) rate of 21%. Interestingly, there was only one restenosis (proximal to stent) out of the ten patients treated for restenosis lesions (10%). It is possible that a lower stent activity could be effective in restenosis lesions if the proliferating target tissue derives from the recently formed neointima rather than from the adventitia, as is likely for *de novo* lesions. An example of the 6-month angiographic follow-up of a restenosis lesion treated with the radioisotope stent from the IRIS trial is shown in Fig. 5.35. There was an 18% restenosis rate for patients receiving stents >0.75 μCi. There were no further TVR events between 6 months and 12 months. Of note, in the *de novo* subgroup, the mean reference vessel diameter was 2.85 mm, and seven of 22 reference vessels in this subgroup were <2.50 mm. One stent was implanted in a vessel with a reference vessel size of 1.95 mm. Quantitative angiographic follow-up at 6 months demonstrated a lesional late loss of 0.94 mm for the group as a whole and 0.70 mm for the restenosis subgroup. These data are similar to late loss data from contemporary stent trials with nonradioactive stents. It should be emphasized that this was a small feasibility trial and was not intended to detect differences in restenosis with these very low activity stents.

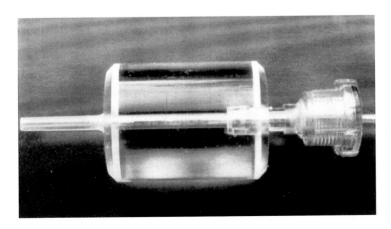

FIG. 5.34. The photograph is showing the lucite shield covering the radioisotope (Palmaz-Schatz) stent as used in the Phase 1 IRIS Trial. This shield completely blocks the escape of beta-particles from the stent.

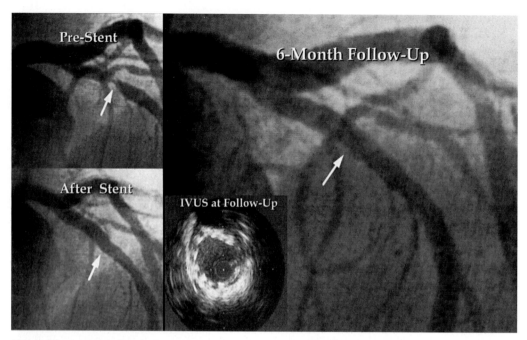

FIG. 5.35. Angiographic and intravascular ultrasound 6-month follow-up of high-grade LAD restenosis lesion treated with radioisotope stent. Stent activity was approximately 0.75 μCi at time of implant. **Left panels:** LAD restenosis lesion prior to and immediately after stenting. **Right panels:** 6-month angiographic and IVUS follow-up at lesion site, showing minimal neointimal hyperplasia within stent.

The Phase 1 IRIS trial (1B) has been expanded to test the safety of higher activity (0.75 to 1.5 mCi) stents at five additional medical centers. Twenty-five patients have been enrolled in this extension of the Phase 1 trial, with a mean stent activity of 1.14 μCi at the time of implantation. All 25 cases were performed successfully, without reported adverse events at 1-month safety follow-ups. The late follow-up in the 1B was similar to the 1A and did not suggest either increased or decreased neointimal responses to this range of activities.

Dr. Antonio Colombo is completing the 6-month follow-ups of a cohort of approximately 30 patients with 3.0- to 6.0-μCi BX stents (15-mm length). The early IVUS and QCA core laboratory data suggest that this activity is associated with diminished late loss within the stents. Among these patients, however, there were a number of restenosis lesions at the edges of the stent. The final results from this safety–feasibility trial are pending. These preliminary observations regarding diminished in-stent late loss are

encouraging and are in line with the observations from the *in vitro* studies regarding dose rate, and with the rabbit model. Interestingly, these observations in the ''human'' model stand in sharp contrast to the porcine model, in which these same activities (3 to 6 μCi) caused a significant increase in late loss. These clinical data are critical to our understanding of dose response and shed doubt on the predictive power of the porcine model in evaluating intravascular brachytherapy with the radioisotope stent.

Based on these encouraging data, further dose-response and feasibility testing at higher activities is underway. In Milan, another cohort of 19 patients have had 6.0- to 12.0-μCi BX stents implanted. At a mean follow-up of approximately 3 months, there have been no major adverse cardiac events reported. Longer term follow-up is pending.

CONCLUSIONS

Recent clinical data support the notion that radiation therapy may be effective in the prevention of restenosis. The early clinical results with more than 200 implants of low-activity ^{32}P Palmaz-Schatz and BX radioactive stents have demonstrated excellent procedural and 30-day event-free survival. Animal models, *in vitro* data, and now early clinical data suggest that significantly higher activities than were used in the initial safety trials may be required to find the "therapeutic window" of correct dosing with a ^{32}P beta-particle–emitting radioisotope stent. Further dose finding safety trials were underway in 1998 and will continue in 1999. Implementation of a large-scale, randomized, clinical trial will commence if and when early safety and efficacy data suggest a therapeutic effect from this technology. Thus, future studies will focus on optimal stent design and delivery and will evaluate more aggressive dosing strategies.

REFERENCES

1. Serruys PW, De Jaegere P, Kiemeneij F, et al., for the Benestent Study Group. A comparison of balloon-expandable-stent implantation with balloon angioplasty in patients with coronary artery disease. *N Engl J Med* 1994;331:489–495.
2. Fischman DL, Leon MB, Baim DS, et al., for the Stent Restenosis Study Investigators. A randomized comparison of coronary-stent placement and balloon angioplasty in the treatment of coronary artery disease. *N Engl J Med* 1994;331:496–501.
3. Painter JA, Mintz GS, Wong SC, et al. Serial intravascular ultrasound studies fail to show evidence of chronic Palmaz-Schatz stent recoil. *Am J Cardiol* 1995;75: 398–400.
4. Hoffmann R, Mintz G, Dussaillant G, et al. Patterns and mechanisms of in-stent restenosis: a serial intravascular ultrasound study. Circulation 1996;94:1247–1254.
5. Edelman ER, Rogers C. Hoop dreams: stents without restenosis. *Circulation* 1996;94:1199–1202.
6. Komatsu R, Ueda M, Naruko T, Kojima A, Becker A. Neointimal tissue response at sites of coronary stenting in humans: macroscopic histological and immunohistochemical analyses. Circulation 1998;98:224–233.
7. Laird JR, Carter AJ, Kufs W, et al. Inhibition of neointimal proliferation with a beta particle emitting stent. *Circulation* 1996;93:529–536.
8. Carter AJ, Laird JR, Bailey LR, et al. The effects of endovascular radiation from a b-particle emitting stent in a porcine restenosis model: a dose response study. Circulation 1996;94:2364–2368.
9. Hehrlein C, Gollan C, Dönges K, et al. Low-dose radioactive endovascular stents prevent smooth muscle cell proliferation and neointimal hyperplasia in rabbits. *Circulation* 1995;92:1570–1575.
10. Hehrlein C, Stintz M, Kinscherf R, et al. Pure b-particle emitting stents inhibit neointima formation in rabbits. Circulation 1996;93:641–645.
11. Waksman R, Robinson KA, Crocker IR, et al. Intracoronary radiation before stent implantation inhibits neointima formation in stented canine coronary arteries. *Circulation* 1995;92:1383–1386.
12. Tierstein PS, Massullo V, Jani S, et al. Radiotherapy reduces coronary restenosis; late follow-up. J Am Coll Cardiol 1997;129:397A.
13. Fischell TA, Kharma BK, Fischell DR, et al. Low-dose, b-particle emission from stent wire results in complete, localized inhibition of smooth muscle cell proliferation. Circulation 1994;90:2956–2963.
14. Rivard A, Leclerc G, Bouchard M, et al. Low-dose B-emitting radioactive stents inhibit neointimal hyperplasia in porcine coronary arteries; an histological assessment. *J Am Coll Cardiol* 1997;29:238A.
15. Waksman R, Robinson KA, Crocker IA, et al. Intracoronary low dose B-irradiation inhibits neointima formation after coronary artery balloon injury in the swine restenosis model. *Circulation* 1995;92:3025–3031.
16. Waksman R, Robinson KA, Crocker IA, Gravanis MB, Cipolla CD, King SB III. Endovascular low dose irradiation inhibits neointima formation after coronary artery balloon injury in swine: a possible role for radiation therapy in restenosis prevention. *Circulation* 1995;91: 1553–1559.
17. King SB, Williams DO, Chougule P, et al. Intracoronary beta irradiation inhibits late lumen loss following balloon angioplasty: results of the BERT-1 Trial. *Circulation* 1997;96:I-219.
18. Janicki C, Duggan DM, Coffey CW, Fischell DR, Fischell TA. Radiation dose from a phosphorous-32 impregnated wire mesh vascular stent. *Med Phys* 1997;24: 437–445.

H. Coronary Ultrasound Thrombolysis: State-of-the-Art and Clinical Perspective

Uri Rosenschein

Catheterization Laboratory, Department of Cardiology, The Tel Aviv Sourasky Medical Center, Tel Aviv 64239, Israel

The Priests blew their horns . . . and the wall fell down flat
  Joshua VI:20

Sound waves are a class of mechanical waves that consist of vibrations of the atomic or molecular particles of a substance about the equilibrium position of those particles. These waves propagate ideally through solids and, to a lesser extent, through liquids and gases. The range of sound audible to the human ear is from 20 to 18,000 Hz. Sound waves above the audible range lie in the ultrasound range. There are roughly two classes of ultrasound applications: those of low power and those of high-power. The low-power class includes instruments that perform diagnostic tests and measurements, while the high-power class includes devices that change the physical and/or chemical state of the material on which they operate. Classically, the ultrasound employed in cardiology for diagnostic echocardiology is a low-power class device. Recently, high-power ultrasound has been harnessed for ultrasound surgery and percutaneous transluminal lysis of arterial clots.

EXPERIMENTAL DATA

Transient acoustic cavitations are produced in liquid media subjected to high-power acoustic irradiation when the negative acoustic pressure during the rarefaction phase of the cycle becomes so great that the tensile strength of the water is not sufficient to maintain continuity. The liquid is then disrupted and vapor-filled microbubbles form. When the positive-pressure phase begins, the cavitation collapses violently. During the final stage of collapse, transient cavitations generate shock waves (1). One bubble was calculated to deposit about 300×10^6 eV of energy upon collapse (2). These forces are sufficient to induce depolymerization in a variety of polymers (3).

We have studied *in vitro* the relationships between ultrasound ablation, cavitation, and tissue elasticity. These investigators found that ultrasound thrombolysis is evident only when the cavitation threshold has been exceeded, suggesting that the cavitation effect is involved in the mechanism of ultrasound thrombus ablation. Above the cavitation threshold, there was a good correlation between the thrombolysis efficiency and ultrasound power (4). A negative correlation between ultrasound ablation and tissue elasticity was observed. The high elasticity of the arterial wall makes it resistant to the disruptive effects of ultrasound, while the low elasticity of the thrombus makes it sensitive to ultrasound ablation. The data suggest that the differences in elasticity between arterial wall and thrombi delineate the wide margins of safety of ultrasound angioplasty. Indeed, the experience with the ultrasound scalpel showed that blood vessels are very resistant to ultrasound, while soft tissue such as liver or brain were found to be very sensitive to ultrasound ablation (5).

This inherent selective ablation of high-power ultrasound led us to the hypothesis that high-power ultrasound can induce the selective injury required for successful transluminal intervention. Ultrasound had potential for ablating the occlusion without damaging the ultrasound-resistant arterial wall.

Coronary ultrasound thrombolysis (CUT) was studied by Hartnell et al. (6) using *in vitro* apparatus to simulate the geometric configuration and physical conditions of intracoronary thrombolysis. They found that ultrasound can induce very effective thrombus ablation. The majority of debris was of subcapillary size, and only infrequently were debris found on a 5μ filter. Muller et al. (7) studied the potential risk of embolization by ultrasound-lysed clots. They have measured the coronary flow and perfusion *in vivo* at baseline, after intracoronary injection of ultrasound-lysed clot and after intracoronary injection of control mechanically ablated clots. Following injection of ultrasound-lysed clots, a significant increase in coronary flow and perfusion was observed. After the injection of the mechanically ablated clot, there was significant reduction in flow.

We have studied ultrasound thrombolysis in thrombotically occluded dog femoral arteries (8). In each dog, a thrombotic occlusion was generated in both femoral arteries. The left femoral artery was sonicated, while the right femoral artery was mechanically "dottered." There was dramatic reduction in clot mass after ultrasound thrombolysis, while dottering did not change the degree of clot burden.

Thus, the experimental studies suggest that a thrombus-rich lesion is the ideal lesion to be treated by ultrasound. Thrombus is very sensitive to ultrasound, while the arterial wall is resistant to ultrasound; thus, a desired selective injury can be excepted. Experimental data suggest that effective thrombolysis is induced by ultrasound and not by dottering. There was potentially low-risk embolization.

DEVELOPMENT OF A CORONARY DEVICE

The device consists of a solid-metal, flexible ultrasound probe coupled at its proximal end to an ultrasound transducer in the hand-piece. The transducer consists of piezoelectric crystals that convert electrical energy, supplied by a small portable power generator, to high-power, 42-kHz ultrasonic energy. The ultrasound is transmitted by the ultrasound probe to the target le-

sion in the arterial system (Fig. 5.36). Among all current ultrasound angioplasty devices, whether for peripheral or coronary applications, this design is classic. It differs from the design of intravascular ultrasound imaging devices. In the latter, the piezoelectric crystals generate low-power, high-frequency ultrasound and are mounted at the tip of the catheter that carries only the electrical signal.

In the development of a coronary device, several technologic challenges had to be addressed:

1. To attain acceptable levels of miniaturization, the diameter of the transmission wire needs to be reduced to optimal dimensions. This will invariably increase compressional and tensile forces, which may lead to catheter fatigue problems.

2. Ultrasound is best transmitted in a solid-metal wire, in proportion to the cross-sectional area of the wire. Thus, the issue of the flexibility of the wire versus the quantity of usable energy had to be dealt with in the development of a coronary device.

3. Acoustic waves, like any wave, are attenuated at curves of the waveguide—the ultrasound probe. This theoretically may result in loss of acoustic energy and unacceptable heat generation.

There are a variety of coronary ultrasound angioplasty devices (6,9,10). The device we use to investigate coronary ultrasound angioplasty consists of an ultrasound probe (140 cm long) with a distal, flexible, multiwire segment connected to a 1.6 mm tip designed specially to optimize the cavitation effect (Acolysis, Angiosonics, Morrisville, NC). The multiwire flexible segment uses solid-metal wire for effective ultrasound transmission but is still able to maintain the desired flexibility. The multiwire flexible segment behaves acoustically in a manner similar to that of fiberoptics, which effectively transmit light waves through glass and yet maintain their flexibility. The device fits into a standard 7 Fr angioplasty guide catheter and accepts, in a "monorail" fashion, a 0.014 in. angioplasty guidewire.

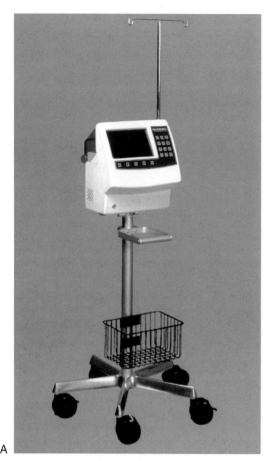

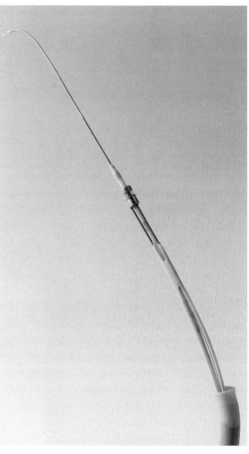

A   B

FIG. 5.36. The ultrasound thrombolysis device consists of a controller, which is an electric signal generator with sophisticated computer controls and safety circuitry. An external transducer converts electrical energy into ultrasonic energy **(A).** The coronary ultrasound angioplasty probe has a 1.6-mm tip and can be inserted in a 7 Fr guide catheter in a "monorail" fashion over a 0.014-in. high-torque guidewire. The multifire flexible element allows the tip of a solid-metal wire for effective ultrasound transmission while maintaining the designed level of flexibility needed for coronary use. The tip is designed specially to optimize the cavitation effect **(B).**

CLINICAL EXPERIENCE

The clinical investigational plan for the assessment of intracoronary ultrasound thrombolysis started with the acute myocardial infarction study (ACUTE Study) and was followed by a registry (Acolysis Registry).

In the ACUTE Study (11,12), we have studied consecutive patients with first infarct, only acute anterior myocardial infarction, and occluded left anterior descending artery. Ultrasound thrombolysis achieved effective reperfusion in 97% of the patients; final flow of TIMI grade 3 was achieved in 93% of the patients (Fig. 5.37). Dur-

ing the procedure, there were no clinical (death, ventricular fibrillation, cardiac arrest, pulmonary edema, cardiogenic) or angiographic (dissection, perforation, embolization, spasm, no reflow) adverse events. During hospitalization, there was no need for urgent target vessel revascularization in 13% of the patients. Adjunct percutaneous transluminal coronary angioplasty (PTCA) and stent were used in 94% and 22% of the patients, respectively. Abciximab was used in only 3% of the patients. There was no need for adjunct thrombolytic therapy. Preliminary data from the 6-month follow-up showed

mer degradation and release of incorporated substances. *Proc Natl Acad Sci U S A* 1989;86:7663–7666.

4. Rosenschein U, Frimmerman A, Laniado S, Miller HI. Study of the mechanism of ultrasound angioplasty from human thrombi and bovine aorta. *Am J Cardiol* 1994; 74:1263–1266.

5. WJB Hodgson. Ultrasonic surgery. *J R Coll Surg Edinb* 1980;62:459–461.

6. Hartnell GG, Saxton JM, Friedl SE, et al. Ultrasonic thrombus ablation: In–vitro assessment of a novel device for intracoronary use. *J Intervent Cardiol* 1993;6: 69–76.

7. Muller DWM, Moncur J, Rosenschein U, et al. Ultrasound thrombolysis: ablated thrombus does not impede microcirculatory flow or impair regional left ventricular wall motion. *Aust N Z J Med* 1998;28:1288(abst).

8. Rosenschein U, Bernstein J, DiSegni E, et al. Experimental ultrasonic angioplasty: disruption of atherosclerotic plaques and thrombi in vitro and arterial recanalization in vivo. *J Am Coll Cardiol* 1990;15:711–717.

9. Philippe F, Drobinski G, Bucherer C, et al. Effects of ultrasound energy on thrombi in vitro. *Cathet Cardiovasc Diagn* 1993;28:173–178.

10. Steffen W, Luo H, Nita H, et al. Catheter delivered therapeutic ultrasound recanalizes thrombotically occluded canine coronary arteries. *J Am Coll Cardiol* 1993;21: 228A (abst).

11. Rosenschein U, Roth A, Rassin T, et al. Analysis of coronary ultrasound thrombolysis endpoints in acute myocardial infarction (ACUTE Trial): results of the feasibility phase. *Circulation* 1997;95:1411–1416.

12. Rosenschein U, Herz I, Tenenbaum-Koren E, et al. Coronary ultrasound thrombolysis in acute myocardial infarction: Results from the ACUTE Study. *J Am Coll Cardiol* 1998;31:192A(abst).

13. Fajadet J, Calderon L, Thomas M, et al. Coronary ultrasound thrombolysis in acute coronary syndromes: the first 100 patients from the Acolysis Registry. *Circulation* (in press).

14. Rosenschein U, Gaul G, Erbel R, et al. Percutaneous transluminal therapy of occluded saphenous vein grafts: can the challenge be met with ultrasound thrombolysis? *Circulation* January 1999.

15. Rosenschein U, Ellis SG, Yakubov SJ, Haudenschild CC, Dick RJ, Topol EJ. Histopathologic correlates of coronary lesion angiographic morphology: lessons from a directional atherectomy experience. *Coron Artery Dis* 1992;3:953–961.

16. Coller BS. GPIIb/IIa antagonist: pathophysiologic and therapeutic insights from studies of c7E3 Fab. *Thromb Haemost* 1997;78:730–735.

17. Merlini PA, Bauer KA, Oltrona L, et al. Persistent activation of coagulation mechanism in unstable angina and myocardial infarction. *Circulation* 1994;90:61–68.

18. Meyer BJ, Badimon JJ, Chesebro JH, et al. Dissolution of mural thrombus by specific thrombin inhibition with r-hirudin: comparison with heparin and aspirin. *Circulation* 1998;97:681–685.

19. Kyrle PA, Chesebro JH, Hayes RM, et al. Antithrombo-

tic effect of PEG-hirudin compared to heparin and heparin plus c7E3. *Circulation* 1997;97(Suppl): 1:1-41(abst).

20. Gregorini L, Marco J, Fajadet J, et al. Ticlopidine and aspirin pretreatment reduces coagulation and platelet activation during coronary dilation procedures. *J Am Coll Cardiol* 1997;29:13–20.

21. Steinhubl SR, Lauer MS, Mukerjee DP, et al. Pretreatment with ticlopodine reduces non Q-wave myocardial infarctions following intracoronary stenting. *J Am Coll Cardiol* 1998;31:100A(abst).

22. Leon MB, Baim DS, Gordon P, et al. Clinical and angiographic results from stent anticoagulation regimen study (STARS). *Circulation* 1996;94:I-685(abst).

23. Kornowski R, Stein G, Miller HI, Laniado S, Keren G. Angiographic morphology following heparin and aspirin therapy in patients with acute coronary syndromes and intracoronary thrombus. *J Thromb Thrombol* 1998; 5:159–164.

24. Ambrose JA, Almeida OD, Sharma SK, et al. Adjunctive thrombolytic therapy during angioplasty for ischemia rest angina: results of the TAUSA trial. *Circulation* 1994;90:69–77.

25. Mehran R, Ambrose JA, Bongu RM, et al. Angioplasty of complex lesions in ischemia rest angina: results of the thrombolysis and angioplasty in unstable angina (TAUSA) trial. *J Am Coll Cardiol* 1995;26:961–966.

26. Khan MM, Ellis SG, Aguirre FV, Weisman HF, et al. Does intracoronary thrombus influence the outcome of high risk percutaneous transluminal coronary angioplasty? Clinical and angiographic outcomes in a large multicenter trial. *J Am Coll Cardiol* 1998;31:31–36.

27. Brener SJ, Barr LA, Burctenal JRB. Randomized placebo-controlled trial of platelet glycoprotein iib/iia blockade with primary angioplasty for acute myocardial infarction. *Circulation* 1998;98:734–741.

28. The EPIC Investigators. Use of monoclonal antibody directed against the platelet glycoprotein IIb/IIIa receptor in high-risk coronary angioplasty. *N Engl J Med* 1994;330:956–961.

29. The EPILOG Investigators. Platelet glycoprotein IIb/IIIa receptor blockade and low-dose heparin during percutaneous coronary revascularization. *N Engl J Med* 1997;336:1689–1696.

30. The CAPTURE Investigators. Randomized placebo-controlled trial of abciximab before and during coronary intervention in refractory unstable angina: the CAPTURE study. *Lancet* 1997;349:1429–1435.

31. The TIMI IIIB Investigators. Effects of tissue plasminogen activator and a comparison of early invasive and conservative strategies in unstable angina and non Q-wave myocardial infarction. *Circulation* 1994;89: 1545–1556.

32. Fishman DL, Leon MB, Baim D, et al. A randomized comparison of coronary stent placement and balloon angioplasty in the treatment of coronary artery disease. *N Engl J Med* 1994;331:496–501.

33. Serruys PW, de Jaegere P, Kiemeneij F, et al. A comparison of balloon expandable stent implantation with balloon angioplasty in patients with coronary artery disease. *N Engl J Med* 1994;331:489–495.

SECTION II

Clinical Problems

6

Evaluating Stenosis Severity: Quantitative Angiography, Coronary Flow Reserve, and Intravascular Ultrasound

David Hasdai, *David R. Holmes, Jr., and *Amir Lerman

*Department of Cardiology, Rabin Medical Center, 49100 Petah Tikva, Israel; *Division of Cardiovascular Diseases and Internal Medicine, Mayo Clinic and Mayo Foundation, Department of Medicine, Mayo Medical School, Rochester, Minnesota 55905*

Intermediate coronary artery stenoses are a challenge to physicians performing coronary angiography. The lesion may seem to be significant in one planar view but not in other views. Moreover, it is often difficult to determine based on the angiographic result whether the lesion is of physiological significance—i.e., whether it compromises coronary blood flow (CBF) to the extent that it impairs myocardial perfusion at rest or during stress.

In addition, after percutaneous coronary revascularization, the interventional cardiologist often faces the challenge of deciding whether the procedural result is optimal or suboptimal. A suboptimal result may be associated with increased rates of restenosis as well as adverse cardiac events such as acute vessel closure. It is now well-documented that after coronary interventions the angiographic result may be deceiving, and thus the patient may be unknowingly left with a suboptimal result.

The aim of this chapter is to describe the currently available techniques for evaluating the anatomy and physiology of coronary artery lesions before and after coronary interventions.

EVALUATION OF LESIONS BEFORE INTERVENTIONS

Anatomic Evaluation

Quantitative Coronary Angiography

Generally, there is good agreement among interventional cardiologists who visually estimate stenosis severity regarding the severity of mild or severe stenoses. In contrast, there is a great deal of intraobserver and interobserver variability regarding intermediate stenoses. In addition, there is some variability in the visual estimate of vessel dimensions (1). Computer-assisted methods have been developed to provide a more accurate and unbiased assessment of absolute and relative coronary artery dimensions during angiography, a technique termed quantitative coronary angiography (QCA). QCA entails digitization of the film, image calibration, arterial contour editing, and observer editing. In addition to the inherent shortcomings of individual QCA systems, there are errors common to all systems at each stage. For example, image acquisition and analyses may be performed during systole, thus skewing the results. Moreover, observer editing may render this objective technique operator-dependent and susceptible to bias.

To compare lesion severity in serial angiographic procedures or before and after interventions, the angles, skew rotation, and table height must be kept constant for each view. In addition, the distances between the image intensifier, the X-ray tube, and the patient must be kept constant. Slight shifts in position may substantially alter the results. Failure to fully separate the artery of interest from overlapping or bifurcating branches or vessel foreshortening may also introduce errors in measurement.

The major advantage of coronary angiography over the other techniques of intravascular ultrasound and Doppler is the ability to assess the severity of the lesion without the need to cross the lesion with a guidewire or other devices. Although uncommon, there have been reports of complications such as guidewire or catheter trauma during the assessment of lesion severity using these newer devices. However, given the shortcomings of coronary angiography described above, the information gleaned from these other techniques clearly can impact therapeutic strategies in specific patients and thereby improve patient outcome by either sparing the patient of complications associated with unnecessary percutaneous coronary interventions or from suboptimal interventions. Thus, the interventional cardiologist must weigh the possible complications of more invasive assessment techniques against the risk of complications from unnecessary percutaneous coronary interventions or from suboptimal interventions. Moreover, since coronary atherosclerosis is a diffuse disease that involves the vessel wall, it is reasonable to get a good look at both the lumen and the vessel wall when developing therapeutic strategies.

Intravascular Ultrasound

As documented above, the angiographic assessment of coronary artery lesions is based on the comparison of radio-contrast dye opacification of the lesion relative to a presumed normal reference segment. Thus, if the lumen diameter of the reference segment is 2 mm and the mean luminal diameter of the lesion is 1 mm, then the mean diameter stenosis is 50%. However, the true lumen diameter of the reference segment may be inaccurately measured because it is diffusely and concentrically diseased. For instance, a true lumen diameter of 4 mm may be measured as 2 mm. In this case, the calculated mean diameter stenosis would be 75%, and the lesion would be incorrectly considered hemodynamically significant (Fig. 6.1). Likewise, if the true dimensions of the vessel are underestimated, undersized balloon catheters might be chosen for use during a subsequent coronary intervention. Given the importance of achieving an optimal

minimal luminal diameter without causing vessel wall injury by using oversized balloons, this is an important pitfall of angiography.

It should be stressed that, due to vascular remodeling, the vessel dimensions at the site of stenosis may change over time relative to the reference segment. The vessel may either shrink or grow in diameter focally at the site of stenosis. In this case, the reference segment does not accurately represent the actual dimensions of the artery at the site of stenosis.

Another pitfall of coronary angiography may stem from the eccentricity of the lesion (2). Even using multiple planar views it is often difficult to fully delineate the lesion, especially in the presence of ostial or bifurcation lesions or overlapping branches. Therefore, the lesion may be much more severe then appreciated angiographically.

Coronary angiography may also fail to accurately characterize the composition of the atheroma (3), which is an important factor in the choice of the device used in a possible intervention. For example, calcifications and intracoronary thrombi often produce the same angiographic picture. A heavily calcified lesion may be more suitable for rotational atherectomy, whereas a lesion with a large thrombus burden would contraindicate rotational atherectomy.

Intravascular ultrasound (IVUS) has become the gold standard for the delineation of the vessel wall anatomy and plaque morphology (4). IVUS catheters with an outer diameter of between 2.9 and 3.5 Fr are most often introduced using 7 or 8 Fr guiding catheters. The catheter is placed distal to the segment of interest and is gradually pulled back. Motorized pull-back devices are now available, enabling the three-dimensional reconstruction of the vessel wall. In two large prospective series, in approximately 20% of examinations before coronary interventions, IVUS changed the treatment strategy, by demonstrating more severe or milder coronary artery disease than appreciated by angiography (5,6).

Physiologic Evaluation

Coronary Flow Reserve Measurement

The coronary angiogram or images derived from IVUS are merely a ''road map'' of the

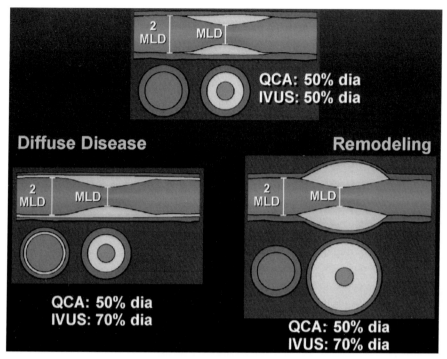

FIG. 6.1. Comparison of lesion assessment by QCA and intravascular ultrasound. This figure demonstrates the concept of discrepancy between QCA and intravascular assessment of lesion severity. The degree of coronary artery stenosis is dependent also on the degree of coronary arteriosclerosis in the adjacent segment such as demonstrated in the left coronary (diffuse disease) and also by the process of coronary artery modeling as demonstrated in the right coronary (remodeling). QCA, quantitative coronary angiography; IVUS, intravascular ultrasound; DIA, diameter.

coronary epicardial tree, offering no information regarding the coronary microcirculation, nor of the physiologic significance of lesions. Regardless of the anatomic appearance of the lesion, it must be remembered that the purpose of the coronary arteries is to nourish the myocardium at rest, and more so during stress. A physiologically significant lesion impairs CBF at rest, or more commonly during stress.

At rest, myocardial demand is low, and accordingly CBF is at its lowest level. Coronary resistance vessels have a high basal vasomotor tone in this state. Under conditions of increased stimulation, the normal physiologic response to an increase in myocardial demand is enhanced CBF (7); this enhancement is achieved by vasodilation of epicardial and resistance vessels (8). The ability to increase CBF by reducing vasomotor tone to meet myocardial demand is called

coronary flow reserve (CFR). Normal individuals can increase CBF four to six fold to meet the increased myocardial demand.

In the presence of a physiologically significant lesion, the resistance vessels compensate for the impaired CBF by vasodilating. In case of a severe lesion, the resistance vessels are fully dilated. Thus, in response to a physiological or pharmacological stimulus that increases myocardial demand, the resistance vessels are not capable of further vasodilating, constituting a state of impaired CFR. In experimental animal studies, increasing the stenosis of a conduit artery to about 60% artery diameter narrowing produces a predictable decline in CFR. Gould and Lipscomb (9) demonstrated that the CFR is attenuated beginning with coronary artery stenosis of more than 50% of the diameter. Compensatory vasodilation of the distal coronary vascular bed maintains near normal resting flow for lesions between 60% to 85% diameter stenosis, but adaptive vasodilation fails to compensate for lesions greater than 85% diameter stenosis. These important findings have served as the reference for our current definition of obstructive coronary artery disease. Thus, it is widely accepted that ≥70% stenosis of an epicardial artery constitutes significantly obstructive coronary artery disease. However, it is clear that lesions estimated to be 50% to 70% diameter stenosis may also be physiologically significant, and hence may merit further evaluation. Using physiological assessments of intermediate lesions, it has been demonstrated that it is possible to safely defer an intervention in patients with normal physiological parameters (10). The importance of physiological assessment of the lesion is particularly useful in cases where the culprit lesion needs to be determined in the absence of noninvasive functional tests. Thus, physiological assessment of coronary artery disease may be determined ''on-line'' in the catheterization laboratory and may emerge as a last effort method.

Physiologic assessment of coronary arteries was previously performed using the readily available end-hole catheters. However, even the smallest end-hole catheter may introduce gross errors into the measurements. For example, the cross-sectional area of the 0.018-in. guidewire causes only a 15% reduction in area of a circular lumen of 1.2 mm in diameter, whereas a 1 mm diameter end-hole catheter would induce a 70% reduction. Currently, there are two major techniques for the evaluation of CFR in the cardiac catheterization laboratory using transducers mounted on guidewires: intracoronary Doppler and fractional flow reserve (FFR).

Intracoronary Doppler

The availability of a 0.014- or a 0.018-inch intracoronary Doppler guide wire has made the measurement of CBF with good correlation to actual flow easily available in the cardiac catheterization laboratory (11). CBF blood flow is calculated using the formula $\pi D^2 \times APV \div 8$, where D represents the coronary diameter mea-

sured 5 mm distal to the tip of the Doppler wire (by quantitative angiography or IVUS) and APV equals the average peak velocity from the Doppler tracing (12). The CFR is calculated by the ratio of peak-to-baseline CBF in response to drug infusion or injection. When coronary artery diameter is presumed to remain unchanged in response to drug manipulation, the CFR is calculated by the ratio of peak-to-baseline flow velocities (APV).

Specific pharmacological tools are currently used to discern abnormalities in CFR. Adenosine is thought to act on the coronary vasculature via stimulation of the adenosine A2 receptor on smooth muscle cells (13). At pharmacological doses, such as given in the cardiac catheterization laboratory, adenosine can cross the endothelial barrier and stimulate the receptor on the smooth muscle directly in an endothelium-independent mechanism (14). Adenosine acts predominantly on vessels less than 150 μm in diameter (13) and, therefore, mainly assesses changes in the coronary resistance vessels as reflected by changes in coronary flow. The administration of adenosine provides mainly an endothelium-independent evaluation of the coronary microvasculature (altered endothelium-dependent vasomotor regulation has been shown in response to the increase in flow induced by adenosine). Adenosine may cause bradyarrhythmias including sinus bradycardia and atrioventricular block, facial flushing, and bronchoconstriction. Due to the short half-life of adenosine, the duration of these side effects is very brief.

Papaverine and dipyridamole are alternative agents to adenosine. Although some investigators have reported variability in values of CFR using different pharmacological agents (15,16), others have reported similar values (17,18). These differences may be attributed, at least in part, to differences in doses and routes of administration of the different drugs. In contrast to the minimal effect of adenosine on epicardial arteries, papaverine may affect epicardial arteries; in fact, papaverine may even cause epicardial vasoconstriction after vascular injury (19). In addition, papaverine may prolong the QT-interval, thus causing ventricular dysrhythmias (17). For these reasons, it is not commonly used.

The following is our protocol for the evaluation of the hyperemic response of the coronary microcirculation distal to the stenosis. A 0.014-inch Doppler guide wire (Cardiometrics, Santa Anna, California) is advanced via a 6 Fr to 8 Fr guiding catheter into the coronary artery in question distal to the lesion. The wire should not be placed in proximity to a bifurcation, which may alter CFR measurements. Baseline APV is recorded, followed by intracoronary injection of adenosine (18 to 36 μg; solution of 6 mg adenosine in one liter of saline) into the guiding catheter seated at the ostium of the coronary artery. Because adenosine has a negligible effect on coronary artery diameter, the CFR is simply calculated by dividing the APV after adenosine injection by the baseline APV. We consider a CFR ratio of more than 2.5 in response to adenosine as being normal (20) (Fig. 6.2).

It is important to recognize several possible pitfalls in the measurement of CFR using the Doppler wire. Basal CBF and the CFR may be adversely affected by a guiding catheter seated deeply in the ostium of the coronary artery. Systemic conditions that may affect systemic hemodynamics such as thyrotoxicosis and anemia may also affect basal CBF and the CFR, and thus they should be corrected if possible before proceeding with the examination. The microvasculature in infarcted areas of the myocardium may be functionally impaired. Thus, it is important to ascertain that the territory interrogated is not infarcted. In addition, because the signal analyzed is obtained 5.2 mm beyond the transducer (to minimize distal flow-velocity distortion caused by the guidewire), caution should be exercised in placing the tip of the guidewire. The guidewire tip should not abut the vessel wall, should not be grossly distorted in shape after manipulating it across the stenosis, and should not be placed in proximity to a major bifurcation. It is therefore vital to recognize a normal Doppler signal. In the left coronary artery system the blood flow velocity in diastole is greater than in systole, perhaps because of the greater compression of the left ventricle during systole, whereas for the right coronary artery, the flow velocities are fairly similar during both phases. Although the basal CBF may be highest in the left anterior

descending coronary artery and lowest in the right coronary artery (with a wide range of values for basal CBF in each vessel among control subjects), the CFR is fairly similar for all three major epicardial arteries. However, due to the increased sensitivity of the right coronary artery to the pharmacological agents used, especially the chronotropic effects of adenosine, lower doses are recommended initially for injections to the right coronary artery. In the absence of untoward side effects higher dose may be used serially until the CFR measurements do not change with increased doses.

Coronary microvessels may have reduced vasodilating abilities due to structural or functional abnormalities, resulting in the inability to decrease vasomotor tone during stress. Therefore, in case of a low CFR ratio, we recommend measuring the CFR in a similar manner in another angiographically normal coronary artery. If the CFR is abnormally low in the control artery, coronary microvessel disease or another pathology should be sought. If the CFR in the control artery is normal, it is reasonable to assume that the lesion in question is physiologically significant. Calculation of CFR as the ratio of the CFR of the target lesion divided by the CFR of the reference normal segment may be a more accurate assessment of the physiological assessment of the culprit lesion (21).

Fractional Flow Reserve

A novel method for assessing indeterminate coronary artery stenoses based on pressure-flow analysis during maximal flow was recently introduced (22–24). The concept of myocardial FFR, defined as the maximal blood flow to the myocardium in the presence of a stenosis in the supplying coronary artery, divided by the theoretical normal maximal flow in the same distribution, has been developed as an index of physiologic severity of the lesion (23). FFR represents the fraction of the normal maximal myocardial flow that can be achieved despite the coronary stenosis. This index can be calculated from the ratio of the mean distal coronary-artery pressure to the aortic pressure during hyperemic maximal vasodilation, and is independent of changes in

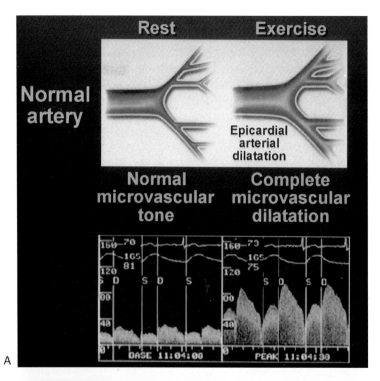

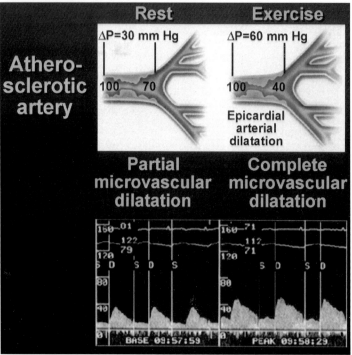

FIG. 6.2. Shown here is coronary flow reserve in response to intracoronary adenosine. (Adopted with permission from ref. 32.) **A:** A normal response to intracoronary adenosine results in an increase in intracoronary Doppler velocity resulting in normal coronary flow reserve of 3.5. This response simulates the normal microvascular dilatation in response to increased myocardial demand such as exercise. **B:** An abnormal response to intracoronary adenosine resulted in attenuated increase in increased intracoronary Doppler velocity, representing an abnormal coronary flow reserve of 1.4. This abnormal coronary flow reserve represents attenuated microvascular dilatation secondary to hemodynamically significant lesion in the epicardial vessels.

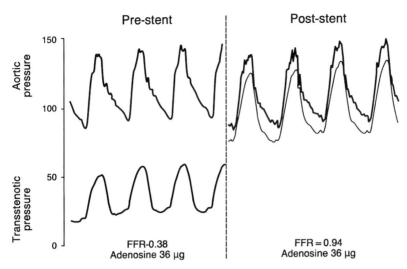

FIG. 6.3. Aortic and transstenotic pressure in a 72-year-old man. The patient has a moderate severe stenosis in the left anterior descending artery. The pressure recordings on the left side were obtained with the pressure wire located distal to the stenotic segment. Intracoronary adenosine at 36 μg was administered, and this resulted in a maximum hyperemia and abnormal fraction of flow reserve of 0.38, indicating a significant hemodynamical lesion. On the right, pressure recordings following a successful stent implantation resulted in normalization of the fraction of flow reserve to 0.94. FFR, fractional flow reserve

systemic blood pressure and heart rate. Moreover, the FFR takes into account the collateral blood supply. Per definition, the normal value of the FFR is 1.0 for any vessel investigated. Based on prior studies, it is accepted that an index value of less than 0.75 is abnormal and correlates well with pathological findings using noninvasive techniques (22–24).

After calibration at zero the wire is positioned distal to the lesion at question, and adenosine is administered (18 to 36 μg) into the ostium of the coronary artery through the guiding catheter. The distal coronary pressure is monitored; maximal CBF is achieved with minimal coronary distal pressure. When the coronary distal pressure reaches a new steady state, the FFR is calculated by dividing the mean distal intracoronary pressure (measured by the guide wire) by the mean arterial pressure (measured by the guiding catheter positioned in the ostium of the coronary artery) (Fig. 6.3).

The utilization of CFR in cases with microvascular disease is still controversial. The inability of the microcirculation to respond to adenosine may result in inaccurate results. However,

the ability of the Doppler wire to assess the microcirculation may be considered an advantage in certain circumstances. For example, an impaired CFR measured in more than one epicardial artery may indicate coronary microvessel disease that may account for the patient's symptoms.

EVALUATION OF LESIONS AFTER INTERVENTIONS

Quantitative Coronary Angiography

After coronary angioplasty, it is well-documented that the visual estimation of residual stenosis by the performing operator is frequently better than lesion severity measured by QCA. Therefore, in clinical trials rigorously evaluating percutaneous interventions, QCA has supplanted visual estimations. However, even using QCA, lesion severity after balloon angioplasty is not accurately assessed. Nakamura et al. (25) reported that whereas superficial vessel wall injuries are similarly imaged by angiography and IVUS, deep injuries to the plaque produce a difference in measurements between the two modalities. When angiography reveals a dissection, there is a high probability that IVUS will demonstrate a plaque fracture extending to the media. Thus, the contrast dye may fill areas of dissections rather than the true lumen.

Intravascular Ultrasound

IVUS is a gold standard for the anatomical assessment of arterial wall changes and of lesion severity after percutaneous coronary interventions (4). As mentioned above, coronary angiography often fails to reveal suboptimal procedural results. In case of intracoronary stent placement, Nakamura et al. (26) demonstrated that in 88% of cases with an optimal angiographic result, IVUS revealed incomplete stent strut apposition or residual stenosis within or in proximity to the stented segment, which were not appreciated by angiography. Albiero et al. (27) demonstrated that using IVUS, short-term results after intracoronary stent placement were better than with angiographic guidance, owing to the greater improvement in luminal diameter using the former technique. Moreover, IVUS can be used to better localize stent deployment. Indeed, in the recent CRUISE trial, IVUS-guided intracoronary stent placement resulted in 44% lower target vessel revascularization and 23% greater cross-sectional area achieved acutely (unpublished). A recent randomized study found a much more modest effect of IVUS: The use of IVUS guidance in stent deployment produced a nonsignificant 6.3% absolute reduction in the 6-month restenosis rate and a nonsignificant difference in the 6-month minimal lumen diameter (28). It is worth mentioning that the use of high-pressure balloon inflations after intracoronary stent placement (Palmaz-Schatz stents) was introduced into clinical practice only after serial IVUS studies were performed after stent placement, clearly demonstrating the suboptimal stent tine apposition to the vessel wall until increasingly high pressures were deployed.

Coronary Flow Reserve Measurement

QCA and IVUS offer an anatomic assessment of procedural results, but do not address the physiological aspect. The CFR as measured by the intracoronary Doppler wire is often still impaired after balloon angioplasty. There are data indicating that after the placement of intracoronary stents, the CFR is normalized in a higher proportion of patients than after balloon angioplasty (29). This may reflect a greater acute gain in lumen diameter after stent deployment (29). Moreover, the geometric configuration of the lesion after stent placement may be more conducive to blood flow. Others claim that the placement of intracoronary stents favorably affects the microcirculation (30).

The recently published Doppler Endpoints Balloon Angioplasty Trial Europe (DEBATE) study emphasized the importance of normalized CFR after percutaneous coronary interventions (20). In 225 with angiographically successful coronary angioplasty, postprocedural CFR and percent diameter stenosis (angiographic) were correlated with subsequent clinical and angiographic outcome. A CFR of more than 2.5 and residual diameter stenosis of 35% identified lesions with a low incidence of recurrence of symptoms at 1 and 6 months, a low need for reintervention, and a low restenosis rate. These data suggest that physiological parameters may complement anatomic evaluations of lesion severity after coronary interventions. These findings also have immediate clinical ramifications; patients with a normalized CFR after balloon angioplasty may not require stent placement.

One may also use the Doppler wire for the estimation of the residual stenosis of the dilated lesion after balloon angioplasty or stent placement (31). As the Doppler wire is gradually pulled back into the guiding catheter, the flow velocities within the stent and immediately proximal to the stented segment are recorded. Using the continuity equation, the ratio of the flow velocity in the proximal reference segment to the velocity within the stent denotes the residual stenosis within the stent.

In summary, the evolution of technology over the last decade allows us to better determine the functional and structural abnormalities of coronary artery disease (32). The measurement of CFR, FFR, and IVUS should be regarded as complementary methods and should be inte-

Coronary angiography

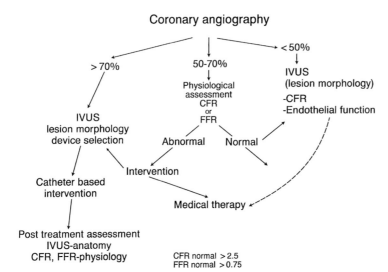

FIG. 6.4. Schematic flow chart illustrating the concept of the use of physiological and anatomical assessment of coronary artery disease for decision making in the cardiac catheterization laboratory. As indicated in the text, the use of intravascular ultrasound, Doppler wires, and wave-pressure wires contribute to decision making, the assessment of the significance of coronary artery disease, and the assessment of interventional procedures.

grated to better access the physiological and anatomical characteristic of coronary artery disease (Fig. 6.4).

REFERENCES

1. Saucedo JF, Lansky AJ, Ito S, Pompa JF. A practical approach to quantitative coronary angiography. In: Beyar R, Keren G, Leon MB, Serruys P (eds). *Frontiers in interventional cardiology.* London: Martin Dunitz Publishers, 1997:281–296.
2. Mintz GS, Pompa JJ, Pichard AD et al. Limitations of angiography in the assessment of plaque distribution in coronary artery disease. A systematic study of target lesion eccentricity in 1446 lesions. *Circulation* 1996; 93:924–931.
3. Mintz GS, Pompa JJ, Pichard AD et al. Patterns of calcification in coronary artery disease. A statistical analysis of intravascular ultrasound and coronary angiography in 1,155 lesions. *Circulation* 1995; 91:1959–1965.
4. Di Mario C, Gorge G, Peters R et al. Clinical application and image interpretation in intracoronary ultrasound. *Eur Heart J* 1998;19:207–229.
5. Lee DY, Nishioka T, Tabak SW, Forrester JS, Siegel RJ. Effect of intracoronary imaging on clinical decision making. *Am Heart J* 1995;129:1084–1093.
6. Mintz GS, Pichard AD, Kovach JA et al. Impact of pre-intervention intravascular ultrasound imaging on trans-catheter treatment strategies in coronary artery disease. *Am J Cardiol* 1994;73:423–430.
7. Drexler H, Zeiher AM, Wollschlager H, Meinertz T, Just H, Bonzel T. Flow-dependent coronary artery dilatation in humans. *Circulation* 1989;80:466–474.
8. Zeiher AM, Drexler H, Wollschlaeger H, Saurbier B, Just H. Coronary vasomotion in response to sympathetic stimulation in humans: Importance of the functional integrity of the endothelium. *J Am Coll Cardiol* 1989;14: 1181–1190.
9. Gould KL, Lipscomb K. Effects of coronary stenoses on coronary flow reserve and resistance. *Am J Cardiol* 1974;34:48–55.
10. Kern MJ, Donohue TJ, Aguirre FV et al. Clinical outcome of deferring angioplasty in patients with normal translesional pressure-flow velocity measurements. *J Am Coll Cardiol* 1995;25:178–187.
11. Doucette JW, Corl PD, Payne HM et al. Validation of a Doppler guide wire for intravascular measurement of coronary artery flow velocity. *Circulation* 1992;85: 1899–1911.
12. Ofili EO, Labovitz AJ, Kern MJ. Coronary flow velocity dynamics in normal and diseased arteries. *Am J Cardiol* 1993;71:3D–9D.
13. Hori M, Kitakaze M. Adenosine, the heart, and coronary circulation. *Hypertension* 1991;18:565–574.
14. Liang BT. Adenosine receptors and cardiovascular function. *Trends Cardiovasc Med* 1992;2:100–108.
15. Holdright DR, Lindsay DC, Clarke D, Fox K, Poole-Wilson PA, Collins P. Coronary flow reserve in patients with chest pain and normal coronary arteries. *Br Heart J* 1993;70:513–519.
16. Rossen JD, Quillen JE, Lopez AG, Stenberg RG, Talman CL, Winniford MD. Comparison of coronary vaso-dilation with intravenous dipyridamole and adenosine. *J Am Coll Cardiol* 1991;18:485–491.
17. Kern MJ, Deligonul U, Tatineni S, Serota H, Aguirre F, Hilton TC. Intravenous adenosine: continuous infusion and low dose administration for determination of coronary flow reserve in patients with and without coronary artery disease. *J Am Coll Cardiol* 1991;18: 718–729.
18. Wilson RF, Wyche K, Christensen BV, Zimmer S, Laxson DD. Effects of adenosine on human coronary arterial circulation. *Circulation* 1990;82:1595–1606.
19. Holdright DR, Clarke D, Poole-Wilson PA, Fox K, Collins P. Endothelium dependent and independent responses in coronary artery disease measured at angioplasty. *Br Heart J* 1993;70:35–42.
20. Serruys PW, di Mario C, Piek J et al. Prognostic value

of intracoronary flow velocity and diameter stenosis in assessing the short- and long-term outcomes of coronary balloon angioplasty: the DEBATE Study (Doppler End-points Balloon Angioplasty Trial Europe). *Circulation* 1997;96:3369–3377.

21. Kern MJ, de Bruyne B, Pijls NH. From research to clinical practice: current role of intracoronary physiologically based decision making in the cardiac catheterization laboratory. *J Am Coll Cardiol* 1997;30:613–620.

22. Pijls NHJ, de Bruyne B, Peels K et al. Measurement of fractional flow reserve to assess the functional severity of coronary-artery stenoses. *N Engl J Med* 1996;334: 1703–1708.

23. de Bruyne B, Paulus WJ, Pijls NHJ. Rationale and application of coronary transstenotic pressure gradient measurements. *Cathet Cardiovasc Diagn* 1994;33:250–261.

24. Pijls NHJ, van Son JAM, Kirkeeide RL, de Bruyne B, Gould KL. Experimental basis of determining maximum coronary, myocardial, and collateral blood flow by pressure measurements for assessing functional stenosis severity before and after percutaneous transluminal coronary angioplasty. *Circulation* 1993;87:1354–1367.

25. Nakamura S, Mahon DJ, Maheswaran B, Gutfinger DE, Colombo A, Tobis JM. An explanation for discrepancy between angiographic and intravascular ultrasound measurements after percutaneous transluminal coronary angioplasty. *J Am Coll Cardiol* 1995;25:633–639.

26. Nakamura S, Colombo A, Gaglione A et al. Intracoro-

nary ultrasound observations during stent implantation. *Circulation* 1994;89:2026–2034.

27. Albiero R, Rau T, Schluter M et al. Comparison of immediate and intermediate-term results of intravascular ultrasound versus angiography-guided Palmaz-Schatz stent implantation in matched lesions. *Circulation* 1997; 96:2997–3005.

28. Schiele F, Meneveau N, Vuillemenot A et al. Impact of intravascular ultrasound guidance in stent deployment on 6-month restenosis rate: A multicenter, randomized study comparing two strategies—with and without intravascular ultrasound guidance. *J Am Coll Cardiol* 1998;32:320–328.

29. Kern MJ, Dupouy P, Drury JH et al. Role of coronary artery lumen enlargement in improving coronary blood flow after balloon angioplasty and stenting: a combined intravascular ultrasound Doppler flow and imaging study. *J Am Coll Cardiol* 1997;29:1520–1527.

30. Wilson RF, Johnson MR, Marcus ML et al. The effect of coronary angioplasty on coronary flow reserve. *Circulation* 1988;77:873–885.

31. Lerman A, Higano ST, Garratt KN, Rihal CS, Hasdai D, Holmes DR Jr. Measuring percent stenosis with intracoronary Doppler and the continuity equation: correlation with intracoronary ultrasound and angiography. *Circulation* 1997;96:I-79.

32. Wilson RF. Assessing the severity of coronary artery stenoses. *N Engl J Med.* 1996;334(26):1735–1737.

7

Management of the Calcified Lesion

Stuart T. Higano, Charles R. Cannan, Nelson A. Araujo,
and *David R. Holmes, Jr.

*Cardiovascular Division, Mayo Clinic, *Division of Cardiovascular Diseases and Internal
Medicine, Mayo Clinic and Mayo Foundation, Department of Medicine, Mayo Medical School,
Rochester, Minnesota 55905*

CORONARY CALCIFICATION AND OUTCOME

Calcification is an important component of the atherosclerotic plaque. It is related to plaque burden and to the degree of luminal compromise, with more severe calcification being associated with tighter stenoses. Despite a growing number of coronary revascularization tools, such as stents, laser, and atherectomy, the calcified plaque has remained difficult to treat. The response of plaque to interventional devices is critically dependent on its morphology, with calcium being one of the most important components. Acute success rates with PTCA are lower in lesions that are calcified (1,2). Heavy calcification also increases the potential for dissection and other acute complications and may be associated with increased rates of restenosis following PTCA (3,4). Heavily calcified vessels may prevent the delivery of stents or may prevent complete and full expansion of the stent. Laser angioplasty may be useful for ablating moderate amounts of calcification, but is less effective for severe calcification. Superficial calcification prevents directional atherectomy from cutting into the plaque, thus yielding lower amounts of tissue removal. Conversely, rotational atherectomy has shown efficacy in removing calcified plaque with a high acute success rate. Thus, it is important for the interventionalist to be aware of the presence and extent of target lesion calcification and the effect it may have on device-specific therapies. This chapter will review the detection of target lesion calcium, the effect of calcium on interventional devices, and the current management of the calcified lesion.

DETECTION OF TARGET LESION CALCIFICATION—IVUS VERSUS ANGIO

The detection of the calcified plaque is important for deciding optimal management strategy when planning percutaneous coronary intervention. Clinical indicators can be helpful, because lesion calcification is more prominent in the elderly, multivessel disease, patients with prior CABG, renal disease, and smaller vessels. Both angiography and intracoronary ultrasound can detect coronary calcification. Angiography detects calcium with a sensitivity of only 40% to 48%, a specificity of 82% to 89%, and an overall accuracy of only 59% (5,6). However, intracoronary ultrasound has higher sensitivity for detecting calcium and can further localize the calcium within the plaque. Calcified plaque is the simplest tissue subtype to identify with intravascular ultrasound. The bright echo reflection with signal attenuation and shadowing beyond, often with reverberations, is readily recognizable. Two large series in over 1,000 lesions have shown that target lesion calcium is seen in 75% of all lesions interrogated. In contrast, angiography only identified calcium in one-third of these lesions (5,7). Patients with angiographically vis-

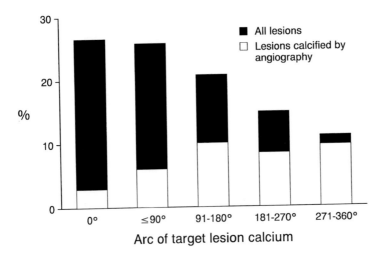

FIG. 7.1. Bar graphs demonstrating the frequency of calcification by IVUS grade of calcification, or number of quadrants involved, in 1155 lesions. Also shown is the number of lesions that were calcified by angiography. Lesions with minimal calcification (0, 1 quadrant) were usually not seen by angiography, while those with severe calcification (3, 4 quadrant) were seen about three quarters of the time by angiography (from ref. 7, with permission).

ible calcium had greater amounts of plaque calcium on intracoronary ultrasound.

The sensitivity of angiography increased with increasingly severe degrees of calcification. In fact, with severe calcification by intracoronary ultrasound, the sensitivity of angiography increases to 63% for more than 180 degrees calcium arc and 85% for four-quadrant calcium (Fig. 7.1) (7). Angiography was more likely to be abnormal when the calcification was superficial in location (52% vs. 21%, $p < .001$) (5). The predictors of angiographically visible calcium were the arc of target lesion calcium, the arc of superficial calcium, the length of reference segment calcium, and the location of calcium. Therefore, angiography is most likely to detect the lesions with the most severe forms of calcification, i.e. more than 180 degrees and superficial in location. Conversely, patients without angiographically visible calcium are not likely to have severe calcification, as only 13% had more than 180 degrees of calcium (grades 3 and 4), only 2% had more than 180 degrees of superficial calcium (grades 3 and 4), and only 1% had more than 270 degrees of calcium (grade 4). Thus, the probability of significant superficial target lesion calcium without any angiographic calcification is small. Of all variables analyzed, however, the presence of angiographic calcium at a nontarget lesion site was the only predictor of ultrasound detected calcium in patients without angiographic target lesion calcium. Of note, coronary angiography also had a false positive rate of 11% for detecting target lesion calcium (7). Coronary calcification by intravascular ultrasound correlated with plaque burden but not lumen compromise (8). Whether intracoronary ultrasound is needed to assist with interventional procedures, especially of the calcified lesion, is still a matter of debate. However, the data would suggest that intracoronary ultrasound is not mandatory for identifying the most severe forms of coronary calcification, but is certainly far more accurate.

PATHOPHYSIOLOGY OF CALCIFIED PLAQUE INTERVENTIONS

Having identified the presence and extent of target lesion calcium, the effect on subsequent catheter-based intervention needs to be considered. In theory, atherosclerotic coronary plaques respond to catheter-based interventions in predictable ways based upon the biomechanical properties of the plaque and the mechanism of lumen enlargement of the device used (9–13). For example, PTCA results in lumen enlargement by a combination of plaque compression, or displacement, and vessel stretch (14). In soft plaques, there is more plaque compression than vessel stretch, while in hard or calcified plaques, there is more vessel stretch (15–17). In both cases, the dilating force of the balloon results in plaque disruption, with fissures or tears occurring in most lesions. The location and severity of PTCA-induced plaque disruption can be predicted by analyzing the magnitude of wall stress induced by the dilating pressure within the lumen (9). Increased wall stress will occur when there are circumferential layers of varying mechanical properties in the arterial plaque, such as between plaque and adventitia or between soft plaque and calcium (13). The wall stress is concentrated near these regions and PTCA generally causes a fissure or tear from the lumen to this point of high wall stress, typically at an area of calcification. Lesions with calcium are much more prone to dissection and have larger dissection tissue planes (18). In addition, higher balloon pressures are needed which can result in an increased risk of vessel trauma. Large dissections are more likely to result in acute complications following PTCA, such as abrupt closure.

Although calcium results in larger dissections following PTCA, coronary stenting may not provide a solution. The important relationships between lesion calcification and stent implantation must be kept in mind (19). Although these are often the very lesions that need to be stented due to large dissections, there is a strong relationship between the degree of calcification and outcome of stent deployment. Hoffmann et al evaluated the outcome in 303 patients undergoing Palmaz-Schatz stent implantation (20). Lesions were divided into 4 groups depending upon the number of quadrants that were calcified by intravascular ultrasound examination. In heavily calcified lesions, despite the use of higher pressure for deployment, the final stent result had a smaller minimal lumen diameter (MLD), small minimal luminal cross-sectional area (MLA), and less acute gain compared with mildly calcified lesions. In addition, stent expansion was more apt to be eccentric, or noncircular. In a smaller series of patients receiving an intracoronary Palmaz-Schatz stent, clinical and ultrasound variables were examined and correlated with the final stent expansion and symmetry (21). The number of quadrants with calcium, the arc of calcium in degrees, and the presence of superficial calcium at baseline were the most significant predictors of poor outcome. Although both series did not

examine the long-term clinical outcome, the smaller minimal lumen area (MLA) seen in calcified lesions following stent placement likely results in higher restenosis rates and target lesion revascularization. Certainly other studies of PTCA and stent placement have demonstrated that no matter what technique is used, the final MLD, MLA, and acute gain have the most dramatic effect on long term outcome (22,23).

This is most important in the presence of severe calcification where final lumen dimensions may be restricted. Thus, removal or debulking of the calcified plaque before PTCA or stent placement may play an important role. A number of debulking devices are presently available. Directional atherectomy (DCA) has essentially no role in treating the calcified lesion, especially when there is superficial calcium. Superficial calcium prevents the atherectomy cutter from cutting the plaque, resulting in much reduced weight of excised tissue and success rates are as low as 50% (24–29). When the calcium is located deep in the plaque, DCA can be successful at debulking the superficial portion of the lesion. In very large calcified vessels, DCA can be used as an adjunct to PTCRA after removal of the superficial calcium (30). In many cases it is difficult to deliver the atherectomy catheter to the calcified plaque.

Excimer laser coronary angioplasty (ELCA), while initially promising for complex lesion subsets, appears to result in increased rates of dissection (31). Coronary dissections were present 39% of the time following ELCA, with most occurring in superficial calcium. The calcified deposits took on a characteristic "shattered" or "fragmented" appearance with newly created, sharp-edged gaps with previously solid calcified masses. In lesions with deep calcium or no calcium, dissection occurred only 14% and 23% of the time, respectively (32). Another concern relates to the inability and failure of ELCA to ablate plaque in heavily calcified lesions (33). A recent multicenter trial evaluating the holmium:YAG laser found that calcium within a lesion was associated with reduced procedural success and calcified lesions required significantly more energy pulses than noncalcified lesions (34).

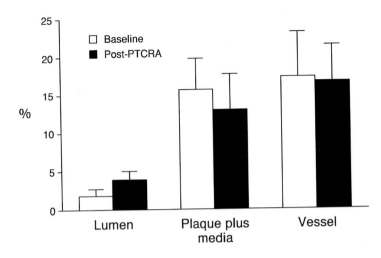

FIG. 7.2. Effect of PTCRA on lumen, plaque plus media (P + M), and vessel dimensions. The improvement in lumen dimension came entirely from plaque removal, not from vessel stretch (from ref 38, with permission).

Rotational atherectomy (PTCRA) is ideally suited to the calcified lesion as it selectively removes hard or calcific elements of the plaque (35–37). PTCRA is also well suited to traverse calcific tortuosity proximal to the lesion site. Intracoronary ultrasound imaging before and after PTCRA has shown that plaque removal accounts for most of the lumen enlargement (Fig. 7.2) (38). The arc of calcium is reduced following PTCRA indicating that calcium is selectively removed. Dissections were infrequent after PTCRA, occurring in 6% of lesions as evident by angiography and in 29% of lesions as evident by ultrasound, far less frequent than after PTCA (39). The pattern of dissection was also much different than after PTCA, originating within calcific deposits rather than adjacent to them. Furthermore, a large clinical series has demonstrated equivalent clinical success rates with PTCRA in both calcified and noncalcified lesions (40).

Debulking with PTCRA would be expected to improve the effectiveness of PTCA or stenting. The law of Lamaze describes dilating force exerted on the vessel wall as a function of the dilating pressure, lumen diameter, and wall thickness (Fig. 7.3). Debulking increases the lumen diameter and decreases the wall thickness, thereby increasing the force of dilation and thereby facilitating subsequent PTCA and possible stent placement (41).

Compared to stent placement alone, rotational atherectomy prior to stent placement clearly improves the acute lumen dimensions in lesions with moderate to severe and severe calcification (grade III to IV, or over 180 degrees) (20,42). The acute lumen gain and final percent diameter stenosis by QCA are improved with rotational atherectomy prior to stent placement compared to stent placement alone (1.94 vs. 1.72 mm, and 4% vs. 9%). By intravascular ultrasound, the acute diameter gain (1.35 vs. 1.02 mm), acute CSA gain (5.41 vs. 4.57 mm2), final percent diameter stenosis (12% vs. 17%), and eccentric-

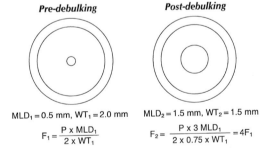

Pre-$debulking$ $Post$-$debulking$

$MLD_1 = 0.5$ mm, $WT_1 = 2.0$ mm $MLD_2 = 1.5$ mm, $WT_2 = 1.5$ mm

$$F_1 = \frac{P \times MLD_1}{2 \times WT_1} \qquad F_2 = \frac{P \times 3\,MLD_1}{2 \times 0.75 \times WT_1} = 4F_1$$

FIG. 7.3. Demonstration of the Law of Lamaze. When debulking improves the lumen and wall thickness dimensions, there is increased dilating force at a given balloon inflation pressure. In this example, plaque debulking has increased the diameter threefold and decreased the wall thickness by 25%, resulting in a fourfold higher dilating force. D, lumen diameter; WT, wall thickness; P, dilating pressure, or inflation balloon pressure; F1 and F2, the dilating force exerted on the wall.

sus intravascular ultrasound. *J Am Coll Cardiol* 1996; 27:832–838.

6. Mintz GS, Douek P, Pichard AD et al. Target lesion calcification in coronary artery disease: an intravascular ultrasound study. *J Am Coll Cardiol* 1992;20: 1149–1155.

7. Mintz GS. Popma JJ. Pichard AD et al. Patterns of calcification in coronary artery disease. A statistical analysis of intravascular ultrasound and coronary angiography in 1,155 lesions. *Circulation* 1995;91:1959–1965.

8. Mintz GS. Pichard AD. Popma JJ et al. Determinants and correlates of target lesion calcium in coronary artery disease: a clinical, angiographic and intravascular ultrasound study. *J Am Coll Cardiol* 1997;29:269–274.

9. Lee RT, Loree HM, Cheng GC, Lieberman EH, Jaramillo N, Schoen FJ. Computational structural analysis based on intravascular ultrasound imaging before in vitro angioplasty: prediction of plaque fracture locations. *J Am Coll Cardiol* 1993;21:777–782.

10. Lee RT, Grodzinsky AJ, Frank EH, Kamm RD. Schoen FJ. Structure-dependent dynamic mechanical behavior of fibrous caps from human atherosclerotic plaques. *Circulation* 1991;83:1764–1770.

11. Lee RT, Loree HM, Fishbein MC. High stress regions in saphenous vein bypass graft atherosclerotic lesions. *J Am Coll Cardiol* 1994;24:1639–1644.

12. Cheng GC, Loree HM, Kamm RD, Fishbein MC, Lee RT. Distribution of circumferential stress in ruptured and stable atherosclerotic lesions. A structural analysis with histopathological correlation. *Circulation* 1993;87: 1179–1187.

13. Richardson PD, Davies MJ, Born GV. Influence of plaque configuration and stress distribution on fissuring of coronary atherosclerotic plaques. *Lancet* 1989;2: 941–944.

14. Braden GA, Herrington DM, Downes TR, Kutcher MA, Little WC. Qualitative and quantitative contrasts in the mechanisms of lumen enlargement by coronary balloon angioplasty and directional coronary atherectomy. *J Am Coll Cardiol* 1994;23:40–48.

15. Gil R, Di Mario C, Prati F et al. Influence of plaque composition on mechanisms of percutaneous transluminal coronary balloon angioplasty assessed by ultrasound imaging. *Am Heart J* 1996;131:591–597.

16. Baptista J, di Mario C, Ozaki Y et al. Impact of plaque morphology and composition on the mechanisms of lumen enlargement using intracoronary ultrasound and quantitative angiography after balloon angioplasty. *Am J Cardiol* 1996;77:115–121.

17. Baptista J, Umans VA, di Mario C, Escaned J, de Feyter P, Serruys PW. Mechanisms of luminal enlargement and quantification of vessel wall trauma following balloon coronary angioplasty and directional atherectomy. *Eur Heart J* 1995;16:1603–1612.

18. Fitzgerald PJ, Ports TA, Yock PG. Contribution of localized calcium deposits to dissection after angioplasty. An observational study using intravascular ultrasound. *Circulation* 1992;86:64–70.

19. Albrecht D, Kaspers S, Fussl R, Hopp HW, Sechtem U. Coronary plaque morphology affects stent deployment: assessment by intracoronary ultrasound. *Cathet Cardiovasc Diagn* 1996;38:229–235.

20. Hoffmann, R, Mintz GS, Popma JJ et al. Treatment of calcified lesions with Palmaz-Schatz stents: an intravas-

cular ultrasound study. *Eur Heart J* 1998;19: 1224–1231.

21. Cannan CR, Fehrenbach MC, Williams DO. The deployment of stents in calcified lesions: are we between a rock and a hard place? *Circulation* 1997;96:3264(abst).

22. Kuntz RE, Gibson CM, Nobuyoshi M, Baim DS. Generalized model of restenosis after conventional balloon angioplasty, stenting, and directional atherectomy. *J Am Coll Cardiol* 1993;21:15–25.

23. De Jaegere, Mudra H, Figulla H et al. Intravascular ultrasound guided optimized stent deployment: immediate and 6 month clinical and angiographic results from Multicenter Ultrasound Stenting In Coronaries Study (MUSIC). *Eur Heart J* 1998;19:1214–1223.

24. Fitzgerald PJ, Yock PG. Mechanisms and outcomes of angioplasty and atherectomy assessed by intravascular ultrasound imaging. *J Clin Ultras* 1993;21:579–588.

25. Kimura BJ, Fitzgerald PJ, Sudhir K, Amidon TM, Strunk BL, Yock PG. Guidance of directed coronary atherectomy by intracoronary ultrasound imaging. *Am Heart J* 1992;124:1365–1369.

26. Yock PG, Fitzgerald PJ, Sudhir K, Linker DT, White W, Ports A. Intravascular ultrasound imaging for guidance of atherectomy and other plaque removal techniques. *Intern J Card Imaging* 1991;6:179–189.

27. Yock PG, Fitzgerald PJ, Linker DT, Angelsen BA. Intravascular ultrasound guidance for catheter-based coronary interventions. *J Am Coll Cardiol* 1991;17(6)[Suppl B]:39B–45B.

28. Yock PG, Yock CA, Fitzgerald PJ. Ultrasound-guided atherectomy: the vision for the future? *Coron Artery Dis* 1996;7:299–303.

29. Safian RD. Coronary atherectomy: directional and extraction techniques. In: Topol EJ, ed. *Textbook of Interventional Cardiology*. Philadelphia: WB Saunders, 1999:501–522.

30. Mintz GS, Pichard AD, Popma JJ, Kent KM, Satler LF, Leon MB. Preliminary experience with adjunct directional coronary atherectomy after high-speed rotational atherectomy in the treatment of calcific coronary artery disease. *Am J Cardiol* 1993;71:799–804.

31. Bittl JA, Sanborn TA, Tcheng JE, Siegel RM, Ellis SG. Clinical success, complications and restenosis rates with excimer laser coronary angioplasty. The Percutaneous Excimer Laser Coronary Angioplasty Registry. *Am J Cardiol* 1992;70(20):1533–1539.

32. Mintz GS, Kovach JA, Javier SP et al. Mechanisms of lumen enlargement after excimer laser coronary angioplasty. An intravascular ultrasound study. *Circulation* 1995;92:3408–3414.

33. Buchwald AB, Werner GS, Unterberg C, Voth E, Kreuzer H, Wiegand V. Restenosis after excimer laser angioplasty of coronary stenoses and chronic total occlusions. *Am Heart J* 1992;123:878.

34. Topaz O, Melvor M, Stone GW et al. Acute results, complications, and effect of lesion characteristics on outcome with the solid state, pulsed wave, mid-infrared laser angioplasty system: Final multi-center report. *Lasers Surg Med* 1998;22:228–239.

35. Ahn SS, Auth D, Marcus DR, Moore WS. Removal of focal atheromatous lesions by angioscopically guided high-speed rotary atherectomy. Preliminary experimental observations. *J Vasc Surg* 1988;7:292–300.

36. Hansen DD, Auth DC, Hall M, Ritchie JL. Rotational

endarterectomy in normal canine coronary arteries: preliminary report. *J Am Coll Cardiol* 1988;11:1073–1077.

37. Dussaillant GR, Mintz GS, Pichard AD et al. Effect of rotational atherectomy in noncalcified atherosclerotic plaque: a volumetric intravascular ultrasound study. *J Am Coll Cardiol* 1996;28:856–860.

38. Kovach JA, Mintz GS, Pichard AD et al. Sequential intravascular ultrasound characterization of the mechanisms of rotational atherectomy and adjunct balloon angioplasty. *J Am Coll Cardiol* 1993;22:1024–1032.

39. Hodgson JM. Graham SP. Savakus AD et al. Clinical percutaneous imaging of coronary anatomy using an over-the-wire ultrasound catheter system. *Intern J Card Imaging* 1989;4:187–193.

40. MacIsaac AI, Bass TA, Buchbinder M et al. High-speed rotational atherectomy: outcome in calcified and non-calcified coronary artery lesions. *J Am Coll Cardiol* 1995;26:731–736.

41. Lee RT, Kamm RD. Vascular mechanics for the cardiologist. *J Am Coll Cardiol* 1994;23:1289–1295.

42. J. Moussa I, Di Mario C, Moses J et al. Coronary stenting after rotational atherectomy in calcified and complex lesions. Angiographic and clinical follow-up results. *Circulation* 1997;96:128–136.

43. Hoffmann R. Mintz GS. Kent KM et al. Comparative early and nine-month results of rotational atherectomy, stents, and the combination of both for calcified lesions in large coronary arteries. *Am J Cardiol* 1998;81:552–527.

44. Serruys PW, Deshpande NV. Is there MUSIC in IVUS guided stenting? Is this MUSIC going to be a MUST? Multicenter Ultrasound Stenting in Coronaries Study. *Eur Heart J* 1998;19:1122–1124.

8

The Long Lesion

A. The Mayo Clinic Perspective

David R. Holmes, Jr. and *Kirk N. Garratt

*Division of Cardiovascular Diseases and Internal Medicine, *Adult Cardiac Catheterization Laboratory, St. Mary's Hospital, and Mayo Clinic and Mayo Foundation, Department of Medicine, Mayo Medical School, Rochester, Minnesota 55905*

Long lesions and diffuse disease represent significant problems for interventional cardiology. The definition of long and/or diffuse disease varies. Lesion length judged angiographically has been arbitrarily divided into lesions <10 mm (short); lesions from 10 to 20 mm (tubular); and lesions >20 mm (long). Diffuse disease, in addition to being long, usually involves segments where there is no apparent normal reference vessel. Intravascular ultrasound has shown that arterial segments that appear normal angiographically are often involved with atheromatous disease, making the ultrasonic definition of long lesions problematic. While intravascular ultrasound is of great utility in guiding coronary therapy, definition of lesion length still depends primarily on angiography.

Lesion length has several implications for procedural performance. These include:

1. Involvement of side branches. This is particularly a problem for circumflex and left anterior descending lesions in which case the branches may be large and may supply a substantial amount of left ventricular myocardium. For the right coronary artery, this is less of a problem, as the free wall right ventricular branches do not supply a large amount of myocardium. Even if these occlude, the occlusions rarely cause clinically significant problems, although they may result in enzyme elevation.

2. Increased plaque burden. This predisposes the lesion to dissection, inadequate dilatation because of plaque mass, inadequate stent expansion, and acute stent thrombosis (1). In addition, this predisposes to increased restenosis (2).

3. Lesion calcification. Diffusely diseased vessels are often calcified. This imparts its own degree of difficulty and complications. The combination of lesion length and calcification produces a significant challenge, since insertion of equipment requires a certain amount of compliance on the part of the vessel being traversed. Under some circumstances, passage of equipment through long, calcified (i.e., noncompliant) vascular segments may be impossible.

4. Increased potential for no reflow during attempts at ablation.

5. Taper of the vessel. This has important implications. Angiographic studies have documented that approximately 20% of blood vessels taper from 0.5 to 0.9 mm over a 20-mm segment length and approximately 25% of the vessels taper 1 mm over the same distance (3). This results in a difficult dilemma: balloon selection based upon proximal reference diameter may result in increased risk of dissection, whereas balloon sizing based upon the distal reference segment may yield a suboptimal result. Accordingly, over very long lesions, balloon and possibly stent size needs

to vary to avoid the oversizing problem. In the past, tapering balloons were available; they tapered 0.5 mm over 30 mm and were found to give excellent results (4). These, however, are no longer available.

Choosing an interventional strategy depends on several of these factors and includes presence of side branches, length of the lesion, presence and extent of calcium at the segment to be treated, and the size of the distal vasculature bed. Options include dilatation with conventional-length balloons, dilatation with longer balloons, debulking with rotational atherectomy or excimer laser angioplasty, and long stents.

CONVENTIONAL-LENGTH BALLOONS

Approaching long or diffuse lesions with conventional balloons often results in inadequate outcome. This approach results in longer procedure times than necessary because of the need to make repeated adjustments in the balloon position. In addition, the junction of the inflated balloon with the diseased arterial segment may increase mechanical shear stress and result in a dissection. For this reason this approach is not widely used.

LONG BALLOONS

Balloons are available commercially in lengths of up to 40 mm and under special circumstances have been available in lengths of up to 60 mm. These balloons usually do not track as well and have a larger profile than some more recent conventional length balloons. They do have the advantage that they can be used to cover the entire length of diseased segment. These balloons often conform well to the vessel contour, particularly if a soft guidewire is used. Placement of these balloons can be difficult depending upon the length of the balloon and the location of the balloon markers. Proximal and distal balloon markers would be ideal so that the lesion could be straddled with these markers. This is of particular importance for the 40-mm long and even longer balloons. If just a proximal and mid-

marker is present, it may be difficult to make certain that the balloon spans the lesion. Due to the potential for dissection, long balloons should be inflated slowly and high pressure should be avoided. This is particularly important in preventing balloon rupture, which can severely damage the vessel wall. We typically also maintain inflation as long as the patient's ischemia allows it to improve the initial result. We typically start with a short inflation and then perform angiography to document that we have adequately spanned the diffusely diseased segment and then proceeded with a longer inflation.

In our initial series of 14 high-risk patients and 19 treated coronary segments using a 60 mm-long balloon, the results were excellent. Angiographic success was achieved in all patients. While intimal dissection occurred in four of the 19 treated segments, in each it was less than 50% and no patient required stent implantation. In such long lesions at high risk for complications, a IIb/IIIa agent should be given at the beginning of the procedure. Long balloons are also helpful for treatment of very long dissections, particularly involving the right coronary artery, which can extend from the ostium down to the posterior descending coronary artery. In these cases, it may be desirable to avoid stenting the entire length because of an increased incidence of restenosis (see below). Accordingly, long balloons may be very helpful here.

DEBULKING

Debulking long lesions or diffuse disease is an attractive concept. Two technologies were developed in part to address this: laser angioplasty and rotational atherectomy. Initially, there was substantial interest in the former. FDA approval was based in part on the lack of decremental success rates with increasing lesion complexity with laser angioplasty in contrast to conventional dilatation and indeed the common characteristic making the laser-treated lesions complex was lesion length. Improvement in initial results within this patient subgroup was a key benefit of laser therapies (5). However, both ultraviolet and infrared laser systems are associated with an increased risk of coronary dissection and perforation, and have not proven to be consistently effective in treating calcified vessels (5,6). Since long lesions and diffuse disease are often calcified, this limits the utility of laser angioplasty for these lesions. Laser may still be useful, however, for debulking long in-stent restenotic lesions. Typically, these lesions are not calcified.

Rotational atherectomy has some specific advantages because it can treat calcification and fibrocalcific plaques. It has been studied in two completed randomized trials of patients with unfavorable lesion anatomy and has been found to result in improved success rates compared with conventional PTCA. Unfortunately, rotational atherectomy has the disadvantage of no reflow. This is a particular problem in long lesions that require long ablation runs or in lesions which have poor distal vascular beds, both of which are common in long diffuse disease. Rotational atherectomy still plays a role in this setting, but it must be performed slowly with time between ''runs'' to let the particulate debris filter. Liberal use of intracoronary adenosine and calcium channel antagonists will vasodilate the distal microvascular bed and optimize flow. Following ablation, the artery must be treated with either balloon inflation, with stent implantation, or with both. Currently, the burr size or the laser fiber size are inadequate to completely debulk lesions as a stand-alone procedure.

STENT IMPLANTATION

Stents are used in 60% to 80% of all interventional procedures. Their role in long diffuse lesions is evolving. Now that stents are available in variable lengths up to 40 mm, they are being used to treat longer lesions. Despite the availability of long stents, diffusely diseased segments are often treated with two or more stents to achieve the desired final result. When treating long lesions with multiple stents it is best to use a single stent type, since use of multiple stent designs in the same vessel may be associated with an increased risk of abrupt closure (7).

There are also concerns about the durability of stent therapy for long lesions. While stent placement for long lesions usually enjoys good early success, late outcomes are often poor. A strong correlation between length of stent material placed and late adverse events, including restenosis, was found in the randomized study of outcomes after Gianturco-Roubin-II (Cook, Inc., Bloomington, NJ) and JJIS (Johnson and Johnson International Systems, Warren, NJ) stents (data on file, Cook Inc). In a study done by the Mayo Clinic, virtual reconstruction of coronary arteries using three or more coronary stents was associated with the need for further intervention within 6 months in more than three quarters of treated patients (8). It is not clear whether stent placement in long lesions fares worse because of the additional stent material *per se*, or if lesion length is simply a reflection of greater plaque burden or intimal injury (dissection) at the time of intervention. Further, it is unknown whether use of fewer, longer stents will substantially improve results. At least one study reports no difference in outcomes between use of multiple short stents versus single long ones (9). Thus, when diffuse disease is present in which the need for multiple contiguous stents is anticipated, intervention must be undertaken with the expectation that further revascularization therapies will most likely be necessary.

This has led to the concept of spot stenting for these long lesions. The goal of this approach is to minimize the stent length within the segment and rely on conventional dilatation if the results appear acceptable for the remainder of the diffusely diseased target segment. For this approach, a long balloon, matching the lesion length, would be used with a balloon/artery ratio of approximately 1.1:1. Following inflation, stenting would only be performed in the portion of the segment which did not appear to be adequately dilated. The adequacy of dilatation result could be evaluated by either angiography or ultrasound. Preliminary communications about the use of this strategy have documented good results.

There also appears to be a relationship between reference vessel diameter and outcomes among patients who are treated with stents for long lesions. As mentioned, tapering of the treated vessel challenges the operator to select an appropriate balloon or stent size. In a recent study, distal reference diameter <2.5 mm was associated with a significant increase in the risk of adverse events after stenting of long lesions (10). It is unclear whether this is true because of the smaller minimal lumen diameter (MLD) achievable in small vessels or if difficulties in properly matching a stent to both the proximal and distal reference segments influence outcome in long lesions.

When treating long lesions it is very important to optimize the MLD throughout the length of the stent. Intravascular ultrasound may be very helpful in this regard (2), although quantitative coronary angiographic systems work well, especially when the reference MLD is >3.0 mm and high-pressure angioplasty of stents is conducted (11). In the case of long lesions, optimizing stent size throughout the length of the stent is likely to be very important in reducing adverse event rates. This can be accomplished readily by using shorter, high-pressure-tolerant balloon catheters with moderate compliance properties for poststent dilatation purposes. Use of higher pressures at the proximal end of the stent will increase the final MLD to a greater degree than lower pressure angioplasty at the distal end.

In the future, radiation therapies may play an important role in therapy for long lesions. Although none of the brachytherapy protocols active at this time permit treatment of *de novo* long lesions or diffuse disease, there is enthusiasm for study of these problematic patients. Because an essential premise behind this concept holds that radiation is beneficial because it passivates the intimal surface after intervention (12), brachytherapy of diffuse disease as an initial therapy may make a lot of sense, because it is relatively easy to treat a long vascular segment. If brachytherapy fails to improve initial results of intervention, the potential of brachytherapy to improve secondary outcomes after treatment of in-stent restenosis may prove very important in the long-term management of long lesions. Intravascular ultrasound studies show that significant intimal hyperplastic tissue remains protruding through the stent and into the lumen after conventional dilatation of restenosis lesions, and this is especially true for long lesions treated with stents (13). Radiation therapy to quell the metabolic activity of this tissue may be of great benefit in improving long-term outcome in these patients.

CONCLUSION

Long segments of diffuse disease remain problematic, both from the standpoint of achieving an adequate initial result without complication and from the standpoint of achieving a longer lasting, good outcome. Selection from a number of options is dependent on the specific vessel treated, length of segment involved, presence of side branch, degree of calcification, and the size of the target vessel and the distal bed.

REFERENCES

1. Werner GS, Gastmann O, Ferrari M et al. Risk factors for acute and subacute stent thrombosis after high-pressure stent implantation: a study by intracoronary ultrasound. *Am Heart J* 1998;135:300–309.
2. Gorge G, Ge J, Erbel R. Role of intravascular ultrasound in the evaluation of mechanisms of coronary interventions and restenosis. *Am J Cardiol* 1998;81(12A):91G–95G.
3. Javier SP, Mintz GS, Popma JJ, Pichard AD, Kent KM, Satler LF, Leon MB. Intravascular ultrasound assessment of the magnitude and mechanism of coronary artery and lumen tapering. *Am J Cardiol* 1995;75(2):177–180.
4. Laird JR, Popma JJ, Knopf WD et al. Angiographic and procedural outcome after coronary angioplasty in high-risk subsets using a decremental diameter (tapered) balloon catheter. Tapered Balloon Registry Investigators. *Am J Cardiol* 1996;77(8):561–568.
5. Bittl JA, Sanborn. Excimer laser-facilitated coronary angioplasty. Relative risk analysis of acute and follow-up results in 200 patients. *Circulation* 1992;86(1):71–80.
6. Topaz O, McIvor M, Stone GW et al. Acute results, complications, and effect of lesion characteristics on outcome with the solid-state, pulsed-wave, mid-infrared laser angioplasty system: final multicenter registry report. Holmium: YAG Laser Multicenter Investigators. *Lasers Surg Med* 1998;22(4):228–239.
7. Moussa I, Di Mario C, Reimers B, Akiyama T, Tobis J, Colombo A. Subacute stent thrombosis in the era of intravascular ultrasound-guided coronary stenting without anticoagulation: frequency, predictors, and clinical outcome. *J Am Coll Cardiol* 1997 29(1):6–12.
8. Mathew V, Hasdai D, Bell MR et al. Clinical outcomes of patients undergoing endoluminal coronary arterial reconstruction with three or more stents. *J Am Coll Cardiol* 1997;30:676–681.
9. De Scheerder IK, Wang K, Kostopoulos K, Dens J, Desmet W, Piessens JH. Treatment of long dissections by use of a single long or multiple short stents: clinical and angiographic follow-up. *Am Heart J* 1998;136(2):345–351.

10. Kerr AJ, Stewart RAH, Low CJS, Restieaux NJ, Wilkins GT. Long stenting in native coronary arteries: relation between vessel size and outcome. *Cathet Cardiovasc Diagn* 1998;44:170–174.

11. Blasini R, Neumann FJ, Schmitt C, Bokenkamp J, Schomig A. Comparison of angiography and intravascular ultrasound for the assessment of lumen size after coronary stent placement: impact of dilatation pressures. *Cathet Cardiovasc Diagn* 1997;42(2):113–119.

12. King SB III, Williams DO, Chougule P et al. Endovascular beta-radiation to reduce restenosis after coronary balloon angioplasty: results of the beta energy restenosis trial (BERT). *Circulation* 1998;97(20):2025–2030.

13. Shiran A, Mintz GS, Waksman R, Mehran R, Abizaid A, Kent KM, Pichard AD, Satler LF, Popma JJ, Leon MB. Early lumen loss after treatment of in-stent restenosis: an intravascular ultrasound study. *Circulation* 1998; 98(3):200–203.

B. The University Hospital Gasthuisberg Perspective

Patrick Coussement and Ivan De Scheerder

Department of Cardiology, University Hospital Gasthuisberg, B-3000 Leuven, Belgium

Since the early days of percutaneous intervention, indications for percutaneous transluminal coronary angioplasty (PTCA) continue to extend. Where complex, long and diffuse lesions were initially a contraindication for PTCA, this is nowadays no longer the case, due to progression of the angioplasty technique, operator experience, and catheter-based technology. However, long coronary stenoses in diffusely diseased, atherosclerotic coronary arteries remain challenging for percutaneous revascularization.

CONVENTIONAL BALLOON ANGIOPLASTY

Studies in the early and middle 1980s recognized the influence of lesion length on procedural success. Meier and Grüntzig reported a complication rate twice as high in eccentric lesions longer than 5 mm compared to short, concentric lesions (24% vs. 12%, $p < .05$) (1). Analysis of the NHLBI-PTCA registry recognized a "diffuse or multiple discrete" lesion morphology as an independent risk factor for peri-procedural coronary occlusion (2). In a retrospective analysis, Ellis et al. identified a lesion length twice or more the lumen diameter as one of the seven independent preprocedural factors related to abrupt vessel closure (AVC) (3).

According to the ACC/AHA Task Force report (1988), subtotal lesions exceeding 20 mm in length remained a relative contraindication for percutaneous revascularization (4).

In contrast with the earlier reports, lesion length had no predictive value on the acute outcome in the Multi-Hospital Eastern Atlantic Restenosis Trial (M-Heart). This was probably due to the technical advantages of steerable, low-profile catheter systems (5).

In contrast with other reports (6,7), longer lesions correlated with a higher incidence of restenosis in this trial ($\leq$4.6 mm, 33% restenosis rate (RR); >4.6 mm, 45% RR; $p = .001$) (8).

In the early 1990s, Goudreau et al. reported a retrospective analysis of 98 patients who underwent angioplasty of at least one diffusely diseased coronary artery. The patient population was divided into three groups: group I, narrowing $\geq$50% that involved the entire vessel, group II, long lesions $\geq$2 cm in length, and group III, three or more lesions in the same vessel. The overall immediate angiographic success (93%) and the clinical recurrence rates (31%) were comparable with angioplasty for discrete lesions. Only in group I, which included patients with disease that involves the entire length of the artery, was the complication rate significantly higher (17.5%), compared to group II patients (2.5%), and group III patients (0%) ($p < .002$) (9).

In a 1993 analysis of the Cleveland Clinic Interventional Cardiology Database including more than 3,000 patients, Ellis et al. found that lesion length, among other factors, still increased the risk of complications (odds ratio 1.4; $p = .004$). Even lesions between 5 and 9 mm in length correlated with a higher risk for dissection-mediated closure than those shorter than 5 mm in length (10).

The EPIC (Evaluation of c7E3, for the Prevention of Ischemic Complications) data, however, showed that treatment with abciximab (ReoPro, Malvern, PA) benefited all high risk patients with complex lesion morphology (35% reduction in acute complications from 12.8% [placebo] to 8.3% (c7E3); $p = .008$) (11).

More recently, Kaul et al. reported angiographic and clinical success rates of 99% and 96%, respectively, in patients with long (11 to 20 mm) or diffuse (longer than 20 mm) lesions. In the group with diffuse lesions, long balloons and rotational atherectomy were used more frequently (12).

Progress in catheter technology led to the introduction of long balloons of 30, 40 and even 60 mm, which improved the acute results in this setting by distributing the inflation pressure more evenly across the diseased vessel segment and decreasing the shear forces at the endpoints of the lesion. In an observational study in patients with long lesions (>10 mm), Zidar et al. reported that long balloons significantly improved procedural success and reduced the incidence of abrupt vessel closure and major dissections, compared to standard 20-mm balloons (success: 89.9% vs. 97.8%; AVC: 14.1% vs. 5.6%; and dissection: 18.1% vs. 8.9%) (13). This finding was also confirmed by Savas et al. in a study including 109 patients with long lesions (mean length 38 mm) using a 40-mm-long balloon; here the procedural success was 90% and the incidence of AVC was 7% (14).

In a randomized trial, selecting 44 patients with long (15 to 25 mm) or tandem (<25 mm overall length) lesions, Brymer et al. reported a high overall primary success rate (95%). Treatment with a 30-mm-long balloon required less inflations and resulted in fewer moderate or severe dissections compared to a standard 20-mm-balloon ($p = .0001$ and $p = .028$, respectively) (15). Tenaglia et al. also reported a high procedural success rate (97%) and an acceptable rate of acute vascular closure (AVC) (6%) and major dissection (11%). In this study, however, the use of a long balloon did not appear to influence the risk of restenosis (50% angiographic restenosis; however, only 76% of the patients underwent follow-up angiography) (16). A very long (60 mm) balloon was used in a small study of 14 high-risk patients, reported by Harris and Holmes from the Mayo Clinic, with a comparable high clinical success rate (93%) and low complication rate (21% dissections, none of them were obstructive). At a mean follow-up of 9 months, only three patients (21%) required a reintervention and one patient (7%) had undergone surgical revascularization (17).

Another problem with long lesions, especially in the left anterior descending artery, is tapering of the vessel. In a study by Banka et al., selecting 100 coronary arteries, the incidence of significant tapering (>0.5 mm along 20 mm in length) was found in 42% of the cases. The use of a balloon catheter with a decremental diameter, to minimize oversizing of the distal segment, was proposed, resulting in an overall angiographic success rate of 98% (18). Laird et al also described a procedural success rate of 96% with a tapered balloon catheter in 115 patients of the multicenter Tapered Balloon Registry. Major complications occurred only in three patients (2.7%) (19).

In conclusion, conventional balloon angioplasty of long lesions can be performed with a success and complication rate comparable to that of short, concentric lesions. A long balloon, or in some cases a tapered balloon, is preferable to a standard balloon. Although the data on restenosis are controversial, the risk of restenosis in this patient population seems to be significantly higher.

NEW INTERVENTIONAL DEVICES

Rotational Atherectomy

Although high-speed rotational atherectomy (HSRA) has been proposed as an alternative treatment in patients with complex, long, calcified lesions, who are poor candidates for balloon angioplasty, initial studies with this device in this patient population were discouraging. Teirstein et al. reported a procedural success of HRSA in only 70% of patients with lesions >10 mm in length (compared to 92% success rate in patients with lesions ≤10 mm; $p < .01$). Non-Q-wave myocardial infarction due to embolization of particles, which occurred in 19% of the patients, was associated with longer lesions. Furthermore, the overall angiographic restenosis rate in this study was 59%. In patients with long lesions, >10 mm, the restenosis rate was 75%, compared to 22% for short lesions; ($p < .05$) (20).

To optimize the immediate results of HRSA, adjunctive PTCA was proposed. In a larger study with 316 patients, Ellis et al. reported that the procedural success of HRSA followed by adjunctive PTCA (performed in 82% of the cases) was higher (89.8%). Major ischemic complications were seen in 8.9% of the patients. Multivariate analysis of these data showed an independent correlation between ischemic complications and lesion length (defined as ≥50% narrowing) ≥4 mm (complication rate, 12%; odds ratio, 3.6; $p = .005$) (21).

In the Rotablator (Heart Technology Inc., Bellevue, WA) multicenter registry, procedural success of HSRA, when combined with balloon angioplasty, was achieved in 95% of patients with lesions <10 mm, in 97% of patients with lesions from 11 to 15 mm and in 92% of patients with lesions of 15 to 25 mm ($p = $ NS). Compared to short lesions (<10 mm) the incidence of non-Q-wave MI and Q-wave MI was slightly higher in the group with longer lesions (4.0% vs. 6.2%, respectively, and 0.7% vs. 2.8%, respectively) (22). Stertzer et al. also reported a high procedural success rate of 94% in a large single-center study in 242 patients, of which 92.5% were ACC/AHA classification Type B or

C. Major complications occurred in only 4.3% of the patients and the estimated incidence of restenosis using clinical and angiographic criteria was 37.4% (23).

In conclusion, procedural success of rotational atherectomy, whether or not combined with adjunctive balloon angioplasty, in patients with long lesions seems to be comparable to conventional balloon angioplasty. This device should be preferred in patients with diffuse, calcified lesions. The use of small burrs and slow passes could be important to minimize "slow reflow" and ischemic complications in this setting.

Directional Atherectomy

Directional coronary atherectomy (DCA) was developed to treat short (≤10 mm), noncalcified, eccentric lesions in proximal segments of the coronary artery tree or at bifurcations with large side branches. Although DCA has been used successfully in lesions >10 mm in length, results from several large randomized DCA trials (CAVEAT-I, CCAT, BOAT and OARS) indicate an adverse outcome (24–30).

Mooney et al. reported in a selected group of 88 patients with LAD lesions longer than 10 mm and favorable morphology (≥3 mm vessel diameter, noncalcified, absence of angulation) a high procedural success rate of DCA (99%) with a 4.6% incidence of abrupt closure and 1.0% rate of emergency surgery (31).

In conclusion, DCA is usually not performed in patients with long lesions, due to a mismatch between the window length of the cutter and the lesion length. However, in selected cases the outcome is comparable to that of standard balloon angioplasty.

Laser Atherectomy

Analysis from the excimer laser coronary angioplasty (ELCA) registry, which included 3,000 patients, showed a high procedural success rate of 90% with an acceptable complication rate (3.8% in-hospital bypass surgery, 2.1% Q-wave myocardial infarction, 0.5% death and

1.2% coronary perforation). The latter complication declined significantly to 0.4% in the last 1,000 patients. Procedural success or complication rates were not influenced by lesion length or complexity (32). However, in subsequent randomized trials like the Amsterdam Rotterdam (AMRO) trial and the Excimer Laser, Rotational Atherectomy, and Balloon Angioplasty Comparison (ERBAC) Study, a trend toward a higher incidence of binary restenosis was observed in the ELCA group compared to the balloon angioplasty (BA) group (AMRO: 53% in ELCA group vs. 41% in BA group; p = .058 and ERBAC: 46% in ELCA group vs. 31.9% in BA group; p = .013) (33,34). This could be explained by a more intense vessel wall injury during laser intervention.

In conclusion, the procedural success of ELCA in long, complex lesions is compared to standard balloon angioplasty. However the long term outcome with this technique is disappointing.

Coronary Stents

Although elective stent implantation has shown to significantly reduce angiographic restenosis rate, this favorable result was obtained in highly selected patients with short ($\leq$15 mm) lesions in large ($\geq$3.0 mm) vessels (35,36). Only few data are available on coronary stenting in patients with long lesions.

Maiello et al. reported a high procedural success of 93% of Palmaz-Schatz (PS) stent (Johnson and Johnson International Systems, Warren, NJ) implantation in 89 patients with 108 long lesions (>20 mm) with an acceptable rate of procedure-related complications, including myocardial infarction in 3%, emergency bypass surgery in 3%, and elective bypass surgery in 1%. There was only one acute stent thrombosis (1.2%) (37). In a small study, reported by Shaknovich et al., including 54 patients with very long lesions or dissections (mean length 50.3 ± 17.8 mm) who received three or more PS stents per vessel, the procedural success was very high (98.2%). Procedure-related complications occurred in 11% of patients (38).

Ellis et al. reported, in an observational study with 206 consecutive patients with PS stent implantation, a significantly higher incidence of angiographic restenosis ($\geq$50% diameter stenosis at follow-up) after implantation of multiple, overlapping stents compared to implantation of a single stent (64% vs. 30% respectively; p < .001). This was explained by the increase in thrombogenicity of the larger metal surface of multiple stents, which possibly induces more neointimal proliferation. Also repeated stent-on-stent trauma with overlapping stents might impair passivation of the stent surface, promote thrombus formation, and increase the risk of restenosis (39). This finding was supported by several other studies (40,41). In a study by Eccleston et al. including 481 consecutive patients (receiving 684 stents), a trend toward increased incidence of major cardiac events at 180 days follow-up was seen in patients receiving multiple stents (MS), compared to the single stent (SS) group (21.8% vs. 17.9%, respectively; p = .043) (42).

The impact of lesion length on restenosis after stent implantation is not clear. Wong et al. concluded, in a study with 248 patients, that lesion length had no influence on restenosis after implantation of a single PS stent. The overall angiographic restenosis rate was 30% (43). On the other hand, several other investigators reported that the incidence of restenosis increased with increasing lesion length (44–46). In a study reported by Hall et al., longer lesion length, rather than the number of stents, was one of the three strongest predictors of restenosis; the study included 359 patients with 429 lesions in which successful intravascular, ultrasound-guided PS stent implantation was performed. The overall incidence of restenosis in this study was only 21% (47).

Recently, long ($\geq$20 mm) stents became available for clinical use (Figs. 8.1, 8.2). To compare implantation of a single long stent (SS) with multiple overlapping short stents (MS), we performed an observational study including 107 patients and 113 vessels with long ($\geq$20 mm) lesions. In 53 vessels a single long stent was implanted. The other 60 vessels were treated with multiple overlapping short (16 mm) stents. In the single stent group there were four (8%)

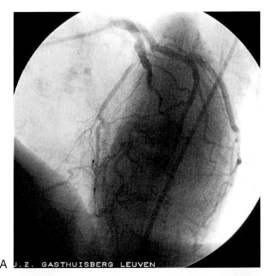

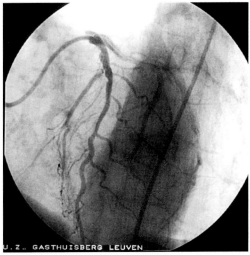

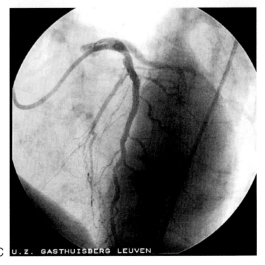

FIG. 8.1. Treatment of a long, suboptimal mid LAD lesion. **A:** Angiographic view before PTCA. **B:** Angiographic result after PTCA with a 40 mm, 3.0 mm balloon. **C:** Angiographic result after stenting with a 36 mm Freedom (Global Therapeutics, Broomfield, CO) coronary stent.

implantation failures, successfully managed by multiple overlapping short stents. The in-hospital complication rate was low: three patients suffered myocardial infarctions (one in the SS group, and two in the MS group) related to long lasting ischemia during the procedure. Subacute stent thrombosis was not observed. We observed no significant differences in late outcome and restenosis between the groups (restenosis rate 29% in SS group vs. 35% in MS group; p = NS) (48).

This study confirmed what was known from previous data. It is not the number of stents used,

but the total length of the stented segment, that correlates with restenosis. However, implantation of a single long stent, when technically feasible, reduces catheterization time, dye volume, for the patient, and radiation exposure for both operator and patient.

In conclusion, stenting of long lesions or dissections can be performed with high procedural success and acceptable complication rates. If technically feasible, a single long stent is preferable to multiple overlapping short stents. Although the incidence of restenosis increases with increasing lesion/stent length, the overall reste-

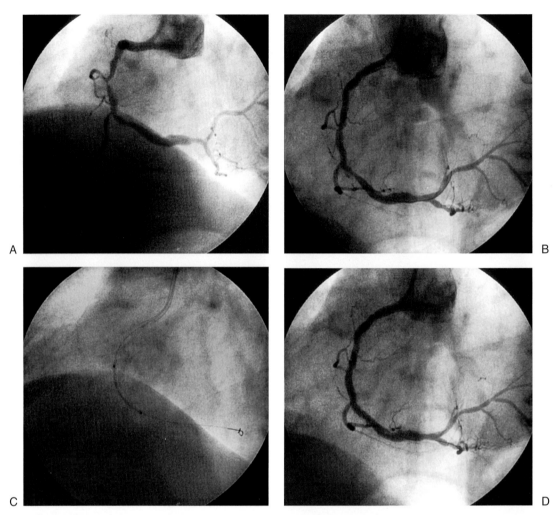

FIG. 8.2. Treatment of a diffusely diseased mid RCA. **A:** Angiographic view before PTCA. **B:** Angiographic result after PTCA with a 20 mm, 3.0 mm balloon. **C:** Implantation of a 36-mm Freedom (Global Therapeutics) coronary stent. **D:** Angiographic result after stenting.

nosis rate after stenting of long lesions is quite favorable when compared to other new devices or balloon angioplasty alone.

PRACTICAL APPROACH FOR TREATMENT OF LONG CORONARY LESIONS

In our center, we promote the provisional stenting theory. When we treat a long lesion (≥10 mm) we first try to properly open the vessel using a well-sized balloon, taking care that the balloon length covers the whole diseased segment. When the vessel is tapered, we use a semi-compliant balloon with the size of the distal segment. Tapered balloons are not commonly used in our center. In case of severe calcifications suitable for rotational atherectomy, we first perform some passes with a small burr before additional ballooning. When a suboptimal angioplasty result is achieved with balloon angioplasty (DS > 20%, visual dissections, visual haziness or any combination of these indications) we stent the whole diseased vessel segment, using, preferably, a single long multicellular coronary stent. When the vessel is severely tapered we use a stent mounted on a balloon with the size of the distal part of the vessel. The proximal stent deployment is consequently optimized using a larger balloon. When the angiographic result remains suboptimal, we perform stent deployment optimization using IVUS control.

REFERENCES

1. Meier B, Gruentzig A, Hollman J, Ischinger T, Bradford J. Does length or eccentricity of coronary stenoses influence the outcome of transluminal dilatation? *Circulation* 1983;67:497–499.
2. Detre K, Holmes D, Holubkov R et al. and coinvestigators of the National Heart, Lung and Blood Institute's Percutaneous Transluminal Coronary Angioplasty Registry. Incidence and consequences of periprocedural occlusion. *Circulation* 1990;82:739–750.
3. Ellis S, Roubin G, King III SB et al. Angiographic and clinical predictors of acute closure after native coronary angioplasty. *Circulation* 1988;77:372–379.
4. Ellis S, Vandormael M, Cowley M et al., and the Multivessel Angioplasty Prognosis Study Group. Coronary morphologic and clinical determinants of procedural outcome with angioplasty for multivessel coronary disease. Implications for patient selection. *Circulation* 1990;82:1193–1202.
5. Savage M, Goldberg S, Hirshfeld J et al., for the M-Heart Investigators. Clinical and angiographic determinants of primary coronary angioplasty success. *J Am Coll Cardiol* 1991;17:22–28.
6. Ryan T, Faxon D, Gunnar R et al. Guidelines for percutaneous transluminal coronary angioplasty. A Report of the American College of Cardiology/American Heart Association Task Force on Assessment of Diagnostic and Therapeutic Cardiovascular Procedures. *Circulation* 1988;78:486–502.
7. Ellis S, Roubin G, King III SB, Douglas J, Cox W. Importance of stenosis morphology in the estimation of restenosis risk after elective percutaneous transluminal coronary angioplasty. *Am J Cardiol* 1989;63:30–34.
8. Hirshfeld J, Schwartz S, Jugo R et al., and the M-Heart Investigators. Restenosis after coronary angioplasty: A multivariate statistical model to relate lesion and procedure variables to restenosis. *J Am Coll Cardiol* 1991; 18:647–656.
9. Goudreau E, DiSciascio G, Kelly K, Vetrovec G, Nath A, Cowley M. Coronary angioplasty of diffuse coronary artery disease. Am Heart J 1991;121:12–19.
10. Ellis S. Coronary lesions at increased risk. Am Heart J. 1995;130:643–646.
11. The EPIC Investigators. Use of monoclonal antibody directed against the platelet glycoprotein IIb/IIIa receptor in high risk coronary angioplasty. *N Eng J Med* 1994; 330:956–961.
12. Kaul U, Upasani P, Agarwal R, Bahl V, Wasir H. In-hospital outcome of percutaneous transluminal coronary angioplasty for long lesions and diffuse coronary artery disease. *Cathet Cardiovasc Diagn* 1995;35:294–300.
13. Zidar J, Tenaglia A, Jackman JJr et al. Improved acute results for PTCA of long coronary lesions using long

14. Savas V, Puchrowicz S, Williams L, Grindes C, O'Neill W. Angioplasty outcome using long balloons in high-risk lesions. *J Am Coll Cardiol* 1992;19:34A.
15. Brymer J, Khaja F, Kraft P. Angioplasty of long or tandem coronary artery: lesions using a new longer balloon dilatation catheter: a comparative study. *Cathet Cardiovasc Diagn* 1991;23:84–88.
16. Tenaglia A, Zidar J, Jackman J et al. Treatment of long coronary artery narrowings with long angioplasty balloon catheters. *Am J Cardiol* 1993;71:1274–1277.
17. Harris W, Holmes D. Treatment of diffuse coronary artery and vein graft disease with a 60-mm-long balloon: Early clinical experience. *Mayo Clin Proc* 1995;70: 1061–1067.
18. Banka V, Baker III H, Vermuri D, Voci G, Maniet A. Effectiveness of decremental diameter balloon catheters (Tapered balloon). *Am J Cardiol* 1992;69:188–193.
19. Laird J, Popma J, Knopf W et al., for the Tapered Balloon Registry Investigators. Angiographic and procedural outcome after coronary angioplasty in high-risk subsets using a decremental diameter (tapered) balloon catheter. *Am J Cardiol* 1996;77:561–568.
20. Teirstein P, Warth D, Haq N et al. High speed rotational coronary atherectomy for patients with diffuse coronary artery disease. *J Am Coll Cardiol* 1991;18:1694–1701.
21. Ellis S, Popma J, Buchbinder M et al. Relation of clinical presentation, stenosis morphology, and operator technique to the procedural results of rotational atherectomy and rotational atherectomy-facilitated angioplasty. *Circulation* 1994;89:882–892.
22. Reisman M, Cohen B, Warth D, Fenner J, Gocka I, Buchbinder M. Outcome of long lesions treated with high-speed rotational ablation. *J Am Coll Cardiol* 1993; 21:443A.
23. Stertzer S, Rosenblum J, Shaw R et al. Coronary rotational ablation: initial experience in 302 procedures. *J Am Coll Cardiol* 1993;21:287–295.
24. Robertson G, Selmon M, Hinohara T et al. The effect of lesion length on outcome of directional coronary atherectomy. *Circulation* 1990;82:III-623.
25. Popma J, Topol E, Hinohara T, et al. Abrupt vessel closure after directional coronary atherectomy. *J Am Coll Cardiol* 1992;19:1372–1379.
26. Lincoff A, Ellis S, Leya F et al. Are clinical and angiographic correlates of success the same during directional coronary atherectomy and balloon angioplasty? The CAVEAT Experience. *Circulation* 1993;88:I-601.
27. Adelman A, Cohen E, Kimball B et al. A comparison of directional atherectomy with balloon angioplasty for lesions of the left anterior descending coronary artery. *N Eng J Med* 1993;329:228–233.
28. Baim D, Cutlip D, Sharma S et al., for the BOAT Investigators. Final results of the Balloon vs Optimal Atherectomy Trial (BOAT). *Circulation* 1998;97:322–331.
29. Simonton C, Leon M, Baim D et al. Optimal directional coronary atherectomy. Final results of the Optimal Atherectomy Restenosis Study (OARS). *Circulation* 1998; 97:332–339.
30. Hinohara T, Rowe M, Robertson G et al. Effect of lesion characteristics on outcome of directional coronary atherectomy. *J Am Coll Cardiol* 1991;17:1112–1120.
31. Mooney M, Mooney J, Nahhas A, Lesser J, Madison J.

Directional atherectomy in long lesions: improved acute results. *Cathet Cardiovasc Diagn.* 1993;29:83.

32. Litvack F, Eigler N, Margolis J et al., for the ELCA Investigators. Percutaneous excimer laser coronary angioplasty: results in the first consecutive 3000 patients. *J Am Coll Cardiol* 1994;23:323–329.

33. Foley D, Appelman Y, Piek J, for the AMRO group. Comparison of angiographic restenosis propensity of excimer laser coronary angioplasty (ELCA) and balloon angioplasty (BA) in the AMsterdam ROtterdam (AMRO) Trial. *Circulation* 1995;92:I-477.

34. Reifart N, Vandormael M, Krajcar M et al. Randomized comparison of angioplasty of complex coronary lesions at a single-center. Excimer Laser, Rotational Atherectomy, and Balloon Angioplasty Comparison (ERBAC) Study. *Circulation* 1997;96:91–98.

35. Serruys P, De Jaegere P, Kiemeneij F et al., for the BENESTENT Study Group. A comparison of balloon-expandable-stent implantation with balloon angioplasty in patients with coronary artery disease. *N Eng J Med* 1994;331:489–495.

36. Fischman D, Leon M, Baim D, et al., for the Stent Restenosis Study Investigators. *N Eng J Med* 1994;331:496–501.

37. Maiello L, Hall P, Nakamura S et al. Results of stent implantation for diffuse coronary disease assisted by intravascular ultrasound. *J Am Coll Cardiol* 1995; 25:156A.

38. Shaknovich A, Moses J, Undemir C, Cohen N, Higgins E, Strain J, Kreps E. Procedural and short-term clinical outcomes of multiple Palmaz-Schatz stents in very long lesions/dissections. *Circulation* 1995;92:I-535.

39. Ellis S, Savage M, Fischman D et al. Restenosis after placement of Palmaz-Schatz stents in native coronary arteries. Initial results of a multicenter experience. *Circulation* 1992;86:1836–1844.

40. Pulsipher M, Baker W, Sawchak S et al. Outcomes in patients treated with multiple coronary stents. *Circulation* 1996;94:I-332.

41. Lablanche JM, Danchin N, Grollier G et al. Factors predictive of restenosis after stent implantation managed by ticlopidine and aspirin. *Circulation* 1996;94:I-256.

42. Eccleston D, Belli G, Penn I, Ellis S. Are multiple stents associated with multiplicative risk in the optimal stent era? *Circulation* 1996;94:I-454.

43. Wong S, Rocha-Singh K, Teirstein P, Schatz R. Lesion length does not influence restenosis following placement of single Palmaz-Schatz coronary stents. *Circulation* 1992;86:I-512.

44. Tamura T, Kimura T, Nosaka H, Nobuyoshi M. Predictors of restenosis after Palmaz-Schatz stent implantation. *Circulation* 1994;90:I-324.

45. Hamasaki N, Kimura N, Nakagawa Y, Yokoi H, Tamura T, Nobuyoshi M. Influence of lesion length on late angiographic outcome and restenotic process after successful stent implantation. *J Am Coll Cardiol* 1997;29:239A.

46. Kobayashi Y, DeGregorio J, Reimers B, DiMario C, Finci L, Colombo A. The length of the stented segment is an independent predictor of restenosis. *J Am Coll Cardiol* 1998;366A.

47. Hall P, Nakamura S, Maiello L et al. Factors associated with late angiographic outcome after intravascular ultrasound guided Palmaz-Schatz coronary stent implantation: a multivariate analysis. *J Am Coll Cardiol* 1995; 25:36A.

48. De Scheerder I, Wang K, Kostopoulos K, Dens J, Desmet W, Piessens J. Treatment of long dissections by use of a single long or multiple short stents: Clinical and angiographic follow-up. *Am Heart J* 1998;136:(in press).

9

Management of Angulated Lesions

Stephen G. Ellis

Sones Cardiac Catheterization Laboratories, Department of Cardiology, The Cleveland Clinic Foundation, Cleveland, Ohio 44195-5066 and Department of Medicine, Ohio State University, Columbus, Ohio 43210

OVERVIEW

Flow disturbances associated with changes in coronary direction predispose to atheroma formation, and it has been long recognized that the resultant angulated lesions are predisposed to dissection when treated with balloon angioplasty (1). Stenting, however, has revolutionized the approach to angulated lesions, rendering them far less dangerous. In fact, in the 1994 to 1997 Cleveland Clinic experience, angulated lesions were no longer an independent risk factor for complications of coronary intervention (Fig. 9.1). Nonetheless, some aspects of their management may still be treacherous. This chapter briefly reviews options for the percutaneous treatment of angulated lesions.

BALLOON ANGIOPLASTY

In the middle 1980s, standard balloon angioplasty of lesions associated with a >45 degree angle at end-diastole was associated a 13% risk of major complications, compared to a 3.5% risk with nonangulated lesions (1). In the latter part of the 1980s, development and use of >30 mm balloons in this setting reduced the risk of complications somewhat, especially for lesions with <60 degree angle. However, in the Cleveland clinic experience, use of long balloons without Rotablator or stenting of highly angulated lesions (>60 degrees) was still associated with a 21% risk of major complications.

If one is forced to use balloon angioplasty alone, by virtue of vessel size, inability to deliver a stent, or risk with Rotablator (Heart Technol-

ogy Inc., Bellevue, WA), a long balloon should be chosen. Ideally the balloon should be long enough such that there is a 10-mm margin of balloon extending beyond the bulk of the atheroma. Balloon diameter should be matched to the normal adjacent reference dimension. Balloon characteristics (compliant vs. noncompliant) that are optimal in this regard have not been well characterized. Balloon inflation pressure should be enough to achieve an adequate result (<30% diameter stenosis), but not overly aggressive. The guide catheter and wire should be chosen so that a stent (even if somewhat oversized) can be placed if necessary.

ROTABLATOR

Rotational atherectomy may be a useful technique for selected nonstentable 45- to 60-degree angle lesions, except when the bulk of the atheroma lies on the inside of the curve or when the lesion is actively flexing. Both of the latter anatomic conditions predispose to vessel perforation, as does lesion angle >60 degrees. However, the role of Rotablator use in treatment of angulated lesions has not been rigorously studied. Data from the ERBAC (2) and COBRA (3) trials, while demonstrating fewer complications in complex lesions and more restenosis with Rotablator use than balloon angioplasty, simply have too few patients with small-diameter angulated lesions to be useful. Despite obvious limitations, a careful, nonrandomized comparison of well-characterized results may be helpful. The Cleveland Clinic 1992 to 1997 experience in this

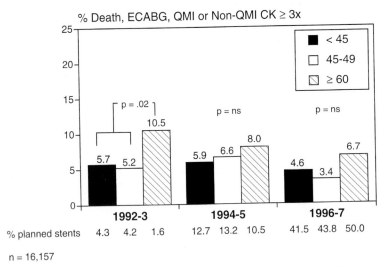

FIG. 9.1. Cleveland Clinic Foundation experience with angulated lesions, 1992 through 1997. Excess risk attributable to ≥60 degree lesions has diminished considerably.

regard is characterized in Figure 9.2. These data would suggest that the Rotablator should not be used for noncalcified, small, angulated lesions. Conclusions regarding calcified lesions are more difficult to draw.

The role of rotational atherectomy for stent-

able and otherwise eligible 45- to 60-degree angle lesions, with the intent of optimizing stent deployment, is likewise unclear. Recent Cleveland Clinic data are provided in Figure 9.3, but must be regarded as inconclusive.

When used for angulated lesions, the initial

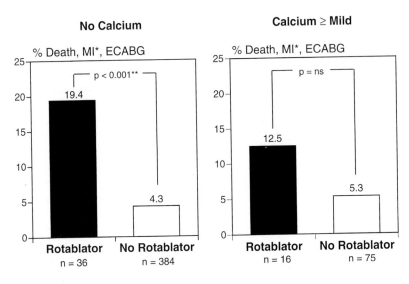

FIG. 9.2. Cleveland Clinic Foundation experience with Rotablator treatment for angulated lesions in small vessels. Although nonrandomized, a heightened risk, especially for noncalcified lesions, appears to be present.

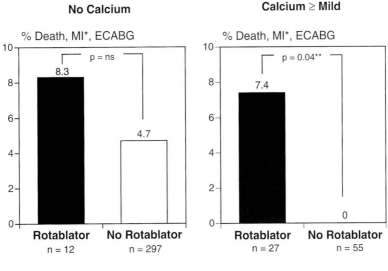

FIG. 9.3. Cleveland Clinic Foundation experience with "Rotastenting" angulated lesions. Possible risk with no apparent acute benefit.

burr should be chosen conservatively—i.e. with burr-artery size <0.7. To avoid wire bias, a floppy wire should be used. Burr advancement should be slow and the duration of burring limited to <30 seconds at a time. Special attention should be paid to avoid burr decelerations >5000 rpm. Depending on vessel size, a second burr may be used, but the burr-artery ratio should be kept to <0.8 and the risk of perforation kept in mind.

When utilizing Rotablator for angulated lesions, the use of ReoPro (Malvern, PA) and other glycoprotein IIb/IIIa inhibitors is relatively contraindicated because they make management of perforation-induced tamponade far more difficult.

STENTING

The capacity to stent a dissection resultant from balloon inflation has revolutionized the percutaneous treatment of angulated lesions.

Guide Catheter and Guidewire Selection

A guide catheter should be chosen that provides maximal support. It should fit coaxially into the appropriate coronary ostium and provide either firm passive support (8 Fr) or be able to be placed deeply and atraumatically into the proximal vessel (6 Fr). In most cases a moderately firm guidewire is appropriate. A very firm guidewire passed through a heavily calcified and angulated lesion may occasionally "bias" the stent against the wall of the lesion and make stent passage difficult.

Predilatation

With most currently available stents it is still advisable to predilate the lesion. Generally a somewhat undersized balloon (usually a 2.5-mm balloon is sufficient) should be chosen to minimize the risk of a lengthy dissection. Calcified lesions should definitely be predilated, whereas depending on the stent available, predilatation of noncalcified and not greatly angulated or severe lesions may not be necessary.

Choosing a Stent

Any of a number of currently available stents can be used to obtain excellent results in angulated lesions. Coil stents (due to lack of vessel wall support) and slotted-tube stents (due to lack of flexibility) should be avoided. We generally prefer the AVE, GFX II (Arterial Vascular Engineering, Santa Rosa, CA), Multi-Link (Guidant Corp, Indianapolis, IN), or NIR (Medinol/Boston Scientific, Jerusalem, Israel) stents. Early versions of the Multi-Link stent tended to slip on the delivery balloon; if that has been the experience in your laboratory, these stents should also be avoided in this setting. Stent diameter should be chosen to match the normal vessel diameter. Stent length should be chosen so that the stent ends extend at least 5 mm beyond the bulk of the atheroma.

Stent Delivery

Stent delivery should be similar to stent delivery other settings, with special attention paid to make sure that the stent does not catch in the lesion and back out the guide catheter. The optimal implantation pressure is not known. An ongoing, randomized trial is presently addressing this issue in general. It is the author's current practice to use 12 to 14 atm for noncalcified lesions and 14-18 atm for calcified angulated lesions. High-pressure delivery of slotted tube stents, particularly with the use of GP IIb/IIIa inhibitors, appears to predispose to microperforation and cardiac tamponade.

Troubleshooting

Crossing Recently Deployed Stents

Occasionally it may be difficult to recross a stent with a balloon to postdilate it or approach a more distal lesion. Several issues should be considered:

1. Some currently available high-pressure balloons have a very stiff tip that may not be flexible enough to make the turn through the lesion. In this case, choose a different balloon.
2. Sometimes a very stiff guidewire will "force" the balloon against a portion of the stent. In this case, if possible, change to a more flexible guidewire. Guidant also makes a "Wiggle" wire to use in the situation, but I have had little experience with this wire.
3. Sometimes the stent placed in the angulated lesion will need to be somewhat overdilated to allow passage of a second stent more distally, when that is required.

Pseudostenoses

"Pseudostenoses" are caused when a stiff guidewire straightens a tortuous or angulated coronary segment, invaginating a segment of its outer well and creating an iatrogenic stenosis. These may be troublesome in that they can obstruct passage of stiff balloons or stents, and can be mistaken for true obstructions. The guidewire should be partially withdrawn such that its floppy tip lies across the area in question and the angiogram should be retaken to distinguish with certainty between a pseudostenosis and a real one.

REFERENCES

1. Ellis SG, Topol EJ. Results of percutaneous transluminal coronary angioplasty of high-risk angulated stenoses. *Am J Cardiol* 1990;66:932–937.
2. Reifart N, Vandormael M, Krajcar M et al. Randomized comparison of angioplasty of complex coronary lesions at a single center. Excimer laser, rotational atherectomy, and balloon angioplasty comparison (ERBAC) Study. *Circulation* 1997;96:91–98.
3. Hamm CW. Percutaneous transluminal coronary angioplasty versus rotablation (the COBRA study). Presented at the XIXth Congress of the European Society of Cardiology, Stockholm, Sweden, August, 1997.

10

The Bifurcation Lesion

A. The Role of Stents

Bernhard Reimers and Antonio Colombo

Cardiac Catheterization Laboratory, Centro Cuore Columbus, 20145 Milano, Italy

Coronary bifurcations are reported to be at high risk to develop an atherosclerotic plaque due to turbulent flow and increased shear stress (1,2). Lesions situated at a bifurcation account for up to 16% of coronary angioplasty procedures (3). A true bifurcation lesion is characterized by the presence of a significant ≥50% diameter stenosis involving both a main vessel and a side branch. For practical reasons we consider a bifurcation lesion a stenosis located in the major branch close to the origin of a side branch where the treatment of the main branch may compromise the side branch. A classification of bifurcation lesions with regard to the threat of side-branch occlusion during coronary angioplasty has been proposed by Koller and Safian (3) and recently modified by Aliabadi et al. (4) for coronary stenting (Fig. 10.1). These authors identified side branches at risk for occlusion when diseased at the side branch's origin and when the disease in the major branch was very close to the ostium of the side branch, with possible plaque shift at the time the major branch was being dilated or stented. All other types were classified as nonthreatened. Besides the risk of side-branch occlusion, the operator should consider the size of the side branch and its angle of origin.

Balloon angioplasty for coronary bifurcation lesions has been associated with increased complication rates (5–7), suboptimal immediate and long-term results (8). There is frequently an ineffective lumen expansion in both the main vessel and the side branch due to plaque shift and lesion recoil. Treatment of bifurcations with directional atherectomy was shown to improve the procedural outcome but the incidence of restenosis remained high (9,10). Coronary stents reduce lesion recoil, achieving effective lumen scaffolding, but coronary stents may also compromise side branches (4,11,12) and the incidence of procedural complications in case of stenting bifurcations, especially when both the main and the side branch were stented, has been up to 9% (13). Thanks to increased operator experience and recent technical developments, a success rate of 98% can now be achieved when stenting bifurcations (14). To date there are only limited data, based on single-center experiences, on the incidence of restenosis after the stenting of bifurcations. The available results report an incidence of restenosis up to 36%, indicating that stenting a bifurcation results in a higher risk of restenosis compared to stenting a lesion not involving a bifurcation (14,15).

DECISION-MAKING BEFORE THE TREATMENT OF BIFURCATION LESIONS

Any side branch of >2.0 mm should be preserved; therefore, the very first step treating a bifurcation is to decide: Does the side branch need wire protection? Does the side branch need

1: Side branch morphologies at risk for occlusion during stent implantation in the main branch.

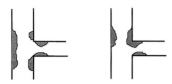

Presence of disease at the origin of the side branch and presence of disease in the major branch with possible plaque shift at the time the major branch is being dilated or stented.

2: Side branch morphologies <u>not</u> at risk for occlusion after stent implantation in the main branch.

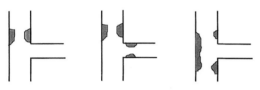

All other morphologies.

FIG. 10.1. Side branch morphologies.

balloon dilatation? Does the side branch need a stent? Does the lesion need debulking ? Our approach to this decision making follows (Table 10.1).

Does the Side Branch Need Wire Protection?

Side branch protection can comprise the positioning of a second wire into the daughter branch before starting the treatment of the main branch. The decision to protect the side branch depends on the risk of closure while treating the main branch and on the size of the side branch. In the experience of Aliabadi et al. (4) only 4% of ≥1-mm side branches with a nonthreatened morphology occluded after stenting the major branch, while 67% of threatened side branches occluded. Thus, nonthreatened side branches should not be wired. Daughter branches of small size (<2.0 mm) need not be protected from the beginning of the procedure, but only in the case of important compromise after dilatation of the main branch. Side branches of ≥2.0 mm at risk for closure should be protected. In doubt, we always prefer to protect a side branch rather than to face its closure without a wire already in place.

Does the Side Branch Need Balloon Dilatation?

We distinguish between elective side branch treatment with balloon dilatation followed by conditional stenting and bailout treatment of a side branch compromised following dilatation of the main branch. Side branches of ≥2.5 mm in diameter with ostial disease or at risk for plaque shift should, in our opinion, be treated with elective balloon dilatation. This may prevent side-branch occlusion following stent placement on the major branch and may facilitate rewiring the side branch through the struts

TABLE 10.1. *Strategic approach to bifurcational lesions: Treatment of the side branch*

Side branch	<2.0 mm	>2.0 mm <3.0 mm	>3.5 mm
Threatened side-branch occlusion	• Wire protection	• Wire protection • Predilate before stenting the main branch	• Wire protection • Predilate and/or debulk • Plan to stent both branches
Nonthreatened side branch Side branch significantly compromised after main branch balloon dilatation Side branch significantly compromised after main branch stenting	• No wire protection • Only if clinically indicated wire and predilate before stenting the main branch • Only if clinically indicated wire and dilate	• No wire protection • Wire and predilate • If >2.5 mm consider to stent both branches • Especially if flow impaired or closed try to wire and dilate • If >2.5 mm consider stenting for bailout through struts.	• No wire protection • Wire and predilate • Plan to stent both branches • Stent both branches

of the stent. The dilatation of the side branch should be performed avoiding oversized balloons To prevent dissections which will commit the operator to side branch stenting, the use of oversized balloons in the dilatation of the side branch should be avoided.

Does the Side Branch Need a Stent?

In our opinion, true bifurcational stenting with elective stent implantation of both the main and the side branch should be performed only if the side branch is ≥3.0 mm in diameter. In <3.0 mm side branches, stent should possibly be avoided. The incidence of restenosis appears higher after stenting both branches, compared to single-stent implantation followed by side-branch dilatation, when the size of the side branch is <3.0 mm. In a retrospective evaluation of bifurcations treated between 1996 and 1997 at our institution, the restenosis rate of 90 lesions treated with double stents and 92 lesions treated with single-stent and side-branch dilatation were 39% and 28%, respectively. This finding emerged independently of the size of the side branch. It is easy to imagine how the problem is amplified when the side branch is small.

If during the dilatation procedure the side branch occludes, dissects, or has an impaired flow, the threshold for stenting lowers significantly. Bailout stenting of the occluding side branch appears reasonable if its diameter is 2.5 mm or larger.

When both branches have been treated with directional atherectomy in our practice, both branches should almost always receive a stent.

Do We Need to Debulk the Bifurcation Lesion?

When treating bifurcations (as with any coronary procedure) the interventionist should aim for the best possible procedural result in terms of minimum lumen diameter and minimum lumen area. Directional atherectomy has been applied in the treatment of bifurcations, with improvement limited to short-term results (7,8,16,17). The very large plaque burden of a bifurcation can be reduced by directional atherectomy, as

shown by intravascular ultrasound, to a residual plaque area smaller than 50%. Atherectomy prior to stenting allows complete stent expansion, reduces plaque shift, and maximizes the lumen (17). In a recent experience of 90 consecutive cases of directional atherectomy followed by stenting, a 7.9% target lesion revascularization rate appears promisingly low (18). Unfortunately, the current catheter platform for performing directional atherectomy is not very friendly and limits its applicability to large vessels with favorable anatomy. In the presence of calcium, the use of rotational atherectomy may become necessary to debulk some of the plaque, change its compliance, and allowing a better stent expansion (19).

Guiding Catheters and Wires

A guiding catheter and wires must be chosen according to the planned approach. In any case of bifurcational interventions requiring kissing balloon inflation, an 8 Fr guiding catheter should be used to allow comfortable balloon and wire handling and to guarantee reasonable contrast injections. When positioning two stents simultaneously (for example, as in the modified "T" technique, described below) a new, big lumen 8 Fr catheter is wide enough to accommodate two premounted stents with low-profile shaft and balloons. For debulking procedures, adequate catheter sizes are needed. New 6 Fr guiding catheters with large inner lumens combined with very low-profile dilatation balloons and usage of a fixed wire system may allow "kissing" inflations, as described below. The gain from the small access site with the usage of a 6F guiding catheter is negated by the increased friction and reduced visualization.

For bifurcation lesions, any regular PTCA wire and support wire can be used. For procedures with directional atherectomy that require the use of two wires, Nitinol wires prevent accidental wire cutting. We have also been successful and remained free from wire cutting by performing directional atherectomy on a platform of two Platinum Plus 0.014-in. wires (Scimed-Boston Scientific, Inc. Minneapolis, MN). Specific steerable or coated wires or balloons with fixed wires might be useful in crossing previously implanted stents or in crossing stent struts.

STENTING OF BIFURCATIONAL LESIONS

In the following, we present different techniques of stent implantation in bifurcations as performed in our laboratory (20–23) (Table 10.2).

Stenting the Main Branch and Dilating the Side Branch Through the Struts

The easiest way to stent a bifurcation is to stent the main branch covering the ostium of the side branch. However, several precautions should be considered. Debulking of the main branch reduces the risk of plaque shift with side-branch compromise. In situations considered at high risk for occlusion of the side branch, the vessel side branch should be wired and eventually predilated. In some cases, a hydrophilic-coated wire can be left in the side branch while stenting the main branch. In case of occlusion, this wire can be a valuable landmark to re-cross with another wire into the side branch. If the stent was released at 6 to 8 atm without an oversized balloon, a stent expansion sufficient to allow wire removal from underneath the struts without resistance should have been achieved. Side branches that are not significantly compromised (angiographic diameter stenosis ≤50%) might not need to be dilated. When there is a significant lumen compromise (≥70%) of a small side branch (≤2.0 mm) with reasonable TIMI flow and no signs of ischemia, the operator should resist the temptation to do anything else but calling the case finished. It is known that excellent long-term patency rate is present when a side branch is even modestly patent at the end of the stenting procedure on the major branch (11,12).

When necessary, the struts of most stents are easily crossed with a wire. It is not yet clear whether side-branch wiring is easier after low-pressure stent implantation (with possibly less plaque shift), or after high-pressure stent implantation with wider expanded struts. In our institution, generally, the stent is implanted directly at medium or high pressure. Any type of wire might be used to cross stent struts. The wire should be shaped to approximately 90 degrees; after the tip is engaged within the struts at the origin of the side branch, a slight backward movement with careful steering allows crossing into the side branch. In case of no success, reshaping of the tip with a wider, ≥90-degree curve should be attempted. Newly developed, short transition wires with prolapsing tips can be helpful because they can be easily advanced through the proximal part of the stent and then withdrawn in the manner described above. Hydrophilic-coated wire might find less friction in crossing the struts, but the risk of dissecting the side branch is increased. In some difficult situations, we find helpful the use of an intermediate or standard wire, keeping in mind all the precautions and risks involved. In case of no success, a 1.5-mm, over-the-wire balloon or an open-end catheter can be advanced close to the origin of the side branch to increase the support of the wire crossing the struts. This technique is especially useful for a reverse (>90 degrees) angle of origin of a side branch.

After wire crossing, a balloon needs to be advanced into the side branch. This can be very easy but sometimes the use of a new, unexpanded, small-diameter and low-profile balloon is necessary. Over-the-wire balloons, which are easier to push than are monorail balloons, might be used. Repeated, quick forward and backward movement ("Dottering") of the balloon, adjusting the guiding catheter position by intubation from time to time, can be attempted. Some patience with this may lead to success. Generally the balloon should not be advanced completely through the stent into the side branch for inflation because this increases the risk of balloon entrapment. The inflation pressure should also be kept well under the rated burst pressure because balloon rupture within a stent strut can also cause balloon entrapment.

Another alternative for crossing the stent strut is a balloon with a fixed wire. The fixed wire has a transition between wire and balloon with low profile, preserving optimal "pushability," which allows comfortable strut crossing. Furthermore, this method is quick, because only one

TABLE 10.2. *Stenting of bifurcations: Techniques*

Technique	Angle of origin of side branch	Advantages	Disadvantages	Suitable Stents
Stent the main branch and dilate side branch through struts	20–120 degrees	• Less complex and less expensive compared to double stenting • Described lower complication rate and lower incidence of restenosis compared to double stenting	• Sometimes difficult to wire side branch and/or to cross struts with balloon • Lesion coverage only of the main branch • Often suboptimal result in case of disease at origin of side branch	• Slotted-tube: all, preferably with struts which allow creation of a wide side lumen • Coil stents: all, often easier side branch access compared to slotted-tube but higher risk of stent distortion and less scaffolding
"Culottes" Stent Technique	30–90 degrees	• Optimal lesion coverage in the main branch and the side branch • Second stent implantation only if necessary	• Access to both branches not always maintained (possible difficulties in rewiring) • Possible difficulties in crossing struts with second stent	Premounted, low-profile: • slotted-tube with wide expandable struts or ring design: ACS Duet, mini Crown, CrossFlex LaserCut, AVE gfx • coil stents require less scaffolding: CrossFlex, Wiktor
"Modified T Stent" Technique	close to 90 degrees	• Access to main branch always maintained • A good solution for 90-degree bifurcations	• Only for close to 90-degree bifurcations • Possible imperfect lesion coverage at ostium of side branch	Preferably premounted: • for side branch: AVE gfx or ACS Duet • for main branch: any slotted-tube
"V Stent" Technique	≤75 degrees	• Access to both branches always maintained • Safe and quick method for two large branches	• Creation of a metallic neocarina not in contact with the vessel wall	• All slotted-tube or ring design stents
"Y Stent" Technique	30–75 degrees	• Access to both branches always maintained	• Complex technique • Possible gaps in lesion coverage • Need for 3 stents	For branches: AVE gfx, ACS Duet Proximal stent: visible: NIR Royal, ACS Duet.
Creating a proximal funnel	30–75 degrees	• Creates wide "inflow" into the bifurcation • Avoids stenting of side branches especially if small sized • Ideal in presence of disease only proximal to the bifurcation	• Lesion coverage only of the main branch • Often need for a second, distal stent	Visible slotted-tube: NIR Royal; ACS Duet

device needs to be inserted. However, when a fixed-wire balloon is used, the operator should be very careful because of the increased risk of side-branch dissection The final balloon for side-branch inflations should be adequately sized, but not oversized, because side branch ruptures, especially of diagonal branches, might occur. Final "kissing" balloon inflations in the stented main branch and in the side branch should be performed liberally, because stent deformation after side branch dilatation might have occurred.

The simplest, most predictable way to perform side-branch dilatation through a stent is to use a coil stent or a ring design stent (Fig. 10.2). The three most frequently used coil stents are: the Wiktor stent (Medtronic Inc, Minneapolis, MN), the CrossFlex (Cordis, Johnson and Johnson Inc., Warren, NJ) stent and the Gianturco Roubin II (Cook Inc, Bloomington, IN) stent. Despite the fact these stents do not provide the same scaffolding of the slotted tubular stents, they leave easier access to the side branch. We tend to use one of these stents when there are multiple branches originating from the bifurcation, when the plaque burden is not very large and/ or when the bifurcation involves a bend or a sharp curve.

A problem with use of a coil stent without a longitudinal spine is the risk of stent deformation during stent crossing or during balloon withdraws.

A very reasonable compromise between optimal support and easy recrossing is the use of a ring-design stent, such as the GFX II stent (AVE Inc. Santa Rosa, CA), or the new slotted tubular design with larger struts, such as the CrossFlex LC (Cordis, Johnson and Johnson Inc., Warren, NJ), the ACS Multi-Link Duet (Guidant Inc. Santa Clara, CA) or the Mini Crown (Cordis, Johnson and Johnson Inc., Warren, NJ).

The "Culottes" Technique

This kissing stent technique was first described by Chevalier et al. (24) and is in our view the most elegant method for stenting both

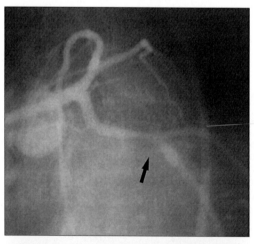

A

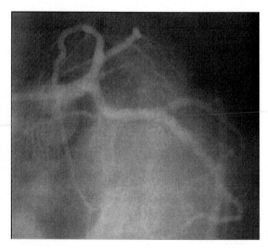

B

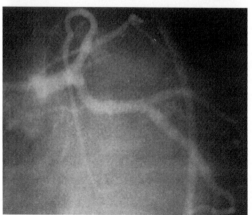

C

FIG. 10.2. Example of stent implantation in the main branch and balloon dilatation of the side branch through the struts. **Panel A:** a lesion in the mid left circumflex artery involving the origin of an obtuse marginal branch. A stent (Wiktor) was deployed in the circumflex artery covering the ostium of the marginal branch (**panel B**). A wire crossed into the marginal branch. **Panel C:** The result after kissing balloon inflation of the circumflex artery and the marginal branch. Kissing inflation was performed to prevent stent distortion during side branch dilatation.

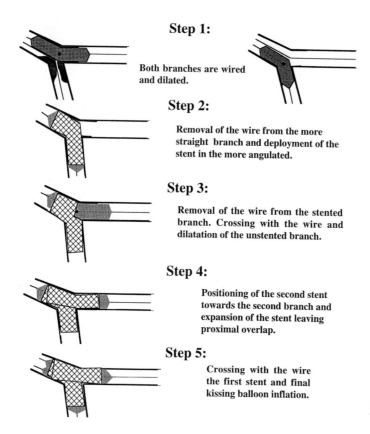

Step 1:

Both branches are wired
and dilated.

Step 2:

Removal of the wire from the more
straight branch and deployment of the
stent in the more angulated.

Step 3:

Removal of the wire from the stented
branch. Crossing with the wire and
dilatation of the unstented branch.

Step 4:

Positioning of the second stent
towards the second branch and
expansion of the stent leaving
proximal overlap.

Step 5:

Crossing with the wire
the first stent and final
kissing balloon inflation.

FIG. 10.3. The "Culottes"
Technique.

branches of a bifurcation. The technique is performed in five steps and is described in Figure 10.3.

Step One

Both branches are wired and predilated alternately.

Step Two

The wire is removed from the straighter branch and the more angulated branch is stented. Obviously, if an important dissection or occlusion occurred in one branch, this branch should be stented first because wire removal might be risky.

Step Three

The wire is removed from the stented branch and used to rewire the nonstented branch through the struts of the stent just deployed. The stent struts should now be dilated toward the nonstented branch with the already-used balloon. In case the balloon does not cross a small diameter (1.5 mm), a low-profile balloon can be used.

Step Four

A second stent is advanced and expanded into the not stented branch maintaining the proximal part of the stent within the previous deployed stent.

Step Five

Finally, the first stented branch is rewired and final kissing balloon inflation is performed.

Discussion of "Culottes" Technique

With this five-step technique, the vessel proximal to the bifurcation is covered by two over-

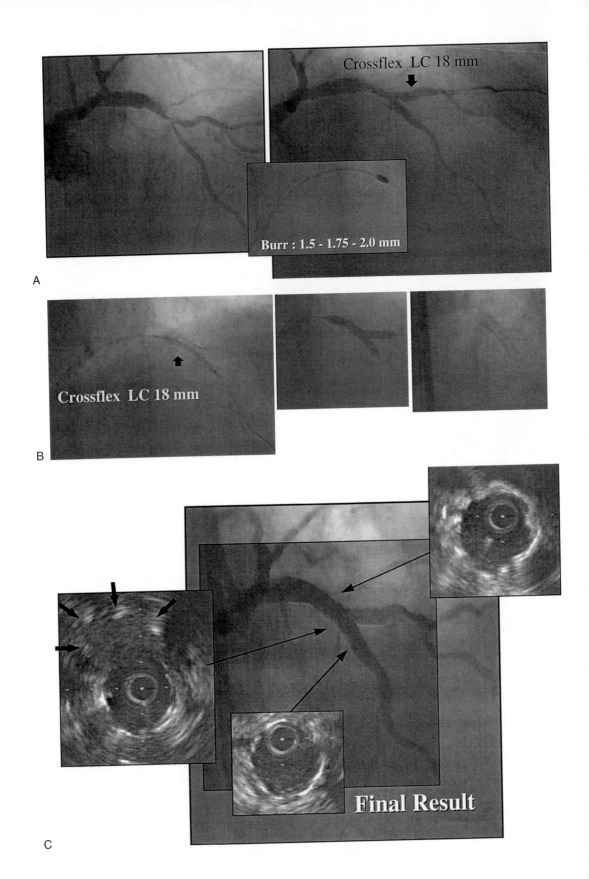

A

Crossflex LC 18 mm

Burr : 1.5 - 1.75 - 2.0 mm

B

Crossflex LC 18 mm

C

Final Result

lapping stents and each branch is covered by a single stent. This technique is particularly suitable for angles of bifurcation between 30 and 90 degrees but can also be performed for reverse >90-degree angles. This technique can also be used when the initial plan was to stent only one vessel, but the result on the second branch deteriorated to such a level as to suggest stenting the second branch as well. When using this technique, the operator does not need to equally overlap the stents proximally. If necessary, one of the two stents can be asymmetrically advanced into one branch, as long as the bifurcation is covered. A possible drawback of this approach is that it may be difficult to rewire and redilate in steps three and five and to cross the second stent through the struts of the first stent in step four. However, these difficulties occur less frequently with new low-profile, pre-mounted stents with large expandable strut areas.

Initially, coil stents were used for this technique; however, new slotted-tube or ring design stents such as the ACS Duet, the CrossFlex LaserCut and the AVE GFX are ideal for this approach, providing excellent scaffolding of the entire bifurcation. Using these designs, large side lumens can be created, and because of the round or smoothed strut edges, balloon ruptures should not occur (Fig. 10.4).

The Modified "T" Stent Technique

This technique with kissing stents can be employed when the side branch originates with an

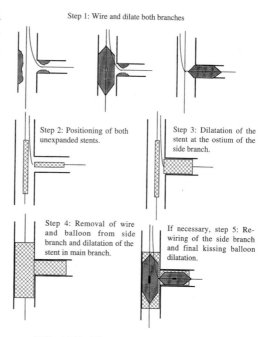

Step 1: Wire and dilate both branches

Step 2: Positioning of both unexpanded stents.

Step 3: Dilatation of the stent at the ostium of the side branch.

Step 4: Removal of wire and balloon from side branch and dilatation of the stent in main branch.

If necessary, step 5: Rewiring of the side branch and final kissing balloon dilatation.

FIG. 10.5. The modified "T" technique.

angle of 90 degrees or close to 90 degrees (22,25) and can be described in five steps (Fig. 10.5).

Step One

Both branches are wired and alternately dilated.

Step Two

A first stent is advanced into the side branch, but not expanded, and a second stent is advanced

---

FIG. 10.4. Example of the "Culottes" technique. **A:** The left panel shows a lesion at a bifurcation of the left anterior descending artery with a diagonal branch. Due to angiographic evidence of calcifications, rotational atherectomy with 1.5, 1.75 and 2.0 mm burrs was performed in the left anterior descending artery. Subsequently the diagonal branch was wired and both branches predilated. A stent (18-mm CrossFlex Laser Cut) was positioned (**right panel**) in the diagonal branch. **B:** After expansion of the stent in the diagonal branch the wire was removed and advanced into the left anterior descending artery. The struts of the stent just deployed into the diagonal branch were dilated and a second stent (18-mm CrossFlex LaserCut) was positioned in the left anterior descending artery with proximal overlap of both stents (**left panel**). After stent deployment the diagonal branch was crossed again with a wire and kissing balloon inflation was performed (**mid panel**). The right panel shows the expanded stents. **C:** The final result as seen at angiography and with intravascular ultrasound performed in the left anterior descending artery. Note the stented lumen of the diagonal branch (*arrows*) visible on the left ultrasound image. On the right ultrasound image the two overlapping proximal stents are more evident compared to the less evident single stent on the ultrasound image in the middle.

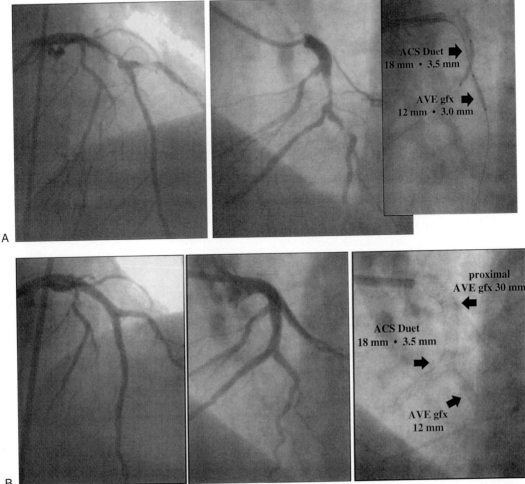

FIG. 10.6. The modified "T" technique. **A:** Presence of diffuse disease of the left anterior descending artery and of the diagonal branch (**left and mid panel**). After wiring and predilation of both branches a short stent (AVE gfx 12 mm) was positioned in the diagonal branch and a second stent (ACS Duet 18 mm) was positioned in the left anterior descending artery covering the ostium of the diagonal branch (**right panel**). At first the stent in the diagonal was inflated followed by removal of the balloon and the wire from the branch. Subsequently the stent in the left anterior descending artery was deployed. Another stent was implanted to treat the proximal disease in the left anterior descending artery. **B:** The final result and the radiographic evidence of the expanded stents are shown.

in the main branch, covering the ostium of the side branch.

Step Three

The first stent is carefully positioned at the ostium of the side branch and expanded.

Step Four

The balloon and wire are removed from the side branch and then the stent in the main branch is expanded.

Step Five

The side branch is rewired and kissing balloon dilatations of both branches are performed.

Discussion of the Modified "T" Stent Technique

This technique is very safe, because both stents are positioned before inflation, eliminating the difficulties that arise in crossing a second stent. The technique allows exact positioning of the first stent at the ostium of the side branch. In case of slight protrusion of the first stent into the main branch while dilating the second stent, the first stent might be pushed into the side branch. For this reason, we prefer to use for the side branch a ring-design stent, allowing it to be pushed into the side branch. In addition, the smooth, round edges of this stent minimize the risk of balloon rupture. The AVE gfx stent is ideal for this approach (Fig. 10.6). The second stent can be any slotted-tube stent, possibly with large struts to facilitate rewiring and dilatation of the side branch. An 8 Fr guiding catheter is needed for this technique. Disadvantages of this procedure are that it is limited to near-90-degree bifurcations and that if the stent in the side branch is implanted too distal, an uncovered gap might remain at the ostium of the side branch.

The "V" Stent Technique

This is a kissing stents technique suitable for bifurcations of two large side branches with a

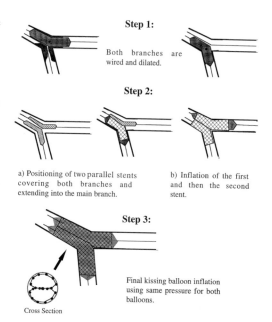

Step 1:

Both branches are wired and dilated.

Step 2:

a) Positioning of two parallel stents covering both branches and extending into the main branch.

b) Inflation of the first and then the second stent.

Step 3:

Final kissing balloon inflation using same pressure for both balloons.

Cross Section

FIG. 10.7. The "V" stent technique.

large diameter of the vessel proximal to the bifurcation. As the name implies, this technique is best suited for branches, which originate with a narrow angle (less than 70 degrees, Fig. 10.7).

This technique can be resumed in three steps.

Step One

Both branches are wired and alternately predilated.

Step Two

The two unexpanded stents are positioned close to the ostium of the branches with a slight abutment into the main vessel. It is better to expand the two stents alternately to avoid dislodgment of one balloon during simultaneous inflations. High pressure inflation with eventually short balloons might be performed alternately.

Step Three

The final inflation should be simultaneous ("kissing"), using the same pressure and appropriately sized balloons.

Discussion of the "V" Stent Technique

Using this technique, a metallic neocarina is created within the vessel proximal to the bifurcation. Theoretical concerns about this carina, regarding an increased risk of thrombosis, have not been confirmed in our experience. The most appropriate stents for this technique are two slotted-tube stents of equal design with good radial strength to preserve the best configuration of the proximal carina. This technique is safe as access to both branches is always maintained. The lesion coverage is also complete. However, compared to the "Culottes" technique the "V" technique has more limited applications. This technique is best suited for very large branches with a narrow angle of origin. Quick performance and easy execution are the major advantages of the "V" technique (Fig. 10.8). A minimum 8 Fr guiding catheter is needed for this technique. The use of intravascular ultrasound to control expansion of both stents is recommended. Alternative "V" techniques, stenting only the ostium of the two branches without creating a neocarina, have been described (26,27).

In one description, the articulation of a Palmaz-Schatz stent is bent and the two half-stents are mounted on two balloons and advanced on two wires until the articulation reaches the carina of the bifurcation. If an additional stent is placed in the vessel proximal to the bifurcation, the "V" technique is converted to a "Y" technique.

The "Y" Stent Technique:

This technique implies the use of multiple stents and was probably the first technique used for true bifurcation stenting (28). The technique can be summarized in three steps (Fig. 10.9).

Step One

Both branches are wired and predilated.

Step Two

In each ostium a stent is deployed and expanded with kissing dilatations (separate inflations).

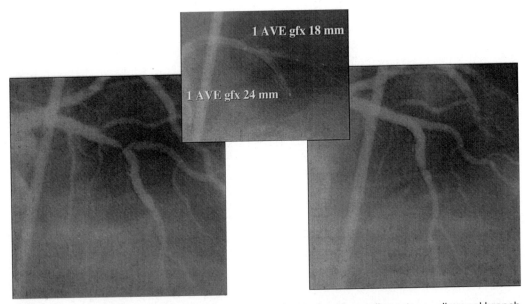

FIG. 10.8. The "V" stent technique. A bifurcational left anterior descending artery—diagonal branch lesion (**left panel**). After wiring and predilatation of both vessels, two stents were positioned in the branches leaving proximal overlap in the main vessel (**small panel**). Subsequently the stents were inflated separately. The final result is shown in the **right panel**.

TABLE 10.3. *Side lumen creation and stent distortion during simulated side-branch dilatation*

Balloon diameter	AVE gfx	beStent	Crown	ACS Multi-Link	NIR[a]
		Mean Side Lumen Diameter (mm)			
2.5 mm	2.7	2.7	2.3	2.5	2.0
3.0 mm	3.1	2.9	2.5	3.0	2.0
3.5 mm	3.6	3.0	3.0	3.5	2.2
4.0 mm	4.1	3.8[b]	3.7	3.7	3.6[b]
		Distal Diameter Stenosis (%)			
2.5 mm	17	18	16	28	4
3.0 mm	25	42	25	38	36
3.5 mm	25	43	31	48	46
4.0 mm	50	64	38	55	58

[a] Cell number not specified;
[b] Strut rupture;
From ref. 30, with permission.

achieving an optimal result has created interest on the part of the industry in developing stent design dedicated to use in the treatment of bifurcations. The NIR side (Scimed, Maple Grove, MN), the Jostent B (Jomed International AB, Drottninggatan, Sweden), and the Devon Side-arm stent (Devon Medical, Hamburg, Germany) are all characterized by the presence of larger struts in the central part of the stent and normal-sized struts at the extremities. This is to facilitate the passage of a wire, a balloon, and/or a stent into the side branch after stent expansion. We could define this approach as "provisional side branch stenting." The "Carina stent," developed by BARD Inc. (Billerica, MA), is a unique stent design. This stent uses the design of the Bard XT stent, creating a Y-shaped stent mounted on a special balloon system. The delivery system consists of two monorail balloons with the shafts jointed into a single shaft proximally to the entrance site of the wires (Bard XT Bifurcate Stent Delivery System) (Fig. 10.13).

This system allows advancement of the stent into the main and side branch at the same time. Care has to be taken to avoid wire criss-crossing. In our experience, this stent system is best applied to large proximal bifurcations because of the large profile of the system. Bard has in development a lower profile variant of this stent, with thinner struts, to be used for smaller-sized and more distal bifurcations.

PHARMACOLOGICAL THERAPY

When dealing with a bifurcation, it must be kept in mind that the double trauma created by the dilatation in two branches and the shear stress induced by the new angle formed by the single or double stent, will create a more thrombogenic environment. Therefore it is important to pay the utmost attention to antiplatelet therapy. If possible, Ticlopidine should be started three days before the procedure and the use of abciximab should be quite liberal.

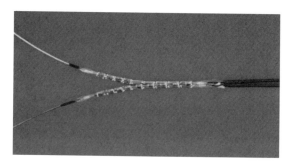
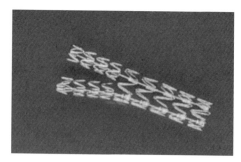

FIG. 10.13. A stent specially designed for bifurcations (The Bard XT Bifurcate Stent Delivery System).

In practice, we almost always use abciximab when we perform debulking before bifurcational stenting.

We also believe there are good reasons to use abciximab routinely when dealing with bifurcational stenting to improve patency of the side branch during any maneuver which could compromise the lumen and flow. Recent data from the EPISTENT trial may favor this approach (31).

CONCLUSIONS

Bifurcational stenting demands an appropriate balance of the need to achieve an optimal result, the procedural risk, and the long-term outcome. Coronary stenting has made it possible to achieve superb immediate results, which too frequently are not maintained at follow-up. The operator should always be aware of this gap.

The approach we would like to suggest is the use of the simplest possible technique, such as stenting the major branch and dilatation of the side branch. On the other hand, directional atherectomy and stenting, which can be considered the most complex but most rewarding approach (18), should be utilized when dealing with large bifurcations.

REFERENCES

1. Pinkerton CA, Slack JD. Complex coronary angioplasty: a technique for dilatation of bifurcation stenosis. *Angiology* 1985:543–548.
2. Renkin J, Wijns W, Hanet C et al. Angioplasty of coronary bifurcation stenoses. *Cathet Cardiovasc Diagn* 1991;22:167–173.
3. Koller P, Safian RD. Bifurcation Stenosis. In: Freed M, Grines C, Safian RD, eds. *The new manual of interventional cardiology*. Birmingham, MI: Physicians Press, 1996:233–243.
4. Aliabadi D, Tilli FV, Bowers TR et al. Incidence and angiographic predictors of side-branch occlusion following high-pressure intracoronary stenting. *Am J Cardiol* 1997;80:994–997.
5. Meier B, Gruentzig AR, King SB III et al. Risk of side branch occlusion during coronary angioplasty. *Am J Cardiol* 1984;53:10–14.
6. Arora RR, Raymond RE, Dimas AP, Bhadwar K, Simpfendorfer C. Side-branch occlusion during coronary angioplasty: incidence, angiographic characteristics and outcome. *Cathet Cardiovasc Diagn* 1989;18:210–212.
7. Mathias DW, Mooney JF, Lange HW, Goldenberg IF,

Fredarick LG, Mooney MR. Frequency of success and complications of coronary angioplasty of a stenosis at the ostium of a branch vessel. *Am J Cardiol* 1991;67:491–495.
8. Weinstein JS, Baim DS, Sipperly ME, McCabe CH, Lorell BH. Salvage of branch vessels during bifurcation lesion angioplasty: acute and long-term follow up. *Cathet Cardiovasc Diagn* 1991;22:1–6.
9. Adelman AG, Cohen EA, Kimball BP et al. A comparison of directional atherectomy with balloon angioplasty for lesions of the left anterior descending artery. *N Engl J Med* 1993;329:228–233.
10. Boehrer JD, Ellis SG, Pieper K et al. Directional atherectomy versus balloon angioplasty for coronary ostial and non-ostial left anterior descending artery lesions: results from a randomized multicenter trial. *J Am Coll Cardiol* 1995;25:1380–1386.
11. Fischman DL, Savage MP, Leon MB et al. Fate of lesion-related side branches after coronary artery stenting. *J Am Coll Cardiol* 1993;22:1641–1646.
12. Pan M, Medina A, Suarez de Lezo J et al. Follow-up patency of side branches covered by intracoronary Palmaz-Schatz stent. *Am Heart J* 1995;129:436–440.
13. Colombo A, Maiello L, Itoh A. Coronary stenting of bifurcation lesions: immediate and follow-up results. *J Am Coll Cardiol* 1996;27:277A (abstract).
14. LefËfre T, Louvard Y, Morice MC et al. Should we stent a bifurcation lesion? A single-center experience. *Eur Heart J* 1997;18:26 (abst).
15. Kobayashi Y, Colombo A, Reimers B, Di Mario C. Coronary stenting in bifurcational lesions: immediate and follow up results. *Circulation* 1997;96 [Suppl]:I-693 (abst).
16. Spokojny AM, Sanborn TA. The bifurcation lesion. In: Ellis SG, Holmes DR Jr, eds. *Strategic approaches in coronary intervention*. Baltimore: Williams and Wilkins, 1996: 286–291.
17. Di Mario C, De Gregorio J, Kobayashi Y, Colombo A. Atherectomy for ostial LAD stenosis: a cut above. *Cathet Cardiovasc Diagn* 1998;43:101–104.
18. Moussa I, Moses J, Di Mario C et al. The stenting after optimal lesion debulking registry (SOLD): Angiographic and clinical outcome. *Circulation* 1998; in press.
19. I Moussa, C Di Mario, J Moses et al. Coronary stenting after rotational atherectomy in calcified and complex lesions: angiographic and clinical follow-up results. *Circulation* 1997;96:128–136.
20. Di Mario C, Colombo A. Trousers-stents: how to choose the right size and shape? *Cathet Cardiovasc Diagn* 1997;41:197–199.
21. Colombo A, Gaglione A, Nakamura S, Finci L. ''Kissing'' stents for bifurcational coronary lesions. *Cathet Cardiovasc Diagn* 1993;30:327–330.
22. Nakamura S, Hall P, Maiello L, Colombo A. Technique for Palmaz-Schatz stent deployment in lesions with a large side branch. *Cathet Cardiovasc Diagn* 1995;34:353–361.
23. Kobayashi Y, Colombo A, Akiyama T, Reimers B, Martini G, Di Mario C. Modified ''T'' stenting: a technique for kissing stents in bifurcational coronary lesions. *Cathet Cardiovasc Diagn* 1998;43:323–326.
24. Chevalier B, Glatt B, Royer T. Kissing stenting in bifurcation lesions. *Eur Heart J* 1996;17:218 (abst).
25. Carrie D, Karouny E, Chouairi S, Puel J. ''T''-shaped

stent placement: a technique for the treatment of dissected bifurcation lesions. *Cathet Cardiovasc Diagn* 1996;37:311–313.

26. Schampaert E, Fort S, Adelman AG, Schwartz L. The V-stent: a novel technique for coronary bifurcation stenting. *Cathet Cardiovasc Diagn* 1996;39:320–326.

27. Khoja A, Ozbek C, Bay W, Heisel A. Trouser-Like stenting: a new technique for bifurcation lesions. *Cathet Cardiovasc Diagn* 1997;41:192–196.

28. Baim DS. Is bifurcation stenting the answer? *Cathet Cardiovasc Diagn* 1996;37:314–316.

29. Pomerantz RM, Ling FS. Distortion of Palmaz-Schatz

geometry following side-branch balloon dilatation through the stent in a rabbit model. *Cathet Cardiovasc Diagn* 1997;40:422–426.

30. Ormiston JA, Webster MWI, Ruygrok PN, Scott D, Stewart JT. Stent distortion during simulated side-branch dilatation. *J Am Coll Cardiol* 1998;37:18A (abst).

31. The EPISTENT Investigators. Randomised placebo-controlled and balloon-angioplasty-controlled trial to assess safety of coronary stenting with use of platelet glycoprotein-IIb/IIIa blockade. *Lancet* 1998; 352: 87–92.

B. The Role of Coronary Atherectomy

Charles A. Simonton III

The Sanger Clinic, P.A., Charlotte, North Carolina 28203-5866

BACKGROUND

Directional coronary atherectomy (DCA) was FDA approved in 1990 following submission of registry data that showed promising results of DCA in over 1000 patients (1). However, the "minimalist" technique of DCA at that time—minimal atherectomy with no adjunctive percutaneous transluminal coronary angioplasty (PTCA)—did not prove to be superior to PTCA in the first randomized trials of CAVEAT, CAVEAT-II and CCAT (2–4). Multivariable analysis of the relationship of procedural factors to long-term outcome in these trials subsequently showed that the larger the lumen achieved at the lesion site, the lower the restenosis rate (5,6). This finding initiated the era of "maximalist" DCA, or "optimal" DCA. The Optimal Atherectomy Restenosis Study (OARS) and the Balloon vs Optimal Atherectomy Trial (BOAT) (7,8) confirmed this theory in prospective models. In the BOAT study (8), DCA was shown to have a lower angiographic restenosis rate than PTCA at six months without an increase in procedural complications. In fact, the need for "bailout" stent-

ing was significantly less for DCA than PTCA in this study.

Soon after "optimal" DCA was adopted, however, coronary stents were introduced and also showed superior results over PTCA (9,10). The ease of use for coronary stents made them preferable to DCA and hence the practice of DCA has declined since 1995.

LESION SELECTION FOR DCA

Presently, DCA continues to have a role in certain lesion types which are difficult to treat or have higher complication rates with PTCA or stents (Table 10.4). Aorto-ostial and branch ostial lesions are excellent for DCA, since PTCA usually fails due to plaque recoil and stents are very difficult to place in these locations without overlapping the adjacent vessel or missing the lesion. Lesions near side-branches fall in the same category, with PTCA often causing compromise of the side-branch due to dissection or plaque-shifting, and stents often result in "jailing" or pinching of the side-branch. DCA is highly effective in debulking these lesions, al-

TABLE 10.4. *Lesions made easier with DCA*

1. Bifurcation lesions, particularly eccentric lesions involving one branch more than the other, in vessels ≥3.0 mm.
2. Aorto-ostial lesions, particularly left main, saphenous vein graft, and noncalcified right coronary ostial lesions.
3. Lesions near large side branches
4. Bulky, eccentric lesions in proximal or mid-segment vessel locations.
5. Branch ostial lesions, such as ostial LAD, ostial left circumflex, or ostial diagonal/obtuse marginal lesions.

lowing subsequent PTCA or stenting without side-branch compromise.

DCA aids in the treatment of bulky, eccentric lesions by reducing the plaque burden prior to either adjunctive PTCA or stenting. Recent intravascular ultrasound (IVUS) studies such as the GUIDE II trial (11,12) have shown that plaque burden (plaque area) is predictive of late restenosis, even with coronary stents. Thus, an effort to debulk lesions with DCA may improve late outcomes. This approach is currently being tested in a randomized trial examining late restenosis following DCA versus PTCA prior to stenting.

DCA FOR BIFURCATION LESIONS

The approach to bifurcation coronary lesions in the interventional lab depends on the type of bifurcation lesion being treated. A working knowledge of the various types of bifurcation lesions is essential to selecting the appropriate device and technique for dealing with these complex lesions. The primary goal in treating these lesions is to take the approach which will offer the best chance of achieving acute procedural success (<50% residual stenosis in both branches) without a major complication. Since there are presently no studies showing a lower late restenosis rate with one device versus another (e.g., DCA or stents versus PTCA), the operator should choose the approach which he/she feels most comfortable with performing to achieve a safe, successful result.

Classification of bifurcation lesions

The major types of bifurcation lesions are classified as either *true* bifurcation lesions, defined as beginning proximal to the carina of the bifurcation and involving both branches, or other types of lesions (Table 10.5). Of the true bifurcation lesions, some are symmetric (or balanced), involving both branches equally, and some are asymmetric (unbalanced or eccentric), involving one branch much more than the other. Other considerations include the size of each branch, degree of angulation of the carina, tortuosity, and calcification.

Other types of bifurcation lesions (nontrue) include *trunk lesions* (proximal to the carina in the parent vessel and not involving ostia of branches), *completely eccentric lesions* beginning proximal to carina and extending into only one of the two branches, and *double-ostial lesions* with the lesion involving the ostium of each branch without involvement of the trunk (parent vessel) proximal to the carina.

Device Selection and the Role of DCA

The acute and long-term success rates of PTCA, DCA, rotational atherectomy, or stents for bifurcation lesions are not well known due to a paucity of data available from small studies

TABLE 10.5. *Classification of bifurcation lesions*

I. True Bifurcation Lesions:
   Lesion begins proximal to carina (in parent vessel) and extends into *both* branches
   a. Symmetric: balanced lesions involve both branches equally
   b. Asymmetric: unbalanced; eccentric lesions involve one branch more than the other
II. Other Types of Lesions
   a. Trunk lesions: proximal to carina
   b. Completely eccentric lesions: trunk lesion extending into one branch
   c. Double-ostial lesions: no trunk involvement; ostia of both branches involved
III. Other Considerations
   a. Angle of bifurcation at carina (shallow versus wide angle)
   b. Degree of calcification
   c. Tortuosity
   d. Trifurcation lesions (third branch involved and large enough to preserve)

(13–20). The studies of PTCA with "kissing" balloon techniques have reported lower procedural success rates (<85%) than other lesions with relatively high restenosis rates (>50%). Small studies with DCA (13–15) have reported somewhat higher acute success but with little data available on restenosis. No significant improvement in these outcomes has been reported in comparative clinical trials with rotational atherectomy or coronary stent techniques. Thus, the choice of a catheter-based intervention (as opposed to coronary bypass surgery) should take into account the somewhat lower procedural success and higher restenosis following these procedures.

Device selection for bifurcation lesions depends upon the morphology of the lesion, as outlined in Table 10.5. The following general guidelines are often helpful in deciding which device to use:

1. True bifurcation lesions almost always require either debulking (DCA, rotational atherectomy) or stenting rather than PTCA alone.
2. The more eccentric the lesion morphology (unbalanced), the more debulking with DCA is helpful to prevent plaque shifting and compromise of the less-involved branch.
3. Completely eccentric and double-ostial lesions are well-suited for DCA debulking to prevent plaque-shifting during final PTCA or stent deployment.
4. The wider the angle of the carina (>45 degrees and ideally 90 degrees), the easier the approach with stents, allowing the "T"-stent approach with a stent in the side branch and a stent covering the trunk and the main branch without overlapping stents.

C. DCA Technique for Bifurcation Lesions

The DCA technique for bifurcation lesions begins with an assessment of the relative size of the branches involved. If one branch is less than 2.5 mm in diameter, PTCA of this branch is preferable followed by DCA of the proximal trunk lesion and the lesion in the larger branch. If both branches are >2.5 mm, then sequential DCA of both branches may be preferable to provide greater debulking. A 6 Fr GTO AtheroCath (Guidant Corp., Santa Clara, CA) should be used for vessel diameters of 2.5–3.0 mm, a 7 Fr GTO device for 3.0–4.0 mm, and 7 FG (graft) catheter for >4.0 mm.

The sequence of procedures for bifurcation lesion DCA is as follows:

1. Use 10 Fr guiding catheters (DVI, ACS Tourguide [ACS, Santa Clara, CA], Medtronic Sherpa, [Medtronic, Inc., Minneapolis, MN] or ACS Viking [ACS]) for left coronary and 9 Fr or 9.5 Fr for right coronary procedures. A 9 Fr guide is large enough to accept a 6 Fr AtheroCath, but 9.5 Fr or 10 Fr are required for 7 Fr devices.
2. Place 0.014-in., medium-stiffness, floppy-tip coronary guidewires into each branch, taking care not to twist or wrap wires around each other while torquing into the branches.
3. Predilate (PTCA) the smaller branch with a 2.0-mm balloon to improve its ostium, then remove the balloon and guidewire from this branch. If both branches are large (>2.5 mm), predilate each with a 2.0-mm balloon and remove the wire from one branch. This will help preserve the ostial lumen of one branch (prevent "snow-plowing") during DCA of the other branch.
4. Perform DCA on one branch, then, if satisfactory, remove the coronary guidewire and redirect down the other branch. Perform DCA on the other branch.
5. Rewire both branches and finish with either "kissing" balloons or stents plus "kissing" balloons (simultaneous balloon inflations in both branches).

Other Directives

1. Always finish bifurcations with "kissing" balloon inflations to ensure even expansion of each lumen and prevent compromise of a branch ostium. If adjunctive stents are used, final "kissing" balloon inflations are essential to prevent displacement of a strut

into one branch after dilating the other branch.

2. Use a glycoprotein IIbIIIa platelet receptor antagonist (e.g. abciximab, tirofiban, eptifibatide) with weight-adjusted heparin to achieve ACT 200–250 seconds.

3. DCA cuts can be made in the direction of the carina in each branch at low balloon pressures (<30 psi) without increasing risk, given proper device sizing.

4. Nitinol coronary wires can be left in one branch while performing DCA on the other branch, but only a 5 Fr or 6 Fr GTO AtheroCath will fit in the standard 10 Fr guide with a wire remaining alongside the device (7 Fr device is too large).

CONCLUSIONS

DCA continues to have a role in the treatment of certain lesions which are unfavorable or difficult to treat with PTCA or stents. The most recent clinical trials of DCA (OARS and BOAT) show that DCA can be performed safely and with excellent acute procedural results and competitive late revascularization rates (<20%). Bifurcation lesions are complex and challenging, but debulking plaque with DCA followed by either PTCA or stenting can aid in achieving a large lumen in both involved branches.

REFERENCES

1. Baim DS, Hinohara T, Holmes D et al. and the U.S. Directional Coronary Atherectomy Group. Results of directional coronary atherectomy during multicenter preapproval testing. *Am J Cardiol* 1993; 72:6E–11E.

2. Topol EJ, Leya F, Pinkerton CA et al., for the CAVEAT study group. A comparison of directional atherectomy with coronary angioplasty in patients with coronary artery disease. *New England J Med* 1993:329(July 22): 221–227.

3. Holmes D, Topol E, Califf R et al. A multicenter randomized trial of coronary angioplasty versus directional atherectomy for patients with saphenous vein bypass graft lesions. CAVEAT-II Investigators. *Circulation* 1994[(7):1966–1974.

4. Adelman A, Cohen E, Kimball B et al. A comparison of directional atherectomy with balloon angioplasty for lesions of the left anterior descending coronary artery. *New England J Med* 1993;329:228–233.

5. Kuntz RE, Gibson MC, Nobuyoshi M, Baim DS. Generalized model of restenosis after conventional balloon angioplasty, stenting and directional atherectomy. *J Am Coll Cardiol* 1993;21:15–25.

6. Kuntz R, Hinohara T, Safian R, Selmon M, Simpson J, Baim D. Restenosis after directional coronary atherectomy. Effects of luminal diameter and deep wall excision. *Circulation* 1992;86:1394–1399.

7. Simonton CA, Leon MB, Baim DS et al. "Optimal" directional coronary atherectomy. Final results of the Optimal Atherectomy Restenosis Study (OARS). *Circulation* 1998;97:332–339.

8. Baim D, Cutlip DE, Sharma SK et al., for the BOAT Investigators. Final Results of the Balloon vs Optimal Atherectomy Trial (BOAT). *Circulation* 1998;97: 322–331.

9. Fischman DL, Leon MB, Baim DS et al. A randomized comparison of coronary stent placement and balloon angioplasty in the treatment of coronary artery disease. *N Engl J Med* 1994;331:496–502.

10. Macaya C, Serruys P, Ruygrok P et al. Continued benefit of coronary stenting versus balloon angioplasty: One-year clinical follow-up of BENESTENT Trial. *J Am Coll Cardiol* 1996;27(2):255–261.

11. The GUIDE Investigators: IVUS-determined predictors of restenosis in PTCA and DCA: final report from the GUIDE trial, phase II. *J Am Coll Cardiol* 1996;27: 156A.

12. Mintz GS, Popma JJ, Pichard AD et al. Intravascular ultrasound predictors of restenosis after percutaneous transcatheter coronary revascularization. *J Am Coll Cardiol* 1996;27:1678–1687.

13. Mansour M, Fischman RF, Kuntz RE, Carrozza JP. Feasibility of directional atherectomy for the treatment of bifurcation lesions. *Cor Art Dis* 1992;3:761–765.

14. Eisenhauer AC, Clugston RA, Ruiz CE. Sequential directional atherectomy of coronary bifurcation lesions. *Cathet Cardiovasc Diagn* 1993;[Suppl 1]:54–60.

15. Lewis B, Leya F, Johnson S et al. Acute procedural results in the treatment of 30 coronary artery bifurcation lesions with a double-wire atherectomy technique for side-branch protection. *Am Heart J* 1994;127: 1600–1607.

16. Metz D, Nazeyrolla P, Maillier B et al. Coronary angioplasty of bifurcational lesions with the protecting branch technique using 6 French guiding catheter. *Cathet and Cardiovasc Diagn* 1995;35(4):343–347.

17. de Groote P, Bauters C, McFadden E, Lablanche J, Leroy F, Bertrand M. Local lesion-related factors and restenosis after coronary angioplasty. *Circulation* 1995; 91(4):968.

18. Fischman D, Savage M, Leon M, Schatz R, Ellis S et al. Fate of side-branches after stenting. *J Am Coll Cardiol* 1993;22:1641–1646.

19. Colombo A et al. Kissing stents. *Cathet and Cardiovasc Diagn* 1993;30(4):327–330.

20. Teirstein P, Kissing Palmaz-Schatz Stents for coronary bifurcation stenoses. *Cathet and Cardiovasc Diagn* 1996;3:307–310.

C. The Role of Excimer Laser Coronary Angioplasty

Martin J. Sebastian, *Frank Litvack, and Neal Eigler

Cardiovascular Intervention Center, °Catheterization Laboratory, Cedars-Sinai Medical Center, Los Angeles, California 90048-1865

The first applications of laser technology to the cardiovascular system were in the early 1980s, using continuous-wave lasers. These devices produce visible light (argon laser) or infra-red energy (carbon dioxide and neodymium-YAG lasers) and create tissue effects by the generation of intense local heat. However, it became apparent that excessive thermal injury was created by these lasers; histologic examination of athero-sclerotic plaque treated by continuous wave-lasers demonstrates concentric zones of carbonized material, eosinophilic coagulum, and vacuolization (1,2). A new phase of optimism was ushered in with the advent of the excimer laser. *Excimer* is a term derived from the words excited dymer; a high voltage electrical discharge is placed across a mixture of gases, producing high-energy light of a uniform wavelength. These lasers are characterized by pulsed-wave emissions in the ultraviolet spectrum from 193–351 nanometers (nm). The precise wavelength of emission depends on the exact nature of the gas mixture from which the photons are generated. Experience in the cardiovascular field has involved the xenon chloride (XeCl) 308-nm laser, which became available in 1983. *In vitro* studies of the excimer laser focused in air or saline on segments of vascular tissue demonstrated a much more precise method of tissue ablation than continuous-wave lasers; histological examination revealed effects ranging from well-defined craters to relatively small zones of thermal and blast injury (3,4). In recognition of this the excimer laser was dubbed the "cool laser."

EVOLUTION OF EXCIMER LASER TECHNOLOGY

The encouraging preclinical results and the maturation of excimer laser technology led to the introduction of excimer laser coronary angioplasty (ELCA) in 1988. Over the last decade, catheter design has become more sophisticated to adapt to the clinical challenge. The diameter of individual fiberoptics was able to be decreased from 600 to about 50 microns, resulting in increased flexibility, enabling catheters to negotiate the coronary vasculature.

Both blood and angiographic contrast media are strong absorbers of excimer light at 308 nm. This results in the formation of insoluble gas and rapidly expanding and imploding cavitation bubbles ("fast bubbles"). These bubbles generate intense pressure pulses which are believed to contribute to arterial complications such as perforation and dissection (5–6). This also helps explain the observation that severe dissections are more frequently seen in focal lesions compared to long diffuse lesions (where there is less blood at the laser tip). Knowledge of this deleterious interaction led to the development of the saline flushing technique, which has substantially reduced the severity of coronary dissections, and is now a routine part of the procedure (7,8).

One disadvantage of multifiber catheters is the presence of ablative "dead space" between adjacent laser fibers, which results in an inhomogeneous or stippled ablation effect. Some researchers have demonstrated that this may result in less efficient tissue penetration, necessitating excessive energy densities which in turn predispose to fast bubble formation and complications. This has led to attempts to "homogenize" the laser beam as it exits the catheter (9). Another promising technology is "multiplexing;" with this system, rapid sequential firing of different sections of the multifiber catheter enables a decrease in the pulse energy. Experimental results have shown reduced photoacoustic effects on tissue (10,11).

Traditional laser catheters have incorporated a concentric design in which the laser fibers are arranged symmetrically around a central guidewire lumen. With clinical experience it became apparent that this configuration is not well suited to eccentric or bifurcation lesions, and an arrangement with eccentric positioning of the fibers in relation to the guidewire lumen was developed. One variation included a protective tip extending past the laser-tissue interface. The eccentric fiber-array provides directional control, enabling the ablative surface to be rotated into contact with the eccentric plaque, while sparing the nondiseased arterial wall opposite the lesion. The concentric catheters range in diameter from 1.4 to 2.0 mm, while the directional (eccentric) catheter is available in 1.7 mm and 2.0 mm diameters (Fig. 10.14). They require 7, 8 or 9 Fr guide catheters depending on which size is chosen.

CLINICAL EXPERIENCE WITH EXCIMER LASERS

Most of the clinical experience in the United States has been obtained using devices from two manufacturers. Our group was involved in the development and early clinical application of the Advanced Interventional Systems (AIS) (Irvine, CA) excimer laser. The registry experiences with this device and the Spectranetics (Colorado Springs, CO) device comprise the largest body of clinical data available. We have reported the results of the first 3000 patients treated at 33 sites with the AIS system (12). This group was 75% male with a mean age of 62 ± 10 years. There was a wide selection of cases including complex disease, with 20% long lesions (>20 mm) and about 8% aortoostial lesions amongst the 3,592 lesions treated. There are several salient features from the analysis. Firstly, adjunctive percutaneous transluminal coronary angioplasty (PTCA) was performed in 79% overall, but in the last 1,000 cases this figure was 95%, reflecting the recognition over time that laser alone was not resulting in adequate luminal gain. Secondly,

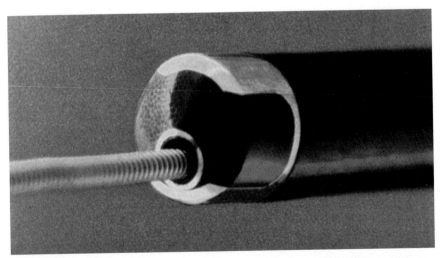

FIG. 10.14. Photograph of directional laser catheter. The eccentric fiber bundle may be torqued to appose the lesion, giving the operator directional control, and the radiolucent "window" facilitates accurate alignment (reproduced by courtesy of Spectranetics).

procedural success was high, about 90%, and remained stable over the period of the registry. Lesion analysis by subgroup suggested that with this technology, lesion length, and morphology were not strong predictors of success, in contrast to previous experience with PTCA. Thirdly, with respect to complications, rates for in-hospital death, Q-wave myocardial infarction and in-hospital bypass surgery were 0.5%, 2.1%, and 3.8% respectively. The laser perforation rate was 1.6% for the first 2,000 patients, although in the last 1,000 patients this figure was reduced to 0.4%, indicating better case selection as operators became more cognizant of relative contraindications. Laser perforation is a serious complication, and was associated with a 5.4% in-hospital mortality rate. Dissection was noted in 13% of cases; this too was associated with poorer outcome with major ischemic complications occurring in 15% of patients who suffered dissection versus 4.1% for those who did not have dissection.

One subgroup of the ELCA registry which was specifically studied were aortoostial lesions. A series of 209 stenoses (59% in the RCA, 28% in vein grafts, 12% in the left main coronary) were treated with laser, with adjunctive PTCA in 72%. Major complications were uncommon (0% death, 0.5% Q-wave MI, 3.4% bypass surgery). Procedural success was 90%, and the restenosis rate (defined as >50% diameter stenosis) was 39% overall and only 35% in the RCA, but 64% in the left main coronary artery (13).

The PELCA (Percutaneous Excimer Laser Coronary Angioplasty) registry monitored the experience using the Spectranetics laser, and described a 3% perforation rate in 764 patients. Risk factors for perforation included bifurcation lesions, diabetes mellitus, and female gender, each of which carried approximately three times the risk of this complication (14).

The New Approaches to Coronary Intervention (NACI) registry recently reported a series of 1,000 lesions in 887 patients, using both the AIS and the Spectranetics excimer laser systems (15). The majority of these patients had complex lesions. Again, while procedural success rate was quite high (84%), there were significant dissections in up to 23.4% of lesions and perfora-

tion occurred in 2.6%; in-hospital mortality was 1.2%. At 1-year follow-up, the combined incidence of death, Q-wave MI or target lesion revascularization was 42.3%. In this group, no specific lesion characteristics were found to be predictive of complications.

The ERBAC (Excimer Laser, Rotational Atherectomy, and Balloon Angioplasty Comparison) Study was a prospective, single-center, randomized trial conducted in Germany. It comprised 685 patients assigned to one of three interventional strategies: either balloon angioplasty alone or in conjunction with one of the debulking methods, rotational atherectomy (Rotablator, Heart Technology, Redmond, WA) or excimer laser (16). When interpreting the results it is important to remember that patients with total occlusions and long lesions (two groups of complex disease which do relatively well with excimer laser) were excluded from this cohort. As conducted, this study showed higher procedural success in rotational atherectomy than excimer laser or balloon angioplasty groups, no difference in major in-hospital complications, and higher 6-month target-lesion revascularization rates in the two debulking groups (42.4% for Rotablator, 46.0% for ELCA, and 31.9% for balloon angioplasty, $p = .013$). Once again, a propensity for dissections was found with ELCA; severe dissections (resulting in TIMI flow <3, residual stenosis ≥50%, length >10 mm) were seen in 6.9% of ELCA-treated lesions versus 0.9% for the Rotablator ($p < .001$). However it must also be noted that the saline infusion technique was not in use at this time.

Another small randomized trial, the Amsterdam-Rotterdam (AMRO) trial, compared excimer laser coronary angioplasty (with adjunctive balloon dilatation in 98% of cases) to balloon angioplasty in 308 patients with lesions more than 10 mm in length and stable angina (17). Although ELCA appeared safe in this study, there was no reduction in the long-term clinical adverse event rate compared to balloon angioplasty, and angiographic follow-up suggested a tendency for higher restenosis rates (52% for ELCA versus 41% for PTCA, $p = .13$). Subsequent subgroup analysis did not suggest any advantage of ELCA over balloon angioplasty in long (>20 mm) lesions, small vessels (<2.5 mm), calcified lesions or total coronary occlusion—some of the categories that were believed to be potential niches for excimer laser angioplasty (18).

Thus, the overall results obtained to date with excimer laser angioplasty have been less impressive than originally hoped; this realization, coupled with the explosion in stenting has seen waning use of ELCA. In our center only 2.6% of interventions in 1997 involved the excimer laser; by comparison this figure was in the 11% to 14% range from 1988 until 1993. This trend has also been reported in other centers (19). However, before abandoning this treatment modality, it is important to recognize that most of the published results were obtained using developing techniques and equipment, both of which have subsequently undergone refinement. There are certain subsets of complex lesions which remain vexatious to treat and may still benefit from ELCA. Currently we consider using it most for aortoostial disease, total occlusions, lesions >20 mm long, vein graft lesions, restenotic lesions, and lesions which are uncrossable or undilatable with a balloon catheter. With the emergence of the new disease entity of in-stent restenosis, laser angioplasty may have a new indication. A recent report of 107 patients suggests ELCA is safe, and demonstrates a trend to lower target-vessel revascularization compared to balloon angioplasty (21% versus 38%, $p = .08$) when treating this difficult category of patients (20).

THE BIFURCATION LESION: A ROLE FOR THE EXCIMER LASER?

The bifurcation lesion has long been the bête-noir of interventional cardiologists, with a lower primary success rate, higher complication rate, and higher restenosis rate than other lesion subtypes (21). None of the technological advances in the two decades since the inception of the specialty have made much impact on this shortcoming, and many operators regard bifurcation disease as an indication for coronary bypass surgery rather than percutaneous therapies. The intrinsic problem in the true bifurcation lesion is the adjacency of the two target vessels; when

any expansile maneuver is applied to one lesion, plaque-shifting occurs with resulting impingement on the other vessel. Stenting, the savior of many difficult interventional situations, has not altered the risk of adverse early events due to the difficulty in positioning side-by-side stents or one stent through another without leaving excessive metal surface area in the bloodstream, thereby increasing the risk of acute or subacute thrombosis (22). Moreover, the branch vessels involved in bifurcation disease, while large enough to be clinically significant, are often below the optimal size for stenting. Coupled with the exaggerated intimal hyperplastic response seen with stents, restenosis rates have been high where stenting has been employed in bifurcation disease (23).

The seemingly logical mechanical solution to the geometric challenge of bifurcation disease would be to remove as much of the plaque as possible rather than merely displacing it outwards. It follows that "debulking" strategies such as excimer laser angioplasty and rotational atherectomy offer a theoretical advantage over the predominantly "stretching" strategies of balloon angioplasty and stenting.

During the early period of excimer laser coronary angioplasty, the laser catheters used had a concentric fiber array. This was not able to selectively target eccentric plaque, and adequate branch vessel protection with a second guidewire was not possible. Furthermore the saline flushing technique was not in routine use. In this setting, excimer laser angioplasty was found to have a prohibitively high perforation rate and risk of side-branch occlusion. With the advent of the directional catheter, both the safety and precision of the procedure improved. In a series of 53 patients with 57 complex lesions (including 12% bifurcation lesions) treated at our institution with a prototype directional device containing a protective hood, there were no perforations and no laser-related deaths. Angiographic follow-up was obtained for 30 lesions with a 37% incidence of restenosis defined as >50% diameter stenosis (24). An example of one such case is shown in Figure 10.15. Unfortunately, this device was discontinued when the two major laser companies merged. The current Spectranetics eccentric catheter does not have

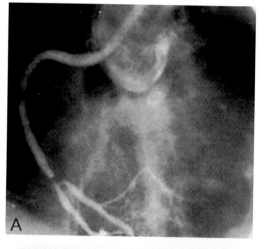
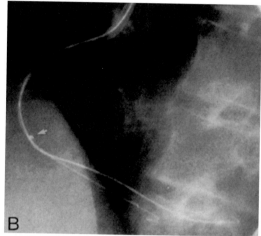
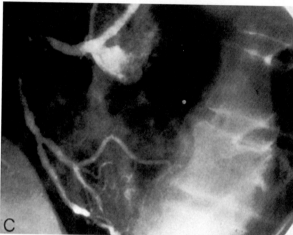

FIG. 10.15. Use of the directional catheter in bifurcation disease. **A:** Baseline LAO/cranial view of RCA. A severe, highly-eccentric lesion involves the bifurcation. **B:** Separate guidewires have been placed in the posterior descending branch and ongoing RCA, and a 1.8-mm directional excimer laser catheter has been advanced over the guidewire for the continuing RCA *(arrow)*. The tip marker is aligned so that the laser fibers are oriented to the eccentric atheroma mass; the protective tip (not visible) will shield the region of the vascular carina. **C:** Appearances after excimer laser atherectomy of the main lesion and adjunctive balloon angioplasty of both branches, showing a widely patent bifurcation with very little recoil.

the protective tip, but does have a refined system for aligning the ablative surface with the lesion.

TECHNICAL APPROACH TO THE BIFURCATION LESION

1. The most desirable lesion morphology involves a lesion either just distal or just proximal to the bifurcation. Native vessels should be 2.5 to 3.5 mm in diameter.

2. The eccentric (directional) laser catheter is appropriate, allowing ablation of plaque on the outer walls of the vessels without jeopardizing the carina. The 1.7-mm catheter is the initial choice, up-sizing to the 2.0-mm unit is possible in very large vessels.

3. Always use a well-supported guiding catheter, to avoid any back-and-forth movement of the laser catheter during ablation, minimizing the risk of trauma (dissection, perforation).

4. Cross the target lesion with a conventional or extra-support guidewire; we recommend free-wiring the lesion. Always keep the tip as far distal as possible to allow catheter tracking over the stiffer body of the wire. Protect the side branch with a second wire.

5. Machine settings: use energy densities between 45 and 60 mJ/ mm² at frequencies of 25 to 50 Hz.

6. Position the laser catheter in direct contact with the lesion before ablation; contact of

the laser surface with blood or normal arterial wall increases the risk of acoustic shock and associated complications. The current Spectranetics system (Vitesse-E) has a tip configuration with a radiolucent "window" that enables more precise fluoroscopic alignment of the eccentric laser bundle and the lesion.

7. Check the alignment of the catheter in two views to be sure that the fibers are pointed away from the carina.

8. Flush saline through the guide catheter via a control syringe. The saline should be warmed to 37°C. An initial bolus of approximately 8 mL at 2mL/sec is given to replace the optically absorbent fluids in the region of the catheter tip with crystalloid. A continuous infusion of approximately 1 to 2 mL/sec is given during laser use. One should always initiate flushing prior to laser use and terminate flushing after laser energy delivery has been stopped.

9. Laser energy should be applied for up to 5 seconds (1 to 2 seconds is desirable), with a "waiting" of 5 seconds between delivery trains.

10. Forward movement of the catheter should not exceed 1 mm/sec. Always keep the guidewire taut while advancing the laser catheter.

11. Perform only one pass and then withdraw the laser catheter to assess luminal patency. If a lumen diameter equal to the size of the laser catheter has been achieved, no further lasing should be performed. If a sufficient diameter has not been achieved and the operator is sure that there is no luminal dissection, another laser pass may be performed.

12. If the branch lesion is also eccentric and vessel caliber is suitable for ELCA then debulking of both disease loci can be performed by repeating the above steps, again taking particular care to align the fiber away from the carina.

Troubleshooting

1. Guidewire motion is "freezing" in the catheter: remove catheter and vigorously flush lumen and wet wire again.

2. Laser catheter does not fully cross lesions around a bend: the problem here may be inability of the laser catheter to flex round the bend—do not use force as this may result in vessel perforation.

3. No-flow in distal artery following laser pass: unless there is obvious dissection or guide catheter obstruction, attempt use of intracoronary nitroglycerin if clinically appropriate. If microcirculatory dysfunction is suspected then intracoronary verapamil may also be of benefit (watch carefully for conduction disturbance).

4. If flow-limiting dissection is diagnosed: adjunctive PTCA with or without stenting is generally appropriate. *Never* apply further laser energy in this setting.

Avoiding and Managing Complications

Excimer laser angioplasty is a procedure that requires careful attention to case selection and technical detail. The best results occur when the laser catheter crosses the lesion with minimum force and resistance. If resistance is encountered that is not readily overcome within the parameters mentioned above, then the laser component of the procedure should be terminated. Applying excessive laser energy in one location where a catheter is not crossing a lesion is associated with dissection and/or acute occlusion. Maintaining absolute catheter/plaque contact and meticulous saline flushing are important to avoid dissections caused by acoustic transients caused when blood absorbs laser energy.

Perforation, a serious but not universally catastrophic complication, should occur in well under 0.5% of cases. In the application of bifurcation lesion excimer laser angioplasty, perforation is more likely to occur in certain situations: (a) use of a concentric catheter (Fig. 10.16), (b) use of a catheter that is equal to or greater than the vessel diameter (c), failure to align an eccentric catheter with a very eccentric lesion, particularly if on a tight bend, (d) applying laser energy in a previously dissected vascular segment, and (e) failure to "back off" when the laser catheter is not successfully crossing the lesion. Perforation may result in hemodynamic compromise in

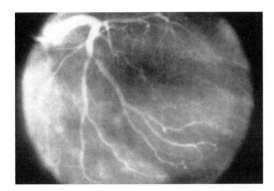

FIG. 10.16. Example of a lesion now regarded as unsuitable for laser angioplasty using the concentric catheter. This RAO/caudal view shows a bifurcation lesion involving the circumflex and a large obtuse marginal branch. Due to inability to selectively target the eccentric plaque, perforation at the vascular carina occurred resulting in pericardial tamponade requiring emergency pericardiocentesis.

approximately one-third of cases, depending on flow-rate, underlying heart disease and status of the pericardium. When it does occur, hemodynamic compromise can develop in less than 1 minute. Tamponade is best treated by inflating a balloon at the perforation site, supportive medical therapy, and pericardiocentesis if necessary. If dye extravasation is noted, make sure to maintain guidewire position and rapidly inflate a conventional or perfusion balloon to seal the perforation. Cardiac surgery should be considered in these patients, even if stabilized and no further extravasation is noted. Although not uniform, delayed hemodynamic compromise (48 hours) has been reported following apparent stabilization. The patients that may be "safest" from this complication are those with previously opened pericardium and those with intramuscular dye extravasation. Those that may be at highest risk for delayed compromise are those with pericardial extravasation and intact pericardium.

SUMMARY

The past fifteen years have seen the evolution of excimer laser therapy from an untested concept into a clinically-approved treatment for obstructive coronary artery disease. While ongoing refinements have reduced the risks of device-related complications, the cost of the equipment and lack of clear-cut superiority over other techniques has limited its applicability. However there remain potential "niche" applications, one of which is treatment of bifurcation disease, which responds poorly to other interventional modalities. We have experienced procedural success with the newer eccentric catheter for bifurcation lesions. While these results are encouraging, the number of patients treated to date is insufficient to draw any firm conclusions as to whether this lesion subset derives incremental long-term benefit from ELCA compared to other interventional techniques.

REFERENCES

1. Litvack F, Grundfest WS, Papaioannou T, Mohr FW, Jakubowski AT, Forrester JS. Role of laser and thermal ablation devices in the treatment of cardiovascular diseases. *Am J Cardiol* 1988;61:81G–86G.
2. Sanborn TA, Faxon DP, Haudenschild CC, Ryan TJ. Experimental angioplasty: distribution of laser thermal injury with a laser probe. *J Am Coll Cardiol* 1985;5: 934–938.
3. Grundfest WS, Litvack F, Forrester JS et al. Laser ablation of human atherosclerotic plaque without adjacent tissue injury. *J Am Coll Cardiol* 1985;5:929–933.
4. Isner JM, Donaldson RF, Deckelbaum LI et al. The excimer laser: gross, light microscopic and ultrastructural analysis of potential advantages for use in laser therapy of cardiovascular disease. *J Am Coll Cardiol* 1985;6: 1102–1109.
5. van Leeuwen TG, van Ervin L, Meertens JH, Motamedi M, Post MJ, Borst C. Origin of arterial wall dissections induced by pulsed excimer and mid-infrared laser ablation in the pig. *J Am Coll Cardiol* 1992;19:1610–1618.
6. Hamburger JN, Gijsbers GHM, Verhoofstad GGAM et al. Excimer laser coronary angioplasty: a physical perspective to clinical results. In: Topol EJ and Serruys PW, eds. *Current review of interventional cardiology*, 2nd ed. Philadelphia: Current Medicine 1995:159–172.
7. Tcheng JE. Development of a new technique for reducing pressure pulse generation during 308-nm excimer laser coronary angioplasty. *Cathet Cardiovasc Diagn* 1995;34:15–22.
8. Deckelbaum LI, Natarajan MK, Bittl JA et al. Effect of intracoronary saline infusion on dissection during excimer laser coronary angioplasty: a randomized trial. The Percutaneous Excimer Laser Coronary Angioplasty (PELCA) Investigators. *J Am Coll Cardiol* 1995;26: 1264–1269.
9. Gijsbers GH, Hamburger JN, Serruys PW. Homogeneous light distribution to reduce vessel trauma during excimer laser angioplasty. *Seminars in Interventional Cardiology* 1996;1:143–148.
10. Deckenbaum LI. Coronary laser angioplasty. *Lasers in Surgery and Medicine* 1994;14:101–110.

11. Haase KK, Rose C, Duda S, Baumbach A, Oberhoff M, Athanasiadis A, Karsch KR. Perspectives of coronary excimer laser angioplasty: multiplexing, saline flushing and acoustic ablation control. *Lasers in Surgery and Medicine* 1997;21:72–78.

12. Litvack F, Eigler N, Margolis J, Rothbaum D, Bresnahan JF, Holmes D. Percutaneous excimer laser angioplasty: results of the first consecutive 3,000 patients. *J Am Coll Cardiol* 1994;23:323–329.

13. Eigler N, Weinstock B, Douglas JS et al. Excimer laser coronary angioplasty of aortoostial stenoses: results of the excimer laser coronary angioplasty (ELCA) registry in the first 200 patients. *Circulation* 1993;88: 2049–2057.

14. Bittl JA, Ryan TJ, Keaney JF, Tcheng JE, Ellis SG, Isner JM, Sanborn TA for the PELCA Registry. Coronary artery perforation during excimer laser coronary angioplasty. *J Am Coll Cardiol* 1993;21:1158–1165.

15. Holmes DR Jr, Mehta S, George CJ et al. Excimer laser coronary angioplasty: the new approaches to coronary intervention (NACI) experience. *Am J Cardiol* 1997; 80(10A):99K–105K.

16. Reifart N, Vandormael M, Krajcar M et al. Randomized comparison of angioplasty of complex coronary lesions at a single center: ERBAC study. *Circulation* 1997;96: 91–98.

17. Appelman YEA, Piek JJ, Strikwerda S et al. Randomized trial of excimer laser angioplasty versus balloon angioplasty for treatment of obstructive coronary artery disease. *Lancet* 1996;347:79–84.

18. Appelman YEA, Piek JJ, Redekop WK et al. Clinical events following laser angioplasty or balloon angioplasty for complex coronary lesions: subanalysis of a randomised trial. *Heart* 1998;79:34–38.

19. Hasdai D, Berger PB, Bell MR, Rihal CS, Garrat KN, Holmes DR. The changing face of coronary interventional practice: the Mayo Clinic experience. *Arch Intern Med* 1997;157:677–682.

20. Mehran R, Mintz GS, Satler LF, Pichard AD, Kent KM et al. Treatment of in-stent restenosis with excimer laser coronary angioplasty: mechanisms and results compared to PTCA alone. *Circulation* 1997;96:2183–2189.

21. Meier B, Gruentzig AR, King SB III, Douglas JS Jr, Hollman J, Ischinger T et al. Risk of side branch occlusion during coronary angioplasty. *Am J Cardiol* 1984; 53:10–14.

22. Pomerantz RM, Ling FS. Distortion of Palmaz-Schatz geometry following side-branch balloon dilatation through the stent in a rabbit model. *Cathet Cardiovasc Diagn* 1997;40:422–426.

23. Colombo A, Martini G, Di Francesco L, Finci L. Coronary stenting of bifurcation lesions: immediate and follow-up results. *J Am Coll Cardiol* 1996;27:277A.

24. Rechavia E, Federman J, Shefer A, Macko G, Eigler N, Litvack F. Usefulness of a prototype directional catheter for excimer laser coronary angioplasty in narrowings unfavourable for conventional excimer or balloon angioplasty. *Am J Cardiol* 1995;76:1144–1146.

D. The Role of Rotational Atherectomy[1]

Charanjit S. Rihal

Division of Cardiovascular Diseases and Internal Medicine, Mayo Clinic and Mayo Foundation, Mayo Medical School, Department of Medicine, Rochester, Minnesota 55905

Atherosclerotic lesions, in both the coronary and systemic circulations, frequently occur at vessel bifurcations. Following the inception of percutaneous transluminal coronary angioplasty (PTCA), it was recognized that such lesions were difficult to treat and were associated with a relatively high incidence of procedural complications, such as myocardial infarction and emergent coronary artery bypass surgery (1,2). Various balloon and wire techniques were developed, including double wiring with single or double guide catheters, "kissing" balloon inflations, sequential balloon inflations, and the use of fixed-wire systems in side branches (3–10). Operators attempting balloon angioplasty of bifurcation lesions frequently encounter the problem of alternate branch compromise—PTCA is performed down one limb of the bifurcation and the other is compromised. Simultaneous, or "kissing," balloon inflations are associated with limited success and suboptimal results, with dissections or tissue prolapse often occurring. The risk of complications with balloon angioplasty, particularly acute vessel occlusion, has remained high and in many reports is greater than 15% (1,2,11,12).

New technologic devices directed primarily

---

[1]Cases 1 and 2 are from ref. 19, with permission by Elsevier Science Ireland.

at debulking atherosclerotic lesions with directionally targetable catheters, such as directional atherectomy (13–17) and directional laser fibers (18), have also been used. Directional atherectomy catheters are bulky devices and frequently cannot be advanced across heavily calcified or sharply angulated lesions, which bifurcation lesions tend to be. Laser catheters are now used infrequently and are not commonly available in catheterization laboratories. Although stent deployment is used in more than 50% of interventional cases, it is technically difficult in bifurcation lesions and prone to problems such as stent entrapment, stripping, and balloon rupture. As yet, no widely applicable stent design has emerged for treating most bifurcation lesions.

ROLE OF ROTATIONAL ATHERECTOMY

Rotational atherectomy, which uses the principle of differential cutting, has been proposed as a first-line treatment for bifurcation coronary artery stenoses (19). This technique has several advantages that we believe make it particularly suitable for bifurcations. First, rotational atherectomy allows controlled treatment of calcific lesions. Bifurcation lesions tend to be calcified, presumably a reflection of their chronicity. Although they can occur in any age group, they are frequent among elderly patients with multivessel disease, in whom a strategy of culprit lesion revascularization is often considered. Second, rotational atherectomy allows effective lesion debulking. Bifurcation points are associated with a large volume of atheroma, especially after arterial remodeling has occurred. The volume of atheroma present at bifurcations makes it difficult to attain good results after balloon angioplasty. Debulking may allow more predictable preservation of side branches, even when treatment of the branch is not contemplated or possible. Third, rotational atherectomy devices are relatively inexpensive and are in the repertoire of most busy catheterization laboratories. A high level of training and experience, however, are requisite to consistently obtain good results without complications.

CLINICAL RESULTS

Few published reports on rotational atherectomy for bifurcation lesions exist. We examined the outcomes of bifurcation rotational atherectomy procedures performed in 15 patients. The clinical and angiographic characteristics are listed in Table 10.6. The mean age was 64 years, and 14 were men. Five patients previously had experienced myocardial infarction, and 13 were symptomatic with chest pain. The cohort included three patients with diabetes mellitus and seven with hypertension; six were former or current smokers. The majority of lesions involved the left anterior descending (LAD) artery and its diagonal branches. The procedure outcomes are listed in Table 10.7. A successful angiographic result was achieved in all patients and arterial segments (final residual stenosis was 30% or less in all limbs) after a combination of rotational atherectomy, balloon angioplasty, or stenting, as needed. Rotational atherectomy of both limbs of the bifurcation was performed in seven cases and of one limb in eight. Of the 22 bifurcation limbs treated with rotational atherectomy, only three required no further treatment after rotational ath-

TABLE 10.6. *Clinical and angiographic characteristics of 15 patients undergoing rotablation of coronary bifurcation lesions[a]*

Characteristic	Patients	
	No.	%
Male	14	93
Diabetes mellitus	3	20
Hypertension	7	47
Total cholesterol >250 mg/dL	8	53
Current or former smoker	6	40
Previous myocardial infarction	5	33
Previous coronary artery bypass	2	13
No. of vessels diseased[b]		
1	9	60
2	4	27
3	2	13
Culprit lesion		
L anterior descending artery	11	73
L circumflex artery and branches	3	20
R coronary artery and branches	1	7

[a] Ejection fraction (mean % ± SD), 55 ± 19;
[b] Stenosis of ≥70% was considered a significant lesion;
From ref. 19, with permission by Elsevier Science Ireland.

TABLE 10.7. *Complications among 15 patients who had rotational atherectomy*

Complication	Patients No.	%
Death	0	
Q-wave myocardial infarction	0	
Non-Q-wave myocardial infarction	1	7
Coronary artery bypass surgery	0	
Ventricular tachycardia or fibrillation	0	
Transient hypotension	3	20
Transient bradycardia	2	13
Branch occlusion	1[a]	7
Occlusion outside laboratory	0	
Congestive heart failure	0	
Intra-aortic balloon pump	0	
Vascular bleeding or repair	0	
Renal failure	0	

[a] Asymptomatic;
From ref. 19, with permission by Elsevier Science Ireland.

erectomy; follow-up balloon angioplasty was performed in 16. Five Gianturco-Rubin (Cook, Inc., Bloomington, IN) and four Palmaz-Schatz (Johnson and Johnson Interventional Systems) stents were deployed in seven patients (two patients received stents in both limbs of the bifurcation). Two patients had transient severe spasm; one patient experienced hypotension that required vasopressors. One non-Q-wave myocardial infarction occurred, with a peak serum level of creatine kinase of 800 IU/L. Asymptomatic occlusion of the contralateral limb occurred in one patient, and no attempt was made to open it. When rotational atherectomy was used in only one limb of the bifurcation (generally, the more severely diseased limb), in no case did compromise of the contralateral limb occur.

In a consecutive series of patients with bifurcation lesions, 40 patients treated with mechanical debulking with directional or rotational atherectomy had superior acute and midterm results compared with 30 patients treated with balloon angioplasty alone (20). In this study, patients treated with debulking experienced superior acute procedural success rates (97% versus 73%, debulking versus PTCA groups, respectively; $p = .01$) and required repeat procedures less often (28% target vessel revascularization at 1 year versus 53%; $p = .05$). However, only six of these patients had debulking with rotational ath-

erectomy. These data and others, based primarily on debulking with directional atherectomy (13–17), support the importance of mechanical debulking in the treatment of bifurcation stenoses.

TECHNIQUE

Diagnostic Study

A carefully performed diagnostic angiogram is crucial for a successful procedure. Special attention should be directed at assessing the size and geometric configuration of the lesion, the proximal and distal reference segments, and the degree of lesion calcification. With modern radiographic equipment, calcification frequently can be assessed better with high-resolution fluoroscopy than with cineangiographic film. Atherosclerotic bifurcation lesions may have several different geometric configurations, and particular attention must be paid to the location of the tightest lesions and side branch involvement. Bifurcation lesions often can be considered tandem ostial branch lesions with or without proximal vessel involvement. The location of the bulk of the lesion in relation to the takeoff of both limbs should be assessed. If the bulk of the lesion is anatomically opposite the origin of a limb, the likelihood of compromise is less. If the lesion is located immediately adjacent to, or circumferentially involves the origin of one or both limbs, a very careful assessment must be made of the lumen. On occasion, atheromatous plaque may prolapse over the origin of a limb and render wire passage almost impossible. Care must be taken to distinguish a very tight lumen from an overlying small branch, collateral, or linear calcification. For extremely tight complex lesions, no attempt should be made to pass a wire into the limb unless it is clear where the lumen is in two orthogonal angiographic views.

Bifurcation angles can vary markedly, from relatively mild 45-degree bifurcations (often seen with LAD-diagonal combinations) to 90 or more degrees (typical of right posterior descending and posterolateral arteries). It is more difficult to pass a rotational atherectomy wire into a sharp side-branch takeoff, and the possibility of vessel perforation is increased. The likelihood of branch occlusion, whether sacrificing a small branch is acceptable, and other alternatives (such as bypass surgery) should be assessed. Options for back-up must be considered because opportunities for stent deployment may be significantly limited (21). Reference segment calibers and the anticipated final caliber of each diseased limb should be assessed carefully, because this will determine the subsequent selection of equipment.

Equipment Selection

Vascular sheaths should be chosen to allow passage of the largest anticipated final guiding catheter size. Usually, 8 Fr or 9 Fr arterial access is required. Many operators prefer to place a temporary pacemaker wire at the start of a procedure, especially if the right coronary artery is involved. Generally, we place a temporary wire if the right coronary artery is being treated, obtain venous access only if the left circumflex is being treated, and do neither if the LAD is being treated.

Rotational atherectomy rarely is used as the sole procedure. Nearly always, another technique such as balloon angioplasty or stenting is needed. The final burr size for each limb and follow-up technique should be determined before initiating the procedure. Although we have occasionally passed 1.5-mm and 1.75-mm burrs through 7 Fr guiding catheters, an 8 Fr to 10 Fr guiding catheter is usually required, depending on final anticipated burr size. For patients in whom lower extremity access was not available, we have performed rotational atherectomy from brachial and radial access sites, with pacemaker wires from the internal jugular vein. If potential exists for subsequent simultaneous balloon or stent inflations, a guiding catheter with sufficient caliber to accommodate two balloon shafts should be chosen. Lack of guide catheter support is not a problem generally encountered with rotational atherectomy. Judkins curves generally suffice and provide sufficient support for rotational atherectomy and follow-up procedures.

Rotational Atherectomy Technique

Various wires are available for rotational atherectomy. We prefer to use rotational atherectomy wires at the outset instead of first using a standard angioplasty wire and then exchanging it for a rotational atherectomy wire. Care must be taken not to compromise the lumen of sharply angulated branches when first passing the wire. Generally, we wire the largest and most important limb first and perform rotational atherectomy with a small burr (for example, a 1.5-mm burr into a 3.0-mm limb) to secure a reliable lumen. If the lumen of the second limb is readily accessible, it can usually be accessed by withdrawing the burr just proximal to the bifurcation, placing it on "Dynaglide," and manipulating the wire directly into the branch. This maneuver is not recommended if the lumen of the second limb appears difficult to wire. After the lumen of the second limb has been secured with rotational atherectomy, a decision has to be made about the next burr size. We generally try to achieve a final burr-to-artery ratio of 0.6 or 0.7. Care must be taken not to oversize the burr used in the smaller limb because of the risk of perforation. Wire bias in pulling or pushing a burr into or out of a lesion must be taken into account. A small burr pulled up into a lesion by a guide wire will ablate much more tissue than a small burr directed away from the same lesion. If a second burr is required, an exchange can be performed and further rotational atherectomy performed. Because of the volume of atheroma present in many bifurcation lesions, care must be taken not to overwhelm the capacity of the microcirculation to clear microparticulate matter; coronary flow should be monitored closely.

Subsequent Procedures

After debulking with rotational atherectomy, widely patent lumens are frequently obtained in both limbs. At this point, we often wire both limbs of the lesion with soft-tipped angioplasty wires and dilate each bifurcation limb with balloon catheters inflated to low pressures (less than 4 atm). Simultaneous inflations usually are not necessary. This maneuver often results in very acceptable angiographic results. If not, strong consideration should be given to stent deployment. We would stent the larger of the two limbs first, using a stent design that would allow access to the side branch. If effective debulking has been performed, gaining access to the second limb usually is not a problem. If stenting of the branch is also needed, extreme care must be taken not to entrap either the stent or the balloon. Predilation and use of a sheathed or covered delivery system minimize this possibility.

Adjunctive Therapy

During the procedure, anticoagulation with unfractionated heparin given intravenously is standard. Because of the complexity and bulk of a typical lesion, the patients may benefit from concomitant abciximab, which is given at the operator's discretion. Liberal doses of intracoronary vasodilators, systemic atropine, and systemic vasopressors are used as needed. After the procedure, we administer antiplatelet therapy with clopidogrel or ticlopidine for 2 weeks and aspirin indefinitely.

ILLUSTRATIVE CASES

Case 1: Bifurcation Rotational Atherectomy Followed by Balloon Angioplasty

A 51-year-old man with progressive angina and rest pain had a non-Q-wave myocardial infarction. Electrocardiography on presentation at his local hospital revealed ST-segment depression in precordial leads V_3V_6 and a peak level of creatine kinase of 400 IU/L. Cardiac catheterization and angiography revealed normal left ventricular function, a 60% stenosis of the ostium of the circumflex artery, and a severe, calcified bifurcation stenosis involving the LAD and first diagonal arteries (Fig. 10.17A). After angiography, the patient was transferred to the author's institution for further treatment. Five days after presentation, the patient had bifurcation rotational atherectomy, with adjunctive administration of abciximab because of the recent non-Q-wave infarction. The origin of the diagonal had progressed to occlusion. With the use of

a 9 Fr left Judkins guiding catheter, the distal LAD artery was cannulated with a type C rotational atherectomy wire and rotational atherectomy was performed with 1.50-mm and 1.75-mm burrs (Fig. 10.17B). After this, the diagonal branch was cannulated with the same type C guidewire and also treated with 1.50-mm and 1.75-mm burrs. Follow-up balloon angioplasty was performed with two 3.0-mm balloon catheters (Fig. 10.17C). This resulted in an excellent angiographic appearance (Fig. 10.17D). The procedure was well tolerated, and coronary blood flow remained normal during the procedure. The patient was dismissed the next day.

Case 2: Bifurcation Rotational Atherectomy to Facilitate Stenting

A 48-year-old man was admitted with chest pain and ST-segment elevation in leads I, aVL, and V_5V_6. He received treatment with tissue plasminogen activator, and the creatine kinase level subsequently peaked at 600 IU/L. Q-waves did not develop; however, significant ST-segment depression was noted on an exercise test 4 days after admission. Coronary angiography revealed severe stenosis at the bifurcation of a large intermediate artery with two major marginal branches (Fig. 10.18A). The ejection fraction was 48%, with inferolateral hypokinesis. The patient was transferred to the author's institution for further treatment. Approximately 2 weeks after his infarction, the patient underwent rotational atherectomy of both limbs of the bifurcation stenosis, with 1.5-mm and 2.0-mm burrs placed over a type C guidewire and through a 9 Fr left Judkins guiding catheter. After rotational atherectomy, angioplasty was performed on both vessel limbs with a 3.0-mm SciMed NC Bandit balloon catheter (Maple Grove, MN). A 3.0-mm Palmaz-Schatz stent (Johnson and Johnson International Systems, Warren, NJ)was placed in the inferior branch from its origin and dilated to high pressures. A 3.0-mm Gianturco-Rubin stent (Cook, Inc., Bloomington, IN) was placed across this stent into the anterior branch. Following postdilation, an excellent angiographic appearance was achieved (Fig. 10.18B). Heparin was

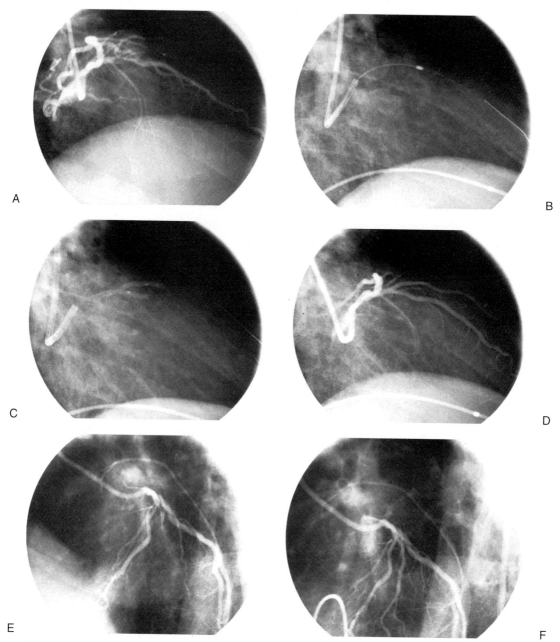

FIG. 10.17. Representative images from case 1. **A:** Baseline right anterior oblique angiographic views of a very complex heavily calcified stenosis involving the left anterior descending artery and first diagonal branch. The first diagonal branch became occluded during the 5-day interval between presentation and rotational atherectomy, but the patient was asymptomatic. **B:** Rotational atherectomy with 1.50-mm and 1.75-mm burrs over a type C guidewire was performed on the left anterior descending artery and diagonal branch, in that order. **C:** A second guidewire (0.012-mm USCI Silk) was then passed alongside and both limbs dilated with 3.0-mm balloon catheters (Medtronic Evergreen) in a "Y" configuration. **D:** The angiographic result after intervention was excellent. **E:** Left anterior oblique view of bifurcation stenosis before intervention. **F:** Left anterior oblique view after rotational atherectomy and percutaneous transluminal coronary angioplasty. (From ref. 19 with permission by Elsevier Science Ireland.)

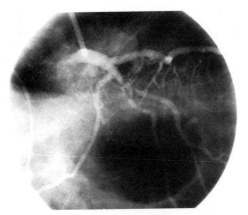
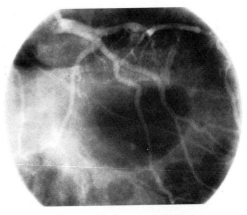

A   B

FIG. 10.18. Representative right anterior oblique angiographic images from case 2. **A:** Severe stenosis involving a large intermediate artery and extending into two large marginal branches. **B:** Rotational atherectomy into both limbs was performed with 1.75-mm and 2.00-mm burrs. After angioplasty with a 3.0-mm balloon, a 3.0-mm Palmaz-Schatz stent was placed in the inferior branch from its origin and a 3.0-mm Gianturco-Rubin stent was placed in the anterior branch, straddling the origin of the inferior branch. An excellent angiographic appearance was achieved. (From ref. 19 with permission by Elsevier Science Ireland.)

administered intravenously and ticlopidine was given orally; abciximab was not administered.

DISCUSSION

Rotational atherectomy has been successfully used to approach lesions that otherwise are associated with unacceptable success or complication rates, such as heavily calcified, ostial, diffuse, and eccentric lesions (22,23). We have found rotational atherectomy to be particularly useful as an initial step in the treatment of complex coronary bifurcation lesions. In our experience, the approach described above has produced acceptable acute procedural results with a relatively low complication rate. Because of the technical success achieved with rotational atherectomy for true bifurcation lesions, it has become an increasingly preferred approach to bifurcation lesions in our laboratory. Potential roles for rotational atherectomy in bifurcation lesions include definitive revascularization of both branches, creation of channels to safely allow balloon angioplasty or stent deployment, and preservation of a side branch. One of the major problems with balloon angioplasty or stenting of bifurcation lesions is shifting of the plaque, with compromise of the contralateral

limb. Often, prolonged double-balloon inflations are required, and they frequently do not yield ideal results. Using the technique described, we observed this complication in only one of 30 bifurcation limbs.

We do not consider any particular caliber of side branch to represent a contraindication to this technique. As long as side branches can be accessed percutaneously, bifurcation rotational atherectomy may be a good therapeutic alternative for branches from 2.0 mm (approachable with 1.25- and 1.50-mm burrs) to 3.5-mm vessels or larger (approachable with 2.0- to 2.5-mm burrs). Because side branch compromise is seen so infrequently after rotational atherectomy, we do not deem "protection" of branches with a second guide wire or predilatation of side branches necessary. Indeed, we try to avoid performing balloon angioplasty before rotational atherectomy, lest the predilatation cause dissection. The low frequency of side branch occlusion is likely related to the debulking nature of rotational atherectomy (as opposed to the plaque shifting or cracking, as may occur with balloon angioplasty). Other approaches to bifurcation lesions continue to evolve and have been the topic of recent reports (21). Stenting (24,25), whether in "T" (26), "Y" (27), or trouser-like configurations (28), holds promise but is still technically challenging, and no widely applicable solution has emerged (25,29,30). True bifurcation stents are under development and will enhance the therapeutic armamentarium of interventional cardiologists with an interest in the treatment of bifurcation lesions.

REFERENCES

1. Meier B, Gruentzig AR, Hollman J, Ischinger T, Bradford JM. Does length or eccentricity of coronary stenoses influence the outcome of transluminal dilatation? *Circulation* 1983;67:497–499.
2. Vetrovec GW, Cowley MJ, Wolfgang TC, Ducey KC. Effects of percutaneous transluminal coronary angioplasty on lesion-associated branches. *Am Heart J* 1985; 109:921–925.
3. Pinkerton CA, Slack JD. Complex coronary angioplasty: a technique for dilatation of bifurcation stenoses. *Angiology* 1985;36:543–548.
4. Zack PM, Ischinger T. Experience with a technique for coronary angioplasty of bifurcational lesions. *Cathet Cardiovasc Diagn* 1984;10:433–443.
5. McAuley BJ, Sheehan DJ, Simpson JB. Coronary angioplasty of stenoses at major bifurcations: simultaneous use of multiple guidewires and dilatation catheters. *Circulation* 1984;70[Suppl 2]:108(abst).
6. Nakhjavan FK, Wertheimer JH, Goldman A. "Crossing balloons:" a new technique for complex angioplasty. *J Am Coll Cardiol* 1986;8:980–981.
7. Laham RJ, Carrozza JP, Baim DS. Treatment of unprotected left main stenoses with Palmaz-Schatz stenting. *Cathet Cardiovasc Diagn* 1996;37:77–80.
8. Oesterle SN, McAuley BJ, Buchbinder M, Simpson JB. Angioplasty at coronary bifurcations: single-guide, two-wire technique. *Cathet Cardiovasc Diagn* 1986;12: 57–63.
9. O'Keefe JH Jr, Holmes DR Jr, Reeder GS, Bresnahan DR. A new approach for dilation of bifurcation stenoses: the dual probe technique. *Mayo Clin Proc* 1989;64: 277–281.
10. Myler RK, McConahay DR, Stertzer SH et al. Coronary bifurcation stenoses: the "kissing" balloon probe technique via a single guiding catheter. *Cathet Cardiovasc Diagn* 1989;16:267–278.
11. Weinstein JS, Baim DS, Sipperly ME, McCabe CH, Lorell BH. Salvage of branch vessels during bifurcation lesion angioplasty: acute and long-term follow-up. *Cathet Cardiovasc Diagn* 1991;22:1–6.
12. Meier B, Gruentzig AR, King SB III et al. Risk of side branch occlusion during coronary angioplasty. *Am J Cardiol* 1984;53:10–14.
13. Leya FS, Lewis BE, Sumida CW et al. Modified "kissing" atherectomy procedure with dependable protection of side branches by two-wire technique. *Cathet Cardiovasc Diagn* 1992;27:155–161.
14. Mansour M, Fishman RF, Kuntz RE et al. Feasibility of directional atherectomy for the treatment of bifurcation lesions. *Coronary Artery Dis* 1992;3:761–765.
15. Lewis BE, Leya FS, Johnson SA et al. Acute procedural results in the treatment of 30 coronary artery bifurcation lesions with a double-wire atherectomy technique for side-branch protection. *Am Heart J* 1994;127:1600–1607.
16. Gambhir DS, Petkar S, Trehan V et al. Directional atherectomy for the dilatation of bifurcation stenoses in the coronary arteries. *Indian Heart J* 1995;47:115–119.
17. Brener SJ, Leya FS, Apperson-Hansen C et al. A comparison of debulking versus dilatation of bifurcation coronary arterial narrowings (from the CAVEAT I Trial). *Am J Cardiol* 1996;78:1039–1041.
18. Ghazzal ZMB, Shefer A, Litvack F et al. The new directional laser catheter (DLC): early results from a multicenter experience. *Circulation* 1992;86[Suppl 1]: 654(abst).
19. Rihal CS, Garratt KN, Holmes DR Jr. Rotational atherectomy for bifurcation lesions of the coronary circulation: technique and initial experience. *Int J Cardiol* 1998;65:1–9.
20. Dauerman HL, Higgins PJ, Sparano AM et al. Mechanical debulking versus balloon angioplasty for the treatment of true bifurcation lesions. *J Am Coll Cardiol* 1998; 32:1845–1852.
21. Baim DS. Is bifurcation stenting the answer? (editorial comment). *Cathet Cardiovasc Diagn* 1996;37:314–316.
22. Bertrand ME, Bauters C, Lablanche J-M. Percutaneous coronary rotational angioplasty with the Rotablator. In: Topol EJ, ed. *Textbook of interventional cardiology.* (vol. 1), 2nd ed. Philadelphia: WB Saunders, 1994: 659–667.
23. Freed M, O'Neill WW. Approach to the high risk patient. In: Roubin GS et al., eds. *Interventional cardiovascular medicine: principles and practice.* New York: Churchill Livingstone, 1994:293–320.
24. Nakamura S, Hall P, Maiello L, Colombo A. Techniques for Palmaz-Schatz stent deployment in lesions with a large side branch. *Cathet Cardiovasc Diagn* 1995;34: 353–361.
25. Colombo A, Gaglione A, Nakamura S, Finci L. "Kissing" stents for bifurcational coronary lesion. *Cathet Cardiovasc Diagn* 1993;30:327–330.
26. Carrie D, Karouny E, Chouairi S, Puel J. "T"-shaped stent placement: a technique for the treatment of dissected bifurcation lesions. *Cathet Cardiovasc Diagn* 1996;37:311–313.
27. Fort S, Lazzam C, Schwartz L. Coronary "Y" stenting: a technique for angioplasty of bifurcation stenoses. *Can J Cardiol* 1996;12:678–682.
28. Khoja A, Ozbek C, Bay W, Heisel A. Trouser-like stenting: a new technique for bifurcation lesions. *Cathet Cardiovasc Diagn* 1997;41:192–196.
29. Teirstein PS. "Kissing" Palmaz-Schatz stents for coronary bifurcation stenoses. *Cathet Cardiovasc Diagn* 1996;37:307–310.
30. Fischman DL, Savage MP, Leon MB et al. Fate of lesion-related side branches after coronary artery stenting. *J Am Coll Cardiol* 1993;22:1641–1646.

11

The Lesion with Thrombus

A. An Approach to the Lesion with Intracoronary Thrombus

Daniel J. Tiede and Guy S. Reeder

Cardiovascular Division, Mayo Clinic, Rochester, Minnesota 55905

The importance and frequency of coronary arterial thrombus has been well documented in the pathophysiology of the acute ischemic syndromes of acute myocardial infarction (MI) and unstable angina. Angioscopy has documented thrombus in the vast majority of those studied. Angiography, although clearly not as sensitive, may often identify coronary thrombus.

There are a variety of settings in which the thrombus occurs: (a) In patients with unstable angina, even if it is not evident at angiography, thrombus is usually present; (b) during acute MI, thrombus is almost universal and is recognized by persistent staining of contrast in a totally occluded vessel; (c) in some patients, angiographically visible thrombus is seen at or just distal to a high-grade stenosis (this is usually in the setting of unstable angina and represents a significant thrombus burden); (d) in patients with acute occlusion secondary to a catheterization procedure, thrombus and dissection often coexist; or (e) in some patients, there is extensive thrombus formation throughout a large segment of the vessel. This is most commonly the right coronary artery or a vein graft. Depending on the clinical setting in which the thrombus occurs and the specific angiographic features, the treatment strategy will vary.

The importance of coronary arterial thrombus for the interventional cardiologist is well recognized. An initial series in 1985 by Mabin et al.

evaluated the outcome of percutaneous transluminal coronary angioplasty (PTCA) in 238 patients. Patients with chronic occlusion and those receiving thrombolytic therapy were excluded from this analysis. The angiograms were reviewed for the presence of predilatation thrombus defined as (a) the presence of an intraluminal filling defect or lucency surrounded by contrast material seen in multiple angiographic views; (b) absence of calcification within the defect, and (c) persistence of contrast within the lumen. (Fig. 11.1). Using these criteria, there were 15 patients (6%) with intracoronary thrombus prior to PTCA. The patients with thrombus had a higher incidence of prior infarction, including within the preceding month, although none of them had an evolving acute infarction. There was a striking difference in outcome. Despite treatment with weak antiplatelet agents (dipyridamole 75 to 100 mg tid or qid, and also aspirin), as well as heparin 5,000 to 10,000 units at the time of the procedure, complete occlusion requiring emergency coronary bypass graft surgery occurred during or immediately after PTCA in 11 (73%) of the 15 patients with intracoronary thrombus and in only 18 (8%) of the patients without angiographic evidence of coronary thrombus. The occlusion was at or immediately adjacent to the stenosis/thrombus in all patients, and dissection was not present angiographically. In patients without thrombus, typically if occlu-

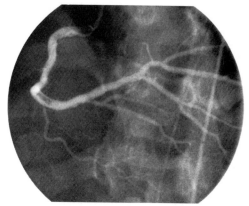

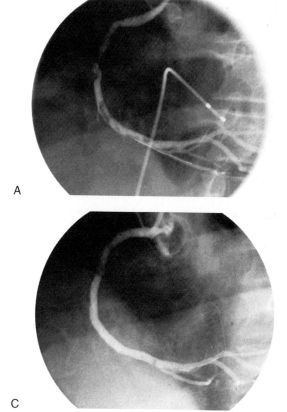

A

B

C

FIG. 11.1. A: Acute inferior wall myocardial infarction. Right coronary artery injection following angioplasty of proximal total occlusion. There are multiple and extensive filling defects in the mid and distal portions of the artery with TIMI-II flow. **B:** After treatment with AngioJet and Reopro infusion, there is still residual thrombus in the distal portion of the artery and the origin of the posterior descending branch. **C:** After stenting of the thrombus-containing segment in the distal portion of the artery, small filling defects are still seen distally. TIMI-III flow is now present.

sion occurred, it was the result of dissection. The authors concluded that they had identified a "small but important subset of patients" at increased risk. Given the ever-increasing emphasis on early dilatation in these patients, the authors had indeed identified a high-risk group of patients. It has evolved, however, into a large and not a small group.

Since that time, there have been multiple other series. A follow-up study by Sugrue et al., in a subsequent group of 297 consecutive patients without acute MI, documented improvement in outcome. However, 24% of patients with angiographic thrombus still had complete occlusion either during or immediately after the procedure, compared with a 13% incidence of complete occlusion in patients without preexisting thrombus. Similar trends have been seen in other series, and the preintervention identification of coronary thrombus continues to define a group of patients at increased risk for acute closure.

Even when thrombus is not visible angiographically, but is present by inference, as in patients with very unstable angina, acute complication rates are increased compared with those of patients with stable angina. In these patients, angiography may not be sensitive enough to identify thrombus. This insensitivity has been previously well described in patients with unstable angina. In the setting of unstable angina, dilation success rates are usually slightly lower than in patients with stable angina. In this setting, failure of dilatation usually results in complications; for example, complete occlusion, compared with failure of dilatation in a stable patient population in whom the failure may be uncomplicated.

Thrombus continues to be a risk factor for adverse events for interventional procedures. Reeder et al. assessed the continued effect over a 7-year period, from 1984 to 1991. The study population included patients undergoing single-

TABLE 11.1. *Approach to the patient with intracoronary thrombus*

- Maximize antiplatelet treatment.
- Use weight-adjusted heparin.
- Optimize PTCA results.
- Utilize new devices and techniques.

lesion dilatation for the first time during those 7 years. Only patients being treated with conventional PTCA were studied. The primary analysis was focused on assessing whether preexisting coronary thrombus remained an independent predictor for angioplasty failure. Of 2,699 patients meeting the study criteria, 1,121 (42%) had angiographic evidence of intracoronary thrombus. Using multivariate analysis, the only factors associated with procedural failure were thrombus, history of congestive heart failure, and multivessel disease. The study was arbitrarily divided into three periods to assess the importance of thrombus over time. Multivariate analysis documented that the risk of angioplasty failure in the setting of coronary arterial thrombus was unchanged from 1984 to 1991.

Given the continued problem with treatment of patients with coronary arterial thrombus, there has been substantial interest in optimizing the results of interventional procedures. There are several tiers of approaches (Table 11.1). Most of these approaches have not been rigorously tested in scientifically controlled trials.

OPTIMIZE ANTIPLATELET AGENTS AND ANTICOAGULATION

Platelet activation and aggregation play a primary role in the formation of the platelet-rich (white) thrombus implicated as the cause of acute coronary syndromes. As this has become increasingly evident, antiplatelet therapy has assumed the forefront in the treatment of these syndromes. Aspirin was originally studied as an agent to decrease restenosis rates; although it was negative in this regard, pretreatment with aspirin reduced acute closure in the catheterization laboratory. Clopidogrel and ticlopidine inhibit ADP-induced platelet inhibition and have been shown to be effective inhibitors of white

thrombus formation. As early as possible prior to dilatation, aspirin 324 mg, well chewed, and clopidogrel 300 mg or ticlopidine 500 mg should be administered. Aspirin should be continued indefinitely. Clopidogrel or ticlopidine should be continued for 14 days. With the latter drug, a remote possibility exists for the development of severe neutropenia. In our experience, neutropenia does not occur with this short duration of use. If longer treatment periods are required, however, white cell counts need to be measured periodically.

The final common pathway of platelet aggregation and thrombus formation occurs via the glycoprotein IIb/IIIa platelet receptor. The EPIC trial was the first to demonstrate that glycoprotein IIb/IIIa receptor inhibition with abciximab concurrently with heparin prior to coronary intervention reduces thrombotic adverse outcomes of high-risk PTCA, both in the short and long terms. In this and other trials, pretreatment of the thrombotic lesion with abciximab bolus and infusion was performed. In many centers, however, it is common practice to administer this agent following the occurrence of a thrombotic complication. Although there are anecdotal data that such "rescue" use of abciximab is effective, no published randomized trials are available. Ongoing trials are evaluating other intravenous and oral specific and nonspecific IIb/IIIa inhibitors.

Heparin has traditionally been an integral part of the antithrombotic regimen used periintervention. Heparin, in conjunction with the cofactor antithrombin III, functions by inactivating activated factor X of the coagulation cascade, and at higher doses can inhibit thrombin's conversion of fibrinogen to fibrin. It also acts to inhibit clot stabilization by inhibiting fibrin cross-linking. Importantly, it does not have any fibrinolytic effects and is only effective on free thrombin, not on thrombin within established clot. In the EPILOG trial, those patients randomized to abciximab and the lowest heparin dose did the best, both in terms of bleeding and with recurrent major adverse cardiac events. Further large trials will be required to assess whether further heparin dose reduction or its elimination altogether will be safe and effective.

To minimize bleeding risk, a weight-adjusted heparin dosing regimen is preferred, as outlined in the EPILOG trial. In the absence of abciximab, a heparin 100 units per kilogram bolus is given. The dose is further titrated to keep the activated clotting time (ACT) to 300 to 350 seconds. Lower heparin doses are used with concurrent abciximab to reduce the risk of bleeding: a 70 U per kilogram bolus titrated to keep the ACT at 200 to 250 seconds. Continuous heparin infusions are generally not used. However, in the setting of severe intracoronary thrombus, prolonged heparin treatment is occasionally desired. A weight-adjusted infusion rate is then employed, usually beginning 4 to 6 hours following sheath removal. Heparin 10 U per kilogram per hour is given in the absence of abciximab, while heparin 7 U per kilogram per hour is given in the setting of concurrent abciximab.

Limited data are available supporting the use of intracoronary heparin given via an infusion catheter directly into the thrombus. As noted, heparin's effect is only on free fibrin and not on established thrombus. Therefore, it may prevent further thrombus growth, but it is unlikely to have a significant effect on thrombolysis.

Increasing interest is emerging in the specific thrombin inhibitors and low-molecular-weight heparins (LMWHs). Specific antithrombins, such as hirudin and hirulog, are in clinical evaluation. These are direct thrombin inhibitors and may be more effective on organized thrombus, in contrast to heparin. Hirudin is a potent, selective, irreversible, and direct thrombin inhibitor, which requires no cofactor. In a pilot study of patients with unstable angina, there was increased inhibition of thrombin activation and more evidence of culprit-vessel clot lysis with hirudin than with heparin. This effect must be carefully monitored; in the GUSTO IIa trial of recombinant hirudin versus heparin for acute coronary syndromes, excessive hemorrhagic stroke with hirudin (1.5%) versus heparin (0.8%) ($p = .11$) occurred. In patients receiving thrombolytic therapy plus hirudin, the incidence of hemorrhagic stroke was highest at 3.6%. A similar increase in hemorrhagic stroke was also seen in TIMI-9a. Both of these studies stopped prematurely and then resumed using a lower

dose of hirudin and heparin. The subsequent doses used have been found to be safe. Very careful titration of doses may be required to decrease the incidence of bleeding. The multicenter international, randomized HELVETICA trial compared two hirudin doses with heparin in a randomized trial of 1,141 patients undergoing PTCA for treatment of unstable angina. In this trial, the event-free survival rate at 7 months was not different between the heparin, the hirudin bolus only, and the hirudin bolus with subcutaneous injection groups (67.3% vs. 63.5% vs. 68.0%, respectively). However, early cardiac events were significantly reduced by hirudin administration with bolus and bolus plus injections, respectively (11.0% vs. 7.9% vs. 5.6%, respectively).

The Organization to Assess Strategies for Ischemic Syndromes (OASIS) trial compared low- and medium-dose hirudin boluses with 72-hour infusion to heparin bolus and infusion in 909 patients with unstable angina or non–ST-segment elevation MI. Significant reduction in cardiovascular death, new MI, or refractory angina was noted in the medium-dose hirudin group, but not in the low-dose group compared with heparin (3.0% vs. 4.4% vs. 6.5%, respectively; $p = .047$) at 7 days. Fewer coronary artery bypass surgeries were required in the medium-dose hirudin group as well. The differences between hirudin and heparin persisted throughout the 180-day follow-up period; however, an increase in ischemic events occurred 24 hours following cessation of the low-dose group and at 5 days in the medium-dose group. Therefore, long-term treatment may be required.

Similarly, the Efficacy and Safety of Subcutaneous Enoxaparin for Non Q wave Coronary Events (ESSENCE) trial showed a significant reduction of the 14- and 30-day incidence of death, MI, and recurrent angina (19.8% vs. 23.3%; $p = .016$) using the LMWH enoxaparin 1 mg per kilogram subcutaneously twice daily versus continuous infusion of unfractionated heparin in 3,171 patients with acute coronary syndromes. Additionally, need for revascularization was reduced at 30 days in the enoxaparin group (27.1% vs. 32.2%). No increased bleeding was found (6.5% vs. 7.0%). A subsequent economic assessment of these patients showed a $1,172 cost saving in the enoxaparin patients. The ongoing TIMI 11B trial will examine the effects of enoxaparin further.

THROMBOLYTIC THERAPY

Given the documented efficacy of thrombolytic therapy for acute myocardial infarction, there has been interest in this approach in patients with unstable angina and coronary arterial thrombus. The results of this approach have been mixed. The largest trial of intracoronary thrombolytic therapy has been the Thrombolysis and Angioplasty in Unstable Angina (TAUSA) trial. A pilot study for this trial had documented that low-dose urokinase reduced angiographic thrombus formation following PTCA for rest ischemia in unstable angina. During the first phase of the full trial, 250,000 U of intracoronary urokinase were administered (150,000 U prior to PTCA and 100,000 U after PTCA) in patients with unstable angina. In the second phase of the study, 500,000 U were used (250,000 U prior to PTCA and 250,000 U after PTCA). The endpoints for this randomized study were angiographic thrombus, acute closure, and in-hospital events of recurrent ischemia, infarction, or coronary bypass graft surgery. In the 469 randomized patients, there was no statistically significant difference in angiographic thrombus between patients treated with placebo and those treated with intracoronary urokinase. In addition, the incidence of acute closure was actually increased at 6.9% in the urokinase group versus 1.7% in the placebo-treated patients. The mechanism of acute closure was thrombotic in 45% and secondary to dissection in 40%.

Based on this randomized trial, routine prophylactic treatment of patients with unstable angina using intracoronary urokinase is probably not indicated. There are still patients with a significant amount of intracoronary thrombus in whom intracoronary lytic therapy may be administered. Typically, urokinase is used, although both r-tissue plasminogen activator (rt-PA) and streptokinase have been administered. For urokinase, typically 500,000 U are adminis-

tered; for rt-PA, 50 mg is used; and for streptokinase, 500,000 U are given. Administering the drug in close proximity to the thrombus with a subselective infusion catheter optimizes the local effect in the segment to be treated.

Rarely in some patients, a more prolonged infusion is administered for 24 to 72 hours. This is typically used in vein grafts with thrombotic occlusion but also may be used in the native coronary artery. For this infusion, urokinase is most commonly used. Multiple side-hole perfusion catheters, currently available, are positioned across the segment with thrombus. Urokinase is then administered by continuous infusion at 50,000 U per hour after an initial bolus. The guiding catheter may be kept in the ostium, particularly if a vein graft is being treated, or may be withdrawn to the descending thoracic aorta. In the former case, urokinase is also administered at 50,000 U per hour through the guiding catheter, or, in the latter case, saline can be used to keep the lumen clear. Guide catheter damping should be particularly avoided if there is a prolonged infusion of the native coronary artery. Nursing care of these patients can be problematic because of the need for continuing infusions and the requirement that the patient be fully immobilized. Vascular access bleeding in our experience is quite common. Following treatment, repeat angiography is required to document the effect.

OPTIMIZE RESULTS OF PTCA

Optimizing the results of PTCA is essential, particularly in high-risk lesions. In patients with a large amount of thrombus (Fig. 11.2), the decision may be made to treat with intravenous abciximab, heparin, clopidogrel, and aspirin and delay intervention. There are limited data to support this, but it does make intuitive sense. Several days, however, may be required, which increases the cost and potential risk of this approach substantially, particularly if the patient requires intensive care unit hospitalization.

At the time of dilatation, matching the balloon size with the artery to be treated is very important. Undersizing and leaving behind a significant residual stenosis may result in acute clo-

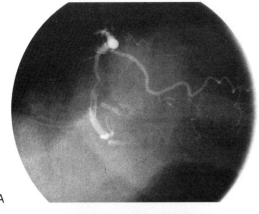

A

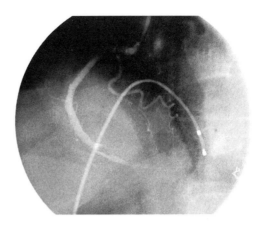

B

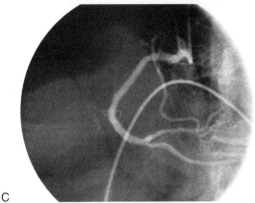

C

FIG. 11.2. A: Acute inferior wall myocardial infarction. Radial artery approach is used because of abdominal aortic occlusion. Extensive thrombus seen in mid right coronary artery with TIMI grade 1 flow. **B:** After administration of Reopro infusion and angioplasty of mid right coronary artery, followed by placement of two stents, there is extensive distal embolization with obstruction of posterior descending and posterolateral branches by a large saddle thrombus. Angioplasty in the region of the thrombus was performed along with continued administration of Reopro, heparin, and intracoronary adenosine and verapamil. **C:** The occluded posterolateral branch was wired, dilated, a dissection noted, and stented. The result demonstrates grade 3 antegrade flow. In all, three stents were placed.

sure. Prolonged inflations, often with perfusion balloons, are used frequently. With prolonged inflations, the initial angiographic result is often improved, although the restenosis rates are typically not affected.

If PTCA alone is desired, an essential part of this strategy is a period of watchful waiting. Typically, we would wait for 10 minutes, sometimes with the dilatation wire across the lesion, but more often after it has been withdrawn. Following this 10 minutes, repeat angiography is performed. If renarrowing has occurred, or if radiolucent filling defects are seen to be accumulating, then repeat dilatation is performed, either for a longer time or sometimes with a slightly larger balloon (either by increasing the pressure in a compliant balloon or changing balloon size). Following repeat dilatation, another 10-minute period of observation is mandated. If the same

sequence of events recurs, the cycle of repeat dilatation can be performed. Abciximab is usually utilized. Alternatively, intracoronary thrombolytic therapy may be administered and may be effective. It is important to treat any outlet stenosis in the vascular bed to enhance vessel flow and decrease stasis. If part of the problem is elastic recoil, decreased flow, and then more thrombus, treatment with another device (e.g., directional coronary atherectomy or intracoronary stenting) may be very helpful.

NEW TECHNOLOGY

Given the problems of conventional dilatation for treatment of thrombus-containing lesions, there has been interest in new technology. Some of these approaches are often useful in selected patients; others have no role to play.

Stents

Previously it was believed that the use of stents was absolutely contraindicated in the presence of thrombus. Early studies showed an increased subacute thrombosis rate following stent implantation in an area of thrombus. However, an increasing body of evidence is becoming available that supports the use of stents in the thrombotic lesion. Better stents, better technique, and better antiplatelet regimens are making stent implantation safer and more effective. The PAMI-Stent Pilot trial involving nine international centers and 312 patients demonstrated a 98% success rate in the 77% patients amenable to stent implantation. Ninety-four percent of these patients were event-free at 30 days, and 83% continued to be event-free at 6 months. Similarly, a randomized trial comparing PTCA versus primary Palmaz-Schatz stent implantation for acute MI was published from the Netherlands. Of the 227 patients enrolled, only 50% were amenable to stent implantation. Ninety-five percent of the stent patients were event-free at 6 months compared with 80% of the PTCA patients ($p < .002$). The MI and TVR rates were significantly reduced in the stent group: 1% versus 7% ($p < .04$) and 4% versus 17% ($p < .002$), respectively. Preliminary data from the 30-day outcome of the EPIStent (Evaluation of IIb/IIIa Platelet Inhibition for Stenting) trial have been presented. This trial enrolled 2,399 patients undergoing elective or urgent revascularization. Unstable coronary syndromes comprised 66% of the population. Acute interventions for MI were excluded. Patients were randomized to stenting plus standard-dose-weight–adjusted heparin versus stenting plus Reopro plus low-dose-weight–adjusted heparin versus PTCA plus Reopro plus low-dose-weight–adjusted heparin. At 30 days, the stent plus Reopro group and the PTCA plus Reopro group showed significant reductions in the primary endpoint of death, MI, and revascularization (5.3%; $p < .001$ vs. 6.9%; $p = .007$ vs. 10.8%). No differences were seen in the major bleeding rates. The ongoing CADILLAC trial involving 90 sites and 2000 patients provides more information on the role of stents and abciximab in acute MI. This is a 2 × 2 factorial design comparing PTCA, PTCA plus abciximab, stent, and stent plus abciximab. Follow-up angiography will be performed in 700 of the patients. Results are expected in 1999. Meanwhile, stenting with abciximab is a rational approach to the lesion with angiographically visible thrombus, and is the most common method employed in our laboratory at present.

Atherectomy

Three types of atherectomy catheters are in use: (a) rotational atherectomy, (b) transluminal extraction catheter (TEC), and (c) directional coronary atherectomy. Rotational atherectomy should not be used in a soft, thrombus-containing lesion. Its mechanism of action is differential ablation of hard fibrous tissue, compared with the more normal elastic arterial wall. The TEC catheter is used infrequently, but may be helpful for treating long thrombotic vein graft lesions. By extracting the thrombus, distal embolization may be decreased. It is most often used in treatment of vein graft disease. Directional coronary atherectomy has been the most commonly used, including in our laboratory. In an initial multicenter report, with thrombus-containing lesions, directional coronary atherectomy resulted in marked improvement in angiographic lumen and a significantly decreased acute closure rate compared with historical cohorts of patients treated with conventional PTCA. In the setting of a large vessel with a bulky lesion and coronary thrombus, we occasionally use directional atherectomy to optimize the initial result and decrease the potential for acute closure.

Laser

At the present time, laser systems for use in the coronary arteries are ablative and designed to treat plaque, not thrombus. The most common systems use an excimer laser with a wavelength of 308 nm. There is a limited amount of information on the use of this laser system in lesions containing thrombus. In the Excimer Laser Coronary Angioplasty Registry (Advanced Interventional Systems, Irvine, CA), 141 lesions with associated thrombus were treated. The success rate in these was 85%; 1.5% of patients developed Q-wave MI, 3.8% required coronary bypass graft surgery, and 4.6% had sustained occlusion. How this would compare with conventional dilatation in a similar subset of patients is not clear. However, there is no particular conceptual reason that excimer laser would be more effective for coronary thrombus.

A second system is the holmium laser angioplasty system (Eclipse Surgical Technologies, Inc., Palo Alto, CA). This is a mid-infrared holmium/YAG laser that can ablate tissue in a blood media by a predominant photothermal effect, compared with excimer laser. The 2-μm wavelength is absorbed by water, both in atherosclerotic plaque and in intracoronary thrombus. This laser may therefore offer some specific advantages in the treatment of thrombus-containing lesions. This laser has been used clinically during acute MI in a small number of cases, as well as in patients with unstable angina, with excellent results. Future randomized trials will be needed to directly compare excimer laser with holmium laser angioplasty.

Rheolytic Thrombectomy (AngioJet)

One of the newest devices to become available in the United States for the removal of intracoronary thrombus is the AngioJet (Possis Medical, Minneapolis, MN). This device functions on the basis of the Venturi effect. As the catheter is slowly advanced, a high-velocity jet of saline is pumped against a dome-shaped cap at the tip of the catheter, which directs a fine spray retrograde and laterally. At the same time, suction is applied through the catheter sheath. This creates a hydrodynamic vortex, which emulsifies fresh thrombus, while the jet creates a Venturi effect, allowing the collection and retrieval of the debris via the vacuum suction. When the AngioJet is used on fresh thrombus, 89% of the thrombus burden can be removed. Firmer, more organized thrombus is more difficult to remove. Histologic studies show minimal endothelial denudation with this device. Approximately 1.8% to 14.0% of the original thrombus volume may embolize distally; however, when this debris was injected into a normal canine renal artery, no adverse effects were noted. In our experience, nearly all patients develop transient heart block, even when the device is used in a nondominant artery. Therefore, it is recommended that a temporary pacemaker be placed in all patients. Because the device is relatively bulky (5 Fr), it may occlude flow in the presence of a significant stenotic lesion. This has led to significant angina and ventricular arrhythmias. Hemolysis is another potential adverse effect. The AngioJet has been approved for use in both native coronary arteries and grafts. The ultimate role of this device in treatment of patients with intracoronary thrombus awaits further study.

SUMMARY

Identification of the importance of coronary arterial thrombus as a marker for an active lesion with the potential for adverse outcome from interventional cardiology procedures has led to continued new approaches to this problem. Selection of the optimal approach involves consideration of clinical circumstances, the location and specific angiographic characteristics of the lesion and the thrombus, and the techniques available. Careful attention to anticoagulation and antiplatelet agents before, during, and after the procedure is essential. New therapeutic drugs, such as potent platelet receptor inhibitors and specific antithrombins, are playing an increasingly important role. Intracoronary thrombolytic therapy may also be used in selected cases, although as routine prophylaxis, it is not indicated. Equally careful attention must be paid to optimizing the result of PTCA. Following treatment, a period of observation to assess the stability of the lesion is mandatory. Stenting may actually improve acute and long-term outcome from intervention in the thrombotic lesion. Newer technology, such as rheolytic thrombectomy, shows the potential to enhance outcome in selected patients.

SUGGESTED READINGS

Ambrose JA, Sharma S, Torro S, et al. Thrombolysis and angioplasty in unstable angina (TAUSA) trial. *Circulation* 1993;88:1113.

Antman EM. Hirudin in acute myocardial infarction: safety report from the Thrombolysis and Thrombin Inhibition in Myocardial Infarction (TIMI) 9A Trial. *Circulation* 1994; 90(4):1624–1630.

Antman EM. TIMI 11B. Enoxaparin versus unfractionated heparin for unstable angina or non-Q wave myocardial infarction: a double-blind, placebo-controlled, parallel-group, multicenter trial. Rationale, study design, and methods. Thrombolysis in myocardial infarction (TIMI) 11B investigators. *Am Heart J* 1998;135: S353–S360.

Bergelson B, Jacobs A, Cupples A, et al. Prediction of risk for hemodynamic compromise during percutaneous transluminal coronary angioplasty. *Am J Cardiol* 1992;70: 1540–1545.

Buchalter M, Seen M, Williams C, Adams R, Reid D. The occurrence of early sudden coronary artery occlusion following angioplasty may be predicted from the clinical characteristics of the patient and their coronary lesion morphology. *Jpn Heart J* 1992;33:295–302.

Cohen M, Demers C, Gurfinkel EP, et al. A comparison of low-molecular-weight heparin with unfractionated heparin for unstable coronary artery disease. Efficacy and Safety of Subcutaneous Enoxaparin in Non-Q-Wave Coronary Events Study Group. *N Engl J Med* 1997;337(7): 447–452.

de Feyter P, van den Brand M, Laarman G, van Domburg R, Serruys P, Suryapranata H. Acute coronary artery occlusion during and after percutaneous transluminal coronary angioplasty. *Circulation* 1991;83:927–936.

de Marchena E, Mallon S, Posada JD, et al. Direct holmium laser-assisted balloon angioplasty in acute myocardial infarction. *Am J Cardiol* 1993;71:1223–1225.

de Marchena E, Mallou S, Topaz O, et al. Unstable angina treated with laser angioplasty. *J Am Coll Cardiol* 1993; 21:196AA.

Detre K, Holmes D Jr, Holubkov R, et al. Incidence and consequences of periprocedural occlusion. *Circulation* 1990;82:739–750.

Ellis S, Roubin G, King S III, et al. Angiographic and clinical predictors of acute closure after native vessel coronary angioplasty. *Circulation* 1988;77:372–379.

The EPIC Investigators. Use of a monoclonal antibody directed against the platelet glycoprotein IIb/IIIa receptor in high-risk coronary angioplasty. *N Engl J Med* 1994; 330:956–961.

The EPILOG Investigators. Effect of the platelet glycoprotein IIb/IIIa receptor inhibitor abciximab with lower heparin dosages on ischemic complications of percutaneous coronary revascularization. *N Engl J Med* 1997;336: 1689–1696.

The Global Use of Strategies to Open Occluded Arteries (GUSTO) IIa Investigators. Randomized trial of intravenous heparin versus recombinant hirudin for acute coronary syndromes. *Circulation* 1994;90:1631–1637.

Harrington RA, Leimberger JD, Serdan L, et al. The ACT index: a method for stratifying likelihood of success and risk of acute complications in coronary intervention. *Circulation* 1993;88:1111.

Hermans W, Foley D, Rensing B, et al. Usefulness of quantitative and qualitative angiographic lesion morphology and clinical characteristics in predicting major adverse cardiac

event during and after native coronary balloon angioplasty. *Am J Cardiol* 1993;72:14–20.

Holmes DR, Klein LW, Lavack F. Lesion morphology and acute outcome after excimer laser angioplasty: a prospective evaluation (*in press*).

Laskey M, Deutsch R, Hirshield J Jr, Kussmaul W, Sarathan E, Laskey W. Influence of heparin therapy or percutaneous transluminal coronary angioplasty outcome in patients with coronary arterial thrombus. *Am J Cardiol* 1990;65: 179–183.

Mabin TA, Holmes DR Jr, Smith HC, et al. Intracoronary thrombus: role in coronary occlusion complicating percutaneous transluminal coronary angioplasty. *J Am Coll Cardiol* 1985;5:198–202.

Maraganore JM, Bourdin P, Jablonski J, Ramachandan KL. Design and characterization of horologes: a novel class of bivalent peptide inhibitors of thrombin. *Biochemistry* 1990;29:7095–7101.

Mark DB, Cowper PA, Berkowitz SD, et al. Economic assessment of low-molecular-weight heparin (enoxaparin) versus unfractionated heparin in acute coronary syndrome patients: results from the ESSENCE randomized trial. Efficacy and Safety of Subcutaneous Enoxaparin in Non-Q-wave Coronary Events [unstable angina or myocardial infarction]. *Circulation* 1998;97(17):1702–1707.

Mooney M, Mochey J, Goldenberg I, Almquist A, Van Tassel F. Percutaneous transluminal coronary angioplasty in the setting of large intracoronary thrombi. *Am J Cardiol* 1990;65:427–431.

Myler R, Shaw R, Stertzer S, et al. Unstable angina and coronary angioplasty. *Circulation* 1990;82:II-88–II-95.

The Organization to Assess Strategies for Ischemic Syndromes (OASIS) Investigators. Comparison of the effects of two doses of recombinant hirudin compared with heparin in patients with acute myocardial ischemia without ST elevation: a pilot study. *Circulation* 1997;96(3):769–777.

Reeder GS, Bryant SC, Suman VJ, Holmes DR. Intracoronary thrombus: still a risk factor for PTCA failure? *Cathet Cardiovasc Diagn* 1995;34:191–195.

Sugrue D, Holmes D Jr, Smith H, et al. Coronary artery thrombus as a risk factor for acute vessel occlusion during percutaneous transluminal coronary angioplasty: improving results. *Br Heart J* 1986;56:62–66.

Surruys PW, Herrman JPR, Simon R, et al. A comparison of hirudin with heparin in the prevention of restenosis after coronary angioplasty. HELVETICA Investigators. *N Engl J Med* 1995;333:757–763.

Topol E. Integration of anticoagulation thrombolysis and coronary angioplasty for unstable angina pectoris. *Am J Cardiol* 1991;68:136B–141B.

Topol EJ, Fuster V, Califf RM, et al. Recombinant hirudin for unstable angina pectoris. A multicenter randomized angiographic trial. *Circulation* 1994;89:1557–1566.

Topol EJ, Leya F, Pinterton CA, et al. (CAVEAT study group). A comparison of directional atherectomy with coronary angioplasty in patients with coronary artery disease. *N Engl J Med* 1993;329:221–227.

Vaikus P, Herrmann H, Laskey W. Management and immediate outcome of patients with intracoronary thrombus during percutaneous transluminal coronary angioplasty. *Am Heart J* 1992;124:1–8.

B. Approach to the Thrombotic Lesion: From Drugs to Devices

Jose A. Silva and Stephen R. Ramee

Cardiac Catheterization Laboratory, Department of Cardiology, Alton Ochsner Medical Institution, New Orleans, Louisiana 70121

Patients with coronary atherosclerosis develop angina pectoris when an atherosclerotic plaque produces hemodynamically significant flow restriction of blood to the myocardium, particularly in circumstances of increased oxygen demand. Some of these individuals may develop sudden and rapid progression of their stable symptoms, a phenomenon that is defined as an "acute coronary syndrome." The pathologic cause of this clinical event is that an atherosclerotic coronary plaque rich in cholesterol, known as a "vulnerable" plaque, suddenly ruptures, leading to the exposure of the highly thrombogenic cholesterol-rich material to the circulating bloodstream (1–4). This induces platelet adhesion and aggregation as well as activation of the coagulation cascade, resulting in thrombus formation. The newly formed thrombus usually sits on the surface of the underlying ruptured or ulcerated plaque. Depending on the size of the thrombus and the intrinsic fibrinolytic system, blood flow may further be impaired and a spectrum of symptoms may ensue, from minimal or no symptoms, to accelerated or unstable angina pectoris, to myocardial infarction (MI), or even sudden death. Although the incidence of complex plaque morphology and coronary thrombi is comparable in native coronary arteries and saphenous vein grafts during acute myocardial ischemia (5), the pathophysiology of acute coronary syndromes in vein grafts appears to be a combination of acute intraluminal obstructive thrombus formation superimposed on a process of chronic thrombosis at the vein surface (6).

The treatment of a coronary or saphenous vein graft stenosis with angiographically evident or suspected thrombus is challenging for the inter-ventionalist, because coronary angioplasty in these circumstances is associated with an increased incidence of procedural complications such as distal embolization, abrupt occlusion, emergent bypass surgery, and death, as well as enhanced late restenosis rate (7–10). In attempting to decrease these complications, strategies aimed at removing thrombus before atherosclerotic plaque intervention have been developed, including pharmacologic and mechanical treatments. In the following discussion, we summarize some of these strategies.

PHARMACOLOGIC APPROACHES

Intracoronary Urokinase Infusion

Chronic Thrombotic Occlusion

Urokinase infusions have been used successfully to recanalize chronic thrombotic occlusion in native coronary arteries and saphenous vein grafts (11,12). In 60 patients with chronically occluded native coronary arteries, urokinase was infused over a mean of 8 hours after failed attempts to recanalize them with standard angioplasty techniques. After urokinase infusion, 53% of the patients were successfully recanalized (11). Similarly, the ROBUST investigators attained successful recanalization in 69% of chronically occluded saphenous vein grafts after a mean infusion dose of 3.7 million units of urokinase over a mean infusion duration of 25.4 hours (12).

Acute Thrombosis

Intracoronary urokinase has been used for thrombus accumulation complicating PTCA

(13,14). In one report (13), urokinase infusion resolved angiographic thrombus in 90% of 48 patients, using a mean dose of 141,000 U during an average period of 34 minutes (90% in native coronary arteries). In contrast, Denardo et al. (15) reported that urokinase infusion in old grafts with angiographic evidence of thrombus undergoing stenting carried an enhanced risk for procedural complications and stent thrombosis.

Although urokinase may have a place in treating angiographic evidence of thrombus, its prophylactic intravenous use in patients with acute coronary ischemia has proved to be deleterious. The TAUSA investigators (16) randomized more than 400 patients with unstable or postinfarction angina to receive intravenous urokinase or placebo. Those that received urokinase had an increased incidence of abrupt occlusion (10.2% vs. 4.3%; $p < .04$), which resulted in an enhanced incidence of the composite of ischemia, MI, or emergent bypass surgery (12.9 vs. 6.3; $p < .02$). Urokinase can also be delivered directly to the thrombus surface, using local infusion catheters or urokinase-coated hydrogel balloons. Although experience is limited, the initial results have been favorable for both devices. Using the Dispatch catheter (Scimed Life Systems, Maple Grove, MN), Glazier et al. (17) showed angiographic resolution of thrombus in both native coronary arteries and saphenous vein grafts. Similarly, the urokinase-coated hydrogel balloon has been shown to inhibit platelet deposition and to cause thrombus lysis in the animal model or thrombus resolution and reversal of abrupt occlusion without evidence of angiographic distal embolization in patients with intracoronary thrombus (18,19). The urokinase-coated hydrogel balloon consists of a standard polyethylene balloon angioplasty catheter covered with a hydrogel compound (Hydro Plus, Mansfield/Boston Scientific Corp). The hydrogel coating consists of a latticework of polyacrylic acid chains that are adhered to the balloon surface. When the hydrogel contacts an aqueous environment, it absorbs water and any agents (urokinase) dissolved in the water.

Platelet Glycoprotein IIb/IIIa Inhibitors

In contrast to the mixed results obtained with the use of intracoronary thrombolytics, the new glycoprotein IIb/IIIa platelet-receptor inhibitors have shown that, when used in conjunction with balloon angioplasty in patients with acute coronary ischemia or MI, they can significantly decrease the procedural complications and the long-term outcome. Two large prospective, randomized trials using abciximab showed a 35% to 50% reduction in the composite of death, MI, and need for target-vessel revascularization at 30 days (20,21). Two prospective, randomized trials using tirofiban showed significant reduction of the composite of death or MI in patients with unstable angina and non–Q wave (22,23). Similarly, the EPILOG investigators demonstrated the favorable effects of abciximab in clinical outcomes in unplanned coronary stenting (24). The mechanism by which these IIb/IIIa platelet-receptor inhibitors "passivate" the complex, thrombus-laden, coronary plaque remains unclear; however, there is some evidence showing partial angiographic resolution of thrombus in patients with acute coronary ischemia (25) or as a complication of coronary angioplasty when these agents are given systemically (26) or even angioscopic disappearance of thrombus when they are locally delivered (27).

Summary

The routine use of intracoronary thrombolytics as prophylactic for thrombus formation in patients with acute coronary ischemia is not indicated. Thrombolytic agents may cause vessel wall hematoma (28) or enhance platelet aggregation (29), leading to deleterious consequences such as abrupt occlusion and recurrence of ischemia, as shown by the TAUSA investigators (16). Intracoronary thrombolysis may be useful as adjunctive treatment prior to attempted percutaneous recanalization of total chronic thrombotic occlusions in native coronary arteries and saphenous vein grafts and in acute thrombosis complicating angioplasty in native coronary arteries. In saphenous vein grafts, especially degenerated grafts, thrombolysis may lead to distal embolization and should be used with extreme caution. The group of platelet glycoprotein IIb/IIIa inhibitors has been shown to significantly decrease the procedural complications after catheter-based revascularization procedures in acute coronary syndromes with angiographically evident or suspected thrombus (20–26). Based on these results, the use of platelet IIb/IIIa inhibitors may be justified in patients with acute coronary ischemia and angiographically suspected thrombus, or in patients with a large thrombus burden as complementary treatment to thrombus-debulking devices.

MECHANICAL APPROACHES

Mechanical intervention in the treatment of thrombus-containing coronary lesions includes mechanical compression with balloon angioplasty or stenting, removal with atherectomy devices, thromboaspiration with the Possis AngioJet and the hydrolyser, and lysis with the ultrasound thrombolysis device.

PTCA and Stenting

Coronary angioplasty of thrombus-containing lesions is considered a high-risk procedure, because it increases procedural complications such as abrupt occlusion, distal embolization, no reflow, and need for emergent revascularization procedures. A study from our institution (7), using coronary angioscopy, found that the presence of thrombus increased the in-hospital composite endpoint of death, MI, or emergent bypass surgery, when compared with target lesions without angioscopic thrombus (14% vs. 2%; $p = .03$). These finding have been confirmed by Waxman et al. (8), also using coronary angioscopy. Furthermore, the presence of thrombus also appears to increase the late restenosis rate (9,10). Consequently, the interventionalist should be prepared to deal with these complications when performing angioplasty in thrombus-laden lesions. As mentioned previously, the group of platelet glycoprotein IIb/IIIa inhibitors appears to significantly decrease these procedural complications and should be considered under these circumstances.

Although the presence of thrombus was considered a contraindication for coronary stenting, particularly in the setting of acute MI, the archetype of the thrombus-containing lesions, experience has shown that when they are optimally deployed, with apposition of the stent struts against the vessel wall and adequate antiplatelet agents, stenting is safe, can be accomplished with a high technical success, and appears to decrease the in-hospital ischemic complication and late restenosis rates (30,31). However, when stenting is performed as a "bailout," the incidence of stent thrombosis is not negligible. Pooled data from 12 studies and 1,150 patients of bail-out stenting in acute MI indicated an incidence of stent thrombosis of 3.4% (32). Similarly, in some trials of stenting in acute MI, patients were excluded when the thrombus burden was considerable (30). As described below, a strategy of thrombus debulking may decrease the incidence of complications in these circumstances.

Atherectomy

Directional Atherectomy

Initial reports of thrombus-containing lesions showed improved procedural success and fewer complication rates of directional coronary atherectomy (DCA) in lesions containing thrombus than in those without thrombus (33). Likewise, some anecdotal reports and small series have shown acceptable results in using DCA in acute MI (34,35). Others, however, have not confirmed these results and have found an increased complication rate when using this device in thrombus-containing lesions (36).

Transluminal Extraction Atherectomy

Removal of thrombus can be accomplished with the transluminal extraction catheter (TEC) device (37). The TEC device excises atherosclerotic plaque and coronary thrombi while extracting the debris by continuous vacuum suction (38). It has been used to treat degenerative thrombus-containing native coronary arteries and saphenous vein grafts (39,40); nevertheless, distal embolization may occur in 12% (39), and severe dissection leading to abrupt occlusion in 11.5% (40). The TEC device does not have any beneficial effect on restenosis, but appears to be of utility as an adjunct to stenting in degenerated and/or thrombotic saphenous vein grafts (41). Also, in one prospective study using this device in 100 patients with acute MI, TIMI 3 coronary flow was obtained in 60% after the use of TEC and in 85% after the use of definitive treatment, with an incidence of distal embolization and abrupt closure of 12% (42).

Mechanical Thrombectomy

Possis AngioJet Catheter

Rheolytic thrombectomy with the AngioJet (Possis Medical, Minneapolis, MN) is a very effective device for removing thrombus by applying the Venturi-Bernoulli vacuum principle. The device is a 5 Fr double-lumen, very flexible catheter that utilizes a 0.014- to 0.018-in. guidewire. Three high-speed saline jets create a low-pressure region at the tip (about -760 mmHg), which acts to pull the thrombus and propel it from the vessel. When we approach a thrombotic filling defect, the AngioJet device is advanced distally and then activated and slowly withdrawn at approximately 0.5 to 1 mm per second. The AngioJet has been shown to be an "assay" for thrombus. Repeat passes are performed with angiography after each pass, until there is no further improvement in the angiographic appearance of the thrombotic lesion (three to five passes on average). Definitive treatment (usually stenting) is then performed, because the majority of the thrombus has been removed. The device

has proved very effective in thrombus-containing lesions in the peripheral and coronary circulation. In the VeGAS I Pilot study (43) the device was tested in 90 patients (91 lesions) with acute coronary ischemia and angiographic evidence of thrombus in native coronary arteries (43%) and saphenous vein grafts (57%) (Fig. 11.3). The AngioJet was successfully delivered in all 91 lesions. Thrombus burden decreased from 81.8 ± 92.8 mm^2 at baseline to 21.4 ± 36.2 mm^2 after rheolytic thrombectomy and to 11.4 ± 37 mm^2 after final treatment ($p < .001$). Procedural success (TIMI 3 flow after final treatment and residual diameter stenosis <50%) was obtained in 87% and clinical success (procedural success and no death, Q-wave MI or emergent bypass surgery during the index hospitalization) in 82%. Distal embolization occurred in 3.3% of the vessels. In the VeGAS-2 trial (44), 346 patients (54% of the cases involved a saphenous vein graft) with angiographically visible thrombus were randomized to receive prolonged urokinase infusion versus a strategy of thrombus aspiration with the Possis AngioJet device. The definitions and endpoints were similar to those in the VeGAS-1 Pilot study. Procedural success was 86% in the AngioJet group and 72.7% in the urokinase group ($p < .05$). Device success was also higher in the AngioJet group (87.4% vs. 75.8%, $p < .05$). Urokinase was associated

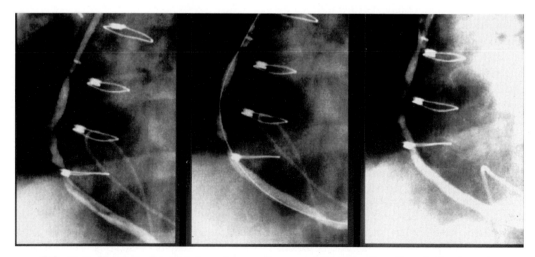

FIG. 11.3. Rheolytic thrombectomy in a saphenous vein graft with a thrombotic stenosis.

with significantly higher in-hospital adverse cardiac events (32.5% vs. 13.9%), bleeding complications (11.8% vs. 5.0%), and vascular complications (17.8% vs. 4.4%). The Possis AngioJet catheter has also been tested in 115 patients with acute MI (13% with cardiogenic shock) and angiographic evidence of large thrombus burden (45) (Fig. 11.4). The device was successfully delivered in all lesions. TIMI 3 coronary flow was present in 25% of the patients at baseline. After rheolytic thrombectomy, TIMI 3 coronary flow was present in 74% of the patients, and after definitive treatment in 89% of the patients ($p < .001$). Thrombus burden also decreased significantly, from 63.1 ± 73.3 mm^2 at baseline to 20.3 ± 34.8 mm^2 after rheolytic thrombectomy ($p < .001$). Due to the excellent angiographic resolution of thrombus, 61% of our patients received coronary stents without complications or stent thrombosis. Distal embolization occurred in 12% of the patients. Nine patients died in the hospital (8%), and one patient suffered a stroke (1%), but none required emergent bypass surgery. At 1-month follow-up, there were no additional deaths, strokes, or need for bypass surgery. MI recurred in 4% of the patients (3% Q-wave MI and 1% non–Q-wave MI). Repeat target-vessel PTCA occurred in 3% of the patients. The 1-month freedom from death or a major adverse cardiovascular event was 88%.

The Cordis Hydrolyser

A new investigational device that is available in Europe is the thrombosuction Cordis Hydrolyser catheter, which has been tested both in the peripheral and coronary circulation (46,47). It applies the Venturi-Bernoulli vacuum principle, similar to the AngioJet system, although the pressure generated is lower than the one generated by the Possis AngioJet. The limited initial experience with this device appears promising.

Ultrasound Thrombolysis

The ultrasound thrombolysis device (Acolysis System, Angiosonics, Morrisville, NC) applies low-frequency ultrasound for rapid mechanical thrombolysis (low-frequency ultrasonic energy disunites the covalent fibrin bonds). Initial experience showed that it is capable of disrupting atherosclerotic plaques and thrombi *in vitro* and recanalizing arteries *in vivo*. The results of the initial experience in treating 15 patients with acute anterior MI have been reported, showing successful TIMI 3 reperfusion in 87% of the patients (device success) with a very low in-hospital complication rate (48) and a low 6-month recurrence of MI or restenosis (49). This device is currently under investigation in the United States in a prospective multicenter trial. The Acolysis during Treatment of Lesions Affecting Saphenous Vein Bypass Grafts (ATLAS) study is a prospective study that will randomize 540 patients with thrombotic stenosis or occlusion in saphenous vein grafts to ultrasound thrombolysis (Acolysis) or the platelet IIb/IIIa inhibitor abciximab in 25 US and Canadian sites. The endpoints are cardiac death, Q-wave MI, emergent bypass surgery, repeat target-vessel revascularization, and disabling stroke. The results will be interesting because, for the first time, a mechanical treatment for thrombus-containing lesions will be tested against a IIb/IIIa platelet inhibitor, a group of drugs known to passivate complex coronary plaques by not well understood mechanisms.

Distal Protection Devices and Covered Stents

Distal embolization is a common occurrence when treating thrombus-containing lesions, particularly in the presence of large thrombus, and/or when intervening in degenerated saphenous vein grafts. The consequences of distal embolization include "no reflow" and periprocedural MI (7,8,39,42,45).

Distal Protection Devices

The Percusurge Guardwire is a latex balloon on a wire, which allows distal occlusion and aspiration of thrombotic and nonthrombotic debris during saphenous vein graft intervention. In a preliminary report, Oesterle et al. (50) tested this device in native porcine coronary arteries. Occlusion times ranged from 2 to 4 minutes in eight

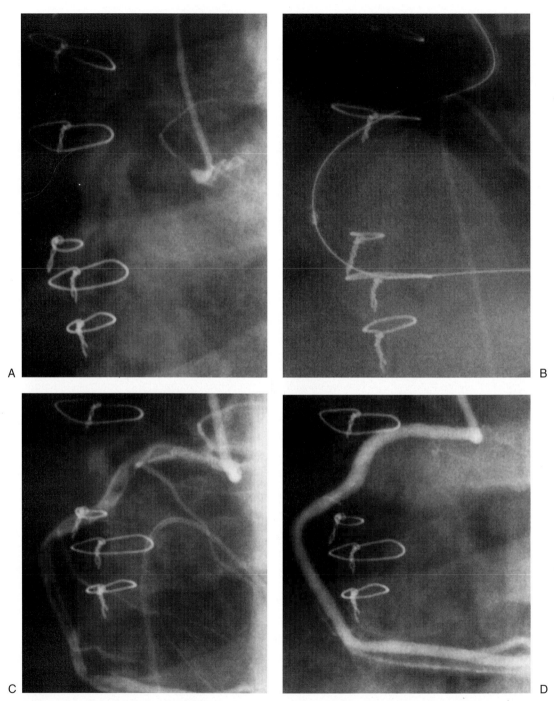

FIG. 11.4. A: Thrombotic occlusion at the origin of the right coronary artery in a patient with acute inferior myocardial infarction. **B:** Possis AngioJet over a guidewire after crossing the thrombotic occlusion. **C:** Angiogram after one pass with the Possis AngioJet, showing still significant amount of thrombus. **D:** Final angiogram with complete resolution of thrombus after several passes with the Possis AngioJet.

animals. The investigators reported no complications, and the histologic analysis showed findings similar to those seen after standard angioplasty. In another preliminary clinical study (51), the Percusurge emboli-containment system was tested in ten patients with degenerated grafts (graft age 10 ± 4 years) undergoing saphenous vein graft intervention. Two of the grafts had a large angiographic thrombus burden and TIMI coronary flow ≤2 was present in five grafts. All the grafts received a stent, and TIMI 3 coronary flow was attained in every case. CK-MB remained within normal limits in nine of ten cases.

Larger studies are needed to assess the efficacy and safety of these kinds of devices.

Covered Stents

A strategy utilizing covered stents, which exclude degenerated or thrombotic material from the vessel lumen, may lead to decreased distal embolization, as recently reported (52–54). Stents may be covered with prosthetic materials (55) or autologous vein or arterial grafts (56,57). A theoretical advantage of autologous tissue over prosthetic material is a potentially decreased incidence of stent thrombosis. Stefanadis et al. (58) reported 100% procedural success and no complications in 13 patients who received autologous vein graft-coated stents in native coronary arteries and saphenous vein grafts. At a mean follow-up of 4.2 ± 1.5 months, all patients were asymptomatic. The same investigators (54) used similar graft-coated stents for treating thrombus-containing coronary lesions in ten patients with acute MI (mean time to treatment of 151 ± 53 minutes). All patients had TIMI 0–1 coronary flow on baseline angiography. TIMI 3 coronary flow, resolution of angiographic thrombus, and absence of distal embolization were obtained in all of the patients after placement of the graft-coated stent. At 10-day angiographic follow-up, all of the stents were patent, and at 1-month clinical follow-up, one patient had recurrence of acute MI. In another study (59), comparing 13 patients who received vein-covered Palmaz-Schatz stents with 15 patients who received regular Palmaz-Schatz

stents, the acute success rate was 100% in both groups (by angiography and intravascular ultrasound). Only one patient (coated stent) developed acute thrombosis. No other complications were reported in this small series of patients.

The experience with these kinds of stents is still limited but appears promising. Whether these kinds of devices will significantly decrease distal embolization will have to be answered in large prospective, randomized trials.

CONCLUSIONS

Intracoronary thrombi are harbingers for increased procedural complications after catheter-based revascularization techniques. Intense investigation is being carried out to resolve the issue of performing angioplasty in thrombus-containing lesions. We have summarized some of the most commonly used strategies and some of the new techniques, which appear promising in light of preliminary results.

A practical approach (Fig. 11.5) is to stratify

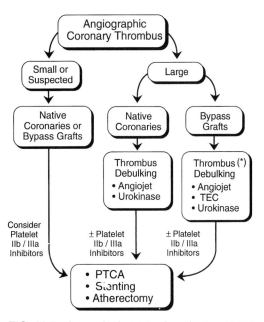

FIG. 11.5. A practical approach to the treatment of the thrombotic lesion. *In degenerated vein grafts, all interventional techniques must be used with caution because of a high risk of embolization and no reflow.

the adjunctive treatment according to thrombus burden. In cases of small or suspected angiographic thrombus in the setting of acute coronary ischemia, the use of platelet IIb/IIIa inhibitors has proved to be beneficial, as discussed previously. Conversely, the use of adjuvant thrombolysis in these circumstances may be detrimental because of enhanced procedural complications. In cases of a large angiographic thrombus burden, a urokinase infusion may be useful for thrombus resolution in native coronary arteries, but it should be used with caution in saphenous vein grafts. In cases of large thrombus burden in native coronary arteries or saphenous vein grafts, the approach that we take at the Ochsner Clinic is mechanical thrombectomy with the Possis AngioJet catheter. In the majority of the cases, we obtain very good results, with total or almost total resolution of angiographic thrombus, after which we immediately proceed with treatment of the underlying lesion. In cases of remaining thrombus after the use of this device, the use of platelet IIb/IIIa inhibitors may be beneficial.

REFERENCES

1. Davies MJ, Thomas AC. Plaque fissuring—the cause of acute myocardial infarction, sudden ischaemic death, and crescendo angina. *Br Heart J* 1985;53:363–373.
2. Davies MJ, Bland JM, Hangartner JR, Angelini A, Thomas AC. Factors influencing the presence or absence of acute coronary artery thrombi in sudden ischemic death. *Eur Heart J* 1989;10:203–208.
3. Fuster VS, Lewis A. Conner Memorial Lecture. Mechanisms leading to myocardial infarction: insights from studies of vascular biology. *Circulation* 1994;90: 2126–2146.
4. Oliver MF, Davies MJ. The atheromatous lipid core. *Eur Heart J* 1998;19:16–18.
5. Silva JA, White CJ, Collins TJ, Ramee SR. Morphologic comparison of atherosclerotic lesions in native coronary arteries and saphenous vein graphs with intracoronary angioscopy in patients with unstable angina. *Am Heart J* 1998;136:156–163.
6. Morasch MD, Zenni GC, Dobrin PB, Mrkvicka R. Intimal hyperplasia following thrombectomy versus thrombolysis in occluded vein grafts. *Ann Vasc Surg* 1997; 11:559–564.
7. White CJ, Ramee SR, Collins TJ, et al. Coronary thrombi increase PTCA risk. Angioscopy as a clinical tool. *Circulation* 1996;93:253–258.
8. Waxman S, Sassower MA, Mittleman MA, et al. Angioscopic predictors of early adverse outcome after coronary angioplasty in patients with unstable angina and non-Q-wave myocardial infarction. *Circulation* 1996; 93:2106–2113.
9. Violaris AG, Melkert R, Herrman JP, Serruys PW. Role of angiographically identifiable thrombus on long-term luminal renarrowing after coronary angioplasty: a quantitative angiographic analysis. *Circulation* 1996;93: 889–897.
10. Bauters C, Lablanche JM, McFadden EP, Hamon M, Bertrand ME. Relation of coronary angioscopic findings at coronary angioplasty to angiographic restenosis. *Circulation* 1995;92:2473–2479.
11. Zidar FJ, Kaplan BM, O'Neill WW, et al. Prospective, randomized trial of prolonged intracoronary urokinase infusion for chronic total occlusions in native coronary arteries. *J Am Coll Cardiol* 1996;27:1406–1412.
12. Hartmann JR, McKeever LS, O'Neill WW, et al. Recanalization of Chronically Occluded Aortocoronary Saphenous Vein Bypass Grafts With Long-Term, Low Dose Direct Infusion of Urokinase (ROBUST): a serial trial. *J Am Coll Cardiol* 1996;27:60–66.
13. Schieman G, Cohen BM, Kozina J, et al. Intracoronary urokinase for intracoronary thrombus accumulation complicating percutaneous transluminal coronary angioplasty in acute ischemic syndromes. *Circulation* 1990;82:2052–2060.
14. Vaitkus PT, Laskey WK. Efficacy of adjunctive thrombolytic therapy in percutaneous transluminal coronary angioplasty. *J Am Coll Cardiol* 1994;24:1415–1423.
15. Denardo SJ, Morris NB, Rocha-Singh KJ, Curtis GP, Rubenson DS, Teirstein PS. Safety and efficacy of extended urokinase infusion plus stent deployment for treatment of obstructed, older saphenous vein grafts. *Am J Cardiol* 1995;76:776–780.
16. Ambrose JA, Almeida OD, Sharma SK, et al. Adjunctive thrombolytic therapy during angioplasty for ischemic rest angina. Results of the TAUSA Trial. TAUSA Investigators. Thrombolysis and Angioplasty in Unstable Angina trial. *Circulation* 1994;90:69–77.
17. Glazier JJ, Kiernan FJ, Bauer HH, et al. Treatment of thrombotic saphenous vein bypass grafts using local urokinase infusion therapy with the Dispatch catheter. *Cathet Cardiovasc Diagn* 1997;41:261–267.
18. Mitchel JF, Fram DB, Palme DF II, et al. Enhanced intracoronary thrombolysis with urokinase using a novel, local drug delivery system. In vitro, in vivo, and clinical studies. *Circulation* 1995;91:785–793.
19. Mitchel JF, Azrin MA, Fram DB, et al. Inhibition of platelet deposition and lysis of intracoronary thrombus during balloon angioplasty using urokinase-coated hydrogel balloons. *Circulation* 1994;90:1979–1988.
20. The EPIC Investigation. Use of monoclonal antibody directed against the platelet glycoprotein IIb/IIIa receptor in high-risk coronary angioplasty. *N Engl J Med* 1994;330:956–961.
21. The EPILOG Investigators. Platelet glycoprotein IIb/IIIa receptor blockade and low-dose heparin during percutaneous coronary revascularization. *N Engl J Med* 1997;336:1689–1696.
22. Platelet Receptor Inhibition in Ischemic Syndrome Management in Patients Limited by Unstable Signs and Symptoms (PRISM-PLUS) Study Investigators. Inhibition of the platelet glycoprotein IIb/IIIa receptor with tirofiban in unstable angina and non-Q-wave myocardial infarction. *N Engl J Med* 1998;338:1488–1497.
23. Platelet Receptor Inhibition in Ischemic Syndrome

Management (PRISM) Study Investigators. A comparison of aspirin plus tirofiban with aspirin plus heparin for unstable angina. *N Engl J Med* 1998;338:1498–1505.

24. Kereiakes DJ, Lincoff AM, Miller DP, et al. Abciximab therapy and unplanned coronary stent deployment. Favorable effect on stent use, clinical outcomes, and bleeding complications. EPILOG Trial Investigators. *Circulation* 1998;97:857–864.

25. Simoons ML, de Boer MJ, van den Brand MJ, et al. Randomized trial of a GPIIb/IIIa platelet receptor blocker in refractory unstable angina. European Cooperative Study Group. *Circulation* 1994;89:596–603.

26. Muhlestein JB, Karagounis LA, Treehan S, Anderson JL. ''Rescue'' utilization of abciximab for the dissolution of coronary thrombus developing as a complication of coronary angioplasty. *J Am Coll Cardiol* 1997;30: 1729–1734.

27. Bailey SR, O'Leary E, Chilton R. Angioscopic evaluation of site-specific administration of ReoPro. *Cathet Cardiovasc Diagn* 1997;42:181–184.

28. Waller BF, Rothbaum DA, Pinkerton CA, et al. Status of the myocardium and infarct-related coronary artery in 19 necropsy patients with acute recanalization using pharmacologic (streptokinase, r-tissue plasminogen activator), mechanical (percutaneous transluminal coronary angioplasty) or combined types of reperfusion therapy. *J Am Coll Cardiol* 1987;9:785–801.

29. Kawano K, Aoki I, Oaki N, et al. Human platelet activation by thrombolytic agents: effects of tissue-type plasminogen activator and urokinase on platelet surface P-selectin expression. *Am Heart J* 1998;135(2 Pt 1): 268–271.

30. Stone GW, Brodie BR, Griffin JJ, et al. Prospective, multicenter study of the safety and feasibility of primary stenting in acute myocardial infarction: in-hospital and 30-day results of the PAMI stent pilot trial. Primary Angioplasty in Myocardial Infarction Stent Pilot Trial Investigators. *J Am Coll Cardiol* 1998;31:23–30.

31. Antoniucci D, Santoro GM, Bolognese L, Valenti R, Trapani M, Fazzini PF. A clinical trial comparing primary stenting of the infarct-related artery with optimal primary angioplasty for acute myocardial infarction: results from the Florence Randomized Elective Stenting in Acute Coronary Occlusions (FRESCO) Trial. *J Am Coll Cardiol* 1998;31:1234–1239.

32. Stone GW. Stenting in acute myocardial infarction: observational studies and randomized trials—1998. J Invas Cardiol 1998;10[Suppl A]:16A–26A.

33. Holmes DR, Ellis SG, Garrats KN. Directional coronary atherectomy for thrombus containing lesions. *Circulation* 1991;84[Suppl II]:II-26(abst).

34. Kurisu S, Sato H, Tateishi H, et al. Directional coronary atherectomy for the treatment of acute myocardial infarction. *Am Heart J* 1997;134:345–350.

35. Saito S, Arai H, Kim K, Aoki N, Sakurabayashi T, Miyake S. Primary directional coronary atherectomy for acute myocardial infarction. *Cathet Cardiovasc Diagn* 1994;32:44–48.

36. Emmi R, Movsowitz H, Manginas A, et al. Directional coronary atherectomy in lesions with coexisting thrombus. *Circulation* 1993;88[Suppl I]:I-596(abst).

37. Kaplan BM, Safian RD, Goldstein JA, Grines CL, O'Neill WW. Efficacy of angioscopy in determining the effectiveness of intracoronary urokinase and TEC atherectomy thrombus removal from an occluded saphe-

38. Popma JJ, Leon MB, Mintz GS, et al. Results of coronary angioplasty using the transluminal extraction catheter. *Am J Cardiol* 1992;70:1526–1532.

39. Safian RD, Grines CL, May MA, et al. Clinical and angiographic results of transluminal extraction coronary atherectomy in saphenous vein bypass grafts. *Circulation* 1994;89:302–312.

40. Safian RD, May MA, Lichtenberg A, et al. Detailed clinical and angiographic analysis of transluminal extraction coronary atherectomy for complex lesions in native coronary arteries. *J Am Coll Cardiol* 1995;25: 848–854.

41. Braden GA, Xenopoulos NP, Young T, Utley L, Kutcher MA, Applegate RJ. Transluminal extraction catheter atherectomy followed by immediate stenting in treatment of saphenous vein grafts. *J Am Coll Cardiol* 1997; 30:657–663.

42. Kaplan BM, Larkin T, Safian RD, et al. Prospective study of extraction atherectomy in patients with acute myocardial infarction. *Am J Cardiol* 1996;78:383–388.

43. Ramee SR, Kuntz RE, Schalz RA, et al. Preliminary experience with the POSSIS coronary AngioJet rheolytic thrombectomy catheter in the VeGAS I pilot study. *J Am Coll Cardiol* 1996;27[Suppl A]:69A(abst).

44. Ramee SR, Baim DS, Popma JJ, et al. A randomized, prospective, multi-center study comparing intracoronary urokinase to rheolytic thrombectomy with the POSSIS AngioJet catheter for intracoronary thrombus: final results of the VeGAS 2 Trial. *Circulation* 1998; 98:I-86(abst).

45. Silva JA, Ramee SR, Kuntz R, Dandreo K, Papma J. Mechanical thrombectomy using the AngioJet catheter in the treatment of acute myocardial infarction. *J Am Coll Cardiol* 1998;31[Suppl A]:410A(abst).

46. Rousseau H, Sapoval M, Ballini P, et al. Percutaneous recanalization of acutely thrombosed vessels by hydrodynamic thrombectomy (Hydrolyser). *Eur Radiol* 1997; 7:935–941.

47. van Ommen VG, van den Bos AA, Pieper M, et al. Removal of thrombus from aortocoronary bypass grafts and coronary arteries using the 6Fr Hydrolyser. *Am J Cardiol* 1997;79:1012–1016.

48. Rosenschein U, Roth A, Rassin T, Basan S, Laniado S, Miller HI. Analysis of coronary ultrasound thrombolysis endpoints in acute myocardial infarction (ACUTE Trial). Results of the feasibility phase. *Circulation* 1997; 95:1411–1416.

49. Agmon Y, Miller HI, Roth A, et al. Coronary ultrasound thrombolysis in acute myocardial infarction (ACUTE Study): 6 month follow-up of the feasibility phase patients. *Eur Heart J* 1997;18[Suppl]:271(abst).

50. Oesterle SN, Baim DS, Hayase M, Ramee SR, Teirstein PS, Virmani R. A coaxial catheter system for prevention of distal embolization. *J Am Coll Cardiol* 1998;31[Suppl A]:236A(abst).

51. Webb JG, Carere RG, Lo K, et al. An emboli containment system for saphenous vein graft angioplasty. *J Am Coll Cardiol* 1998;31[Suppl A]:236A(abst).

52. Gurbel PA, Criado FJ, Curnutte EA, Patten P, Secada-Lovio J. Percutaneous revascularization of an extensively diseased saphenous vein bypass graft with a saphenous vein-covered Palmaz stent. *Cathet Cardiovasc Diagn* 1997;40:75–78.

53. Stefanadis C, Toutouzas K, Tsiamis E, et al. Total reconstruction of a diseased saphenous vein graft by means of conventional and autologous tissue-coated stents. *Cathet Cardiovasc Diagn* 1998;43:318–321.

54. Stefanadis C, Tsiamis E, Vlachopoulos C, et al. Autologous vein graft-coated stents for the treatment of thrombus-containing coronary artery lesions. *Cathet Cardiovasc Diagn* 1997;40:217–222.

55. Malik N, Gunn J, Newman C, Crossman DC, Cumberland DC. Phosphorylcholine coated stents: angiographic and morphometric assessment in porcine coronary arteries. *J Am Coll Cardiol* 1998;31[Suppl A]:414A.

56. Stefanadis C, Toutouzas K, Tsiamis E, et al. Clinical and angiographic follow-up after autologous vein graft-coated stent implantation. *J Am Coll Cardiol* 1998; 31[Suppl A]:351A(abst).

57. Toutouzas K, Stefanadis C, Tsiamis E, et al. Stents coated by an autologous arterial graft: the first application in human coronary arteries. *J Am Coll Cardiol* 1998; 31[Suppl A]:351A(abst).

58. Stefanadis C, Tsiamis E, Toutouzas K, et al. Autologous vein graft-coated stent for the treatment of coronary artery disease: immediate results after percutaneous implantation in humans. *J Am Coll Cardiol* 1996;27[Suppl A]:179(abst).

59. Muramatsu T, Tukahara R, Hou M, Ito S, Inoue T. Immediate results and dilatation effect of the vein-covered Palmaz-Schatz stent assessed by intravascular ultrasound. *Cathet Cardiovasc Diagn* 1998;44:276–282.

C. Management of the Coronary Lesion with Associated Thrombus

John S. Douglas, Jr.

*Division of Cardiology, Emory University School of Medicine and Hospital,
Cardiac Catheterization Laboratory, Atlanta, Georgia 30322*

In the current practice of interventional cardiology, few strategic approaches have been more controversial than the management of patients with intracoronary thrombus. In the individual patient, selection of optimal therapy is encumbered by an evolving understanding of new antithrombotic and fibrinolytic agents, recent availability of stents with variable scaffolding and surface characteristics, limited new techniques for mechanically removing thrombus, and imprecise clinical methods for identifying thrombus.

Quite early in the experience with conventional balloon angioplasty (PTCA), it became apparent that lesion-associated thrombus was a predictor of complications, including distal thromboembolization, thrombus propagation at the angioplasty site, no reflow, and, more commonly, abrupt closure minutes or hours later (1–6). It has not been clear whether it is the thrombus itself, which is a reservoir of clot-bound thrombin, or the underlying unstable plaque surface with exposed subendothelial matrix that plays the major role in the genesis of periangioplasty ischemic complications.

While it is clear that angiographic techniques are insensitive in recognizing thrombus, angiography has been shown by angioscopy to be highly specific for larger thrombi presenting as discrete intraluminal filling defects (7–11). Teirstein et al. (9) reported that when angioscopy was used as a reference standard, the sensitivity of thrombus detection by angiography was only 21%; the specificity was 94%, and the predictive value was 74%. The sensitivity of angiography for the detection of angioscopic intraluminal thrombus (protruding into the lumen) was 100% (six of six), compared with only 10% (four of 42) for mural thrombus (adherent to the wall) ($p < .05$). Of 74 thrombotic lesions identified by angioscopy, White et al. (7) reported that only 24 (32%) were detected angiographically. Thrombus may be suspected angiographically when lesion surfaces are irregular, have a hazy appearance, or have overhanging edges or an unusually abrupt leading or trailing contour. By using these ''softer'' angiographic criteria along with clinical intuition, experienced angiographers can recognize thrombus more frequently, but with lower specificity.

Using angioscopic techniques for diagnosis of thrombus during PTCA, White and colleagues (7) reported that the presence of thrombus was associated with a greater than fivefold increase in major complications of death, myocardial infarction, or coronary bypass surgery (12.2% vs. 2.1%, $p = .04$) and more recurrent ischemia manifest by abrupt closure, repeat PTCA, or recurrent angina (25.7% vs. 10.4%, $p = .03$).

However, in a contemporary multicenter study with a blinded angiographic core laboratory, the impact of angiographically visible thrombus on PTCA outcome was evaluated and found to be less significant than early reports suggested (12). Although abrupt closure was most common in patients with thrombus present, compared with thrombus possible or absent (13%, 10%, and 7.4%, respectively; $p = .04$), the 30-day and 6-month clinical endpoints (death, myocardial infarction, urgent revascularization) were similar. This study, however, included only patients with acute ischemic coronary syndromes and/or complex lesion morphology, and it is likely that a majority of patients had thrombus present, even though it was not visible angiographically. The relatively high rates of abrupt closure experienced would support this impression. Interestingly, White et al. (7) reported that angiographic thrombi were not associated with adverse PTCA outcome, and Violaris et al. (13) had similar findings. These observations emphasize the difficulty of estimating the impact of a variable when the methods for determining its presence are unreliable.

Most patients with intracoronary thrombus have unstable angina or recent myocardial infarction, and the patients with the greatest likelihood of ischemic complications of angioplasty are patients (frequently smokers) with large intraluminal thrombi and refractory unstable angina in spite of medical therapy. Many such patients eventually stabilized on aspirin, heparin, and intensive medical therapy, and intervention, in our experience, was judged to be safer after 5 to 7 days of this therapy (Fig. 11.6), even if some thrombus remained (14). Laskey et al. (15) similarly reported that patients with intracoronary thrombus receiving 5 to 6 days of heparin had a higher angiographic success (94% vs. 61%, $p < .05$) and fewer postprocedure abrupt closures (6% vs. 33%, $p < .05$) than did patients with no heparin or heparin for less than 24 hours.

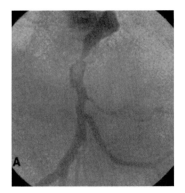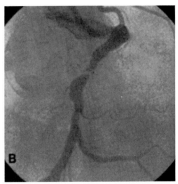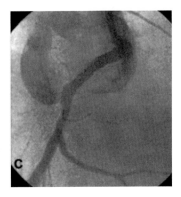

FIG. 11.6. A 57-year-old female smoker with a 3-day history of unstable angina was found to have normal left ventricular function, a normal left coronary artery, and severe stenosis of the right coronary artery. **A:** Right anterior oblique view with a large thrombus just distal to the lesion. The patient was stabilized on intravenous heparin, nitroglycerin, and aspirin, and repeat angiography 6 days later **(B)** revealed persisting severe stenosis but complete resolution of thrombus. Balloon angioplasty yielded an excellent result **(C)**, and the patient was discharged the following day with no complications. In our experience, intravenous heparin for 5 to 7 days is an effective strategy for management of large intracoronary thrombi. (From ref. 14, with permission.) Alternative approaches include direct angioplasty/stenting with use of adjunctive IIb/IIIa platelet receptor inhibition, pretreatment with a thrombolytic agent as described by McKendall et al. (17), or an attempt at thrombectomy (see text).

Importantly, after prolonged heparin therapy, residual lesions in some patients become noncritical and an unnecessary intervention is avoided. Currently, the expense of prolonged hospitalization, a major disadvantage of prolonged intravenous heparin therapy, can be mitigated by a few days of intravenous therapy followed by several days or weeks of outpatient therapy with low-molecular-weight heparin administered subcutaneously. This strategy has considerable utility when large intracoronary thrombi are present.

Thrombolytic agents have been administered via intracoronary or intravenous infusions before and after coronary intervention, or as a bolus to treat intracoronary thrombus, but the optimal strategy is not clear (16–18). An observational study compared intravenous tissue plasminogen activator (TPA), intracoronary urokinase, and intravenous heparin for treatment of intracoronary thrombus and reported more complete and rapid thrombus resolution with TPA (17). Prolonged intracoronary infusions are technically demanding, uncomfortable for the patient, and have some inherent risk of coronary artery trauma and serious bleeding. Local infusion of thrombolytic agent using the Dispatch catheter (Scimed, Maple Grove, MN) shortens the infusion time to 30 to 60 minutes and greatly reduces the amount of thrombolytic agent needed and the risk of bleeding (18,19), but has not been well studied and is not broadly applicable. In many laboratories, including our own, the use of thrombolytic agents to treat intracoronary thrombi has diminished with the availability of new, potent antithrombotic agents.

Atherectomy techniques have had limited success in the presence of thrombus. Intracoronary thrombus remains a predictor of acute complications with the use of the transluminal extraction catheter (TEC), directional atherectomy (DCA), and rotational atherectomy (20). Similarly, use of the excimer laser was associated with reduced success and increased complications when intracoronary thrombus was present (21). Of these FDA-approved, catheter-based techniques, only TEC continues to play a significant role in the treatment of coronary thrombi, and its limited effectiveness and applicability account for its relatively infrequent usage.

Recognition of the benefit of optimal stent expansion and use of antiplatelet agents (aspirin and ticlopidine) in reducing thrombotic stent occlusion ultimately led to the use of stents even when lesion-associated thrombus was present. In 86 consecutive patients with thrombus-laden lesions, Alfonso et al. (22) reported that stenting resulted in angiographic success in 96%, and only 1% experienced subacute stent thrombosis. Although five patients died (6%), four of these had presented in cardiogenic shock. This favorable experience with stenting in the presence of thrombus was mirrored by the report of Schuehlen et al. (23), who noted in almost 3,000 stented patients, most of whom were treated with antiplatelet therapy, that the presence of thrombus did not significantly influence procedural success or the occurrence of major adverse cardiac events. These results contrast with reports of increased complications with stenting in the presence of thrombus prior to use of antiplatelet agents and high-pressure stent expansion (24,25).

Following publication of the positive results with the use of platelet glycoprotein IIb/IIIa inhibitors in high-risk coronary angioplasty (26), use of these agents has become increasingly common when lesion-associated thrombus is identified. Although the magnitude of benefit with abciximab in the EPIC trial was similar in patients with and without angiographic thrombus, most of these high-risk and unstable patients probably had thrombus present, even though it was not detected angiographically (12).

The report of the initial investigative use of the AngioJet thrombectomy catheter (Possis Medical, Inc., Minneapolis, MN) in 87 patients indicated that thrombus removal was effective as assessed angiographically in a majority of patients. The AngioJet catheter removes thrombus by a Venturi effect created by high-pressure saline jets located at the tip of the catheter. Complications were significant, however: in-hospital death in 3.4%, in-hospital bypass surgery in 1%, transient no reflow in 11%, and abrupt closure in 4% (27). Subsequent Japanese reports of the use of the AngioJet catheter in 26 patients with acute myocardial infarction revealed 100% success in 24 patients in which the AngioJet was used as initial therapy to treat massive thrombus, but it failed in two patients when used as a ''bailout'' treatment for distal embolization after balloon angioplasty (28,29). Angioscopy in a single patient with saphenous vein graft occlusion revealed extensive thrombosis prior to AngioJet treatment and no occlusive or partially obstructive thrombus afterward, but some superficial thrombus remained (30). The status of this promising new strategy, however, remains uncertain.

Another new catheter-based technique for the treatment of intracoronary thrombus utilizes low-frequency, high-power ultrasound to selectively disrupt the fibrin matrix of thrombi at a power level one-twentieth of that required to induce arterial damage (see Acolysis in Chapter 5J). Coronary ultrasound angioplasty, which has been shown to be safe and effective in a canine model (31), has been used successfully in acute myocardial infarction (32) and is currently undergoing evaluation in multicenter trials. This technique has considerable promise and may play a significant role in the treatment of intracoronary thrombi in the future.

NATIVE CORONARY ARTERY LESION

Small or Suspected Thrombus

In patients with irregular lesion surface, angiographic lucency, or small filling defects, the availability of potent IIb/IIIa receptor inhibitors has permitted coronary intervention to be performed safely, in our experience, without the need for lengthy preprocedural heparin therapy (14,15,17). Prophylactic use of thrombolytic agents is not recommended based on our experience and the TAUSA trial, which reported increased ischemic complications in unstable angina patients treated with thrombolysis (19). We do not favor use of the TEC or excimer laser in this setting, and avoid use of rotational atherectomy, but utilize stents commonly based on the favorable results reported (22,23) and our own experience. It appears that the optimal lumen imparted by stenting offsets the thrombogenicity of a metal stent. Nonionic contrast agent is avoided in our laboratory in unstable ischemic syndromes and in the presence of suspected or definite intracoronary thrombus (33). Antiplatelet therapy with aspirin and ticlopidine or clopidogrel is carried out routinely following stenting. Postprocedural heparin is rarely administered, except in a patient who cannot receive IIb/IIIa receptor inhibitors.

Large Thrombus

Large intracoronary thrombi, most often observed postinfarction and in smokers, present a formidable clinical problem, the management of which is influenced by multiple factors: size and location of thrombus, degree of underlying stenosis, clinical stability, estimated age of thrombus, availability of thrombectomy devices, and candidacy for aggressive antithrombotic or thrombolytic therapy. Generally, it is desirable to attempt to reduce the thrombus burden as an initial strategy (see Fig. 11.6). Rarely, large proximal thrombi have been aspirated into a guide catheter. On occasion, we have entangled large clots and removed them by wrapping two guidewires (Fig. 11.7). These crude efforts merely emphasize the need for reliable thrombus removal techniques and devices.

Large intracoronary thrombi usually occur at the site of a stenosis and just beyond it. If total vessel occlusion occurs, and especially postinfarction, thrombus may propagate proximal to the stenosis. If the underlying stenosis is insignificant, as occasionally occurs following plaque rupture or in the case of coronary embolization, the main therapeutic effort is simply thrombus removal. In this case, and when the anatomy is suitable (large vessel, absence of extreme tortuosity), use of one of the new devices for thrombus removal, such as the AngioJet or ultrasound catheter, has considerable appeal, but these strategies are only now being evaluated. The TEC has moderate effectiveness in this setting. In patients with excellent coronary flow and stabilized symptoms, we still treat selected patients with prolonged heparin therapy, commonly after administration of a IIb/IIIa receptor inhibitor. After a few days of intravenous heparin, 1 to 4 weeks of outpatient low-molecular-weight hepa-

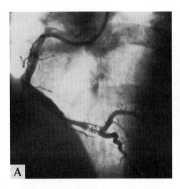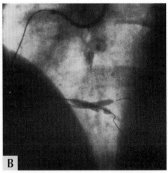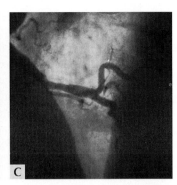

FIG. 11.7. A 53-year-old man presented with recurrent, prolonged chest pain with no evidence of myocardial necrosis. Coronary arteriography revealed single-vessel disease with severe stenosis of the right coronary artery and a large amount of thrombus associated with the lesion. The patient was treated with intravenous heparin for 5 days, with marked clearing of thrombus, but an eccentric, bulky stenosis 3 cm proximal to the posterior descending coronary artery persisted. Balloon angioplasty with a 4-mm-diameter balloon was performed, and a large amount of thrombus was noted immediately thereafter, just proximal to the posterior descending artery **(A)** (left anterior oblique view). This represented shifting of thrombus from the angioplasty site by the balloon inflation. This large thrombus presented a therapeutic dilemma, emphasizing the need for better mechanical thrombectomy devices. We did not believe that this thrombus, which had been present for many days, would respond well to thrombolytic therapy, and we were concerned that administration of thrombolytic therapy would result in an unstable jelly-like mass of thrombus that would occlude flow. **B:** The initial therapy, therefore, was inflation of two balloons at the site of thrombus, in an attempt to compress it. This was only partially effective. Therefore, an attempt at guidewire thrombectomy was made by first twisting a 0.014-in. guidewire and a balloon-on-a-wire to trap fibrin strands and subsequently withdrawing both wires into a deeply seated guide catheter. This maneuver yielded a large amount of thrombus, and subsequent angiography showed an excellent result with no evidence of residual thrombus **(C)**. The patient was treated with heparin for several days and received anticoagulation therapy with warfarin. Recatheterization 14 months later revealed a patent right coronary artery with only minor luminal irregularity at the angioplasty site, and no narrowing at the site occupied by the thrombus **(A)**. Left ventricular function was normal. The patient has remained free of cardiac events, and long-term results have been excellent. (Reprinted with permission from Douglas JS Jr. Percutaneous interventional approaches to specific coronary lesions. In: King SB III, Douglas JS Jr, eds. *Atlas of heart disease: interventional cardiology,* vol. 13. St. Louis: Mosby–Yearbook, 1997:11.10.)

rin administration (the bigger the clot, the longer the treatment) frequently results in complete or quite substantial clot lysis, and intracoronary instrumentation may be completely avoided.

In the more usual case, in which a large intracoronary thrombus is associated with a significant coronary artery stenosis (or an unascertainable degree of stenosis), or in the presence of clinical instability, a more aggressive approach may be necessary. One needs to be aware that administration of thrombolytic agents can lead to deformity and/or fragmentation of large clots, with resultant abrupt closure or ischemia related to distal thromboembolization. If administration of a thrombolytic agent is elected, we have used intravenous TPA (80 to 100 mg), as reported by

McKendall et al. (17), or intracoronary urokinase infusions (50,000 to 100,000 U per hour for 4 to 8 hours) with variable outcome, but sufficiently poor thrombolysis and enough bleeding complications that a thrombectomy approach is preferred when it is possible. In a few carefully selected patients, the Dispatch catheter for local delivery has been used to infuse 150,000 U of urokinase over 30 minutes, and the results have been favorable (18). This approach is not ideal, however, when the underlying stenosis is severe, necessitating predilation (and potential distal thromboembolization), or when there is considerable tortuosity or large side branches, or when a long thrombus is present.

When immediate intervention is required in a

large coronary artery with anatomy suitable for the use of TEC atherectomy, this strategy can achieve significant thrombus removal, but the risks increase when TEC is used in native coronary arteries, and smaller catheters (6 Fr, 5 Fr) are frequently used and case selection should be very conservative. Balloon angioplasty can achieve clot compression and fragmentation, restoring the lumen, and this may be the best option in selected patients, especially when IIb/IIIa receptor inhibitor adjunctive therapy is available. Distal embolization is ubiquitous when this strategy is chosen, but if coronary flow remains good, this redistribution of thrombus away from the lesion may optimize conditions for stenting. It should be remembered that extensive thrombus and complex anatomy may exceed the capability of even the most skilled interventionalist, but present no problems to the cardiac surgeon. When a large LAD is the target and/or multiple arteries are involved, the case for surgery is strengthened.

SAPHENOUS VEIN GRAFT LESIONS

Limited Thrombus

When evaluating saphenous vein graft (SVG) lesions for intervention, the angioplasty operator must consider possible consequences of thromboatheroembolism, considering that the entire lesion and accompanying thrombus may be fragmented, dislodged, and embolized. If the risk of major atheroembolization is acceptable, compared with other therapeutic options, percutaneous intervention may be appropriate. However, the relatively high subsequent coronary event rate and restenosis potential must also be factored into this decision.

Although IIb/IIIa receptor inhibition in patients undergoing vein graft angioplasty in EPIC and EPILOG combined did not significantly reduce complications (perhaps related to the small sample size), the use of these agents seems especially rational in this setting, in which embolization of the microcirculation with thrombus and/or atheroma is more the rule than the exception. Results from the Saphenous Vein De Novo (SAVED) trial support the use of stents in SVGs,

but also emphasize that initial complications and restenosis are common. In-hospital myocardial infarction occurred in 6% of the total group of patients (8% in the balloon group vs. 4% in the stent group, p = NS), and restenosis at 6 months occurred in 41% of patients overall (46% in the balloon group vs. 37% in the stent group, p = .24). At 240 days, however, major cardiac events were less frequent in the stent group compared with the balloon group (26% vs. 39%, p = .04). Only about one-fourth of the patients in the SAVED trial had definite or possible thrombus (thrombus was actually an exclusion criteria), and it might be anticipated that selection of more heavily diseased and thrombotic vein graft lesions would lead to even more complications and a higher rate of late events and occlusion (see Chapters 16A and 16B for more detailed discussion of vein graft lesions) (34). The relatively poor long-term outcome of percutaneous approaches to SVG lesions indicates the need to consider surgery when vein grafts to a large LAD or to multiple coronary arteries are involved. When mildly thrombotic lesions are treated by catheter-based strategies, we may elect pretreatment with TEC if the anatomy is favorable and then deploy stents to cover the lesion. If the lesion is relatively bulky, pretreatment with diltiazem or verapamil in 200- to 300-μg increments intracoronary up to 1 mg seems to minimize slow and no-flow states, but these strategies are of limited effectiveness. It is important to point out that there are no randomized trials that indicate superiority of TEC in this setting or that support the administration of thrombolytic agents.

Extensive Thrombus

Intervention in SVGs with a large amount of thrombus should be undertaken only after careful study of potential risks and benefits (Fig. 11.8). It is rarely appropriate to subject such patients to the procedural risk involved, given the high restenosis and late cardiac event rates expected following manipulation of older SVGs. In some patients, however, the presence of patent grafts to major coronary arteries or other factors makes reoperative surgery unattractive, and

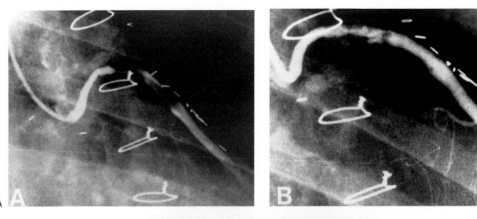

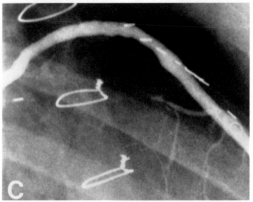

FIG. 11.8. Nine years following coronary bypass surgery, a 61-year-old woman was hospitalized with prolonged chest pain and anterior T-wave changes. A thallium scan revealed a very large area of anterior-septal ischemia with a small scar. Left ventricular angiography showed minimal anterior hypokinesis and a normal ejection fraction. An SVG to the circumflex was patent. The right coronary artery and proximal LAD were occluded. The SVG to the LAD had no effective flow, and a very large thrombus was present **(A)**. There was no antegrade or collateral flow to the distal LAD. Intragraft urokinase was given, with no change in the appearance of the LAD graft. TEC atherectomy removed much of the thrombus **(B)** and restored flow into a large distal LAD that appeared suitable for bypass surgery, but there were no donor veins and both internal mammary arteries were inadequate by angiography. Two 4-mm Palmaz-Schatz stents were deployed in the vein graft, with excellent angiographic results **(C)**. This procedure was complicated by evidence of a small non–Q-wave infarction, and the patient's convalescence was otherwise uneventful. This represented a successful attempt at catheter-based therapy in a difficult situation in which surgery was not an option.

intervention, in spite of the presence of graft thrombus, may be selected over more conservative measures when ischemia cannot be controlled. Although it is clear that reduction of clot burden is a key ingredient to a successful intervention, the optimal technique to achieve this is less certain and is influenced by anatomic and other patient-related factors, as well as available technology.

Catheter aspiration of thrombus is more frequently possible in SVGs than in native vessels, and the concept of simple aspiration has been extended by investigators who have used balloons to distally occlude the SVG while the lesion and associated thrombus are compressed, fragmented, and aspirated, using either conventionally available angioplasty equipment (35) or a specially designed occlusion balloon whose

0.014-in. shaft serves as a rail for subsequent introduction of balloon catheters, stents, and so on (36). Using the latter technique in 24 SVGs, 25% with bulky thrombus, Webb et al. (36) reported that creatine kinase exceeded three times normal in only one patient, and no patient developed new Q wave, required cardiac surgery, or died. Aspirated material included cholesterol clefts, lipid-rich macrophages, fibrous caps, necrotic core, and fibrin. Ischemic times required for distal occlusion, angioplasty, and aspiration, averaging about 2 minutes, were well tolerated. These techniques and the equipment to perform them are evolving, and their place in every day interventional practice is not yet determined.

Currently applied methods to reduce a large SVG clot burden include prolonged anticoagulation, prolonged intragraft infusion of thrombolytic agent, TEC atherectomy, use of the AngioJet or therapeutic ultrasound (Acolysis is discussed in Chapter 5H), and exclusion of thrombus by use of a covered stent (37). All of these strategies have significant limitations but may be indicated in selected patients. Because of the risks and discomfort of prolonged thrombolytic therapy, direct thrombectomy approaches with TEC (see Fig. 11.8) or one of the new devices is more appealing when immediate intervention is required. Adjunctive use of IIb/IIIa platelet receptor inhibitors is virtually routine in this setting in our practice, as is stenting of SVG stenosis.

REFERENCES

1. Mabin T, Holmes D, Smith H, et al. Intracoronary thrombus: role in coronary occlusion complicating percutaneous transluminal coronary angioplasty. *J Am Coll Cardiol* 1985;198–202.
2. Sugrue D, Holmes D, Smith H, et al. Coronary artery thrombus as a risk factor for acute vessel occlusion during percutaneous transluminal coronary angioplasty: improving results. *Br Heart J* 1986;56:62–66.
3. Deligonul U, Gabliani G, Caralis D, et al. Percutaneous transluminal coronary angioplasty in patients with intracoronary thrombus. *Am J Cardiol* 1988;62:474–476.
4. Ellis SG, Roubin GS, King SB III, et al. Angiographic and clinical predictors of acute closure after native vessel coronary angioplasty. *Circulation* 1988;77:372–379.
5. Ellis SG, Vandormael MG, Cowley MJ, et al. Coronary morphologic and clinical determinants of procedural outcome with angioplasty for multivessel coronary disease: implications for patient selection. *Circulation* 1990;82:1193–1202.
6. Tan KH, Sulke N, Taub N, et al. Clinical and lesion morphologic determinants of coronary angioplasty success and complications: current experience. *J Am Coll Cardiol* 1995;25:855–865.
7. White CJ, Ramee SR, Collins TJ, et al. Coronary thrombi increase PTCA risk: angioscopy as a clinical tool. *Circulation* 1996;93:253–258.
8. den Heijer P, van Dijk RB, Hillege HL, et al. Serial angioscopic and angiographic observations during the first hour after successful coronary angioplasty: a preamble to a multicenter trial addressing angioscopic markers for restenosis. *Am Heart J* 1994;128:656–663.
9. Teirstein PS, Schatz RA, DeNardo SJ, et al. Angioscopic versus angiographic detection of thrombus during coronary interventional procedures. *Am J Cardiol* 1995;75:1083–1087.
10. Uretsky BF, Deays BG, Courrihan PC, et al. Angioscopic evaluation of incompletely obstructing coronary intraluminal filling defects: comparison to angiography. *Cathet Cardiovasc Diagn* 1994;33:323–329.
11. White CJ, Ramee SR, Collins TJ, et al. Angioscopically detected coronary thrombus correlates with adverse PTCA outcome. *Circulation* 1993;88[Suppl I]:I-596.
12. Khan MM, Ellis SG, Aguirre FV, et al. Does intracoronary thrombus influence the outcome of high risk percutaneous transluminal coronary angioplasty? Clinical and angiographic outcomes in a large multicenter trial. *J Am Coll Cardiol* 1998;31:31–36.
13. Violaris AG, Melkert R, Herman JR, et al. Role of angiographically identifiable thrombus on long-term luminal renarrowing after coronary angioplasty: a quantitative angiographic analysis. *Circulation* 1996;93:889–897.
14. Douglas JS Jr, Lutz JF, Clements SD, et al. Therapy of large intracoronary thrombi in candidates for percutaneous transluminal coronary angioplasty. *J Am Coll Cardiol* 1988;11:238.
15. Laskey MAL, Deutch E, Hirschfeld JW Jr, et al. Influence of heparin therapy on percutaneous transluminal coronary angioplasty outcome in unstable angina pectoris. *Am J Cardiol* 1990;65:1425–1429.
16. Evans DJ, Pacheco T, Grambow D, et al. Bolus versus prolonged intracoronary urokinase infusion: a therapeutic quagmire? *J Am Coll Cardiol* 1994;185A.
17. McKendall GR, Berman MS, Sharaf BL, Lee B, Williams DO. Comparison of the effectiveness of intravenous heparin, intravenous r-tPA, and intracoronary urokinase for treatment of intracoronary thrombus. *J Am Coll Cardiol* 1993;21:137A.
18. McKay RG, Fram DB, Hirst JA, et al. Treatment of intracoronary thrombus with local urokinase infusion using a new, site-specific drug delivery system: the Dispatch catheter. *Cathet Cardiovasc Diagn* 1994;33:181–188.
19. Ambrose JA, Almeida OD, Sharma SK, et al. Adjunctive thrombolytic therapy during angioplasty for ischemic rest angina: results of the TAUSA trial. *Circulation* 1994;90:69–77.
20. O'Neill WW, Sketch MH Jr, Steenkiste, et al. New device intervention in the treatment of intracoronary thrombus: report of the NACI Registry. *Circulation* 1993;88[Suppl I]:I-595.
21. Estella P, Ryan TJ, Landzberg JS, et al. Excimer laser-

assisted coronary angioplasty for lesions containing thrombus. *J Am Coll Cardiol* 1993;21:1550–1560.

22. Alfonso F, Rodriguez P, Phillips P, et al. Clinical and angiographic implications of coronary stenting in thrombus-containing lesions. *J Am Coll Cardiol* 1997; 29:725–733.

23. Shuehlen H, Kastrati A, Dirschinger J, et al. Intracoronary stenting and risk for major adverse cardiac events during the first month. *Circulation* 1998;98:104–111.

24. Mak K, Belli G, Ellis SG, et al. Subacute stent thrombosis: evolving issues and current concepts. *J Am Coll Cardiol* 1996;27:494–503.

25. Yokoi H, Nobuyoshi M, Nosaka H, et al. Coronary stent thrombosis: pattern, management and long-term follow-up result. *Circulation* 1996;94[Suppl I]:I-332.

26. The EPIC Investigators. Use of a monoclonal antibody directed against the platelet glycoprotein IIb/IIIa receptor in high-risk coronary angioplasty. *N Engl J Med* 1994;330:956–961.

27. Ramee SR, Schatz RA, Carroza, et al. Results of the VeGAS I pilot study of the Possis Angiojet thrombectomy catheter. *Circulation* 1996;94:I-619.

28. Nakagawa Y, Matsuo S, Tamura T, et al. Angiojet thrombectomy catheter for acute myocardial infarction. *J Am Coll Cardiol* 1998;31[Suppl A]:236A.

29. Nakagawa Y, Matsuo S, Yokoi H, et al. Stenting after thrombectomy with the Angiojet catheter for acute myocardial infarction. *Cathet Cardiovasc Diagn* 1998;43: 327–330.

30. Rodes J, Bilodeau L, Bonan, et al. Angioscopic evaluation of thrombus removal by the Possis Angiojet thrombectomy catheter. *Cathet Cardiovasc Diagn* 1998;43: 338–343.

31. Rosenschein U, Rozenszajn LA, Bernheim J, et al. Safety of coronary ultrasound angioplasty: effects of sonication on intact canine coronary arteries. *Cathet Cardiovasc Diagn* 1995;35:64–71.

32. Rosenschein U, Roth A, Rassin, et al. Analysis of coronary ultrasound thrombolysis endpoints in acute myocardial infarction (ACUTE trial): results of the feasibility phase. *Circulation* 1997;95:1411–1416.

33. Grines CL, Schreiber TL, Savas V, et al. A randomized trial of low osmolar ionic versus nonionic contrast media in patients with myocardial infarction or unstable angina undergoing percutaneous transluminal coronary angioplasty. *J Am Coll Cardiol* 1996;27:1381–1386.

34. Savage MP, Douglas JS Jr, Fischman DL, et al. Stent placement compared with balloon angioplasty for obstructed coronary bypass grafts. *N Engl J Med* 1997; 337:740–747.

35. Shaknovich A, Forman S, Parikh M, et al. Prevention of distal embolization and ''no reflow'' during saphenous vein graft and acute infarction coronary interventions: use of a novel occluder balloon-wash out procedure. *J Am Coll Cardiol* 1998;31[Suppl A]:216A.

36. Webb JG, Carere RG, Lo K, et al. An emboli containment system for saphenous vein graft angioplasty. *J Am Coll Cardiol* 1998;31[Suppl A]:236A.

37. Stefanadis C, Toutouzas K, Tsiamis E, et al. Total restruction of a diseased saphenous vein graft by means of conventional and autologous tissue-coated stents. *Cathet Cardiovasc Diagn* 1998;43:318–321.

12

Percutaneous Therapy of Ostial Coronary Disease

Steven B.H. Timmis and *Robert D. Safian

*Division of Cardiology, *Interventional Cardiology, William Beaumont Hospital,
Royal Oak, Michigan 48073*

Percutaneous coronary intervention of ostial coronary stenoses is associated with unique technical challenges. For purposes of coronary intervention, we classify ostial stenoses as (a) aorto-ostial lesions of the left main or right coronary artery (RCA), (b) aorto-ostial stenoses of saphenous vein grafts, and (c) branch-ostial lesions of the left anterior descending (LAD), diagonal branches, left circumflex, obtuse marginal branches, and major branches of the RCA. Our approach depends on this lesion classification, vessel caliber, and extent of calcification.

AORTO-OSTIAL DISEASE

General Considerations

Significant aorto-ostial coronary artery disease is identified in 0.13% to 2.7% of coronary angiograms and is characterized by dense fibro-cellular and calcified atheroma (1–5). These plaque characteristics increase lesion rigidity and elastic recoil, accounting for a greater residual stenosis and more frequent dissection following intervention of ostial lesions compared with nonstial lesions (4,5). We frequently rely on stents and debulking devices to overcome these problems and improve initial results, despite the absence of data from prospective, randomized trials assessing these devices in aorto-ostial lesions.

There is a paucity of high-quality, device-specific data relating to the three types of ostial

lesions described and results. Reports from the early 1990s on outcome of such lesions treated with plain old balloon angioplasty provide a mixed impression. Some (4,6) suggest that initial success rates are only somewhat decreased and that complications are essentially the same as for treatment for lesions with other morphologies. Others (7) suggest that success rates may be as low as 74% and complications as high as 13%. This led, in the early 1990s, to an evaluation of, first, debulking devices and then stents for treatment at these sites. In this regard, Safian et al. (8) and Sabri et al. (9) reported lesser complications and greater acute gain (presumably translating to better long-term outcomes) with debulking devices. Initial reports of stenting of such lesions (10,11) suggest augmented acute gain and lower than previously reported restenosis rates.

Device Selection for Native Aorto-ostial Stenoses

When selecting a device in native aorto-ostial stenoses, we focus on the degree of lesion calcification and the caliber of the target vessel (Fig. 12.1). We perform mechanical rotational atherectomy (MRA) on vessels with any degree of fluoroscopic calcification, regardless of vessel diameter, to facilitate lumen enlargement (6). When significant fluoroscopic calcification is not evident, we recommend intracoronary ultrasound (ICUS) to determine the extent of calcifi-

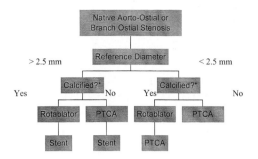

*If the degree of calcification is uncertain, consider intracoronary ultrasound

FIG. 12.1. Treatment strategy for aorto-ostial and branch-ostial coronary stenoses.

cation and estimate vessel size. If the arc of superficial calcium is < 90 degrees, percutaneous coronary angioplasty (PTCA) is sometimes performed without antecedent MRA. If ICUS is unavailable, we recommend MRA prior to stenting in all aorto-ostial native vessels.

Before performing MRA, we cross the target lesion with a 0.014-in. flexible guidewire in virtually all cases. A Tracker or Ultrafuse-X infusion catheter is then employed to facilitate guidewire exchange. We recommend using a 0.009-in. Rotablator (Heart Technology Inc., Bellevue, WA) extra-support wire and a stepped-burr approach. We use a final burr size to achieve a burr-to-artery ratio of 0.7 to 0.8. When MRA is complete, we exchange the Rotablator wire for a 0.014-in. flexible or extra-support guidewire before proceeding with adjunctive PTCA.If the vessel diameter is ≥2.5 mm, we recommend implanting a stent to achieve maximum luminal gain, prevent recoil, and eliminate dissection. A variety of stent designs are available, and stent selection is largely based on operator preference. For aorto-ostial stenoses, we prefer slotted tubular stents, such as the Crown (vessel c ...meter, 3.0 to 5.0 mm) or mini-Crown stent (vessel diameter, 2.5 to 3.0 mm) (Cordis, Johnson and Johnson Inc., Warren, NJ). Although it is more flexible than the Palmaz-Schatz stent (Johnson and Johnson Inc., Warren, NJ), the Crown stent is less flexible than many of the newer stents and requires the use of extra-support guidewires. Alternative stents

include the Nir (Scimed, Maple Grove, MN), GFX, and Duet stents, which are low profile and highly flexible.

Appropriate stent size and position are also important. We employ a stent-to-artery ratio of 1.0 to 1.1. Great care is needed to ensure that the stent covers the entire lesion. Adequate coverage of the ostium must be achieved by positioning the proximal stent margin 1 to 2 mm into the aorta. To adequately visualize the ostium of the RCA during stent placement, we ordinarily choose a 30-degree left anterior oblique (LAO) or lateral projection. When treating the ostium of the left main, a shallow (10 to 20 degrees) LAO or right anterior oblique (RAO) projection with mild (15 to 20 degrees) caudal angulation provides good visualization. During stent deployment, the guide must be retracted to avoid deploying the stent within the catheter and to adequately cover the lesion. After stent implantation, we flare the proximal end with a slightly oversized, noncompliant balloon.

Guide Catheter Selection for Native Aorto-Ostial Stenoses

Despite advancements in balloon, stent, and guidewire technology, stenting at the aorto-ostial location remains a challenge. Success is highly dependent on proper guide catheter selection to avoid proximal or distal misplacement of the stent within the target lesion. Coaxial guide catheter alignment with the ostium is more important than a "power position" to allow the operator to gently advance and retract the guide as needed, ensuring proper stent position and contrast opacification. Aggressive guide support may impair stent deployment at the origin of the artery. We recommend using a conventional or short-tip Judkins Right guide catheter for most ostial RCA narrowings, which usually have a slightly inferior takeoff from the aorta. If the RCA has a superior takeoff, a Hockey Stick or Amplatz Left guide catheter may provide better coaxial alignment. A short-tip Judkins Right, Amplatz Right, or Hockey Stick will provide alignment for a horizontal takeoff. When treating ostial left main stenoses, standard Judkins Left catheters usually provide appropriate support. However, an Amplatz Left 2 or Voda Left guide may be better suited if there is aortic root dilation or an upward orientation of the left main. During stent deployment, it is crucial to retract the guide to facilitate proper stent position 1 to 2 mm in the aorta. When treating aorto-ostial lesions, pressure waveform dampening can be avoided by maintaining coaxial alignment and by using a side-hole catheter. Although side holes can ameliorate pressure dampening, ostial injury may still occur by mechanical trauma.

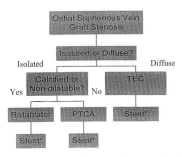

* If the lumen diameter is > 4.5-5.0 mm, a biliary stent should be implanted. If the lumen diameter is <4.5-5.0, a coronary stent with good radial strength should be placed.

FIG. 12.2. Treatment strategy for ostial saphenous vein graft coronary stenoses.

OSTIAL SAPHENOUS VEIN GRAFT DISEASE

General Considerations

Little data exist on the treatment of ostial saphenous vein graft (SVG) lesions, which may be less calcified than native ostial stenoses but are often rigid and elastic. As with native vessels, we frequently rely on stents to improve immediate luminal gain and eliminate elastic recoil and dissection. Conventional balloon angioplasty is seldom employed as a stand-alone device to treat lesions in saphenous vein bypass grafts. Rather, PTCA is usually performed to pre- and postdilate during stent implantation. Because of our expectation of lesion rigidity, we always use a high-pressure, noncompliant balloon to predilate an aorto-ostial lesion. If full balloon inflation cannot be achieved at, or slightly above, nominal inflation pressure, we recommend debulking the lesion with directional coronary atherectomy (DCA) or MRA. For vein grafts >4 mm, DCA may be preferable to MRA to achieve greater debulking. Although MRA is generally avoided in SVG lesions because of concerns of distal embolization, we have not encountered this problem when MRA is restricted to stenoses that cannot be dilated with balloons.

Device Selection for Ostial Saphenous Vein Graft Stenoses

Our initial treatment of an ostial SVG stenosis depends on whether it can be dilated with a balloon (Fig. 12.2). If the ostium is calcified by fluoroscopy, adequate balloon dilation is unlikely without initial MRA. If the lesion has no calcification, a balloon may be gently inflated to nominal pressure to test the distensibility of the stenosis. If the balloon cannot be fully inflated, we perform MRA using a stepped-burr approach, up to a final burr-to-artery ratio of 0.8. After pretreatment with PTCA or MRA, we deploy a stent using a 0.014-in. guidewire. We prefer the Crown stent for vessels 3.0 to 4.5 mm in diameter and the nonarticulated Palmaz biliary stent for vessels 4.5 to 6.0 mm in diameter. A nine-cell Nir stent is also useful for treating ostial lesions in vein grafts 4.0 to 5.0 mm in diameter because of its flexibility and radial strength. We avoid the Palmaz-Schatz biliary stent because of the large articulation gap, and the Wallstent because of unpredictable shortening at the ostium. Frequently, a diffusely diseased, degenerated vein graft is encountered that extends to the ostium. In this setting, we employ TEC atherectomy and stenting in the body of the graft, and PTCA–stenting of the ostium.

Guide Catheter Selection for Ostial Saphenous Vein Graft Stenoses

Selection of a guide catheter with ideal coaxial alignment is crucial for procedural success. A multipurpose guide is ideally suited for the downward takeoff seen in most vein grafts to the RCA. The multipurpose guide permits easy advancement and retraction of the guide during contrast angiography and stent deployment. Right Amplatz or right Judkins catheters may also be used, but are less coaxial than the multipurpose guide. For vein grafts to the left coronary with a superior orientation, a Hockey Stick, El Gamal, or Left Coronary Bypass catheter provides good alignment. A horizontal takeoff in vein grafts to the left coronary artery is best engaged with a standard right Judkins guide. As with native vessels, if dampening is observed, readjust the guide catheter or select one with side holes.

BRANCH-OSTIAL DISEASE

General Considerations

Branch-ostial stenoses are more frequently encountered than aorto-ostial lesions. Elastic recoil is an important cause of PTCA failure at this site. Focal lesions involving the origin of the LAD are generally treated by DCA or coronary artery bypass graft (CABG). We recommend CABG when the artery is <3 mm in diameter, long segments of disease are present, or the vessel is calcified. Focal lesions at the origin of the left circumflex are problematic because of severe angulation from the left main. For ostial circumflex lesions with a gentle takeoff, DCA with a standard or short-window device is possible. We recommend CABG for all others.

Device Selection for Branch-Ostial Stenoses

Our initial assessment of branch-ostial lesions includes determination of the extent of fluoroscopic calcification, the angle of origin of the branch from the parent vessel, and the degree of tortuosity leading to the ostial lesion (see Fig. 12.1). We perform MRA on calcified lesions, using the Rotablator extra-support guidewire and a stepped-burr approach, to achieve a final burr-to-artery ratio of 0.5 to 0.7. To avoid arterial perforation, MRA should be not be employed if the origin of the branch is acutely angled (≥60 degrees) or the parent vessel is excessively tortuous. For lesions without calcium, we usually perform PTCA without MRA.

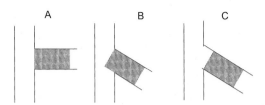

FIG. 12.3. Difficulty of stent placement in an angulated branch-ostial stenosis. **A:** Complete stent coverage in a branch-ostial lesion with a 90-degree takeoff. **B:** Stent protrusion into the parent vessel or **(C)** inadequate ostial coverage in a branch-ostial stenosis with a 90-degree takeoff.

The decision to implant a stent in a branch-ostial lesion depends on the acute angiographic results after PTCA and the angle of origin of the branch from the parent vessel (Fig. 12.3). A 90-degree angle allows complete ostial coverage with a stent (Fig. 12.3A). However, if the angle is not 90 degrees, a stent may protrude into the parent vessel (Fig. 12.3B) or provide inadequate ostial coverage (Fig. 12.3C). As a result, we reserve stent implantation for branch-ostial stenoses when PTCA provides inadequate luminal enlargement.

When a stent is implanted in the branch-ostial location, the most difficult challenge is precise placement. The stent must be deployed directly at the origin of the artery. Unstented ostial disease due to distal stent displacement increases the risk of restenosis, whereas proximal stent displacement encroaches on and endangers the parent vessel. Stents with radiopacity and flexibility, such as the GFX or Duet, may aid in accurate placement. Furthermore, multiple angiographic views and frequent contrast injections will help ensure ideal stent placement. While guide catheter selection is important in any percutaneous intervention, it is less crucial for procedural success in branch-ostial stenoses than in aorto-ostial narrowings.

REFERENCES

1. Pritchard CL, Mudd JG, Barner HB. Coronary ostial stenosis. Circulation 1975;52:46–48.
2. Barner HB, Codd JE, Mudd JG, et al. Non-syphilitic coronary ostial stenosis. Arch Surg 1977;112:1462–1466.

3. Salem B, Terasawa M, Mathur V, Garcia E, de Castro C, Hall R. Left main coronary artery stenosis: clinical marker, angiographic recognition and distinction from left main disease. Cathet Cardiovasc Diagn 1979;5: 125–134.

4. Tan KH, Sulke N, Taub N, Sowton E. Percutaneous transluminal coronary angioplasty of aorta ostial, non-aorta ostial, and branch ostial stenoses: acute and long-term outcome. Eur Heart J 1995;16:631–639.

5. Topol EJ, Ellis SG, Fishman J, et al. Multicenter study of percutaneous transluminal angioplasty for right coronary artery ostial stenosis. J Am Coll Cardiol 1987;9: 1214–1218.

6. Myler RK, Shaw RE, Stertzer SH, et al. Lesion morphology and coronary angioplasty: current experience and analysis. J Am Coll Cardiol 1992;19:1641–1652.

7. Mathias DW, Mooney JF, Lange HW, Goldenberg IF, Gobel FL, Mooney MR. Frequency of success and complications of coronary angioplasty of a stenosis at the ostium of a branch vessel. Am J Cardiol 1991;67: 491–495.

8. Safian RD, Freed M, Reddy V, et al. Do excimer laser angioplasty and rotational atherectomy facilitate balloon angioplasty? Implications for lesion-specific coronary intervention. J Am Coll Cardiol 1996;27:552–559.

9. Sabri MN, Cowley MJ, DiSciascio G, et al. Immediate results of interventional devices for coronary ostial narrowing with angina pectoris. Am J Cardiol 1994;73: 122–125.

10. Zampieri P, Colombo A, Almagor Y, Maiello L, Finci L. Results of coronary stenting of ostial lesions. Am J Cardiol 1994;73:901–903.

11. Rocha-Singh K, Morris N, Wong SC, Schatz RA, Teirstein PS. Coronary stenting for treatment of ostial stenoses of native coronary arteries or aortocoronary saphenous venous grafts. Am J Cardiol 1995;75:26–29.

13

The Simple De Novo Lesion

A. The Case for Provisional Stenting

Carlo Di Mario

Cardiac Catheterization Laboratory, Columbus Clinic and San Raffaele Hospital,
20145 Milano, Italy

The stent revolution has enlarged the indications and simplified the technique of percutaneous treatment of coronary stenoses so that, with the help of long flexible stents, less-experienced interventionalists can approach complex lesions and multivessel disease with a high likelihood of immediate success. The first report of a randomized trial comparing the results of multivessel stent implantation and bypass surgery indicates that the need for bail-out surgery because of percutaneous transluminal coronary angioplasty (PTCA) failure or complications is now reduced to a negligible 0.3% (1). In a consecutive series of 132 patients meeting the inclusion criteria of the GABI trial (German Angioplasty Bypass Investigation) and treated with multivessel stent implantation, bail-out surgery or crossover to surgery was 0%, a striking difference from the 8.7% incidence reported for the multivessel PTCA in the randomized GABI trial, carried out when stents were not practically available (2). Stents have transformed interventional cardiology into a predictable treatment with high immediate success and low complications. The use of aspirin and ticlopidine and the improvement in the technique of deployment have already reduced the risk of subacute stent thrombosis below 1% to 2% (3–5), and new antiplatelet and antithrombotic agents (clopidogrel, IIb/IIIa platelet receptor inhibitors, antithrombin agents, etc.) hold the promise of

similar or greater efficacy, with lower hemorrhagic risk and fewer side effects.

The randomized restenosis trials comparing PTCA and stent implantation were carried out before these more recent technical developments, but they unequivocally showed a reduction in restenosis rate as well as a reduction in the incidence of death, myocardial infarction, and target-lesion revascularization (6–9) (Fig. 13.1). Other trials in specific lesion subsets have confirmed a lower restenosis after treatment with stents of restenotic lesions, lesions in venous grafts, and chronic total occlusions (10–12).

With these premises and with stents implanted in 60% to 90% of all coronary interventions performed in many high-volume centers, the "case for provisional stenting" seems closed. The fear of long-term "foreign body" reactions and the cost issue are still occasionally mentioned by the opponents of stent implantation, but these arguments are now weaker after 10 years of experience (13) and with stents at the price of a balloon in some European countries (14).

In this chapter, we follow a different approach and discuss how we can improve our PTCA results in order to obtain a clinical outcome equivalent to (or better than) the outcome obtained with stent implantation of all suitable lesions. These techniques of aggressive PTCA are certainly not in opposition to the current stent practice, because they are based on knowledge ac-

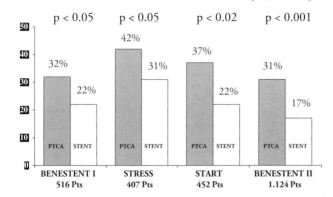

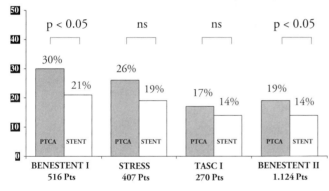

FIG. 13.1. Two histograms showing the results of five randomized trials comparing stent implantation and balloon angioplasty. (Data from refs. 6–9 and 45). **A:** Angiographic restenosis rate (≥50% diameter stenosis). **B:** Incidence of major adverse cardiac events at 6-month follow-up. CABG, coronary artery bypass graft; CVA, cerebrovascular accident; DS, diameter stenosis; IMA, acute myocardial infarction; PTCA, percutaneous transluminal coronary angioplasty.

quired from the process of optimization of stent results and require stent implantation in a large percentage of patients to bail out complications or improve suboptimal results.

INTRACORONARY ULTRASOUND DURING BALLOON ANGIOPLASTY

The diffuse nature of atherosclerotic vascular involvement and the presence of compensatory enlargement in the early phases of atherosclerosis (15–18) explain the discrepancy between angiography and ultrasound, with the detection of moderate-to-severe intimal thickening also in angiographically normal vessel segments. Ultrasound, moreover, does not require calibration, a necessary step with quantitative angiography, which is mostly performed using the guiding catheter, with frequent underestimation of true lumen dimensions (19). Modifications of the dilatation strategy based on intracoronary ultrsound (ICUS) results include changes in balloon size, length, and inflation pressure. If the ultrasound assessment is performed before interventions, the use of alternative treatment modalities (Rotablator [Heart Technology Inc., Bellevue, WA] for severely calcified lesions, directional atherectomy for large, bulky, soft plaques), can facilitate subsequent expansion with the PTCA balloon (20–23). Although various reports have suggested the use of ultrasound for optimal device selection and to judge and eventually improve the final PTCA result, a standardized protocol of PTCA based on ultrasound measurements was only recently proposed and tested in a pilot series in the CLOUT study (Clinical Outcomes with intracoronary Ultrasound Trial) (24). In this study, ICUS was used to guide the balloon selection, with a predefined strategy of balloon oversizing based on the amount of plaque burden. In this protocol, ultrasound was performed only after an initial dilatation with a balloon sized on the angiographic reference diameter. The operator was then required to use a second balloon if the initial balloon diameter was smaller than the average of the mean lumen and mean vessel diameter of the proximal or distal reference segment.

Quarter-size balloons were used routinely for accurate sizing. Upsizing of the balloon was required in 73% of the lesions, ranging from 0.25 mm to 1.25 mm and with a median increase of 0.50 mm, with a balloon-to-vessel ratio measured with quantitative angiography, which increased from 1:1 to 1:1.12 (Fig. 13.2). After balloon upsizing, no increase in incidence and severity of dissections was observed, with a low incidence of abrupt vessel closure (two patients, 1.9%; in one patient after recanalization of a recently occluded artery 4 days after myocardial infarction). The additional dilatation induced an increase in minimal lumen diameter from 1.95 ± 0.49 mm to 2.21 ± 0.47 mm, and a decrease in residual diameter stenosis (DS) from 28.3% ± 14.9% to 18.1% ± 14.4% (both $p < .0001$). Parallel changes were observed in the ultrasound

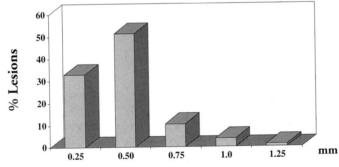

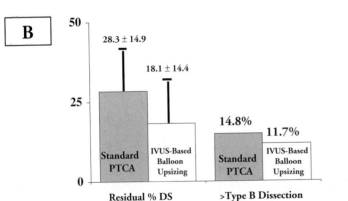

FIG. 13.2. A: Histogram showing the increase in balloon size between angiographic and ultrasound selection in the CLOUT study (24). The balloon initially selected was smaller than the average lumen-vessel diameter in 73% of cases, with balloon upsizing to 1.25 mm. **B:** Effects of the additional dilatation using a balloon sized with ICUS: Note the reduction in residual diameter stenosis from 28% to 18%, with no increase in incidence and severity of dissections. LD, lumen diameter; RD, reference diameter.

measurements after standard balloon angioplasty and after intravascular ultrasound (IVUS)-based balloon upsizing, with an increase in lumen area from 3.16 ± 1.05 mm^2 to 4.56 ± 1.14 mm^2 ($p < .0001$). Interestingly, a large residual plaque burden was still observed at the end of the procedure (reduced from 77.6% ± 6.9% to 69.1% ± 7.5%, $p < .0001$), with a high potential risk of restenosis based on the previously quoted ultrasound observations. Although the CLOUT pilot study demonstrated the safety of IVUS guidance for balloon selection during PTCA, the clinical efficacy of this strategy for restenosis prevention was not directly tested because no long-term angiographic or clinical results were available. Furthermore, based on the ultrasound observations after stent implantation (4,25,26), at the low nominal pressure used in the study (7.3 ± 2.3 atm), it is unlikely that a full balloon expansion was achieved in all lesions because of the resistance of the fibrotic and/or calcified vessel wall.

During the same years, important observations were made using ultrasound for a different type of intervention, stent implantation. The detection of incomplete stent expansion as a major determinant of subacute stent thrombosis was established by the pilot work of the Milan group (4,25,26) and contributed, with the use of the more effective antiplatelet agent ticlopidine (3,5), to a major reduction of this dramatic complication and, consequently, to the rapid growth of the stent implantation procedures. Based on the experience gained during stent implantation, the Washington group (27) developed a strategy of IVUS-guided PTCA with significant methodologic differences from the CLOUT approach. Ultrasound was used before treatment to select the appropriate balloon based on the ultrasound measurements of the media-to-media proximal reference diameter. The large balloons selected (3.5 ± 0.6 mm) were then inflated at high pressure (>10 atm; mean, 13.5 ± 3.3 atm), and ultrasound was used to measure the lumen enlargement. The result was accepted only if the lumen area in the treated segment was >60% of the reference lumen area and no flow limiting dissections were observed. In 94 of 242 lesions (39%), these criteria were fulfilled, with a minimal lumen area of 6.0 ± 2.8 mm^2 and a residual plaque burden of 54% ± 16%. No procedural coronary ruptures or abrupt vessel closures were observed in this group. At a mean follow-up of 8 months, target-lesion revascularization was lower in the group treated with PTCA only (7.8%) than in the group crossed-over to stent implantation (12.9%, $p < 0.08$). The group of Tubingen (28) has used an aggressive approach to balloon angioplasty with some similarities to the Washington study. The balloon was sized on the media-to-media diameter, but the minimal pressure required for full balloon expansion was used (7 ± 2 atm) and no predefined endpoints were required, with stents used as bail-out only in a small minority of patients. With a 78% angiographic follow-up at 1 year, restenosis was observed in 19% of lesions.

Especially considering the unfavorable lesion length and vessel size in the Washington study, the incidence of late recurrence appears low. The main limitation of these studies is the absence of a control group, so the real usefulness of the ultrasound guidance cannot de determined.

The SIPS trial (Strategy of ICUS-guided PTCA and Stenting) was a prospective, randomized comparison of immediate and long-term results of interventional procedures (PTCA–stenting) guided by angiography or by ICUS (29,30). Because of the broad inclusion criteria, vessels with reference diameters between 2.2 and 4.6 mm were included. Among the 286 procedures, stenting was performed in 48% of cases, with exactly the same incidence in the group with and without ultrasound guidance. Despite the additional cost of the ultrasound catheter, the cost of treatment was lower in the ultrasound arm because IVUS guidance was associated with a better clinical and angiographic outcome. In particular, in the lesions treated with PTCA only, the restenosis rate in the ICUS-guided group was 28% versus 38% in the angiographically guided group ($p < .05$).

Our experience in Milan (31) uses some of the guidelines and endpoints defined by the previous studies but differed because the IVUS-guided PTCA strategy was addressed primarily to long lesions (>15 mm) and to lesions located in small vessels (<3.0-mm reference diameter). Balloon angioplasty was initially performed using an angiographically oversized balloon inflated until full balloon expansion was achieved, and then an IVUS examination was performed. IVUS success criteria were defined as the presence of a true minimal lumen area ≥ 5.5 mm² or of a minimal lumen cross-sectional area ≥ 50% of the vessel cross-sectional area at the lesion site.

Dissections were not considered a reason to cross over to stenting as long as the previous two criteria were fulfilled and TIMI 3 flow was present. If the criteria were not met, upsizing of the PTCA balloon was performed by selecting a balloon with a diameter equal to the lesion media-to-media diameter, taking into account balloon compliance. In case of vessel tapering,

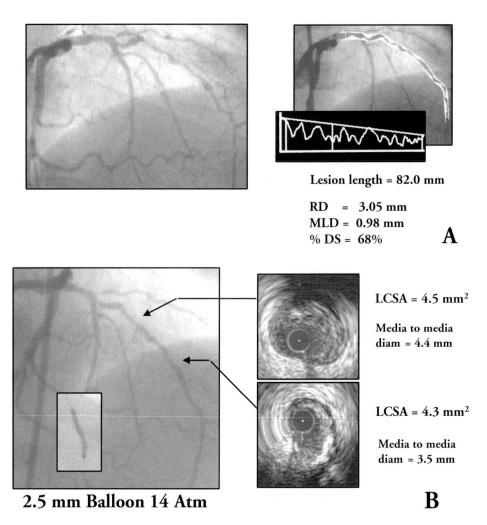

Lesion length = 82.0 mm

RD = 3.05 mm
MLD = 0.98 mm
% DS = 68%   **A**

LCSA = 4.5 mm²

Media to media
diam = 4.4 mm

LCSA = 4.3 mm²

Media to media
diam = 3.5 mm

2.5 mm Balloon 14 Atm   **B**

FIG. 13.3. A: Quantitative angiographic measurements of a long lesion of the mid-distal segment of the left anterior descending coronary artery, with a total length of the stenosis of 8.2 cm and a progressive vessel tapering, with average reference diameter (*RD*) of 3.05 mm, minimum lumen diameter (*MLD*) of 0.98 mm, and percent diameter stenosis (*DS*) of 68%. **B:** After balloon dilatation with a 30-mm-long, 2.5-mm, semicompliant balloon at 14 atm, multiple dissections are evident angiographically. Intracoronary ultrasound **(right panels)** shows a severe residual lumen narrowing (lumen cross-sectional area [*LCSA*], 4.5 mm²), with a vessel diameter media-to-media of 4.4 and 3.5 in the middle and distal segment, respectively. *(Figure continues.)*

regular (20 mm) or short balloons were used to avoid overstretching of the distal vessel. If after high-pressure dilatation (14.5 ± 3.8 atm) with oversized balloon (balloon-to-vessel ratio, 1.29 ± 0.23) the lumen gain was still insufficient and the ultrasound criteria of optimal PTCA were not met, stent implantation was performed using a slotted-tube or modular stent implanted focally at the site where IVUS showed focal recoil (Fig.

13.3). A total of 54 lesions underwent balloon angioplasty alone, while 55 lesions underwent balloon angioplasty and spot stenting. The operator was required to select the shortest stent necessary to cover the segment of severe residual lumen narrowing, but still a total stent length of 19 mm was used. Type B2 and C lesions were present in 75 cases (58% of the total cohort), but type C lesions were more common in the group

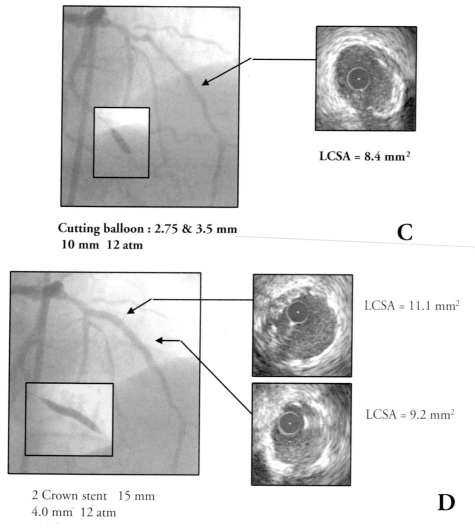

LCSA = 8.4 mm²

Cutting balloon : 2.75 & 3.5 mm
10 mm 12 atm

C

LCSA = 11.1 mm²

LCSA = 9.2 mm²

2 Crown stent   15 mm
4.0 mm   12 atm

D

FIG. 13.3. *Continued.* **C:** The inflation of a cutting balloon 2.75 mm in the distal vessel segment and 3.5 mm in the middle segment achieves a satisfactory result in the distal segment, but severe residual narrowing and large dissections are observed in the middle segment. **D:** Angiographic and ultrasound results after deployment of two 15-mm stents in the middle segment, using a 4-mm balloon inflated at 12 atm.

requiring stent implantation (49% vs. 26%, $p < .04$). Fluoroscopically visible calcification, present in 33 lesions, was also more common in the group undergoing spot stenting ($p < .03$). The final percent DS was 19% $\pm$ 14% in the PTCA group and 2% $\pm$ 13% in the spot-stenting group ($p < .01$), with angiographically visible dissections in 55% of the lesions, without differences between the two groups. Clinical success was achieved in 68 of 71 patients (96%), with procedural complications observed in five patients (one vessel rupture after high-pressure stent implantation, requiring open heart surgery; two patients with Q-wave; and two patients with non–Q-wave myocardial infarction). One patient in the spot-stenting group had subacute thrombosis, and one patient in the optimal PTCA group had sudden death 2 weeks after treatment. At 5 months' clinical follow-up, the cumulative incidence of major cardiac events (death, Q-wave myocardial infarction, target-lesion revascularization) was 28%, with an angiographic restenosis rate ($\geq$50% DS) of 27%.

A common limitation of all of these studies is the absence of a control group treated with conventional stenting (lesion covered from proximal normal to distal normal reference segment). These preliminary results from different centers, however, suggest that the procedural success is higher than the success obtained with conventional PTCA in high-risk lesion subsets (32,33) and, with the application of stents when needed, similar to the success of elective stenting. The fear of an increased risk of acute complications due to the oversized balloons was not confirmed by these initial observations. More difficult is the assessment of the adequacy of medium-term results and especially of the need for target-lesion revascularization and of angiographic restenosis. Although the percentages in the IVUS-guided PTCA patients may appear quite high at first glance, in small vessels and long lesions poor results were observed also after elective ultrasound-guided stent implantation.

INTRACORONARY DOPPLER DURING BALLOON ANGIOPLASTY

Intracoronary Doppler is an appealing alternative to ICUS imaging because this technique can precisely determine the functional severity of the residual coronary stenosis and can be easily integrated in a standard interventional procedure. In the multicenter DEBATE I (34) and II (35) and DESTINI studies (36) (1,600 patients in total), testing the usefulness of intracoronary Doppler during balloon angioplasty, the Doppler guidewire could be used as primary wire to cross the stenosis and advance the balloon or the stent in the great majority of patients.

Balloon angioplasty improves the flow velocity parameters (37–41), but an incomplete normalization is observed in most patients, often despite a good angiographic result. Hemodynamic changes during the procedure, microembolization, or transient or persistent changes of the distal microvascular response may explain part of this discrepancy, as indicated by the late normalization in some lesions (42,43). In other cases, however, the persistent abnormal flow response reflects persistent abnormalities in vessel conductance. The multicenter DEBATE study (Doppler Endpoint Balloon Angioplasty Europe) (34) has shown that impairment in flow reserve after PTCA is associated with a higher incidence of persistence or recurrence of angina, or of a positive exercise test at 1 month and of target lesion revascularization at 6 months. The combination of an optimal angiographic result (<35% DS) and of a flow reserve >2.5 was associated with a favorable clinical outcome at 6 months (16% incidence of major adverse cardiac events [MACEs]). Based on these observations, three independent studies (35,36,44) have randomized patients to elective stenting or a strategy of balloon angioplasty and provisional stenting according to the adequacy of the Doppler and quantitative angiographic measurements after PTCA. The differences in inclusion criteria (single-lesion–single-stent treatment in FROST [French Optimal Stent trial] [44] and DEBATE II [35]; multivessel–multilesions deployment of multiple stents in DESTINI [36]) and in Doppler cutoff criteria (coronary flow reserve [CFR] > 2.0 in DESTINI, >2.2 in FROST, >2.5 in DEBATE II), make these studies highly complementary in addressing the problem of the use of intracoronary Doppler to select the indications to stent implantation.

The largest of these studies is the DESTINI

trial (Doppler Endpoints Stent International Investigation) (36), a randomized study, carried out in 26 centers in Europe, Canada, Australia, Japan, and Korea, and in 36 centers in the United States. At the time enrollment was completed (March 1988), 731 patients were treated and half of them randomized to receive elective stent implantation, using slotted tubular stents in 90% of lesions (mainly Palmaz-Schatz [Johnson and Johnson International Systems, Warren, NJ] and NIR [Scimed, Maple Grove, MN] stents). In the remaining patients randomized to guided angioplasty, all of the following endpoints had to be met: final residual DS, <35%; final CFR measured with a Doppler guidewire distal to the stenosis, >2.0; and absence of dissections at risk of abrupt closure (Figs. 13.4 and 13.5). If all of these criteria were not met, even after additional

dilatation with larger balloons or higher balloon-inflation pressure, the investigators were allowed to perform coronary stent implantation. Because the goal of the study was to evaluate the impact of this strategy on the every-day patient population of a busy catheterization laboratory, the only inclusion criterion was the suitability of all the lesions under treatment for stent implantation. Exclusion criteria were the presence of chronic total occlusion; elective, planned Rotablator or directional atherectomy; recent (<48 hours) myocardial infarction or previous Q-wave myocardial infarction with a-dyskinesia in the territory of distribution of the artery to be treated; graft and ostial stenoses; and second restenosis. Despite these broad inclusion criteria, multivessel treatment was actually performed in 5% of patients, treating angiographically type

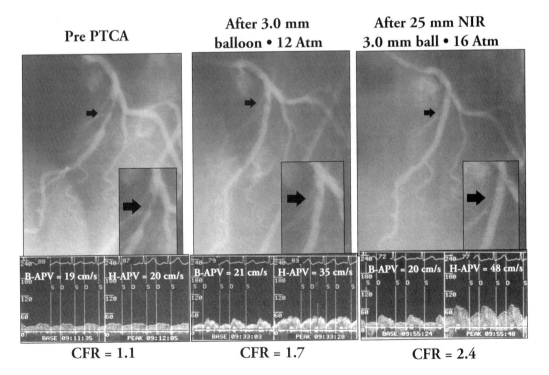

FIG. 13.4. Doppler-guided PTCA and stenting in the DESTINI study (35). **Left panel:** Angiogram showing severe stenosis of the proximal left anterior descending coronary artery (LAD), magnified in the inset. At the bottom, the corresponding Doppler measurements distal to the stenosis, showing absence of velocity increase after adenosine (CFR = 1.1). **Middle panel:** After PTCA, a good lumen improvement is obtained, with a persistent haziness at the treated site. Because an insufficient improvement in CFR was obtained (below 2.0), a stent was implanted. **Right panel:** After stent implantation, normalization of the angiogram and a further increase in CFR. B-APV and H-APV, baseline and hyperemic (after adenosine) time-averaged peak velocities, respectively.

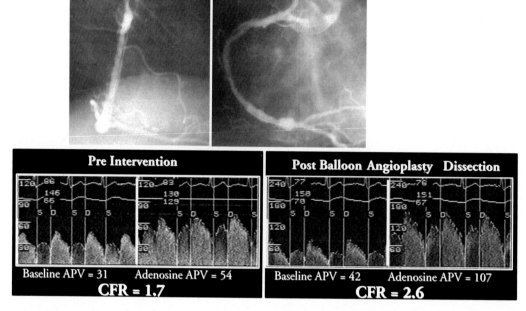

FIG. 13.5. Upper panels: Large dissection of the right coronary artery after dilatation with a 4-mm balloon, which was selected based on the ICUS measurements (media-to-media diameter). **Lower panels**: Note the increase in coronary flow reserve (*CFR*) from preintervention to the post-PTCA result shown above. APV, time-averaged peak velocity.

B2 or C lesions in 59% of cases, with an average lesion length and reference vessel diameter of 12.7 ± 4.2 mm and 3.07 ± 0.3 mm, respectively, similar to the results in the guided-PTCA and stent groups. Of the 386 lesions randomized to guided PTCA, all the predetermined endpoints could be achieved in 167 arteries (43%). The lesions treated with stent implantation had a larger final minimum luminal diameter (2.84 mm and 2.95 mm in the primary and conditional stenting groups, respectively, vs. 2.30 mm in the group treated with PTCA alone; $p < .00001$) and a lower final residual DS (8.8% in the stent groups vs. 26.2% in the group treated with PTCA only, $p < .00001$). At the time of preparation of this chapter, the 6-month follow-up reports of 551 patients (75%) were received and reviewed at the Core Laboratory in Milan. On an intention-to-treat analysis, the early and late cardiac events did not show significant differences between the two groups. The odds ratio (95% confidence intervals) for cumulative MACEs of the stent group versus the optimal

PTCA group was 0.97 (0.55 to 1.76). In particular, overall (PTCA and bypass graft operation) 6-month target-lesion revascularization involving the lesions initially treated was 14.9% in the PTCA group and 14.6% in the stent group (NS). A complete cost analysis was performed only for the US centers and showed a significantly lower catheterization laboratory cost in the guided PTCA than in the stent group ($5,848 vs. $6,269; $p < .05$), due to a lower use of balloons and stents per patient.

The preliminary results of the DESTINI study indicate that when optimal angiographic and physiologic endpoints are met after PTCA, the early and late clinical outcomes are equivalent to the outcome observed after elective stent implantation. In the PTCA group, however, a minority (43%) of patients could achieve the predetermined endpoints and the remaining patients ultimately received a stent. Despite the frequent need to cross over to stenting, initial cost analysis suggests that a provisional stenting strategy still has a lower cost than stenting all suitable lesions. In the most recent and the largest PTCA versus stent trial (BENESTENT II) a significantly lower incidence of major cardiac events and target-lesion revascularization at 6 months in the stent group was observed (45). The conflicting result of the DESTINI trial (almost perfect equivalency of treatment outcome in both groups) can be explained by the implantation of stents in all patients not meeting predetermined angiographic and velocity criteria (57% of patients stented) and not only as bail-out (13% in BENESTENT II). A second explanation can be the inclusion of bifurcation and longer lesions (average lesion length of 12.5 mm in DESTINI and of 8.2 mm in BENESTENT II), which may receive a smaller benefit from stenting.

The FROST study, with a design similar to that of DESTINI but with a smaller sample size (250 patients), showed a lower rate of cross-over to stenting (49.5%), probably due to the more favorable lesion characteristics (44). In FROST, *de novo* lesions treatable with 15-mm-long Palmaz-Schatz 153 stents in >3.0-mm native vessels were enrolled, and only single-vessel treatment was allowed. The similar incidence of repeat revascularization and MACEs was explained also by the results of the quantitative angiographic analysis of the lesions at the compulsory 6-month angiographic follow-up. With 80% of lesions analyzed, a similar minimum lumen diameter was observed in the stent and PTCA groups, with a nonsignificant trend toward a higher binary restenosis rate (>50% DS at follow-up) in the PTCA group. The DEBATE II trial (35), with a total number of patients studied of more than 600, has a more complex design, with a double-randomization process in order to assess, in the group treated with PTCA, the additional value of stent implantation both in the group with optimal angiographic and Doppler measurements (DS < 35%, CFR > 2.5) and in the group with more severe residual stenosis and CFR > 2.5. Preliminary data indicate a significant reduction of MACE in the group with suboptimal PTCA randomized to stenting. The group reaching the physiologic and anatomic endpoints after PTCA had a very low incidence of MACE (8%), similar to the incidence observed in the primary stent group. Preliminary data, however, suggest a further reduction to 2% when a stent is implanted in these patients (difference, nonstatistically significant).

Despite the high expectation that pressure-based indices, unaffected by the changing hemodynamic conditions during interventions, overcome the limitations of intracoronary Doppler and yield better prognostic value of the long-term clinical outcome after PTCA (46,47), the ''unfriendly'' mechanical characteristics of the first-generation pressure wires limited their application to experienced centers and precluded large multicenter trials. Based on this initial clinical experience, a measurement of fractional flow reserve (FFR) >0.90 has been proposed as a cutoff result after PTCA, below which stent implantation should be performed (48).

CONCLUSIONS

The final goal of interventional cardiology is not to cover all significant lesions with stents, but to achieve the most complete and long-lasting relief of patients symptoms and reduction of cardiac adverse events with whatever device is more effective. Conventional balloon dilatation with angiographic guidance is inferior to stent implantation for many indications (6–13), suggesting that different techniques must be used to improve angioplasty results. The advantage of IVUS over intracoronary Doppler is that the former technique can be used not only to confirm the adequacy of the lumen increase after PTCA, but also to select the appropriate balloon size and safely guide it to the achievement of a larger lumen. In case a stent is needed, the same device (IVUS) can be used to optimize the stent expansion and apposition. Limitations of IVUS, however, include the need of a separate insertion of a dedicated, expensive catheter and the absence of firm endpoints, confirmed by large outcome studies. Intracoronary Doppler guidewires can be used as primary wires to perform balloon dilatation and stent implantation, reducing the additional cost and duration of the procedure. CFR after myocardial infarction or in conditions of impaired microvascular response can be misleading, explaining the high incidence of patients in whom CFR remains low despite optimal reconstruction of the vessel lumen with coronary stents. The improved mechanical characteristics and signal reliability of the pressure wires can overcome these limitations, but the experience with FFR after PTCA is still insufficient to draw the firm conclusions of the trial conducted with intracoronary Doppler. In these trials, intracoronary Doppler has always been used in combination with quantitative angiography, although poor angiographic result and low CFR are often associated in the same patient. In clinical practice, there is no need to evaluate a second parameter when one of the two is clearly abnormal after angioplasty, limiting the need of additional confirmation with Doppler or IVUS in those patients with angiographic success. The results of the most recent trials of provisional stenting indicate that the current practice of elective stent implantation of all suitable lesions is not justified (35,36,44). The reasons for this practice is that elective stenting is often easier than a thorough examination of the angiographic, ultrasound, and/or Doppler characteristics of the lesion, and that the decreasing cost of stents makes the economical benefit of PTCA alone smaller. Furthermore, suboptimal PTCA results, in any event, require stent implantation in a large percentage of patients and limit the advantage of a "provisional" stent strategy. These criticisms are valid, especially for BENESTENT-like lesions, because in short lesions the process of restenosis is benign after both PTCA and stenting (49). When longer lesions are treated, the risk is the development of diffuse in-stent intimal hyperplasia, a type of restenosis far more difficult to be treated due to the inadequacy of our current techniques of plaque debulking inside stents and the possible preclusion of surgical alternatives. It is in this setting that the use of new intracoronary techniques can lead to a more careful and complete exploitation of all the potential of PTCA.

REFERENCES

1. Serruys PW, Unger F, van Herwerden L, et al., on behalf of the ARTS Investigators. Arterial revascularization therapy study: the ARTS study, a randomized trial of bypass surgery versus stenting in multivessel disease. *Eur Heart J* 1998;19:137(abst).

2. Baldus S, Reimers J, Kuck KH, et al. The GABI-2 trial: a multicenter prospective study in patients with multivessel disease undergoing percutaneous coronary angioplasty. *Eur Heart J* 1998;19:136(abst).

3. Karrillon GJ, Morice MC, Benveniste E, et al. Intracoronary stent implantation without ultrasound guidance and with replacement of conventional anticoagulation by antiplatelet therapy. Thirty-day clinical outcome of the French Multicenter Registry. *Circulation* 1996;94: 1519–1527.

4. Colombo A, Hall P, Nakamura S, et al. Intracoronary stenting without anticoagulation accomplished with intravascular ultrasound guidance. *Circulation* 1995;91: 1676–1688.

5. Schoemig, Schuhlen H, Blasini R, et al. Prospective randomized trial of antiplatelet vs anticoagulation treatment after intracoronary Palmaz-Schatz stent placement—6 months follow-up. *N Engl J Med* 1996;334:1084–1089.

6. Serruys PW, de Jaegere P, Kiemeneij, et al., on behalf of the Benestent Study Group. A comparison of balloon-expandable stent implantation with balloon angioplasty in patients with coronary artery disease. *N Engl J Med* 1994;331:489–495.

7. Fischman DL, Leon MB, Baim DS, et al. A randomized comparison of coronary-stent placement and balloon angioplasty in the treatment of coronary artery disease. *N Engl J Med* 1994;331:496–501.

8. Masotti M, Serra A, Fernandez-Aviles, et al. Stent versus angioplasty restenosis trial (START). Angiographic results at 6 months follow-up. *Eur Heart J* 1996;17: 120(abst).

9. Penn IM, Ricci DR, Almond DG, et al. Coronary artery stenting reduces restenosis: final results from the Trial of Angioplasty and Stents in Canada (TASC-1). *Circulation* 1995;92:I-279(abst).

10. Erbel R, Haude M, Hopp H, et al., on behalf of the REST study group (Restenosis Stent (REST) study). Randomized trial comparing stenting and balloon angioplasty for treatment of restenosis after balloon angioplasty. *J Am Coll Cardiol* 1996;27:139A(abst).

11. Savage MP, Douglas JS, Fischman DL, et al., for the Saphenous Vein De Novo Trial Investigators (SAVED). Stent placement compared with angioplasty for obstructed coronary bypass grafts. *N Engl J Med* 1997 337: 740–747.

12. Sirnes PA, Golf S, Myreng Y, et al. Stenting in chronic total coronary occlusion (SICCO): a multicenter randomized controlled trial of adding stent implantation after successful angioplasty. *J Am Coll Cardiol* 1996; 28:1444–1451.

13. Eeckhout E, Goy JJ, Stajffer JC, et al. Endoluminal stenting of narrowed saphenous vein grafts: long-term clinical and angiographic follow-up. *Cathet Cardiovasc Diagn* 1994;32:139–146.

14. van den Brand M, on behalf of the European Survey Group. Overview of stent price differences in 21 countries. *Eur Heart J* 1998;19:501(abst).

15. Glagov S, Weisenberg E, Zarins CK, et al. Compensatory enlargement of human atherosclerotic coronary arteries. *N Engl J Med* 1986;316:1371–1375.

16. Ge J, Erbel R., Zamorano J, et al. Coronary artery remodeling in atherosclerotic disease: an intravascular ultrasonic study in vivo. *Coron Artery Dis* 1993;4: 981–986.

17. Hermiller JB, Tenaglia AN, Kisslo KB, et al. In vivo

validation of compensatory enlargement of atherosclerotic coronary arteries. *Am J Cardiol* 1993;71:665–668.

18. Gerber TC, Erbel R, George G, Ge J, Rupprecht HJ, Meyer J. Extent of atherosclerosis and remodeling of the left main coronary artery determined by intravascular ultrasound. *Am J Cardiol* 1993;73:666–671.

19. Di Mario C, Hermans W, Serruys PW. Calibration using the catheter as a scaling device: importance of filming the catheter not filled with contrast medium. *Am J Cardiol* 1992;69:1377–1379.

20. Lee DY, Eigler N, Nishioka T, Tabak SW, Forrester JS, Siegel RJ. Effect of intracoronary imaging on clinical decision making. *Am Heart J* 1995;129:1084–1093.

21. Mintz GS, Pichard AD, Kovach JA, Leon MJ. Impact of preintervention intravascular ultrasound imaging on transcatheter treatment strategies in coronary artery disease. *Am J Cardiol* 1994;73:423–430.

22. Hoffmann R, Mintz GS, Popma JJ, et al. Treatment of calcified coronary lesions with Palmaz-Schatz stents. An intravascular ultrasound study. *Eur Heart J* 1998; 19:1224–1231.

23. Moussa I, Di Mario C, Moses J, et al. Coronary stenting after rotational atherectomy in calcified and complex lesions. *Circulation* 1997;96:128–136.

24. Stone GW, Hodgson JMcB, St. Goar FG, et al., for the Clinical Outcome with Ultrasound Trial (CLOUT) Investigators. Improved procedural results of coronary angioplasty with intravascular ultrasound guided balloon sizing. *Circulation* 1997;95:2044–2052.

25. Nakamura S, Colombo A, Gaglione A, et al. Intracoronary ultrasound observations during stent implantation. *Circulation* 1994;89:2026–2034.

26. Goldberg SL, Colombo A, Nakamura S, et al. Benefit of intracoronary ultrasound in the deployment of Palmaz-Schatz stents. *J Am Coll Cardiol* 1994;24:996–1003.

27. Abizaid A, Pichard AD, Calabuig JN, et al. Can aggressive ultrasound guided balloon angioplasty produce stent-like results? *Circulation* 1997;96:I-582(abst).

28. Haase KH, Athanasiadis A, Mahrholdt H, Treusch AW, Wullen B, Munoz CJ. Acute and 1 year follow-up results after vessel size adapted PTCA using intracoronary ultrasound. *Circulation* 1997;96:I-194(abst).

29. Hodgson McJ, Roskamm H, Frey AW. Target lesion revascularization reduced after ultrasound guided interventions: findings after 6 month follow-up from the Strategy of ICUS guided PTCA and Stenting trial (SIPS). *Circulation* 1997;96:I-582(abst).

30. Frey AW, Grove A, Suciu A, Doerfer K, Hodgson McJ. Reduction of restenosis rate after ICUS guided interventions: QCA results of the SIPS study. *Eur Heart J* 1998; 19:136(abst).

31. Di Mario C, DeGregorio J, Moussa I, et al. Optimal balloon angioplasty. In: Reiber JHC, van der Wall EE, eds. *What's new in cardiovascular imaging?* Dordrecht: Kluwer Academic Publishers, 1998:159–169.

32. Reifart N, Vandormael M, Krajcar M, et al. Randomized comparison of angioplasty of complex coronary lesions at single center. Excimer laser, rotational atherectomy and balloon comparison (ERBAC) study. *Circulation* 1997;96:91–98.

33. Erbel R, Dill T, Dietz U, et al. A randomized study of high speed rotational atherectomy and percutaneous transluminal coronary angioplasty in patients with complex coronary artery stenoses (COBRA study). *Circulation* 1997;I-80(abst).

34. Serruys PW, Di Mario C, Piek J, et al. Prognostic value of intracoronary flow velocity and diameter stenosis in assessing the short and long term outcome of coronary balloon angioplasty. The DEBATE Study (Doppler End-points Balloon Angioplasty Trial Europe). *Circulation* 1997;96:3369–3377.

35. Serruys PW, de Bruyne B, de Sousa JE, et al., on behalf of the DEBATE II Investigators. DEBATE II: a randomized study to evaluate the need of additional stenting after guided balloon angioplasty. *Eur Heart J* 1998;19: 567(abst).

36. Di Mario C, Moses J, Muramatsu T, et al., on the behalf of the DESTINI-CRF Study Group. Multicenter randomized comparison of primary stenting vs balloon angioplasty optimized by QCA and intracoronary Doppler: procedural results in 580 patients. *Eur Heart J* 1998; 19:567(abst).

37. Segal J, Kern MJ, Scott NA. Alteration of phasic coronary artery flow velocity in human during percutaneous coronary angioplasty. *J Am Coll Cardiol* 1992;20: 276–286.

38. Ofili EO, Kern MJ, Labovitz AJ, et al. Analysis of coronary blood flow velocity dynamics in angiographically normal and stenosed arteries before and after endolumen enlargement by angioplasty. *J Am Coll Cardiol* 1993; 21:308–316.

39. Heller LI, Silver KH, Vilegas BJ, Balcom SH, Weiner BH. Blood flow velocity in the right coronary artery: assessment before and after angioplasty. *J Am Coll Cardiol* 1994;24:1012–1017.

40. Donohue TJ, Kern MJ, Aguirre FV, Ofili EO. Assessing the hemodynamic significance of coronary artery stenosis: analysis of translesional pressure-flow velocity relationship in patients. *J Am Coll Cardiol* 1993;22: 449–458.

41. Serruys PW, Di Mario C, Meneveau N, et al. Intracoronary pressure and flow velocity from sensor tip guidewires. A new methodological comprehensive approach for the assessment of coronary hemodynamics before and after interventions. *Am J Cardiol* 1993;71: 41D–53D.

42. Wilson RF, Johnson MR, Marcus ML, et al. The effect of coronary angioplasty on coronary blood flow reserve. *Circulation* 1988;71:873–885.

43. Piek JJ, Boersma E, Serruys PW, on behalf of the DEBATE Investigators Group. The immediate and long-term effect of balloon coronary angioplasty on the distal coronary flow velocity reserve. *Eur Heart J* 1998;19: 566.

44. Steg PG, on the behalf of the FROG Study Group. A multicenter randomized trial comparing systematic stenting to provisional stenting guided by angiography and coronary flow reserve: final results. *Eur Heart J* 1998;19:567(abst).

45. Serruys PW, van Hout B, Bonnier H, et al., on behalf of the BENESTENT II Study Group. Effectiveness, cost and cost-effectiveness of a strategy of elective stenting compared to a strategy of balloon angioplasty allowing bailout stenting in patients with coronary artery disease. *Lancet* 1998 (*in press*).

46. Pijls NHJ, van Son JAM, Kirkeeide RL, Bruyne BD, Gould KL. Experimental basis of determining maximum coronary, myocardial, and collateral blood flow by pressure measurements for assessing functional stenosis se-

verity before and after percutaneous transluminal coronary angioplasty. *Circulation* 1993;86:1354–1367.

47. Pijls NHJ, De Bruyne B, Peels K, et al. Measurement of fractional flow reserve to assess the functional severity of coronary-artery stenoses. *N Engl J Med* 1996;334:1703–1708.

48. Pijls NHJ, Bech GJW, De Bruyne B, et al. Prognostic

value of pressure derived coronary flow reserve to predict restenosis after regular balloon angioplasty. *Circulation* 1997;96:I-649.

49. Reimers B, Moussa I, Akiyama T, et al. Long-term clinical follow-up after successful repeat percutaneous intervention for in-stent restenosis. *J Am Coll Cardiol* 1997;30:186–192.

B. Primary Stenting in Acute Myocardial Infarction

Mandeep Singh

SMH Cardiac Catheterization Laboratory, Mayo Clinic, Rochester, Minnesota 55905

It has been demonstrated unequivocally that time to reperfusion after acute myocardial infarction (AMI) is the single important determinant of myocardial salvage and survival. Traditionally, thrombolytic therapy has been used to achieve this goal. This mode of therapy has been tested in over 250,000 AMI patients with good success rates. There are, however, some limitations to the use of thrombolytic therapy: TIMI 3 flows are achieved in only 50% to 60% of cases; recurrent ischemia or reinfarction is not infrequent; and complications such as hemorrhagic strokes associated with the use of thrombolytic drugs can be life threatening. This has paved the way for primary angioplasty in the setting of AMI. A total of ten randomized trials have been performed comparing thrombolytic therapy with angioplasty in AMI. There were inherent limitations and heterogeneity in the design of trials, number of patients enrolled, dose and duration of heparin given, and the type of thrombolytic therapy administered. Despite these limitations, a meta-analysis documented

significant improvement in the mortality, reinfarction, stroke, and composite endpoints (Table 13.1) (1), all in favor of primary angioplasty. In the largest trial, GUSTO IIb, which included 1,138 patients with AMI randomized to percutaneous transluminal coronary angioplasty (PTCA) and tissue plasminogen activator (tPA), there was significant improvement in the composite endpoint of death, MI, and stroke in the PTCA arm, as compared with thrombolytic arm. (9.6% vs. 13.7%, $p = .033$) (2).

Although primary PTCA results in improved initial outcomes compared with lytic therapy, it is not without problems. These include (Table 13.2) vessel recoil, intimal disruption and consequent platelet activation, and subsequent restenosis. The recurrent ischemia in 10% to 15% of patients and reinfarction in 2% to 5% may in part nullify the short-term gains with PTCA in AMI. In the GUSTO IIb trial, there was no difference in the outcome at 6 months between the two strategies. The restenosis rates after PTCA in AMI have been reported in the range of 40%

TABLE 13.1. *Primary PTCA versus thrombolytic therapy (1)*

Results	PTCA *n* = 1,290 (%)	Thrombolysis *n* = 1,316 (%)	*p* value
Mortality	57 (4.4%)	86 (6.5%)	.02
Mortality + reinfarction	94 (7.2%)	156 (11.9%)	<.001
Total stroke	9 (0.7%)	26 (2.0%)	.007
Hemorrhagic stroke	1 (0.1%)	15 (1.1%)	<.001

TABLE 13.2. *Problems with primary angioplasty*

1. Vessel recoil
2. High restenosis (40%–45%)
3. Intimal disruption and platelet activation
4. High success rates in randomized trials may not be representative at the community level.
5. Target-lesion revascularization: 20%

to 50% (3). This high incidence of restenosis has been associated in some patients with clinical reinfarction. Another problem is that the reported randomized trials may not be representative of the community as a whole.

Stents have been shown to reduce the angiographic and clinical restenosis, as compared with PTCA in elective interventions (4,5). There was an initial apprehension about using a metallic prosthesis in the presence of thrombus-containing lesions. This was the main reason why stents were not used in AMI. With the improvement in stent designs and better poststent antiplatelet regimens, the risks of subacute thrombosis have decreased. Initially there were a few encouraging case reports and small observational studies on the feasibility of stents in the setting of AMI. This led to a spate of trials and registries comparing the efficacy of stents with balloon angioplasty.

In the past year, there have been a number of single-institution studies or multicenter, randomized trials comparing PTCA and primary stenting (6–10) (Tables 13.3 and 13.4). The results of these studies show high procedural success rates (>90%). The in-hospital mortality was lower in the stent group. It did not reach statistical significance in any of the studies mentioned, except in the study reported from Massachusetts General Hospital (10). In this study, there was no death in the stent arm, but the mortality in the PTCA group was very high (11%). This was a nonrandomized, single-institution experience that included a higher risk population in the PTCA group. In the other reported studies, mortality in both groups has been very low. These studies had small numbers and were not powered to detect mortality differences between the two groups. Further, the enrollment of a selected low-risk population after excluding 23% to 50% of patients could have contributed to the low mortality rates. Similarly, reinfarction rates were lower in the stent group. The main difference in the early time period was significantly less recurrent ischemia and less need for target-lesion revascularization in the patients with AMI assigned to the stent arm.

On follow-up, the patients in the stent arm

TABLE 13.3. *Studies and trials on primary stenting published in 1998*

	PAMI stent (6a, 6b)		GRAMI (7)		FRESCO (8)		ZWOLLE (9)		Mahdi et al. (10)	
	PTCA	Stent	PTCA	Stent	PTCA	Stent	PTCA	Stent	PTCA	Stent
Number of patients	72	240	52	52	75	75	115	112	94	53
Study design	Prospective multicenter study		Multicenter randomized trial		Randomization to stent after optimal balloon result, residual stenosis < 30% with TIMI 3 flow		Single-center randomized trial		Single-center, nonrandomized trial	
Primary endpoint	Pilot study to show feasibility of stents in AMI		To compare 30-day composite endpoint and TIMI 3 flow at discharge		Composite clinical endpoints within 6 mo		Clinical endpoints (e.g., death, reinfarction, repeat angioplasty, or emergency bypass surgery)		Immediate and long-term outcome	
Success rates	98%		94.2%	98%	99% before randomization		96%	98%	91.5%	94%

TABLE 13.4. *Clinical and angiographic outcome of patients in primary stenting trials*

	PAMI stent		GRAMI		FRESCO		ZWOLLE		Mahdi et al.	
	PTCA	Stent	PTCA	Stent	PTCA	Stent	PTCA	Stent	PTCA	Stent
Early Events										
(0–30 days)										
Death	0	2 (0.8%)	4 (7.6%)	2 (3.8%)	0	0	3 (3%)	2 (2%)	10 (11%)	0[a]
Reinfarction	0									0 (abrupt
		4 (1.7%)	4 (7.6%)	0	2	0	5 (4%)	1 (1%)	7 (8%)	closure)
Recurrent ischemia	2 (2.9%)	9 (3.2%)	6 (11.5%)	0[a]	11 (15%)	2 (3%)[a]	—	—	—	—
Repeat TLR	5 (6.9%)	1 (0.4%)[a]	5 (9.5%)	1 (1.9%)	9	1[a]	5 (4%)	1 (1%)	13 (14%)	0
Late Events										
TLR at 6 mo–1 yr	—	26 (11%)	21%	14%	10 (16%)	5 (7%)[a]	19	4[a]	29 (37%)	11 (21%)[a]
Event-free survival	—	—	65%	83%[a]	68%	87%[a]	80%	95%[a]	44%	80%
Restenosis	—	27 (5%)	—	—	43%	17%	—	—	—	

[a] $p \le .05$.
TLR, target lesion revascularization.

had significantly less TLR, and event-free survival was improved. Multivariate analysis of predictors of adverse cardiac events included smaller postprocedure minimum lumen diameter (MLD) and assignment to the balloon arm strategy (9). The MLD stent placement was significantly higher as compared with balloon angioplasty (Table 13.5). The restenosis rates in the FRESCO study were 17% in the stent groups versus 43% in the PTCA group (8). Overall, it appears that primary stenting in AMI is a better strategy than is balloon angioplasty alone.

ADVANTAGES OF PRIMARY STENTING IN AMI OVER PRIMARY PTCA

1. Larger postprocedure MLD
2. Lesser vessel recoil
3. Decrease in dissection and abrupt closures
4. Reduced reischemia
5. Less target-lesion revascularization and restenosis

Currently, the PAMI Heparin-Coated Stent trial has enrolled 900 patients from 65 centers to document the effect of heparin-coated stents versus balloon angioplasty. In the reported results, there was a slight increase in mortality in the stent arm, but this was not statistically significant. The incidence of target-vessel revascularization, however, was lower in the stent arm. The CADILLAC trial currently is enrolling patients in a 2 × 2 factorial design. It is enrolling 2,000 patients randomized to primary PTCA alone, PTCA plus abciximab, primary stenting alone, or stenting plus abciximab. The results of this trial will highlight the role of abciximab as an adjunct to either primary PTCA or primary stenting.

The management of AMI continues to evolve rapidly. In selected patients, stents are an attractive option and can decrease the incidence of target-vessel revascularization compared with conventional PTCA, as well as decrease the incidence of restenosis. Problem areas and patient

TABLE 13.5. *Quantitative angiographic results and TIMI flow rates in primary angioplasty and primary stent groups*

QCA	PAMI stent	GRAMI	FRESCO	ZWOLLE	Mahdi et al.
Pre MLD					
PTCA	0.3 ± 0.6	0.3 ± 0.4	—	0.3 ± 0.5	0.2 ± 0.4
Stent	0.2 ± 0.4	0.4 ± 0.4	—	0.2 ± 0.4	0.5 ± 0.5[a]
Post MLD					
PTCA	1.8 ± 0.6	2.33 ± 0.6	3.0 ± 0.4	2.1 ± 0.4	1.9 ± 0.6
Stent	2.7 ± 0.5[a]	2.6 ± 0.6[a]	3.3 ± 0.5[a]	2.5 ± 0.3[a]	2.5 ± 0.5[a]
Residual DS					
PTCA	33 ± 14	—	5 ± 8	28.8 ± 9.1	31 ± 15
Stent	12 ± 16[a]	—	−3 ± 12[a]	17.9 ± 6.8[a]	21 ± 13[a]

[a] $p \le .05$.
MLD, minimal lumen diameter; DS, diameter stenosis.

groups remain. These include patients arriving late after the onset of symptoms, when the potential for myocardial salvage is low, small vessels, diffuse disease, and bifurcation lesions in the infarct-related artery. The future will involve continued efforts to optimize the outcome in these high-risk patients.

REFERENCES

1. Weaver WD, Simes RJ, Betriu A, et al. Comparison of primary coronary angioplasty and intravenous thrombolytic therapy for acute myocardial infarction, a quantitative review. *JAMA* 1997;278:2093–2098.
2. The Global Use of Strategies To Open Occluded Coronary Arteries in Acute Coronary Syndromes (GUSTO IIb) Angioplasty Substudy Investigators. A clinical trial comparing primary angioplasty with tissue plasminogen activator for acute myocardial infarction. *N Engl J Med* 1997;336:1621–1628.
3. Nakagawa Y, Iwasaki Y, Kimura T, et al. Serial angiographic follow-up after successful direct angioplasty for acute myocardial infarction. *Am J Cardiol* 1996;78: 980–984.
4. Serruys PW, de Jaegere P, Kiemeneij F, et al., for the BENESTENT group. A comparison of balloon expandable stent implantation with balloon angioplasty in the treatment of coronary artery disease. *N Engl J Med* 1994;331:489–495.
5. Fischman DL, Leon MB, Baim DS, et al., for the Stent Restenosis Study Investigators. A randomized comparison of coronary stent placement and balloon angioplasty in the treatment of coronary artery disease. *N Engl J Med* 1994;331:496–501.
6a. Stone GW, Brodie BR, Griffin JJ, et al. Prospective multicenter study of the safety and feasibility of primary stenting in acute myocardial infarction, in-hospital and 30 day results of the PAMI Stent Pilot Trial. *J Am Coll Cardiol* 1998;31:23–30.
6b. Stone GW, Brodie BR, Griffin JJ, et al. Clinical and angiographic follow-up after primary stenting in acute myocardial infarction: The PAMI Stent Pilot Trial. *Circulation* 1999;99:1548–1554.
7. Rodriguez A, Bernardi V, Fernandez M, et al. In-hospital and late results of coronary stents versus conventional balloon angioplasty in acute myocardial infarction (GRAMI trial). *Am J Cardiol* 1998;81:1286–1291.
8. Antoniucci D, Santoro GM, Bolognese L, Valenti R, Trapani M, Fazzini PF. A clinical trial comparing primary stenting of the infarct related artery with optimal primary angioplasty for acute myocardial infarction, results from the Florence Randomized Elective Stenting in Acute Coronary Occlusions (FRESCO) Trial. *J Am Coll Cardiol* 1998;31:1234–1239.
9. Suryapranata H, van't Hof AWJ, Hoorntje JCA, deBoer MJ, Zijlstra F. Randomized comparison of coronary stenting with balloon angioplasty in selected patients with acute myocardial infarction. *Circulation* 1998;97: 2502–2505.
10. Mahdi NA, Lopez J, Leon M, et al. Comparison of primary coronary stenting to primary balloon angioplasty with stent bailout for the treatment of patients with acute myocardial infarction. *Am J Cardiol* 1998;81:957–963.

14

The Restenotic Lesion

A. The Restenotic Lesion

Michael Haude, Dietrich Baumgart, Junbo Ge, Thomas Konorza,
Christoph Altmann, and Raimund Erbel

*Division of Internal Medicine, Department of Cardiology, University-Gesamthochschule-Essen,
D-45122 Essen, Germany*

Since the introduction of percutaneous transluminal coronary angioplasty (PTCA) by Andreas Gruentzig more than 20 years ago (1), significant advances in catheter technology, guidewire-systems, adjunctive pharmacotherapy, new device technology, imaging modalities and, last but not least, in operator experience have led to a substantial improvement of the procedure early outcome. Procedural success usually is greater than 90% and overall in-hospital complications are rare (<5%) (2). Nevertheless, long-term outcome of PTCA continues to be limited by the restenotic process causing luminal renarrowing associated with or without angina complaints. These patients require additional revascularization procedures exposing the patients to additional risk and causing substantial health care expenditures. Over the last 2 decades, numerous attempts have been made to limit postinterventional restenosis. Although the complexity of this process has been elucidated more recently, complete understanding of the underlying mechanisms is not yet maintained.

DEFINITION

Because routine follow-up coronary angiography is not performed after coronary interventions, the results of noninvasive tests (stress ECG, Thallium-SPECT or SESTAMIBI, and/or stress echocardiography) are used in addition to patients' symptoms to define the indication for repeat coronary angiography. A restenotic lesion is a coronary luminal renarrowing after a previous coronary intervention, usually documented by repeat coronary angiography or by other intracoronary imaging modalities such as intravascular ultrasound imaging or coronary angioscopy. Different continuous or binary angiographic variables such as minimal luminal diameter or percent stenosis (Table 14.1) are applied to express angiographic restenosis (3,4,5). The most commonly used definition for clinical purposes is that of a more than 50% diameter stenosis at the previously treated vessel site while cumulative frequency curves of minimal luminal diameter before and after intervention and at repeat angiography allow the application of any linear definition of restenosis, which allows more effective comparisons between different interventions (6). Other parameters as the loss index, defined as the late lumen loss divided by the acute gain, more adequately reflect the morphologic extent of postinterventional vessel repair mechanisms causing restenosis (7).

INCIDENCE

The incidence of angiographic restenosis varies widely depending on the definition applied

TABLE 14.1. *Different angiographic definitions of restenosis*

EMORY	Diameter stenosis ≥50% at follow-up
NHLBI I	Increase in diameter stenosis ≥30% at follow-up compared to the postinterventional result
NHLBI II	Residual stenosis post intervention <50% increasing to diameter stenosis ≥70%
NHLBI III	Increase in diameter stenosis at follow-up to within 10% of the diameter stenosis before PTCA
NHLBI IV	More than 50% loss of the initial gain achieved after intervention
Rotterdam	Absolute lumen loss of more than 0.72 mm at follow-up

NHLBI, National Heart, Lung, and Blood Institute; PTCA, percutaneous transluminal coronary angioplasty.

to the lesion previously treated, and the device used during the initial intervention.

Based on the most frequently applied dichotomous definition of a more than 50% diameter stenosis at the site of intervention at follow-up, documented by quantitative coronary angiography, the restenosis rate after PTCA of *de novo* stenoses is reported to range between 20% and 45%, while substantially higher restenosis rates are reported for PTCA of chronic total occlusions, vein graft stenoses, and different subsets of morphologic stenosis criteria (8).

Numerous attempts have been made to limit restenosis by pharmacological interventions. Almost all of them failed, including corticosteroids, cytostatic agents, calcium channel blockers, lipid lowering agents, ACE inhibitors, low molecular weight heparin, high dose vitamin E, and somatostatin analogues (9). Glycoprotein IIb/IIIa receptor blockers provide a reduction in clinical restenosis (10), but angiographic restenosis was not evaluated so far, while probucol (11) was shown to reduce angiographic restenosis as was also suggested for tranilast (12). Nevertheless, no pharmacological intervention for the prevention of restenosis has gained a broad clinical acceptance.

Alternative or adjunct mechanical devices were developed to limit restenosis. Laser angioplasty (13) or high speed rotational angioplasty (13,14) failed to the reduce restenosis rate, while optimal directional coronary atherectomy pro-

vides reduced restenosis rates (15,16). Coronary stents were the first devices with a documented reduction of restenosis compared to balloon angioplasty for the treatment of *de novo* lesions in larger coronary arteries (BENESTENT [17] and STRESS [18] trials). Similar results were also documented for stenting of chronic total occlusions (SICCO trial [19]) and for bail-out stenting of symptomatic dissections or acute vessel closure during coronary intervention (STENT-BY trial [20]).

Stents have shown to limit two of the three major mechanisms of restenosis, namely acute recoil (21) and vessel shrinkage due to remodeling (22), while the response to injury with neointimal proliferation is more pronounced (23). Nevertheless, the net result is associated with a larger lumen at follow-up.

More recently, experimental and first clinical data suggest that the local application of ionizing radiation may favorably impact neointimal proliferation and remodeling after coronary intervention (24,25). Beta or gamma irradiation has been applied.

Finally, vascular gene therapy or local antisense therapy may play a future role to limit the restenosis process.

RISK FACTORS FOR RESTENOSIS

Various studies elucidated different clinical, angiographic and procedural parameters, which are associated with an increased likelihood of developing restenosis, namely: variant or recent onset angina, unstable angina, IDDM, chronic dialysis, long lesions, multiple lesions, lesions in saphenous vein grafts, chronic total occlusions, presence of collaterals supplying the target vessel, ostial and angulated (>45-degree angle) lesions, postinterventional pressure gradient >20 mm Hg, and residual stenosis >30%.

MECHANISMS

The pathophysiological mechanisms underlying the restenotic process are quite complex and presently not fully understood. Three mechanisms have been identified to play a major role in the development of restenosis. First, immediately after balloon deflation, a substantial amount of the lumen created is lost due to the elastic properties of coronary arteries causing elastic recoil (21). Subsequently, the plaque deformation and rupture caused by the balloon is followed by complex local wound-healing processes, including thrombotic, inflammatory, and cell proliferative processes (26). As a result, neointimal formation is causing lumen loss, which previously was thought to be the major contributor to restenosis. Intravascular ultrasound studies in particular elucidated that in addition to acute recoil and neointimal proliferation, a remodeling of the treated vessel segment can be observed as causing shrinkage (22). This restenotic process after PTCA reaches a plateau within 3 to 6 months and is unusual after 12 months.

TREATMENT OF A RESTENOTIC LESION

Since routine follow-up angiography after coronary interventions is not commonly performed nowadays, patients with coronary interventions should be reevaluated with respect to their symptoms and for the detection of ischemia by stress tests (stress ECG, stress echo, TL-SPECT or SESTAMIBI at rest and during effort). If angina pectoris, a documentation of local myocardial ischemia associated to the previously treated coronary artery, or both are present, an indication for repeat coronary angiography is given because of suspected restenosis.

In the case of angiographically documented restenosis, different treatment options exist, depending on patients' characteristics, myocardium at risk, lesion morphology, extent of coexisting coronary artery disease, and left ventricular function. Usually, repeat coronary intervention is preferred over medical therapy. Bypass surgery should be considered if repeat intervention is contraindicated or technically not feasible. Adjunct pharmacological interventions to repeat coronary interventions for the treatment of a restenotic lesion have not been addressed so far in large-scale trials.

Several interventional options exist to treat a restenotic lesion after PTCA. Repeat PTCA of the restenotic lesion is the most frequently ap-

plied intervention. Several studies documented that repeat PTCA can be performed with a high success rate of more than 95% and a low complication rate (<5%) (27,28,29). The long-term outcome with respect to the development of additional restenosis is more or less the same as for the initial procedure. Thereby, a substantial number of patients is left with continuously recurring restenosis. Therefore, alternative interventional techniques were considered as treatment options for restenotic lesions.

Coronary stents have been shown to limit restenosis for the treatment of *de novo* stenosis in native vessels based on their properties to limit elastic recoil and postinterventional remodeling. The Restenosis Stent (REST) trial evaluated the efficacy of stents compared to repeat PTCA for the treatment of restenotic lesions after PTCA (30). This prospective multicenter, randomized trial enrolled 383 patients with at least one episode of restenosis. Morphologic lesion characteristics were similar to the BENESTENT and STRESS trial criteria except that the vessel size had to be >2.5 mm in comparison to >3.0 mm in the other studies. The 15-mm Palmaz-Schatz stent (Johnson and Johnson International Systems, Warren, NJ) was implanted, either as a bare stent or premounted on a stent delivery system. Results documented a restenosis rate of 18% in the stent arm compared to 32% in the repeat PTCA arm at 6 months with less frequent target-lesion revascularization after stenting compared to repeat PTCA. Minimal luminal diameter on an average was 0.19 mm larger at follow-up after stenting compared to repeat PTCA (Fig. 14.1). Event-free survival rate after 250 days was 84% in the stent arm and 72% in the repeat PTCA arm. These positive results in favor of stenting restenotic lesions reached statistical significance. Since adjunct medication after stent placement included aspirin, heparin, and overlapping oral anticoagulation with Coumadin (Du Pont Pharmaceuticals), thrombotic and bleeding complications were found more frequently after stenting compared to repeat PTCA. Today, the application of high-pressure stent dilatation and a more pronounced antiaggregation with aspirin and ticlopidine instead of an oral anticoagulation with Coumadin (Du Pont

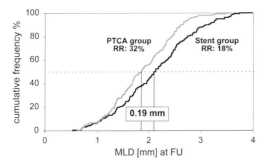

FIG. 14.1. Cumulative distribution curves of minimal luminal diameter at follow-up six months after stent placement or repeat PTCA for the treatment of restenosis after PTCA, according to the results of the STENT RESTENOSIS (REST) trial, showing a larger lumen for the stent arm by 0.19 mm on an average.

Pharmaceuticals, Wilmington, DE) has overcome these serious side effects.

Similar results have been reported by the Canadian TACS I trial (31).

More recently, ionizing radiation is applied to treat restenosis. The SCRIPPS (Scripps Coronary Radiation to Inhibit Proliferation Post-Stenting) trial is a double-blind, randomized, placebo-controlled trial of intracoronary gamma (^{192}Ir) radiation plus stenting in patients with previous restenosis. Results documented a favorable restenosis rate of 17% versus 54% in the control group (24,25).

Other devices have not been tested for the treatment of restenosis after PTCA in prospective randomized trials.

Despite promising results of several stent trials with reduced restenosis rates, the broader application of stenting for nonapproved indications is associated with much higher restenosis rates. Numerous studies identified risk factors for the development of stent restenosis: gender, restenotic lesions, chronic total occlusions, IDDM, multiple stenting per lesion, small balloon-to-artery ratio, low stent-implantation pressure, stent design, postinterventional residual stenosis, stenosis length, small vessel size, calcified lesions, and saphenous vein graft lesions. Since in-stent restenosis theoretically is mainly caused by excessive neointimal proliferation, the treatment of this type of restenotic

lesion is another challenge. Nevertheless, in a series of 113 in-stent restenotic lesions, intravascular ultrasound (but not coronary angiography) documented incomplete stent expansion in 18 cases as the major contributor to stent restenosis, especially in calcified lesions. For these restenotic lesions, high-pressure stent dilation guided by intravascular ultrasound should be performed to achieve complete stent expansion. In the case of excessive neointimal proliferation, repeat PTCA is most frequently performed while atheroablative techniques such as laser angioplasty, rotational atherectomy, or directional atherectomy seem to be more attractive. Lumen enlargement by PTCA of in-stent restenosis is caused by plastic deformation of the neointima with extrusion through the stent struts and by further stent expansion, both inducing excessive response to injury (32). Initial lumen gain is furthermore lost because of early relapse of the extruded neointimal tissue. Restenosis rates after PTCA of in-stent restenosis widely vary between 12% and 85% and are directly related to the restenotic in-stent neointimal plaque burden and lesion length. Additional stent placement (stent-in-stent sandwich), especially in the case of neointimal relapse after balloon angioplasty of in-stent restenosis, can be performed to jail the extruded tissue. In this context, new stent designs and stent grafts (Fig. 14.2) with a PTFE membrane provide attractive options (33,34).

High speed rotational angioplasty (Fig. 14.3), Excimer laser angioplasty (Fig. 14.4), and, rarely, directional coronary atherectomy are applied to ablate or remove neointimal tissue in stent restenosis, theoretically causing a less pronounced response to injury (35,36,37,38). Since available devices are limited, adjunct PTCA usually has to be performed to create an adequate lumen, encountering the above listed mechanisms of tissue extrusion and stent expansion. Early reports tend to show similar restenosis rates after atheroablative techniques for the treatment of focal (<10 mm) in-stent restenosis compared to PTCA alone, while in diffuse in-stent restenosis these techniques tend to provide superior results. Prospective randomized trials are on their way to document the efficacy of

before intervention   after Stent Graft

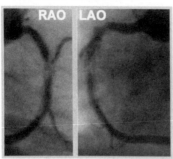
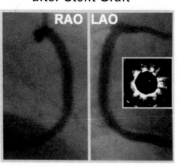

FIG. 14.2. Coronary angiograms in right (RAO) and left (LAO) anterior oblique projections with documentation of a focal in-stent restenosis six months after placement of a 3.5-mm/32-mm NIR stent (Scimed, Maple Grove, MN) before and after implantation of a stent graft because of persisting neointimal relapse after PTCA.

FIG. 14.3. Example of a patient with long diffuse in-stent restenosis after implantation of five 3.0-mm or 3.5-mm/16-mm Pura Vario stents after recanalization of a chronically occluded right coronary artery. Intravascular ultrasound documented excessive neointimal proliferation as the major cause of restenosis. This patient was treated with 2.0-mm laser angioplasty plus adjunct PTCA, showing a reasonable angiographic and intravascular ultrasound result.

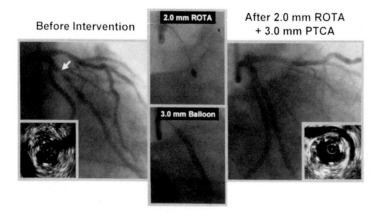

FIG. 14.4. Example of a diffuse in-stent restenosis after placement of a 3.0-mm/24-mm Pura Vario stent because of flow-limiting dissection after PTCA. This restenotic lesion was treated by 2.0-mm rotablation and adjunct PTCA with a 3.0-mm balloon catheter, showing a reasonable post-interventional result.

laser angioplasty (LARS trial) or rotablation (ARTIST and TWISTER trials) in comparison to PTCA for the treatment of in-stent restenosis. Furthermore, the adjunct of local irradiation after PTCA alone or atheroablative techniques plus PTCA is investigated to limit restenosis after treatment of in-stent restenosis.

A CONTEMPORARY APPROACH TO TREAT RESTENOTIC LESIONS

In the case of a symptomatic restenotic lesion with objective signs of ischemia during stress tests, we differentiate among: a stent restenosis or a restenosis after PTCA; laser angioplasty; rotablation; and directional atherectomy. If a patient's clinical and angiographic scenario allows an interventional approach to the restenotic lesion, we follow the flow chart illustrated in Figure 14.5.

For the non-stent restenosis cases we dilate the restenosis and finalize with adjunct stent placement, independent of whether this is the first, second, or so on restenosis based on the results of the REST trial.

For stent restenosis, we perform intravascular ultrasound imaging first, to rule out incomplete stent expansion as the major contributor for stent restenosis. If incomplete stent expansion is present, high-pressure stent dilatation will be performed with noncompliant balloon catheters and a balloon-to-artery ratio of 1.1 to 1, based on the lumen quantification by intravascular ultrasound. In the presence of significant tissue relapse through the stent struts, we try to fix this by another stent, usually a stent graft, if no major side branches will be jailed.

If intravascular ultrasound documents excessive neointimal proliferation as the major contributor to stent restenosis, we measure the length of stent restenosis by quantitative coronary angiography and differentiate between lesions ≤10 mm and those >10 mm.

If stent restenosis is ≤10 mm, we perform PTCA. In the future, we intend to add brachytherapy following a scientific protocol. In the case of significant tissue relapse through the stent struts, we try to fix this by another stent as described before.

If stent restenosis is >10 mm, we first start

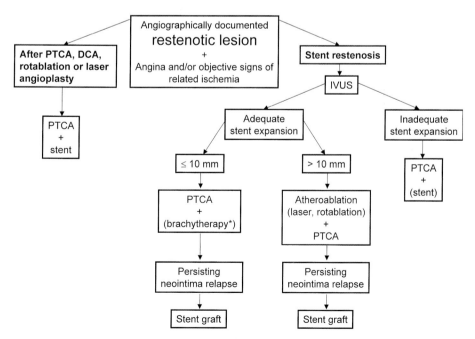

FIG. 14.5. Flow chart of a contemporary treatment strategy for restenotic lesions.

with an atheroablative technique. Our preference at this moment is to start with excimer laser angioplasty and maintain as much neointimal ablation as possible, which can be best documented by repeat intravascular ultrasound runs. If the stiff and bulky laser catheters do not reach the target restenosis or get stuck to the stented vessel wall, we switch to rotablation. Again, we try to use the largest burr size possible to provide maximum neointimal ablation. Then, adjunct PTCA is performed with noncompliant balloon catheters, with a balloon to artery ratio of 1.1 to 1, based on lumen quantification by intravascular ultrasound using nominal pressures. In the future we again intend to add brachytherapy following a scientific protocol. In the case of persisting significant tissue relapse through the stent struts we again try to fix this by another stent as described before.

CONCLUSION

Restenosis still is the "Achilles heel" of coronary interventions with tremendous clinical and health-economical impact. Stents were able to limit restenosis for certain subset of lesions including focal restenotic lesions, but stent restenosis today is the most difficult scenario to treat. Ongoing prospective randomized trials are evaluating different atheroablative techniques, additional stenting or brachytherapy in adjunct to PTCA for the treatment of stent restenosis.

REFERENCES

1. Gruentzig AR. Transluminal dilatation of coronary artery stenoses. *Lancet* 1978;1:263.
2. Ryan TJ, Bauman WB, Kennedy JW et al. Guidelines for percutaneous transluminal coronary angioplasty: a report of the American College of Cardiology/American Heart Association Task Force on assessment of diagnostic and therapeutic cardiovascular procedures (subcommittee on percutaneous transluminal coronary angioplasty). *Circulation* 1993;88:2987–3007.
3. Beatt KJ, Serruys PW, Renseing BJ, Hugenholtz PG. Restenosis after coronary angioplasty: new standards for clinical studies. *J Am Coll Cardiol* 1990;15:491–498.
4. Beatt KJ, Luijten H, de Feyter P, van den Brand M, Reiber J, Serruys PW. Change in diameter of coronary artery segment adjacent to stenosis after percutaneous transluminal coronary angioplasty: failure of percent diameter stenosis measurement to reflect morphologic changes induced by balloon dilatation. *J Am Coll Cardiol* 1988;12:315–323.
5. Rensing BJ, Hermans WM, Deckers JW, de Feyter PJ. Lumen narrowing after percutaneous transluminal coronary balloon angioplasty follows a near gaussian distribution: a quantitative angiographic study in 1,445 successfully dilated lesions. *J Am Coll Cardiol* 1992;19:939–945.
6. Kuntz R, Safian R, Levien M, Reis G, Diver D, Baim D. Novel approach to the analysis of restenosis after the use of three new coronary devices. *J Am Coll Cardiol* 1992;19:1493–1499.
7. Interventional Cardiology Devices Branch, Division of Cardiovascular, Respiratory, and Neurology Devices, Office of Device Evaluation, U.S. Food and Drug Administration. Guidance for the submission of research and marketing applications for interventional cardiology devices: PTCA catheters, atherectomy, laser, intravascular stents. Rockville, MD: U.S. Food and Drug Administration 1993 May:29.
8. Foley DP, Serruys PW. Restenosis after percutaneous coronary interventions, the evolving angiographic perspective. *Coronary Artery Dis* 1994;4:1129–1136.
9. Hillegass WB, Ohman ME, Califf RM. Restenosis: the clinical issues. In: Topol EJ, ed. *Textbook of interventional cardiology*, 2nd ed. Philadelphia: WB Saunders, 1993;415–435.
10. Topol E, Califf R, Weismann H et al. Randomized trial of coronary intervention with antibody against platelet II b/III a integrin for reduction of clinical restenosis: results at six month. *Lancet* 1994;343:881–886.
11. Tardiff JC, Cote G, Lesperance J et al. Probucol and multivitamins in the prevention of restenosis after coronary angioplasty. *N Engl J Med* 1997;337:365–372.
12. Tamai H, Katou K, Hayakawa H et al. The impact of tranilast on restenosis following coronary angioplasty. The second tranilast restenosis following angioplasty trial (TREAT-2). *Circulation* 1996;96:I–620.
13. Reifart N, Vandormael M et al. Randomized comparison of angioplasty of complex coronary lesions at a single center. *Circulation* 1997;96:91–98.
14. Hamm C, Dietz U., Dill T et al. A randomized comparison of balloon versus rotational atherectomy in complex coronary lesions (COBRA-STUDY). *Lancet* 1998 (*in press*).
15. Simonton CA, Leon MB, Kuntz RE et al. Acute and late clinical and angiographic results of directional atherectomy, in the optimal atherectomy restenosis study (OARS). *Circulation* 1995;92:I–545.
16. Baim DS, Kuntz RE, Sharma SK et al. Acute and late results of the Balloon versus Optimal Atherectomy Trial (BOAT). *Circulation* 1995;92:I–544.
17. Serruys PW, de Jaegere P, Kiemeneij F et al. A comparison of balloon expandable stent implantation with balloon angioplasty in patients with coronary artery disease. *N Engl J Med* 1994;331(8):489–495.
18. Fishman D, Leon M, Baim D et al. A randomized comparison of coronary stent placement and balloon angioplasty in the treatment of coronary artery disease. *N Engl J Med* 1994;331:496–501.
19. Sirnes A, Golf S, Myreng Y et al. Stenting in chronic coronary occlusion (SICCO): a randomized, controlled trial of adding stent implantation after successful angioplasty. *J Am Coll Cardiol* 1996;28:1444–1451.
20. Haude M, Erbel R, Hoepp HW, Heublein B, Sigmund

M, Meyer J, and the STENT-BY Study group (1996). STENT-BY Study: a prospective randomized trial comparing immediate stenting versus conservative treatment strategies in abrupt vessel closure or symptomatic dissection during coronary balloon angioplasty. *Eur Heart J* 1996;17[Suppl]:172(abst).

21. Haude M, Erbel R, Issa H, Meyer J. Quantitative analysis of elastic recoil after balloon angioplasty and after intracoronary implantation of balloon-expandable Palmaz-Schatz stents. *J Am Coll Cardiol* 1993;21:26–34.
22. Mintz GS, Popma JJ, Pichard AD et al. Arterial remodeling after coronary angioplasty: a serial intravascular ultrasound study. *Circulation* 1996;94:35–43.
23. Mehran R, Mintz GS, Pichard AD et al. Impact of vessel wall injury on in-stent restenosis: a serial quantitative angiographic and intravascular ultrasound study. *Circulation* 1996;94:I–262.
24. Teirstein PS, Massullo V, Jani S et al. Catheter-based radiotherapy to inhibit restenosis after coronary stenting. *N Engl J Med* 1997;336:1697–1703.
25. Mintz GS, Massullo V, Popma JJ et al. Transcatheter Irridium-192 irradiation reduces in-stent neointimal tissue proliferation: a serial volumetric intravascular ultrasound analysis from the SCRIPPS trail. *J Am Coll Cardiol* 1997;29[Suppl A]:60A.
26. Lafont A, Gunzmann L, PLW. Restenosis after experimental angioplasty. Intimal, medial and adventitial changes associated with constrictive remodeling. *Circ Res* 1995;76:996–1002.
27. Williams DO, Gruentzig A, Kent K, Detre K, Kelsey S, To T. Efficacy of repeat percutaneous transluminal coronary angioplasty for coronary restenosis. *Am J Cardiol* 1984;53:32C–35C.
28. Diams AP, Grigera F, Arora RR et al. Repeat coronary angioplasty as treatment for restenosis. *J Am Coll Cardiol* 1992;19:1310–1314.
29. Meier B, King SBI, Gruentzig AR. Repeat coronary angioplasty. *J Am Coll Cardiol* 1984;4:463–466.
30. Erbel R, Haude M, Höpp H-W et al., for the REST-Study-Group. A comparison of coronary stenting with balloon angioplasty for restenosis after balloon angioplasty. *N Engl J Med* 1998 (*in press*).
31. Penn I, Ricci D, Almond DG et al. Stenting results in increased early complications and fewer late reinterventions: final clinical data from the Trial of Angioplasty and Stents in Canada (TASC) I. *Circulation* 1995;92:I–475.
32. Mehran R, Mintz GS, Popma JJ et al. Mechanism and results of balloon angioplasty for the treatment of in-stent restenosis. *Am J Cardiol* 1996;78:618–622.
33. von Birgelen C, Haude M, Liu F et al. Behandlung eines koronaren pseudoaneurysmas durch stent-graft-implantation. *Dtsch Med Wschr* 1998;123:418–422.
34. Welge D, Haude M, von Birgelen C et al. Versorgung einer koronarperforation nach perkutaner ballonangioplastie mit einem neuen membranstent. *Z Kardiol* 1998 (*in press*).
35. Sharma SK, Duvuri S, Dangas G et al. Rotational atherectomy for in-stent restenosis: acute and long-term results of first 100 cases. *Eur Heart J* 1997;84:497A.
36. Mehran R, Mintz GS, Popma JJ et al. Excimer laser angioplasty in the treatment of in-stent restenosis: an intravascular ultrasound study. *J Am Coll Cardiol* 1996;27:362A.
37. Pathan A, Butte A, Harrell L, Ferell M, Gold HK, Palacios I. Directional coronary atherectomy is superior to PTCA for the treatment of Palmaz-Schatz stent restenosis. *J Am Coll Cardiol* 1997;29:68A.
38. Klues HG, Reffelmann T, vom Dahl J, Hanrath P. High-speed rotational coronary atherectomy for the treatment of restenosis in coronary stents. *J Am Coll Cardiol* 1997;29:313A.

B. In-Stent Restenosis

Joseph R. Califano and *Paul S. Teirstein

Department of Cardiology, Naval Medical Center San Diego, San Diego, California 92134-5000;
**Department of Cardiology, Scripps Clinic, La Jolla, California 92037*

The early randomized trials of coronary stenting versus balloon angioplasty in *de novo* lesions demonstrated that stents reduce the incidence of restenosis in native coronary arteries (1,2). Subsequently, reduced rates of restenosis and/or clinical events were demonstrated for restenotic lesions (3), chronic total occlusions (4,5), and saphenous venous bypass grafts (6). In addition, the use of stents in the setting of failed angioplasty has resulted in a high rate of procedural success, a marked decrease in complications, and favorable long-term outcome (7–10). In recent years, the use of high-pressure inflations and combination antiplatelet therapy have obviated the need for prolonged anticoagulation, and decreased the length of hospitalization. Thus, stents have improved the safety, predictability, and long-term outcome of percutaneous coronary revascularization, and the majority of interventions now involve stents (11).While simple, discrete stenoses are associated with a low rate of target lesion revascularization (7%–11%) (12,13), restenosis is more common when stents are used to treat complex lesion sub-types (20%–35%) (1,2,14). In 1997 the number of lesions treated with stents was estimated to exceed 400,000 worldwide (15). It is also esti-mated that in the same year 100,000 patients were treated for in-stent restenosis (15). Thus the prevention and treatment of in-stent restenosis is a medical as well as a financial imperative.

MECHANISM OF IN-STENT RESTENOSIS

Restenosis is a complex process which is not completely understood. Nevertheless, research-ers have discovered some important differences between in-stent restenosis, and restenosis in nonstented vessels. Gross pathologic studies of stents removed at autopsy, or by surgical exci-sion of saphenous venous grafts, demonstrate proliferating smooth muscle cells and extracel-lular matrix as the predominant components of in-stent restenosis (16–19). Congruent with these histopathological observations, angio-graphic analyses have shown that the implan-tation of Palmaz-Schatz stents (Johnson and Johnson International Systems, Warren, NJ) essentially eliminates recoil and negative re-modeling (20–22). Gordon and colleagues per-formed angiograms of 59 lesions immediately after stent placement and at 6-month follow-up. Although minimum lumen diameter (MLD) de-creased by 0.99 ± 0.87 mm, minimum stent diameter decreased by only 0.03 ± 0.23 mm. (20). A serial quantitative coronary angiography (QCA) analysis of lesions initially treated by balloon angioplasty and then stented for resteno-sis demonstrated the elimination of recoil by stents. Mean elastic recoil following stent place-ment was only 0.10 ± 0.07 mm compared to 0.98 ± 0.5 mm following balloon angioplasty (21).

Using intravascular ultrasound (IVUS), inves-tigators from the Washington Hospital Center showed that 73% of late lumen loss in non-stented lesions was due to arterial remodeling, and only 27% was due to tissue growth. In con-trast, arterial remodeling was essentially elimi-nated in stented vessels. Neointimal hyperplasia was solely responsible for in-stent restenosis (23,24).

One important caveat, however, is that stents appear to affect adjacent vessel segments by a combination of arterial remodeling and tissue proliferation (25). Therefore, the entire coronary segment rather than just the stent should be ana-lyzed at follow-up. For example, in the placebo arm of the Scripps Coronary Radiation to Inhibit Proliferation Post Stenting (SCRIPPS) trial, re-stenosis rates for the stent plus adjacent seg-ments were higher than restenosis rates for the stented segment only (54% versus 36%) (26).

The Use of Intravascular Ultrasound in the Evaluation of In-Stent Restenosis

IVUS provides high quality cross-sectional imaging of coronary arteries *in vivo*. IVUS of-fers several advantages over angiography in the assessment of in-stent restenosis. Stainless steel stents can be difficult to visualize by angiogra-phy; however IVUS provides excellent visualiz-ation of the stent struts which are intensely echo-reflective. Stent borders are clearly demarcated, and stent cross-sectional area can be accurately measured. Unlike angiography, IVUS can depict the vessel wall, and the amount and composition of plaque. The area of the lumen, and the amount of neointimal tissue, can be quantified. IVUS measurements of reference vessel segments, lumen, plaque, and media have been validated (27–30) and are highly reproducible in regions with and without stents (25,31,32). QCA is a two-dimensional method. Thus, errors arise in quantifying disease processes in tortuous three-dimensional vessels. By imaging from within the lumen, IVUS overcomes errors due to pro-jection, such as overlap and tortuosity. QCA lu-minal area is calculated from the luminal diame-ter by assuming that the lumen has a circular morphology. Most lumens are eccentric how-ever, and IVUS is capable of valid quantification of coronary artery diameters and cross-sectional areas even in irregular, eccentric lesions. The assessment of therapies to prevent or treat in-stent restenosis requires an accurate assessment of acute gain, late loss, and binary restenosis rates. Ideally, both IVUS and QCA measurements should be performed.

Risk Factors for In-Stent Restenosis

Clinical and angiographic factors that predict restenosis following stent placement differ somewhat from those following balloon angioplasty. Table 14.2 lists risk factors for restenosis following both angioplasty and stenting.

Most (33–36), but not all (37), large studies with systematic angiographic follow-up have

TABLE 14.2. *Risk factors for restenosis*

PTCA	Stent
Recent onset angina (50,51)	Unstable angina not a factor (36,37,41)
Unstable angina (50,51)	
Severe angina (NYHA Class III or IV) (50,51)	
Diabetes (50,51)	Diabetes (33–36)
Prior restenosis (71–76)	Prior restenosis (14,33, 47,56)
Shorter time intervals between previous procedures and episodes of restenosis (76,77)	Shorter time interval between stent placement and episodes of restenosis (<90 days) (81)
Total occlusion (50)	Total Occlusion (33)
Lesion length (51,78)	Lesion length (37,42,43)
	Multiple stents (14,33,34, 37,44–48)
Left anterior descending lesion (especially if proximal) (50)	Left anterior descending lesion (33,36,37,44,47)
Ostial stenosis (79)	Ostial stenosis (41,43, 45)
More severe stenosis preprocedure (minimal diameter or percent stenosis) (50,51)	Plaque burden by IVUS (41,45), but not preprocedure MLD or percent stenosis (33, 37,41,44)
More severe stenosis postprocedure (minimal diameter or percent stenosis) (50,51)	Postprocedure minimal stent diameter or percent stenosis (33,35,36,41–43)
Postprocedure cross-sectional area (IVUS) (80)	Postprocedure cross-sectional area (IVUS) (41,43,52,55)
Smaller reference vessel size (81)	Smaller reference vessel size (34,35,42,43,45, 82)

NYHA, New York Heart Association.

found that diabetes is an independent risk factor for in-stent restenosis. Late loss and late-loss index have been found to be significantly greater in diabetics (38,39). Serial IVUS studies have demonstrated that this is due to exaggerated intimal hyperplasia (24). This is compounded by the finding that diabetics tend to have smaller reference vessels (40). Although unstable angina is one of the more consistent predictors of restenosis following angioplasty, it has not been shown to be a predictor of in-stent restenosis (36,37,41).

Several studies (37,41,42), have demonstrated that lesion length is an independent predictor of restenosis (42). Many studies have shown that the implantation of multiple stents also increases the probability of restenosis (14,33,34,37, 44–48). Other reports suggest the impact of multiple stents is related to the interaction of lesion length with vessel size, and not the number of stents used (41). In a recent series, 117 lesions were treated with three or more stents. IVUS guidance was used to optimize stent deployment. Despite the use of an average of 3.3 stents per lesion, the TLR rate was only 13.3% (49).

With balloon angioplasty, more severe lesions (by percent diameter stenosis or MLD) have a higher rate of restenosis (50–51). With stents, however, lesion severity has not been shown to predict subsequent restenosis (33,37,41,44). Nevertheless, IVUS studies have shown that plaque burden is a significant independent predictor of in-stent restenosis (41,45).

Studies have consistently demonstrated that smaller reference vessel size is a risk factor for in-stent restenosis (34,35,42,43,45,52). Follow-up IVUS of 177 stented lesions determined that intimal hyperplasia thickness at follow-up is independent of stent size (53). This results in a higher frequency of restenosis when stents are placed in smaller vessels. In addition, restenosis at stent margins tends to occur when stents are implanted into smaller, more diseased arteries (54).

The importance of final stent dimensions is supported by multiple IVUS studies (41,43, 52,55), QCA data (33,35,36), and clinical follow-up (34). Moussa and colleagues studied 921 lesions treated with successful IVUS guided stent placement. Angiographic follow-up was obtained in 75%. A final minimum lumen cross-sectional area of <9 mm^2 was associated with a restenosis rate of 29%; however if this area was ≥9 mm^2, the restenosis rate was only 8% (55).

While some studies have shown that stented lesions in the left anterior descending (LAD) have a higher rate of restenosis (33,36), others have not found vessel location to be a risk factor (37,44,47). Although LAD target vessel may be a predictor of in-stent restenosis, there is ample data to conclude that it is not a powerful predictor (33,44). In a large trial with systematic angiographic follow-up, chronic, but not recent total occlusion was found to be an independent predictor of restenosis (33). Nevertheless, in two prospective, randomized studies of stents versus balloon angioplasty for chronic total occlusions, restenosis was reduced by more than 50% by stenting (4,5).Ostial stenosis is also a predictor of subsequent in-stent restenosis (41,43,45).

Several studies with systematic angiographic follow-up have found that prior restenosis is a risk factor for in-stent restenosis (14,47,56). Nevertheless, Colombo and colleagues recently reported favorable results following stent placement in 139 restenotic lesions. Recurrent restenosis occurred in 25% of cases (57). In addition, a recent randomized trial of stent placement versus balloon angioplasty for restenotic lesions showed a lower rate of recurrent restenosis with stenting (3).

An issue which has not been fully resolved is whether high-pressure inflations influence the risk of in-stent restenosis. Serial dilatations of stents at 12,15, and 18 atm result in progressive increases in minimum stent area (58). However, some studies have suggested that high-pressure inflations, by causing more deep wall injury, evoke a greater amount of intimal hyperplasia. This may increase late loss (59,60). A retrospective analysis in which postprocedure IVUS was performed compared restenosis rates following inflations of ≤16 atm (n = 692), versus >16 atm (n = 489). Optimal IVUS result, rather than maximum deployment pressure, predicted subsequent restenosis (61). Yokoi and colleagues found identical angiographic restenosis rates of 13% in 197 stents deployed with inflations above or below 14 atm (62). Multivariate analysis of 1,650 patients included in the STARS study found that final MLD and vessel size, but not high-pressure dilatation (>16 atm), were associated with subsequent target site revascularization (63). Likewise, follow-up angiography of 1,060 patients following stent placement found that high-pressure inflation did not influence late-loss index (64). In a study of 500 stented lesions, with systematic angiographic follow-up in 81%, the use of high-pressure inflation was associated with *less* late loss (37). In the TASTE registry, 504 patients underwent follow-up angiography. Restenosis was increased when the highest pressure used for stent deployment was <12 atm (43.3% versus 34.3%) (14). Thus, most studies support the concept that achieving optimal stent expansion is essential in preventing restenosis. The safest way to accomplish optimal stent expansion is by the use of high-pressure inflations rather than oversized balloons (65). Currently, a prospective randomized trial is being conducted to attempt to settle this issue. In this study of 900 patients, the rate of early complications was similar in both groups; however a larger acute gain and postprocedure MLD was achieved in the high-pressure group. Six-month follow-up results have not yet been published (66).

Finally, high plasma levels of angiotensin converting enzyme (ACE) have been associated with a marked increase in restenosis rates following stent placement. After vascular injury, the induction of ACE results in local production of angiotensin II. Angiotensin II promotes migration of smooth muscle cells and stimulates cellular proliferation. Plasma ACE level is largely controlled by the insertion/deletion polymorphism of the ACE gene. The D/D phenotype, which is associated with higher levels of ACE, is a powerful predictor of restenosis following stent placement. Recently, Ribichini and colleagues reported that the relative risk of angiographic restenosis for patients with the D/D phenotype was 2.75. The relative risk was 8.2 in the group of patients with high plasma ACE levels. Restenosis occurred in 7.9 % (11/139) of patients with ACE levels below 34 U/L, and 64.9%

occurred in 19% of the rotational atherectomy group and 39% of the angioplasty group ($p = .01$). Routine follow-up angiography was not performed.

The multicenter BARASTER registry includes 172 patients who were treated with rotational atherectomy for in-stent restenosis (106). Many (86%) of the lesions were diffuse (>10 mm in length). Mean burr-to-artery ratio was 0.76 ± 0.15. Adjunctive angioplasty greater than 1 atm was used in 74% of cases (mean of 9 ± 6 atm). Procedural success (<50% residual stenosis without the development of a clinical complication) was achieved in 94% of cases. Procedural complications occurred in 3% of cases, including four dissections, one episode of bradycardia requiring placement of a temporary pacemaker, and one fatal vessel perforation during atherectomy of a separate lesion distal to the stented segment. There were no cases of burr entrapment or slow flow. There were a total of three in-hospital deaths. Clinical follow-up was obtained in all of the patients at a mean of 6 ± 4 months. The TLR rate was 36%. Clinical recurrence, defined as death, myocardial infarction, or target lesion revascularization, occurred in 38% of patients. Routine angiography was not performed, but 50% of patients underwent angiography to evaluate symptoms. In this symptomatic group the angiographic restenosis rate was 73%. The rate of clinical recurrence was significantly lower in the group treated with adjunctive balloon angioplasty to pressures >1 atm than in those treated with rotational atherectomy alone, or inflations ≤1 atm (33% versus 55%).

A single-center, prospective study included 36 consecutive patients who underwent rotational atherectomy for diffuse in-stent restenosis. Success rate was 100%, and there were no complications. Long-term angina-free survival was achieved in 72% of patients (mean follow-up of 277 ± 109 days) (107).

Buttner and colleagues performed rotational atherectomy with adjunctive low pressure angioplasty on 32 patients with diffuse in-stent restenosis. Mean lesion length was 18 ± 5.8 mm. The procedure was successful in all patients without adverse in-hospital events. However, despite an average burr-to-artery ratio of 0.85, angiographic follow-up of 27 patients (84%) revealed a restenosis rate of 56%. The TLR rate was 33% (108).

In summary, rotational atherectomy with adjunctive angioplasty achieves a high rate of procedural success, with few complications. In the treatment of initial episodes of diffuse in-stent restenosis, the ROSTER trial demonstrated a better acute result, and a favorable clinical outcome compared to balloon angioplasty. Issues that remain unresolved include:

1. Is the rate of angiographic restenosis following rotational atherectomy for in-stent restenosis lower than that following balloon angioplasty?
2. What is the optimal method to safely achieve the lowest possible rate of restenosis?
3. What is the optimal burr-to-artery ratio?
4. Should adjunctive PTCA be performed at high or low pressure?

Directional Coronary Atherectomy for In-Stent Restenosis

Little data is available on the use of directional coronary atherectomy (DCA) for the treatment of in-stent restenosis. Initial results with DCA for in-stent restenosis were unfavorable. Between 1991 and 1994, there were four reported cases in which DCA within coil stents (2 Wiktor [Medtronic, Inc., Minneapolis, MN], and 2 Gianturco-Roubin [Cook, Inc., Bloomington, IN]) resulted in stent disruption (101,109–111). Segments of stent wire were cut and removed in each case. In three cases there were no clinical sequelae, however one patient sustained an extensive dissection and required urgent bypass surgery. It was concluded that directional atherectomy should not be used to treat lesions within vascular segments containing coil stents (94). Recently, Cattelaens and associates attempted DCA on 30 patients for in-stent restenosis (various stent types). In 28 patients debulking was successfully performed. In two cases the device could not be advanced to an angulated lesion, despite predilatation. In three patients adjunctive

PTCA was not possible because of balloon rupture. In 19 patients (68%) stent material could be detected macroscopically in the extracted specimen. Siderin staining for stent material was positive in 25 patients (89%). Despite this, there were no major complications (112).

There is little data on long-term outcome following DCA for in-stent restenosis. Strauss and colleagues reported 10 cases, all of which were successful without major complications. Percent diameter stenosis was decreased from 63 ± 9 % to 21% ± 10%. Angiographic follow-up was obtained in five patients, three of whom had recurrent restenosis requiring revascularization (109).

Palacios and associates performed DCA on 45 patients (46 lesions) for restenosis within Palmaz-Schatz stents. Diffuse in-stent restenosis was present in 76% of lesions. Procedural success was 100%. Stent entrapment did not occur in this series. Two patients required additional stents to cover margin dissections from adjunctive PTCA. There were no episodes of acute closure, no reflow, or stent disruption. Postprocedure residual diameter stenosis was 17% ± 10%. Four patients (9%) suffered non-Q-wave myocardial infarctions. Clinical follow-up revealed a TLR of 28.3%. Combined clinical events including TLR, myocardial infarction, and death occurred in 31.1% (90). A small, nonrandomized, retrospective comparison of PTCA (n = 33), rotational atherectomy (n = 23), and DCA (n = 40) for in stent restenosis was performed by the same group. Procedural success without major complications was achieved in 100% with DCA, 96% with rotational atherectomy, and only 85% with PTCA. The group reported that DCA resulted in a larger postprocedure MLD, and a superior event-free survival (defined as freedom from myocardial infarction, death, repeat intervention, or bypass surgery). Angiographic follow-up was not performed. There was a trend toward lower TLR rate with DCA (19.5%) compared with rotational atherectomy (26%) or PTCA (30%) (113).

Additional data is needed to fully establish the safety of DCA for in-stent restenosis. DCA should be avoided in the treatment of restenosis within coil stents. Until further data are available, it may be wise to perform IVUS prior to attempted DCA through slotted tube stents to exclude inadequate stent expansion or strut protrusion into lumen. There is insufficient evidence to conclude that DCA offers any advantage over PTCA or rotational atherectomy for the treatment of in-stent restenosis.

Laser Coronary Angioplasty

Several groups have performed laser angioplasty for in-stent restenosis. Koster and colleagues performed ELCA with adjunctive balloon angioplasty for in-stent restenosis in 70 patients. The average lesion length was 14 ± 6 mm. Procedural success was 94%. There were eight dissections, three perforations, and four non-Q-wave infarctions. No Q-wave infarctions occurred. Postprocedure percent diameter stenosis evident by QCA was 13% ± 13% (114). Subsequently, this group reported 6-month follow-up of ELCA plus PTCA in 73 patients. One episode of sudden death occurred. Recurrent angina ≥Canadian Cardiovascular Society Class II was present in 36 patients (49%). Angiographic follow-up was obtained in 68 patients (93%) and revealed restenosis rate of 52%. Total occlusions were present at follow-up in seven patients (115).

Mehran and associates reported outcomes in 54 patients treated with ELCA plus PTCA for restenosis within Palmaz-Schatz stents. The majority of lesions (52%) were diffuse (>10 mm in length). Procedural success was 98%. Complications included emergency bypass surgery for dissection in one patient and four non-Q-wave infarctions. By IVUS analysis, tissue ablation during ELCA contributed only 29% ± 15% of the overall lumen gain. Tissue extrusion during PTCA contributed 31% ± 14%, and additional stent expansion during PTCA contributed 40% ± 16%. ELCA plus PTCA was only able to achieve 85% ± 18 % of the luminal area that was obtained with initial stent placement. There was significant residual neointima within the stent occupying 25% ± 8% of stent cross-sectional area. Postintervention percent diameter stenosis was 24% ± 12%. Systematic angiographic follow-up was not performed. Target vessel revascularization rate was 21% (116).

The multicenter Laser Angioplasty for Within Stent Restenosis (LARS) study included 414 vessels with in-stent restenosis treated by excimer laser with adjunctive PTCA. Procedural success rate was 92%. Percent diameter stenosis was reduced to 7% ± 12%. Complications from laser angioplasty occurred in 57 patients (13.8%). These included two "minor perforations," and 20 dissections (4.8%). After adjunctive PTCA there were two more perforations and 45 more dissections (10.9%). Pericardial tamponade occurred in two patients. Stent damage also occurred in two patients. Additional stents were placed in 67 patients (16%). In-hospital events included six deaths, two Q-wave myocardial infarctions, and ten non-Q-wave infarctions (117). Follow-up results have not yet been published.

In the only prospective randomized trial to date, Haase and colleagues randomized 96 patients to ELCA plus PTCA versus PTCA alone (118). In-hospital complications included one episode of acute closure in each group. In the laser group, one patient underwent coronary bypass surgery, one underwent repeat PTCA, and one sustained a non-Q-wave infarction. In the PTCA group there was one death, and two major bleeding episodes. Angiographic follow-up was obtained in 77% of patients, and revealed a restenosis rate of 57% in the ELCA plus PTCA group, versus 48% in the group treated with PTCA alone (n.s.).

Based on the data available, it appears that ELCA for in-stent restenosis is associated with a higher rate of complications than PTCA. A reduction of restenosis or clinical recurrence has not been achieved.

Transluminal Extraction Atherectomy

Experience with transluminal extraction atherectomy (TEC) for in stent restenosis is anecdotal (119–122). In 1997, Hara and associates described the results of TEC with adjunctive balloon angioplasty on nine patients with restenosis inside Palmaz-Schatz stents. There were no major complications. Mean percent diameter stenosis was reduced to 11%; however angiographic follow-up revealed restenosis in five of nine cases at 3 months (123).

Stents for In-Stent Restenosis

Investigators at the Washington Hospital Center observed that significant lumen loss occurs soon after the treatment of in-stent restenosis by angioplasty. This early lumen loss also occurs when angioplasty is preceded by debulking with rotational atherectomy or ELCA. In a systematic study of 37 in-stent lesions, the investigators found that there was an average decrease in minimum luminal area of 23% over an average of 42 ± 8 minutes following revascularization. Ten lesions had a greater than 2.0 mm² decrease in minimum lumen CSA (38% ± 3% of acute lumen gain). IVUS demonstrated that this was due to neointimal tissue "reintrusion" into the stent rather than stent recoil (124). They suggest that although ablation does not decrease tissue reintrusion, additional stent implantation appears to prevent it (15).

Initial observations suggest that the placement of additional stents, unlike angioplasty and ablative techniques, appears to fully recover the lumen achieved with original stent implantation. This occurs by extrusion of neointimal tissue out of the stent (15). Mehran and colleagues at the Washington Hospital Center reported results of stent placement to treat focal in-stent restenosis. A total of 56 restenotic segments within Palmaz-Schatz stents, (51 patients), were treated with additional stents. IVUS showed that the placement of additional stents increased lumen area primarily by neointimal tissue extrusion, with little additional stent expansion (change in stent area of 0.9 ± 0.4 mm²). Residual intimal hyperplasia area was 9% ± 2 % of final lumen area. The final angiographic percent diameter stenosis was 10%. The lumen achieved by repeat stenting was greater than the preprocedure area of the original stent. TLR at one year was 27% (125). Since Palmaz-Schatz stents do not usually recoil, this suggests that the placement of additional stents is able to fully recover the lumen achieved at the time of initial stent placement.

TABLE 14.6. *Stents for in-stent restenosis*

	Patients	Diffuse pattern	Procedural success	Follow-up	Recurrence
Mehran (125)	51	None	N.S.	Clinical	TLR rate = 27% at one year
Elezi (127)	84	N.S.	100%	Angiographic: 77.4%	Restenosis: 35.8%
Lefevre (128)	59	73%	100%	Clinical (first 30 patients)	TVR rate = 16.6% at 6 months
Goldberg (129)	48	54%	98%	Angiographic: 53%	Restenosis: 72%

N.S, not stated.

Thus, there is a rationale for using stents to treat in-stent restenosis.

In the placebo arm of the SCRIPPS trial, angiographic restenosis occurred in 83.3% of patients treated with PTCA, versus 33.3% of patients receiving new stents ($p = .13$). MLD at 6-month follow-up was 1.13 ± 0.49 for PTCA and 1.96 ± 0.76 mm for patients receiving additional stents ($p = .049$) (126).

Table 14.6 summarizes the results of stenting for in-stent restenosis. Elezi and colleagues reported on 84 patients in whom stents were placed after failed PTCA for in-stent restenosis. Stent placement was successful in all patients. There were no major complications at 4 weeks. Clinical follow-up at 6 months revealed one myocardial infarction and one cardiac death. Target lesion revascularization rate was 25.4%. Repeat angiography after 6 months was performed in 65 patients (77.4%), and revealed restenosis in 24 lesions (35.8%) (127).

Lefevre and associates reported 59 cases of stent placement for in-stent restenosis. In 73% of cases restenosis was diffuse. Postprocedure percent diameter stenosis was reduced to 4.5% $\pm$ 6.4%. All procedures were successful. There were no major complications at one month. In the first 30 patients TVR was 16.6% at 6 months. Routine follow-up angiography was not performed (128).

Less favorable results were reported by Goldberg and associates. They performed a retrospective analysis of 48 consecutive patients who underwent placement of additional stents for in-stent restenosis. 54% of cases were diffuse. Stents were placed for suboptimal PTCA in 32%, and dissection in 9%. All procedures were successful except for one patient who suffered a guide-catheter-induced dissection, leading to

urgent surgery and death. The postprocedure MLD was equal to the MLD after original stenting. Follow-up at 9 months revealed a clinical event rate (death, myocardial infarction, or TLR) of 40%. Angiographic follow-up was obtained in only 53% of patients and showed a restenosis rate of 72% (129).

To summarize, stenting of in-stent restenosis is associated with a high rate of procedural success, and a low rate of complications. Unlike other interventions, the lumen area achieved at the time of initial stent placement is fully recovered by the placement of additional stents. The long-term benefit of this strategy, however, remains to be proven.

Bypass Surgery

There are no published series of coronary bypass surgeries that focus on patients with in-stent restenosis. Obviously, there must be a sufficient target distal to the stented segment to allow for anastomosis of the graft. Bypass surgery is sometimes the best alternative for patients who are at high risk of recurrence following percutaneous interventions. This includes patients with multiple episodes of in-stent restenosis, shorter intervals between episodes of restenosis, and diffuse pattern of restenosis. Minimally invasive bypass surgery may be particularly well suited for treatment of recurrent in-stent restenosis, especially if the target is the left anterior descending artery.

Pharmacologic Therapy for In-stent Restenosis

Although numerous drugs have successfully prevented recurrence in animal models of restenosis, randomized clinical trials of over 60 medications have shown no benefit or limited benefit in humans. In animal models, most studies attempt to inhibit smooth muscle cell migration and proliferation. The predominance of recoil and remodeling over cellular proliferation in nonstented, restenotic lesions may explain the failure of these drugs in humans. However, in-stent restenosis is a pure model of neointimal tissue proliferation. Thus, pharmacologic approaches to restenosis may succeed when used as an adjunct to stent placement.

Recent double-blind, randomized data from the Multivitamins and Probucol Study Group has shown that probucol begun four weeks prior to PTCA and continued for 6 months postprocedure reduces the incidence of restenosis (130). This finding was confirmed by others (131). Whether similar results can be obtained in patients undergoing stent implantation remains to be seen. Although the EPIC study suggested that abciximab reduced the need for target vessel revascularization (132), this was not confirmed in the EPILOG study (133). In a subgroup of EPILOG, in which routine angiographic follow-up was obtained, there was no difference in restenosis rates between abciximab and placebo treated patients (133,134). Furthermore, the ERASER trial compared abciximab to placebo in patients undergoing stent implantation and found no difference in in-stent restenosis rates as measured by IVUS (135). The use of other glycoprotein IIb/IIIa inhibitors has not reduced target vessel revascularization rates (136,137). Studies are in progress to evaluate whether prolonged use of oral glycoprotein IIb/IIIa inhibitors used after coronary interventions will reduce restenosis rates.

Few studies of medications to reduce restenosis after stenting have been performed. The ISAR study randomized 517 patients undergoing stent implantation to therapy with aspirin and ticlopidine versus aspirin and warfarin. No difference in restenosis rates were seen (138). More promising results have been obtained with cilostazol, a potent antiplatelet agent that also has antithrombotic and vasodilating effects and an inhibitory effect on vascular smooth muscle proliferation. Cilostazol has been shown to reduce

late lumen loss following placement of Palmaz-Schatz stents (139–141). A study of 76 patients randomly assigned to ticlopidine or cilostazol showed a trend towards a reduced angiographic rate of restenosis with cilostazol (19% versus 33%) (141). Another study randomized 70 patients to aspirin versus cilostazol following successful placement of Palmaz-Schatz stents. The restenosis rate was 26.8% in the aspirin group and 8.6% in the cilostazol group ($p < .05$) (139).Cilostazol has also been shown to reduce the rate of restenosis following directional atherectomy compared with aspirin (142). Larger studies are needed to confirm these initial favorable results.

Antiproliferative Therapy For In-Stent Restenosis

Adjunctive antiproliferative therapy, such as intracoronary radiation or gene therapy, may be the ultimate solution for refractory in-stent restenosis. Since cellular and matrix proliferation is the main mechanism of in-stent restenosis, antiproliferative therapies may work best as an adjunct to stent placement.

Intracoronary Radiation For In-Stent Restenosis

Radiotherapy has been used effectively for over 100 years to inhibit cellular proliferation in malignant and benign diseases. In benign proliferative disorders such as keloid scar formation and heterotopic ossification, radiation has effectively prevented fibroblastic activity without impairing the normal healing process. Intracoronary radiation has been shown to reduce intimal proliferation in animal models of restenosis. Wiedermann and colleagues demonstrated that the gamma emitter iridium-192 (^{192}Ir) prevented neointimal proliferation in a swine balloon overstretch model. Neointimal tissue area was significantly reduced compared to control animals both at 30 days and 6 months (143). Waksman and associates used a similar model to demonstrate a dose-response effect with increasing doses of ^{192}Ir (144), and also with the use of the beta-emitter strontium-90/yttrium-90 (145).

Numerous other studies have demonstrated the effectiveness of gamma or beta radiation in animal models of restenosis (146–153). Beta-emitting radioactive stents have also been shown to inhibit neointimal proliferation (154–159). Significant side effects such as necrosis, fibrosis, or aneurysm formation were not observed in these animal models.

Clinical experience with the use of gamma radiation to reduce restenosis is rapidly accumulating. Condado and colleagues treated 21 patients with ^{192}Ir after balloon angioplasty (160). Late angiographic follow-up (>6 months after radiation) was obtained in 19 patients (90%). Although there was no control group, the results were encouraging. The calculated late lumen loss was 0.27 ± 0.56 mm, and the late-loss index was 0.19. Angiographic restenosis occurred in 27.3% of lesions.

The SCRIPPS trial, was a randomized, double-blind trial of intracoronary gamma radiation versus placebo to treat restenotic lesions (26). Criteria for enrollment included a target lesion that either already contained a stent or was suitable for stent placement, reference vessel diameter between 3–5 mm, and lesion length <30 mm. Patients were randomized only after an optimal result was obtained with repeat intervention. They received a 0.03-inch ribbon containing either ^{192}Ir-sealed sources or inactive (placebo) sources at its tip (Best Industries, Springfield, VA). The radiation oncologist and physicist used information from the IVUS image to calculate a dwell time to provide 800 cGy to the internal elastic membrane furthest from the radiation source, provided that no more than 3,000 cGy was delivered to the internal elastic membrane closest to the radiation source. All angiographic and IVUS measurements were performed at an independent core ultrasound laboratory by investigators blinded to procedural information and patient assignment.

A total of 55 patients were randomized: 26 to ^{192}Ir and 29 to placebo. Baseline clinical and angiographic characteristics were similar for both groups. Many study patients had one or more baseline characteristics associated with increased restenosis risk, including multiple epi-sodes of restenosis, lesion length >10 mm, ostial lesion location, vein graft target, and diabetes.

Follow-up angiography and IVUS was obtained in 53/55 patients. Late luminal loss was significantly lower in the ^{192}Ir group (0.38 ± 1.06 mm versus 1.03 ± 0.97 mm; $p = .009$). The late-loss index (late loss divided by acute gain) was also significantly lower in the ^{192}Ir group (0.12 ± 0.63 versus 0.60 ± 0.43; $p = .002$). The binary rate of angiographic restenosis within the stent or adjacent segments covered by the study ribbon was only 16.7% in the ^{192}Ir group, versus 53.6% for placebo ($p = .025$). Restenosis limited to the stented segment occurred in only 8.3% of the ^{192}Ir group compared to 35.7% of placebo patients ($p = .024$). The angiographic results were supported by the independent intravascular ultrasound analysis. By intravascular ultrasound analysis, there was no significant change in stent area or stent volume between the immediate postprocedure and follow-up periods. The decrease in mean lumen area at follow-up was smaller in the ^{192}Ir group (0.7 ± 1.0 mm^2 versus 2.2 ± 1.8 mm^2; $p = .003$). Similar results were obtained for lumen volume (16.4 ± 24.0 mm^3 for ^{192}Ir versus 44.3 ± 34.6 mm^3 for placebo; $p = .008$). The volume of tissue growth within the stent at follow-up was also significantly less in the ^{192}Ir-treated patients (15.5 ± 22.7 mm^3 versus 45.1 ± 39.4 mm^3; $p = .0091$).

Clinical follow-up was obtained for all patients at 24 months after their index study procedure. The difference in angiographic restenosis rates was supported by a reduction in target lesion revascularization in the ^{192}Ir group (15.4% versus 44.8%; $p < .01$). Composite clinical events (death, myocardial infarction, or target lesion revascularization) were also significantly less frequent in ^{192}Ir patients (23.1% versus 48.3%; $p < .01$) (161).

Clinical trials have also been performed with beta-emitters which have a rapid decline in dose rate within millimeters of the actual source. Thus, the exposure to the surrounding tissue and operators can be kept at a minimum and additional shielding is not required. The high intensity of beta-emitters also allows a shorter treatment period than with gamma-emitters. On the other hand, beta radiation may not penetrate deep enough into diseased vessel walls to provide clinical efficacy. Randomized data comparing beta radiation versus placebo are not yet available. In the Beta Energy Restenosis Trial (BERT) (162), patients undergoing balloon angioplasty of *de novo* lesions in native coronary arteries (reference vessel diameter 2.5–3.5 mm), were treated with the beta emitter ^{90}Sr/Y. A recent update has been released (163). Radiation was successfully delivered in 82 of 85 patients enrolled. Follow-up angiography at 6 months revealed a lower than expected late-loss index (9%), with a restenosis rate of 17%. Less favorable results were reported by Verin and colleagues using the beta-emitter yttrium-90 (164). Angiographic restenosis was seen in six of 15 patients (40%), perhaps due to an insufficient radiation dose.

Various new technologies are being developed to deliver radiation in close proximity to the target lesion, and thus minimize exposure to other tissues. Catheter-based delivery systems include line, liquid, gas, and membrane sources. Line sources such as ^{192}Ir, ^{32}P, and ^{90}Sr manufactured in 0.014–0.040 in. diameters can easily pass through intracoronary catheters. Typically, after dilatation and/or stenting of the target lesion, a 3 to 5 Fr catheter containing a blind-end source delivery lumen is advanced over a guidewire and positioned across the target lesion. A "wire" (typically composed of nylon or nitinol) containing radioactive sources at its distal tip is then loaded into the source lumen of the catheter and advanced distally until the radioactive sources span the target lesion. This process, called "afterloading," can either be accomplished manually by the radiation oncologist (165–166) or automatically by a motor-driven unit (167–169). One variation of the line source concept is a hydraulic delivery system (Novoste, Atlanta, GA), where encapsulated sources are injected into a blind-end catheter by a syringe or automated pumping system (162). Radiation delivery with a simple catheter can result in a source placed eccentrically within the vessel lumen. Assuming the target for radiotherapy is the adventitial border, a noncentered source will deliver a high radiation dose to the adventitia

closest to the catheter, and a low radiation dose to the adventitia furthest from the catheter. This dose heterogeneity (maximum/minimum dose) is about 3:1 for most noncentered systems (170). Alternatively, catheter centering systems, using either a segmented balloon (Schneider, Minneapolis, MN) (164) or a helical balloon (147,151) that also allows perfusion while inflated (Guidant, Santa Clara, CA), can reduce dose heterogeneity by maintaining the source in the center of the lumen. Whereas lumen centering does not center the source with respect to the adventitia, in concentric lesions lumen centering can lower dose heterogeneity from a 3:1 to about a 2.5:1 ratio (170).

Several radioactive stent systems have been developed, including ion implantation of phosphorous-32 (P-32) (157,171,172) and activation of a stainless steel stent in a cyclotron, producing a spectrum of radioisotopes (154–156,159,173). Most clinical investigation has been undertaken with the P-32 beta emitting stent. P-32 coated stents contain a specific activity ranging from 0.5–20 microcuries with a 14.3-day half-life, thereby exposing the vessel to beta radiation for about 45 days. These stents are of extremely low activity and can be handled with the aid of a simple 1-cm thick acrylic shield. Establishing safe and effective dosimetry presents a technical challenge to radioactive stent design. As stent struts expand, they separate, increasing the intrastrut distance and creating gaps in dose delivery. Appropriate dosing requires a therapeutic window broad enough to achieve effective inhibition of proliferation in regions where the stent struts are widely spread, without delivering a toxic dose in the region where stent struts come together. Further research in the field of intracoronary radiation is needed to confirm the benefit seen in the SCRIPPS trial, and to determine which isotopes and methods of delivery will yield the best results. Numerous randomized trials versus placebo are underway, and additional data with gamma and beta irradiation will soon be available.

Gene Therapy

Several studies using gene therapy to prevent restenosis in animal models have been successful (174–176). Theoretically, the use of stents to prevent recoil and remodeling, with gene therapy to prevent intimal hyperplasia, is a potent combination. Gene therapy, like intracoronary radiation, may be delivered locally to the arterial wall to limit systemic side effects. However, gene products which interfere with vascular smooth muscle cell replication or metabolism may impair essential functions of the arterial wall. Potential side effects could include aneurysm formation, impairment of vasomotor regulation, and destabilization of atherosclerotic plaques, resulting in acute ischemic syndromes (177). Transfer of the gene for vascular endothelial growth factor (VEGF) has the advantage of preventing restenosis (in animal models), without impairing smooth muscle cell function. Following angioplasty, delays in re-endothelialization have a permissive, if not facilitating effect on smooth muscle cell proliferation. In two separate animal models, transfer of the gene for VEGF accelerated re-endothelialization after balloon injury, leading to significant reductions in neointimal thickening (178–179). Similar results were obtained after deployment of Palmaz-Schatz stents in rabbit iliac arteries (175); however, other results have been less favorable (180). It is encouraging, however, that gene transfer of VEGF in humans with peripheral vascular disease was well tolerated and appeared to promote angiogenesis (181). It remains to be seen whether gene therapy with VEGF, or other molecules, will be effective therapy for restenosis in humans.

CONCLUSIONS

Coronary stents have revolutionized interventional cardiology. Although the use of stents results in reduced rates of restenosis compared to balloon angioplasty, in-stent restenosis remains a common problem. As the number of stents placed continues to rise, so will the number of patients with in-stent restenosis. In-stent restenosis is a new disease, with a different pathophysiology than restenosis in nonstented vessels.

Much uncertainty exists regarding the optimal therapy for in stent restenosis at this time. Large, prospective, multicenter, randomized trials with

systematic follow-up are needed to compare different treatment modalities. Although angioplasty and various forms of atherectomy are effective to varying degrees, refractory cases require more advanced treatment modalities. Fortunately, there are several promising therapies on the horizon.

REFERENCES

1. Fischman DL, Leon MB, Baim DS et al. A randomized study of coronary-stent placement and balloon angioplasty in the treatment of coronary artery disease. *N Engl J Med* 1994;331:496–501.
2. Serruys P, de Jaegere P, Kiemeneij F et al., for the Benestent Study Group. A comparison of balloon expandable stent implantation with balloon angioplasty in patients with coronary artery disease. *N Engl J Med* 1994; 331:489–495.
3. Erbel R, Haude M, Hopp HW et al. REstenosis STent (REST)-Study: randomized trial comparing stenting and balloon angioplasty for treatment of restenosis after balloon angioplasty. *J Am Coll Cardiol* 1996;27: 139A(abst).
4. Sirnes PA, Golf S, Myreng Y et al. Stenting in Chronic Coronary Occlusion (SICCO): a randomized controlled trial of adding stent implantation after successful angioplasty. *J Am Coll Cardiol* 1996;28: 1444–1451.
5. Rubartelli P, Niccoli L, Verna E et al. Stent implantation versus balloon angioplasty in chronic coronary occlusions: results from the GISSOC Trial. *J Am Coll Cardiol* 1998;32:90–96.
6. Savage MP, Douglas JS, Fischman DL et al. Stent placement compared with balloon angioplasty for obstructed coronary bypass grafts. *N Engl J Med* 1997; 337:740–747.
7. Herrmann HC, Buchbinder M, Clemen MW et al. Emergent use of balloon-expandable coronary artery stenting for failed percutaneous transluminal angioplasty. *Circulation* 1992;86:812–819.
8. George BS, Voorhees WD, Roubin GS et al. Multicenter investigation of coronary stenting to treat acute or threatened closure after percutaneous transluminal coronary angioplasty: clinical and angiographic outcomes. *J Am Coll Cardiol* 1993;22:135–143.
9. Hearn AJ, King SB, Douglas JS Jr, Carlin SF, Lembo NJ, Ghazzal ZM. Clinical and angiographic outcomes after coronary stenting for acute or threatened closure after percutaneous coronary angioplasty: initial results with a balloon expandable, stainless steel design. *Circulation* 1993;88:2086–2096.
10. Schomig A, Kastrati A, Mudra H et al. Four year experience with Palmaz-Schatz stenting in coronary angioplasty complicated by dissection with threatened or present vessel closure. *Circulation* 1994;89: 1126–1137.
11. Rankin JM, Milner RA, Carere RG et al. Increasing use of coronary stents is associated with a reduced requirement for repeat intervention in a large unselected population of patients referred for PTCA. *J Am Coll Cardiol* 1988;31:216A(abst).

12. Mudra H, Sunamura M, Figulla H et al. Six month clinical and angiographic outcome after IVUS guided stent implantation. *J Am Coll Cardiol* 1997;29: 171A(abst).
13. Sawada Y, Nosaka H, Kimura T, Nobuyoshi M. Initial and six month outcome of Palmaz-Schatz stent implantation: STRESS/Benestent equivalent versus nonequivalent lesions. *J Am Coll Cardiol* 1996;27:252A(abst).
14. Lablanche JM, Danchin N, Grollier G et al. Factors predictive of restenosis after stent implantation managed by ticlopidine and aspirin. *Circulation* 1996; 94[Suppl I]:I-256.
15. Mintz GS, Hoffman R, Mehran R et al. In-stent restenosis: the Washington Hospital Center experience. *Am J Cardiol* 1998;81(7A):7E–13E.
16. Anderson PG, Bajaj RK, Baxley WA, Roubin GS. Vascular pathology of balloon-expandable flexible coil stents in humans. *J Am Coll Cardiol* 1992;19:372–381.
17. Van Beusekom HMM, Van Der Giessen WJ, Van Suylen RJ, Bos E, Bosman FT, Serruys PW. Histology after stenting of human saphenous vein bypass grafts: observations from surgically excised grafts 3–320 days after stent implantation. *J Am Coll Cardiol* 1993;21: 45–54.
18. Schatz RA, Baim DS, Leon M et al. Clinical experience with the Palmaz-Schatz coronary stent: initial results of a multicenter study. *Circulation* 1991;83:148–161.
19. Komatsu R, Ueda M, Naruko T, Kojima A, Becker AE. Neointimal tissue response at sites of coronary stenting in humans. Macroscopic, histological, and immunohistochemical analyses. *Circulation* 1998;98: 224–233.
20. Gordon PC, Gibson CM, Cohen DJ, Carrozza JP, Kuntz RE, Baim DS. Mechanisms of restenosis and redilatation within coronary stents-quantitative angiographic assessment. *J Am Coll Cardiol* 1993;71: 364–366.
21. Haude M, Erbel R, Issa H, Meyer J. Quantitative analysis of elastic recoil after balloon angioplasty and after intracoronary implantation of balloon-expandable Palmaz-Schatz stents. *J Am Coll Cardiol* 1993;21:26–34.
22. Nunes G, Feres F, Maldonado G et al. Determination of the mechanisms responsible for stent restenosis: a quantitate angiographic study. *J Am Coll Cardiol* 1996; 27:362A(abst).
23. Mintz GS, Popma JJ, Pichard AD et al. Arterial remodeling after coronary angioplasty. A serial intravascular ultrasound study. *J Am Coll Cardiol* 1996;94:35–43.
24. Kornowski R, Mintz GS, Kent KM et al. Increased restenosis in diabetes mellitus after coronary interventions is due to exaggerated intimal hyperplasia. A serial intravascular ultrasound study. *Circulation* 1997;95: 1366–1369.
25. Hoffman R, Mintz GS, Dussaillant GR et al. Patterns and mechanisms of in-stent restenosis: a serial intravascular ultrasound study. *Circulation* 1996;94: 1247–1254.
26. Teirstein PS, Massullo V, Jani S et al. Catheter-based radiotherapy to inhibit restenosis after coronary stenting. *N Engl J Med* 1997;336:1697–1703.
27. Potkin BN, Batorelli AL, Gessert JM et al. Coronary artery imaging with intravascular high-frequency ultrasound. *Circulation* 1990;81:1575–1585.
28. Nishimura RA, Edwards WD, Warnes CA et al. Intravascular ultrasound imaging: *in vitro* validation and

pathologic correlation. *J Am Coll Cardiol* 1990;16: 145–154.
29. Tobis JM, Mallery JA, Gessert J et al. Intravascular ultrasound cross-sectional arterial imaging before and after balloon angioplasty *in vitro*. *Circulation* 1989; 80:873–882.
30. Tobis JM, Mallery J, Mahon D et al. Intravascular ultrasound imaging of human coronary arteries *in vivo*. analysis of tissue characterizations with comparison to *in vitro* histological specimens. *Circulation* 1991;83: 913–926.
31. Mintz GS, Popma JJ, Pichard AD et al. Arterial remodeling after coronary angioplasty: a serial intravascular ultrasound study. *Circulation* 1996;94:35–43.
32. Blessing E, Hausmann D, Sturm M, Wolpers HG, Amende I, Mugge A. Intravascular ultrasound guidance of stent implantation: intra-and interobserver variability. *Circulation* 1996;94[Suppl I]:I-200(abst).
33. Kastrati A, Schomig A, Elezi S et al. Predictive factors of restenosis after coronary stent placement. *J Am Coll Cardiol* 1997;30:1428–1436.
34. Mehran R, Abizaid AS, Hoffman RH et al. Clinical and angiographic predictors of target lesion revascularization after stent placement in native coronary lesions. *Circulation* 1997;96[Suppl I]:I-472A(abst).
35. Dirschinger J, Hausleiter J, Elazi S et al. Predictive factors of restenosis after coronary stent placement. *Circulation* 1997;96[Suppl I]:I-87(abst).
36. Carrozza JP, Kuntz RE, Levine MJ et al. Angiographic and clinical outcome of intracoronary stenting: immediate and long-term results from a large single-center experience. *J Am Coll Cardiol* 1992;20:328–337.
37. Bauters C, Hubert E, Prat A et al. Predictors of restenosis after coronary stent implantation. *J Am Coll Cardiol* 1998;31:1291–1298.
38. Deutsch E, Martin JL, Fischman DL et al. The late benefit of coronary stenting in small vessels is reduced in diabetic patients. *J Am Coll Cardiol* 1998;31: 275A(abst).
39. Carrozza JP, Kuntz RE, Fishman RF, Baim DS. Restenosis after arterial injury caused by coronary stenting in patients with diabetes mellitus. *Annals Of Internal Medicine* 1993;118:344–349.
40. Abizaid A, Mehran R, Bucher T et al. Does diabetes influence clinical recurrence after coronary stent implantation? *J Am Coll Cardiol* 1997;29:188A(abst).
41. Hoffman R, Mintz GS, Mehran R et al. Intravascular ultrasound predictors of angiographic restenosis in lesions treated with Palmaz-Schatz stents. *J Am Coll Cardiol* 1998;31:43–49.
42. Kobayashi Y, DeGregorio J, Reimers B, DiMario C, Finci L, Colombo A. The length of the stented segment is an independent predictor of restenosis. *J Am Coll Cardiol* 1998;31:366A(abst).
43. Kimura T, Takashi T, Yokoi H, Nobuyoshi M. Long-term clinical and angiographic follow-up after placement of Palmaz-Schatz Coronary Stent: a single-center experience. *J Intervent Cardiol* 1994;7:129–139.
44. Baim DS, Levine MJ, Leon MB, Levine S, Ellis SG, Schatz RA. Management of restenosis within the Palmaz-Schatz Coronary Stent (The U.S. multicenter experience). *Am. J Cardiol* 1993;71:364–366.
45. Hoffman R, Mintz GS, Mehran R et al. Predictors of intimal hyperplasia accumulation within Palmaz-Schatz Stents: a serial quantitative angiographic and

intravascular ultrasound study. *J Am Coll Cardiol* 1998;31:387A(abst).

46. Moussa I, DiMario C, Moses J, Reimers B, Blengino S, Colombo A. Single versus multiple Palmaz-Schatz Stent implantation: immediate and follow-up results. *J Am Coll Cardiol* 1997;29:276A(abst).

47. Ellis SG, Savage M, Fischman D et al. Restenosis after placement of Palmaz-Schatz Stents in native coronary arteries. Initial results of a multicenter experience. *Circulation* 1992;86:1836–1844.

48. Haude M, Erbel R, Straub U, Dietz U, Meyer J. Short and long term results after intracoronary stenting in human coronary arteries: monocentre experience with the balloon-expandable Palmaz-Schatz stent. *Br Heart J* 1991;66:337–345.

49. Kornowski R, Mehran R, Hong MK et al. Procedural results and late clinical outcomes after placement of three or more stents in single coronary lesions. *Circulation* 1998;97:1355–1361.

50. Weintraub WS, Kozsinski AS, Brown CL, King SB. Can restenosis after coronary angioplasty be predicted from clinical variables? *J Am Coll Cardiol* 1993;21: 6–14.

51. Rensing BJ, Hermans RM, Vos J et al. Luminal narrowing after percutaneous transluminal coronary angioplasty: a study of clinical, procedural, and lesional factors related to long-term angiographic outcome. *Circulation* 1993;88:975–985.

52. Ziada KM, Tuzcu EM, DeFranco AC et al. Absolute, not relative, post-stent lumen area is a better predictor of clinical outcome. *Circulation* 1996;94[Suppl I]:I-452(abst).

53. Hoffman R, Mintz GS, Mehran R et al. Intimal hyperplasia thickness is independent of stent size: a serial intravascular ultrasound study. *J Am Coll Cardiol* 1998;31:366A(abst).

54. Hoffman R, deVrey EA, Mintz GS et al. Intravascular ultrasound predictors of restenosis at the margins of Palmaz-Schatz stents. *Circulation* 1996;94[Suppl I]:I-199(abst).

55. Moussa I, DiMario C, Moses J, Reimers B, Blengino S, Colombo A. The predictive value of different intravascular ultrasound criteria for restenosis after coronary stenting. *J Am Coll Cardiol* 1997;29:60A(abst).

56. Mittal S, Weiss DL, Hirshfeld JW, Kolansky DM, Herrman HC. Comparison of outcome for *De Novo* versus restenotic narrowings in native coronary arteries. *Am J Cardiol* 1997;80:711–715.

57. Colombo A, Ferraro M, Itoh A, Martini G, Blengino S, Finci L. Results of coronary stenting for restenosis. *J Am Coll Cardiol* 1998;28:830–836.

58. Stone GW, St. Goar F, Fitzgerald P et al. The optimal stent implantation trial—final core lab angiographic and ultrasound analysis. *J Am Coll Cardiol* 1997; 369A(abst).

59. Savage MP, Fischman DL, Douglas JS et al. The dark side of high pressure stent deployment. *J Am Coll Cardiol* 1997;29:368A,(abst).

60. Fernandez-Aviles F, Alonso JJ, Duran JM et al. High pressure increases late loss after coronary stenting. *J Am Coll Cardiol* 1997;29:369A(abst)

61. Akiyama T, DiMario C, Reimers B et al. Does high pressure stent expansion induce more restenosis? *J Am Coll Cardiol* 1997;29:368A(abst).

62. Yokoi H, Nosaka H, Kimura T et al. Influence of high-

pressure stent dilatation on late angiographic and clinical outcome of Palmaz-Schatz Stent implantation. *J Am Coll Cardiol* 1997;29:312A(abst).

63. Mehran R, Popma JJ, Baim DS et al. Routine high pressure post-stent dilation did not influence clinical restenosis in STARS. *J Am Coll Cardiol* 1998;31: 80A(abst).

64. Schofer J, Rau T, Golestani R, Mathey DG. Procedural vessel wall injury is not associated with late tissue proliferation within stents. *Circulation* 1997;96[Suppl I]: I-402(abst).

65. Colombo A, Hall P, Nakamura S et al. Intracoronary stenting without anticoagulation accomplished with intravascular ultrasound guidance. *Circulation* 1995;91: 1676–1688.

66. Dirschinger J, Schuhlen H, Hausleiter J et al. A randomized trial of low versus high pressure for coronary stent placement: analysis of early outcome. *Circulation* 1997;96[Suppl I]:I-653(abst).

67. Ribichini F, Steffenino G, Dellavalle A et al. Plasma activity and insertion/deletion polymorphism of angiotensin i-converting enzyme. A major risk factor and a marker of risk for coronary stent restenosis. *Circulation* 1998;97:147–154.

68. Amant C, Bauters C, Bodart JC et al. *D* allele of the angiotensin i-converting enzyme is a major risk factor for restenosis after coronary stenting. *Circulation* 1997;96:56–60.

69. Ribichini F, Steffenino G, Dellavalle A et al. The pattern (focal/diffuse) of angiographic in-stent restenosis is associated to the i/d polymorphism of the angiotensin converting enzyme gene. *Circulation* 1997;96[Suppl I]:I-87(abst).

70. Bodart JC, Amant C, Bauters F et al. The D allele of the angiotensin I converting enzyme is associated with diffuse in-stent restenosis. *J Am Coll Cardiol* 1998;31: 356A(abst).

71. Mudra H, Regar E, Klauss V et al. Serial follow-up after optimized ultrasound-guided deployment of Palmaz-Schatz Stents. In-stent neointimal proliferation without significant reference segment response. *Circulation* 1997;95:363–370.

72. Williams DO, Gruentzig AR, Kent KM, Kelsey SF, To T. Efficacy of repeat percutaneous transluminal coronary angioplasty for coronary restenosis. *Am J Cardiol* 1984;53:32C–35C.

73. Joly P, Bonan R, Palisaitis D et al. Treatment of recurrent restenosis with repeat percutaneous transluminal coronary angioplasty. *Am J Cardiol* 1988;61:906–908.

74. Quigley PJ, Hlatky MA, Hinohara T et al. Repeat percutaneous transluminal coronary angioplasty and predictors of recurrent restenosis. *Am J Cardiol* 1989;63: 409–413.

75. Glazier JJ, Varrichione TR, Ryan TJ, Ruocco NA, Jacobs AK, Faxon DP. Outcome in patients with recurrent restenosis after percutaneous transluminal balloon angioplasty. *Br Heart J* 1989;61:485–488.

76. Bauters C, McFadden EP, Lablanche JM, Quandalle P, Bertrand ME. Restenosis rate after multiple percutaneous transluminal coronary angioplasty procedures at the same site. A quantitative angiographic study in consecutive patients undergoing a third angioplasty procedure for a second restenosis. *Circulation* 1993;88: 969–974.

77. Teirstein PS, Hoover CA, Ligon RW et al. Repeat coro-

nary angioplasty: efficacy of a third angioplasty for a second restenosis. *J Am Coll Cardiol* 1989;13; 291–296.

78. Meier B, Gruentzig AR, Hollman J, Ischinger T, Bradford JM. Does length or eccentricity of coronary stenoses influence the outcome of transluminal dilatation? *Circulation* 1983;67:497–499.

79. Topol EJ, Ellis SG, Fishman et al. Multicenter study of percutaneous transluminal angioplasty for right coronary artery ostial stenosis. *J Am Coll Cardiol* 1987; 9:1214–1218.

80. Savage MP, Fischman DL, Rake R, Gebhardt S, Goldberg S. Interprocedural interval as a predictor of stent restenosis after previous coronary angioplasty. *Am J Cardiol* 1996;78:683–684.

81. Mintz GS, Popma JJ, Pichard AD et al. Intravascular ultrasound predictors of restenosis after percutaneous transcatheter coronary revascularization. *J Am Coll Cardiol* 1996;27:1678–1687.

82. Hoffman R, Keers B, Borjanca O et al. Predictors of diffuse in-stent restenosis. *Circulation* 1997;96[Suppl I]:I-472.

83. Reimers B, Moussa I, Akiyama T et al. Long-term follow-up after successful repeat intervention for stent restenosis. *J Am Coll Cardiol* 1997;30:186–192.

84. Yokoi H, Kimura T, Nakagawa Y, Nosaka H, Nobuyoshi M. Long-term clinical and quantitate angiographic follow-up after Palmaz-Schatz Stent restenosis. *J Am Coll Cardiol* 1996;27:224A(abst).

85. Bauters C, Banos JL, Van Belle E, McFadden EP, Lablanche JM, Bertrand ME. Six-month angiographic outcome after successful repeat percutaneous intervention for in-stent restenosis. *Circulation* 1998;97: 318–321.

86. Mehran R, Abizaid AS, Mintz GS et al. Patterns of in-stent restenosis: classification and impact on subsequent target lesion revascularization. *J Am Coll Cardiol* 1998;31:141A(abst).

87. Yokoi H, Kimura T, Hamasaki N et al. Coronary stent restenosis; comparison of six different types of stent. *J Am Coll Cardiol* 1998;31:313A(abst).

88. Dauerman HL, Baim DS, Cutlip DE et al. Mechanical debulking versus balloon angioplasty for the treatment of diffuse in-stent restenosis. *Am J Cardiol* 1998;82: 277–284.

89. Sharma SK, Duvvuri S, Kini A et al. Rotational atherectomy for in-stent restenosis: acute and long term results of first 100 cases. *Circulation* 1997;96[Suppl I]: I-88(abst).

90. Mahdi NA, Pathan AZ, Harrell L et al. Directional atherectomy for the treatment of Palmaz-Schatz In-Stent restenosis. *Am J Cardiology: (in press)*.

91. Kastrati A, Schomig A, Dietz R, Neumann FJ, Richardt G. Time course of restenosis during the first year after emergency coronary stenting. *Circulation* 1993;87: 1498–1505.

92. Nibler N, Kastrati A, Elezi S, Walter H, Schuhlen H, Schomig A. Angiographic and clinical follow-up of patients with asymptomatic restenosis after coronary stent implantation. *J Am Coll Cardiol* 1998;31: 65A(abst).

93. Kimura T, Yokoi H, Nakagawa Y et al. Three-year follow-up after implantation of metallic coronary-artery stents. *N Engl J Med* 1996;334:561–566.

94. Macdonald RG, O'Neill BJ, Creighton JE, Brown RIG,

95. Mehran R, Mintz GS, Popma JJ et al. Mechanisms and results of balloon angioplasty for the treatment of in-stent restenosis. *Am J Cardiol* 1996;78:618–622.

96. Schiele F, Meneveau N, Vuillemenot A, Gupta S, Zhang DD, Bassand JP. Intra coronary ultra sound assessment of balloon angioplasty in intrastent restenosis. *J Am Coll Cardiol* 1997;29:240A(abst).

97. Gorge G, Konorza T, Voegele E et al. Incomplete restoration of luminal dimensions after PTCA in restenotic stented segments: an intravascular ultrasound analysis. *J Am Coll Cardiol* 1997;311A(abst).

98. Mehran R, Mintz GS, Popma JJ et al. Treatment of in-stent restenosis: an intravascular ultrasound study of results in 159 stented lesions. *J Am Coll Cardiol* 1997; 29:77A(abst).

99. Sharma SK, Kini A, Duvvuri S et al. Randomized trial of rotational atherectomy versus balloon angioplasty for in-stent restenosis. *J Am Coll Cardiol (in press)*.

100. Eltchaninoff H, Cribier A, Koning R, Tron C, Letac B. *Balloon angioplasty for in-stent restenosis: 6-months angiographic follow-up. Circulation* 1997;96[Suppl I]: I-88(abst).

101. Macander PJ, Roubin GS, Agrawal SK, Cannon AD, Dean LS, Baxley WA. Balloon angioplasty for treatment of in-stent restenosis: feasibility, safety and efficacy. *Cathet and Cardiovasc Diagn* 1994;32:125–131.

102. Schomig A, Kastrati A, Dietz R et al. Emergency coronary stenting for dissection during percutaneous transluminal coronary angioplasty: angiographic follow-up after stenting and after repeat angioplasty of the stented segment. *J Am Coll Cardiol* 1994;23:1053–1060.

103. Bottner RK, Hardigan KR. High speed rotational ablation for in-stent restenosis. *Cathet Cardiovasc Diagn* 1997;40:144–149.

104. Goldberg SL, Shawl F, Buchbinder M et al. Rotational atherectomy for in-stent restenosis: The BARASTER Registry. *Circulation* 1997;96[Suppl I]:I-80(abst).

105. Mehran R, Mintz GS, Abizaid A et al. Mechanistic comparison of rotational atherectomy and excimer laser angioplasty in the treatment of in-stent restenosis: a volumetric intravascular ultrasound study. *J Am Coll Cardiol* 1998;31:103A(abst).

106. Goldberg SL, Shawl F, Buchbinder M et al. Rotational atherectomy in the treatment of intra-stent restenosis: The BARASTER Multicenter Registry. Personal Communication from Steven L. Goldberg.

107. Lee S-G, Lee CW, Cheong S-S et al. Immediate and long-term outcomes of rotational atherectomy versus balloon angioplasty alone for treatment of diffuse in-stent restenosis. *Am J Cardiol* 1998;82:140–143.

108. Buttner HJ, Muller C, Hodgson JMcB, Frey AW, Jander N. Rotational ablation with adjunctive low-pressure balloon dilatation in diffuse in-stent restenosis: immediate and follow-up results. *J Am Coll Cardiol* 1998;31:141A(abst).

109. Strauss BH, Umans VA, van Suylen RJ et al. Directional atherectomy for treatment of restenosis within coronary stents: clinical angiographic and histological results. *J Am Coll Cardiol* 1992;20:1465–1473.

110. Bowerman RE, Pinkerton CA, Kirk B, Waller BF. Dis-

ruption of a coronary stent during atherectomy for restenosis. *Cathet Cardiovasc Diagn* 1991;24:248–251.

111. Meyer T, Schmidt T, Buchwald A, Weigand V. Stent wire cutting during coronary directional atherectomy. *Clin Cardiol* 1993;16:450–452.

112. Cattelaens N, Gerkens U, Mueller R, Gerlach J, Grube E. Directional atherectomy for treatment of stent restenosis-feasibility and histopathological findings in 28 patients. *J Am Coll Cardiol* 1998;31:142A(abst).

113. Mahdi NA, Leon M, Mikulic M et al. PTCA, directional atherectomy and rotational atherectomy in the management of Palmaz-Schatz in-stent restenosis. *J Am Coll Cardiol* 1998;31:275A(abst).

114. Koster R, Hamm CW, Terres W et al. Treatment of in-stent coronary restenosis by excimer laser angioplasty. *Am J Cardiol* 1997;80:1424–1428.

115. Koster R, Hamm CW, Terres W et al. Long term results of laser angioplasty for in-stent restenosis. *J Am Coll Cardiol* 1998;31:141A(abst).

116. Mehran R, Mintz GS, Satler LF et al. Treatment of in-stent restenosis with excimer laser coronary angioplasty. mechanisms and results compared with PTCA alone. *Circulation* 1997;96:2183–2189.

117. Hamm CW, Simon RJ, Gomes S, Sievert C, Macaya C. Laser angioplasty for within stent restenosis-final results of the LARS Surveillance Study. *J Am Coll Cardiol* 1998;31:143A(abst).

118. Haase J, Reifart N, Schwarz F et al. Is excimer laser angioplasty superior to balloon dilatation for the treatment of in-stent restenosis? Results of a prospective single-center study. *J Am Coll Cardiol* 1998;31[Suppl C]:400C(abst).

119. Virk SJS, Bellamy CM, Perry RA. Transluminal extraction atherectomy for stent restenosis in a saphenous vein bypass graft. *Eur Heart J* 1997;18:350–351.

120. Goods CM, Jain SP, Liu MW, Babu RB, Roubin GS. Intravascular ultrasound-guided transluminal extraction atherectomy for restenosis after Gianturco-Roubin Coronary Stent implantation. *Cathet Cardiovasc Diagn.* 1996;37:317–319.

121. Ikari Y, Yamaguchi T, Tamura T, Isshiki T, Saeki F, Hara K. Transluminal extraction atherectomy and adjunctive balloon angioplasty after Palmaz-Schatz coronary stent implantation. *Cathet Cardiovasc Diagn* 1993;30:127–130.

122. Patel JJ, Maedaa R, Cohen M, Adiraju R, Kussmaul WG. Transluminal extraction atherectomy for aortosaphenous vein graft stent restenosis. *Cathet Cardiovasc Diagn* 1996;38:320–324.

123. Hara K, Ikari Yuji, Tamura T, Yamaguchi T. Transluminal extraction atherectomy for restenosis following Palmaz-Schatz Stent implantation. *Am Heart J* 1997; 79:801–802.

124. Shiran A, Mintz GS, Waksman R et al. Early lumen loss after treatment of in-stent restenosis. An intravascular ultrasound study. *Circulation* 1998;98:200–203.

125. Mehran R, Abizaid AS, Mintz GS et al. Mechanisms and results of additional stent implantation to treat focal in-stent restenosis. *J Am Coll Cardiol* 1998;31: 455A(abst).

126. Russo RJ, Massullo V, Jani SK et al. Restenting versus PTCA for in-stent restenosis with or without intracoronary radiation therapy: an analysis of the SCRIPPS Trial. *Circulation* 1997;96[Suppl I]:I-219(abst).

127. Elezi S, Kastrati A, Schuhlen H, Hausleiter J, Alt E,

Wehinger A. Stenting for restenosis of stented lesions: acute and 6 months clinical and angiographic follow-up. *Circulation* 1997;96[Suppl I]:I-88(abst).

128. LeFevre T, Louvard Y, Morice MC. In-stent restenosis: should we stent the stent? A single-center prospective study. *Circulation* 1997;96[Suppl I]:I-88(abst).

129. Goldberg SL, Loussararian AH, Di Mario C et al. Stenting for in-stent restenosis. *Circulation* 1997; 96[Suppl I]:I-88(abst).

130. Tardif JC, Cote G, Lesperance J et al. Probucol and multivitamins in the prevention of restenosis after coronary angioplasty. *N Engl J Med* 1997;337:365–372.

131. Yokoi H, Kuwabara Y, Yamaguchi H. One year follow-up results of the probucol angioplasty restenosis trial. *Circulation* 1996;94[Suppl I]:I-91.

132. Topol EJ, Califf RM, Weisman HF et al., for the EPIC investigators. Randomised trial of coronary intervention with antibody against platelet IIb/IIIa integrin for reduction of clinical restenosis: results at six months. *Lancet* 1994;343:881–886.

133. The Epilog Investigators. Platelet glycoprotein IIb/IIIa receptor blockade and low-dose heparin during percutaneous coronary revascularization. *N Engl J Med* 1997;336:1689–1696.

134. Lefkovits J, Topol EJ. Pharmacological approaches for the prevention of restenosis after percutaneous coronary intervention. *Progress Cardiovasc Dis* 1997;40: 141–158.

135. Ellis SG, Serruys PW, Popma JJ et al. Can abciximab prevent neointimal proliferation in Palmaz-Schatz Stents? The final ERASER results. *Circulation* 1997; 96[Suppl I]:I-87(abst).

136. The IMPACT-II Investigators. Randomised placebo-controlled trial of effect of eptifibatide on complications of percutaneous coronary intervention: IMPACT-II. *Lancet* 1997;349:1422–1428.

137. The CAPTURE Investigators. Randomised placebo-controlled trial of abciximab before and during coronary intervention in refractory unstable angina: the CAPTURE study. *Lancet* 1997;349:1429–1435.

138. Kastrati A, Schuhlen H, Hausleiter J et al. Restenosis after coronary stent placement and randomization to a 4-week combined antiplatelet or anticoagulant therapy. *Circulation* 1997;96:462–467.

139. Kunishima T, Musha H, Eto F et al. A randomized trial of aspirin versus cilostazol after successful coronary stent implantation. *Clinical Therapeutics* 1997; 19:1058–1066.

140. Hara K, Yamasaki M, Kozuma K et al. Cilostazol reduces late lumen loss after Palmaz-Schatz stent implantation. *Circulation* 1996;94[Suppl I]:I-91.

141. Kozuma K, Hara K, Morino Y et al. Effects of cilostazol on restenosis after Palmaz-Schatz coronary stent implantation. *J Am Coll Cardiol* 1998;31:139A(abst).

142. Tsuchikane E, Katoh O, Sumitsuji S et al. Impact of cilostazol on intimal proliferation after directional coronary atherectomy. *Am Heart J* 1998;135:495–502.

143. Wiedermann JG, Marboe C, Amols H, Schwartz A, Weinberger J. Intracoronary irradiation markedly reduces neointimal proliferation after balloon angioplasty in swine: persistent benefit at 6-month follow-up. *J Am Coll Cardiol* 1995;25:1451–1456.

144. Waksman R, Robinson KA, Crocker IR, Gravanis MB, Cipolla GD, King SB III. Endovascular low-dose irradiation inhibits neointima formation after coronary ar-

tery balloon injury in swine. A possible role for radiation therapy in restenosis prevention. *Circulation* 1995; 91:1533–1539.

145. Waksman R, Robinson KA, Crocker IR et al. Intracoronary low-dose β-irradiation inhibits neointima formation after coronary artery balloon injury in the swine restenosis model. *Circulation* 1995;92:3025–3031.

146. Verin V, Popowski Y, Urban P et al. Intra-arterial beta irradiation prevents neointimal hyperplasia in a hypercholesterolemic rabbit restenosis model. *Circulation* 1995;92:2284–2290.

147. Mazur W, Ali MN, Dabaghi SF et al. High-dose rate intracoronary radiation suppresses neointimal proliferation in the stented and ballooned model of porcine restenosis. *Circulation* 1994;90:1–652(abst).

148. Gellman J, Healey G, Chen Q et al. The effect of very low dose irradiation on restenosis following balloon angioplasty. A study in the atherosclerotic rabbit. *Circulation* 1991;84:II-331(abst).

149. Mayberg MR, Lou Z, London S, Gajdusek C, Rasey J. Radiation inhibition of intimal hyperplasia after arterial injury. *Radiat Res* 1995;142:212–220.

150. Shimotakahara S, Mayberg MR. Gamma irradiation inhibits neointimal hyperplasia in rats after arterial injury. *Stroke* 1994;25:424–428.

151. Mazur W, Ali MN, Khan MM et. al. High dose rate intracoronary radiation for inhibition of neointimal formation in the stented and balloon-injured porcine models of restenosis: angiographic, morphometric and histopathologic analyses. *Int J Radiat Oncol Biol Phys* 1996;36:777–778.

152. Waksman R. Intracoronary radiation adjunct therapy to stenting. *J Intervent Cardiol* 1977;10:2133–2136.

153. Waksman R, Robinson K, Crocker I et al. Intracoronary radiation decreases the second phase of intimal hyperplasia in a repeat balloon angioplasty swine model of restenosis. *Int J Radiat Oncol Biol Phys* 1997; 39:475–480.

154. Hehrlein C, Stintz M, Kinscherf R et al. Pure β-particle emitting stents inhibit neointima formation in rabbits. *Circulation* 1996;93:641–645.

155. Hehrlein C, Zimmermann J, Metz J, Fehsenfeld P, von Hodenberg E. Radioactive coronary stent implantation inhibits neointimal proliferation in nonatherosclerotic rabbits. *Circulation* 1993;88:I-651.

156. Hehrlein C, Gollan C, Dönges K et al. Low-dose radioactive endovascular stents prevent smooth muscle cell proliferation and neointimal hyperplasia in rabbits. *Circulation* 1995;92:1570–1575.

157. Fischell TA, Kharma BK, Fischell DR et al. Low-dose, β-particle emission from "stent" wire results in complete, localized inhibition of smooth muscle cell proliferation. *Circulation* 1994;90:2956–2963.

158. Shefer A, Eigler NL, Whiting JS, Litvack FI. Suppression of intimal proliferation after balloon angioplasty with local beta irradiation in rabbits. *J Am Coll Cardiol* 1993;21[Suppl A]:185A(abst).

159. Hehrlein C, Donges K, Gollan C, Metz J, Riessen R, Gehsenfeld P. Low-dose radioactive Palmaz-Schatz stents prevent smooth muscle cell proliferation and neointimal hyperplasia in rabbits. *J Am Coll Cardiol* 1995;9A:(abst).

160. Condado JA, Waksman R, Gurdiel O et al. Long-term angiographic and clinical outcome after percutaneous transluminal coronary angioplasty and intracoronary radiation therapy in humans. *Circulation* 1997;96: 727–732.

161. Teirstein PS, Massullo V, Jani S et al. Two-year follow-up after catheter-based radiotherapy to inhibit coronary restenosis. *Circulation* (*in press*).

162. King SB III, Williams DO, Chougule P et al. Endovascular β-radiation to reduce restenosis after coronary balloon angioplasty. Results of the Beta Energy Restenosis Trial (BERT). *Circulation* 1998;97:2025–2030.

163. Novoste Corporation. Novoste Announces Final Summary Data From BERT Feasibility Trial. Norcross, GA: Novoste Corporation 1998 August 17(press release).

164. Verin V, Urban P, Popowski Y et al. Feasibility of intracoronary β-irradiation to reduce restenosis after balloon angioplasty. A clinical pilot study. *Circulation* 1997;95:1138–1144.

165. Teirstein PS, Massullo V, Jani S. Radiation therapy following coronary stenting—6-month follow-up of a randomized clinical trial. *Circulation* 1996;94[Suppl 1]:1–210.

166. Massullo VM, Teirstein PS, Jani SK et al. Endovascular brachytherapy to inhibit coronary artery restenosis: an introduction to the Scripps Coronary Radiation to inhibit proliferation post stenting trial. *Int J Radiat Oncol Biol Phys* 1996;36:973–975.

167. Henschke UK, Hilaris BS, Mahan GD. Remote afterloading for intracavitary radiation therapy. *Radiology* 1964;83:344–345.

168. Parikh S, Nori D. Endovascular brachytherapy: current status and future trends. *J Brachyther Int* 1997;13: 167–177.

169. Jani SK, Massullo V, Teirstein P. The ^{192}Ir radioactive seed ribbon. In: Waksman R, Serruys PW, eds. *Handbook of vascular brachytherapy*. London: Martin Dunitz, Ltd., 1998:27–32.

170. Arbab-Zadeh A, Russo RJ, Jani SK et al. A comparison of centered versus non-centered source for intracoronary radiation therapy: observations from the SCRIPPS Trial. *Circulation* 1997;96[Suppl I]:I-219(abst).

171. Laird JR, Carter AJ, Kufs WM et al. Inhibition of neointimal proliferation with a beta particle emitting stent. *J Am Coll Cardiol* 1995;287A:773(abst).

172. Fischell TA, Abbas MA, Kallman RF. Low-dose irradiation inhibits clonal proliferation of smooth muscle cells: a new approach to restenosis. *Arterioscler Thromb* 1991;11:1435a(abst).

173. Hehrlein C, Zimmermann M, Metz J, Fehsenfeld P, von Hodenberg E. Radioactive stent implantation inhibits neointimal proliferation in non-atherosclerotic rabbits. *Circulation* 1993;88[Suppl I]:I-651(abst).

174. Varenne O, Sinnaeve P, Gillijns H et al. Comparison of recombinant adenovirus vectors expressing antimigratory and antiproliferative proteins in a porcine coronary restenosis model. *J Am Coll Cardiol* 1998;31: 356A(abst).

175. Van Belle E, Tio FO, Chen D et al. Passivation of metallic stents after arterial gene transfer of phVEGF$_{165}$ inhibits thrombus formation and intimal thickening. *J Am Coll Cardiol* 1997;29:1371–1379.

176. Chang MW, Barr E, Seltzer J et al. Cytostatic gene therapy for vascular proliferative disorders with a con-

stitutively active form of the retinoblastoma gene product. *Science* 1995;267:518–522.

177. DeYoung MB, Dichek DA. Gene therapy for restenosis: are we ready? *Circ Res* 1998;82:306–313.

178. Asahara T, Chen D, Tsurumi Y et al. Accelerated restitution of endothelial integrity and endothelium-dependent function after phVEGF$_{165}$ gene transfer. *Circulation* 1996;94:3291–3302.

179. Asahara T, Bauters C, Pastore C et al. Local delivery of vascular endothelial growth factor accelerates reendothelialization and attenuates intimal hyperplasia in balloon-injured rat carotid artery. *Circulation* 1995;91: 2793–2801.

180. Lazarous DF, Shou M, Scheinowitz M et al. Comparative effects of basic fibroblast growth factor and vascular endothelial growth factor on coronary collateral development and the arterial response to injury. *Circulation* 1996;94:1074–1082.

181. Isner JM, Pieczek A, Schainfeld R et al. Clinical evidence of angiogenesis after arterial gene transfer of phVEGF$_{165}$ in patient with ischaemic limb. *Lancet* 1996;348:370–374.

15

The Chronic Occlusion

A. The Chronic Occlusion

Bernhard Meier

Department of Cardiology, University Hospital, CH-3012, Bern, Switzerland

Chronic total coronary artery occlusions are tackled in about 10% to 20% of angioplasty procedures (1,2) and constitute one of the main criteria when selecting between angioplasty and bypass surgery. Chronic occlusion angioplasty carries a reduced risk for complications but it is technically more intricate and plagued by a reduced success rate when compared with angioplasty of nontotal lesions.

A number of dedicated techniques and materials for chronic occlusion angioplasty have been described and evaluated. They include specific mechanical guidewires such as the ball-tipped Magnum wire (3,4), the laser wire (5), hydrophilic guidewires (6–8), or particularly robust wires (9). Randomized comparisons between these methods are scarce and published results depend heavily on indications and patient selection. A recent short and straight occlusion with a nicely tapered stump in a large and reasonably healthy vessel yields a success rate of over 90% with any method selected. A long occlusion documented to be older than 6 months in a small, tortuous, and diffusely diseased artery, on the other hand, that has already been attempted with a certain technique with determination but in vain, projects a success rate below 30% with any other technique and should be left alone.

Success in chronic total coronary occlusions is firstly a result of the anatomical situation, secondly of the skill of the operator and the material available, and thirdly of the perseverance and the time invested.

PREREQUISITES FOR RECANALIZATION

The indication for a recanalization attempt balances the anticipated benefit of the patient in terms of symptom reduction, improvement of prognosis, and obviation of need for bypass surgery against the technical difficulties and procedural risks. Subjective improvement can only be expected in the presence of symptoms that are based on the occlusion with a high degree of likelihood. Risk reduction can be hoped for based on the hypothesis that the occluded vessel may be needed later to support a vessel not yet occluded. Avoidance (or at least postponement) of bypass surgery, finally, is at stake in patients determined to undergo surgery to better their situation or in patients in whom the total occlusion is the decisive factor between the two revascularization modalities.

The estimate of the technical difficulties had better include trivial things such as the need for travel and absence from work for the intervention and vascular access problems in addition to the attributes of the lesion mentioned above. In other words, an occlusion with a relatively low chance of successful recanalization may be tackled as an ad hoc procedure attached to the diagnostic study or as a supplement to an angioplasty of a different primary target lesion. Per se, it should not be the motive of a long-distance referral or added on to a long waiting list.

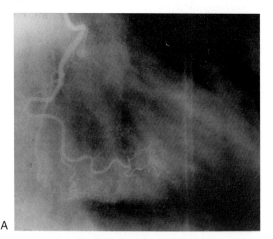

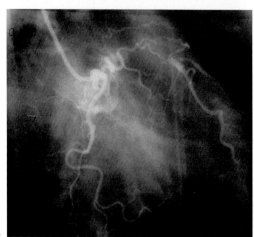

FIG. 15.1. Conal branch, originating in the vicinity of the right coronary artery, as a single collateral to the occluded left anterior descending coronary artery. **A:** Conal branch missed because of too deep an intubation into the orifice of the right coronary artery. **B:** Conal branch visualized after slight withdrawal of the catheter. Only after visualizing the distal part of the left anterior descending coronary artery was the indication for the recanalization attempt of this vessel established.

The presence of collaterals clearly outlining the course, size, and ideally also the state of the distal vessel is the prime prerequisite for any recanalization attempt of chronic occlusions. A myocardial territory devoid of visible blood supply for any prolonged period of time cannot possibly be vital or viable and does not need (or deserve for that matter) costly revascularization attempts. Nor is there hope for reversed collater-

als later, for obvious reasons. It must be mentioned, however, that collaterals can be missed on a diagnostic study. They may be framed out or the film sequences may be too short. In addition, a separately originating conal branch in the right coronary cusp feeding the occluded left anterior descending coronary artery is not uncommon and must be specifically looked for (Fig. 15.1).

BENEFIT IN CASE OF SUCCESS

It is of note that successful recanalization of a chronic total occlusion was the first indication of coronary angioplasty yielding the promise of improved longevity in a carefully analyzed study (10). Nonetheless, improved survival is not the foremost goal of recanalization attempts. The natural course of patients with a chronically occluded coronary artery is rather benign (3% mortality during the first year) with the exception of patients with a recent occlusion of the left anterior descending coronary artery, whose 1-year mortality is 10% (11). A marked reduction of subsequent coronary artery bypass operations is the most conspicuous benefit of the procedure (10,12–14). On the average, a reduction of bypass surgery by two-thirds can be expected (Fig. 15.2).

Improvement in myocardial function after recanalization of a chronic total occlusion has been the focus of numerous studies. While no acute effect has been observed, gradual improvement

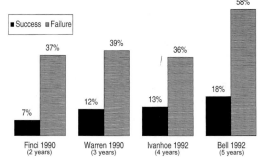

FIG. 15.2. Subsequent need for coronary artery bypass surgery in patients with successful or failed recanalization of chronic total coronary occlusions (10,12–14).

of regional (15,16) and global ejection fraction (16,17) has been conclusively demonstrated, provided long-term patency could be achieved.

Clinical improvement is certainly the driving force for the patient to undergo an attempt to recanalize a chronically occluded coronary artery. As clinical improvement is difficult to quantify, exercise test data serve as a surrogate. They corroborate the impression that patients with successful recanalization have significantly less ischemia during follow-up than those with a failed attempt and medical treatment alone (12).

TECHNICAL CONSIDERATIONS

Prediction of Success

Success or failure can be predicted to a certain degree based on a variety of factors (18). Duration of occlusion emerges from most studies as the key variable with a rapid decline of success already during the first 4 weeks (19–22). The presumed length of the occluded segment is the next important variable (23). The presence of a stump or a tapered segment leading into the occlusion is a favorable attribute (10,24), whereas bridging collaterals exert a strongly negative influence (24) (Fig. 15.3). Only partic-

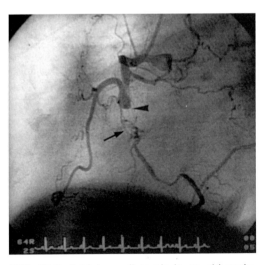

FIG. 15.3. Bridging collaterals in an old occlusion of the right coronary artery. The *arrowhead* indicates the site of occlusion. Tortuous but well-developed "bridging" collaterals (*arrow*) provide complete and prompt filling of the distal artery with contrast medium.

ularly dedicated operators achieve acceptable success rates in the presence of bridging collaterals (25). Chronically occluded bypass grafts are a target to be left alone according to several authors (26–29). Pretreatment with urokinase has been advocated by some. When the respective data are scrutinized, however, the results are rather dismal (29).

Selection of Material

The major drawback of Monorail dilatation systems (Boston Scientific Scimed, Maple Grove, MN) (30) is the inability to reshape or exchange coronary guidewires while securing the attained position in front of the occlusion with the balloon catheter. This may be more important in the setting of chronic total coronary occlusions than in other settings. Hence, some operators retain this indication as their only remaining non-Monorail (over-the-wire) approach. This makes sense for operators starting with a soft wire, because a wire exchange will invariably become necessary unless the initial diagnosis of a chronic occlusion was erroneous. Starting with a robust wire with an intelligently preshaped tip usually succeeds without wire exchange or allows a conclusive enough attempt in case of failure to obviate the need or temptation for immediate further tackling with other wires. A typical time to abandon the procedure is when a long subintimal path has been created that cannot be avoided, in spite of repeated attempts starting sufficiently proximal to the entry.

Hydrophilic guidewires (8) of the stiff variety offer the best potential for crossing a chronic occlusion of any type. Their drawback is that they also harbor the highest risk of subintimal pathways or perforations (31). A wire perforation within the occluded segment typically is clinically irrelevant. It will reclose immediately if the recanalization attempt is terminated or if the true passage is found and the dilatation with or without subsequent stenting is carried out. An unrecognized wire perforation, however, that is enlarged by advancement or even inflation of the balloon catheter, engenders a vessel tear or rupture and may have grave consequences. It is likely to require pericardiocentesis (the harvested blood should be reinjected into a vein), implantation of a (covered) stent, emergency surgery, or a combination thereof. The same holds true for the perforation of a healthy, thin-walled peripheral coronary artery by the tip of a hydrophilic guidewire that had correctly negotiated the occluded segment but was sloppily controlled during subsequent balloon manipulations, catheter exchanges, or stent implantations. Such holes may be multiple and exhibit a low tendency for spontaneous sealing. In addition, the vessel is under pressure through the recanalized segment or, in case of unsuccessful recanalization, through the collaterals. Some authors recommend replacing hydrophilic guidewires with conventional ones, once the occlusion is successfully traversed. This is only feasible with non-Monorail systems and increases cost, an important issue with the clinically, often borderline, indications that are germane to chronic total coronary occlusions (1).

The laser wire has clearly fallen short of expectations in its overall performance in the only randomized trial comparing it to conventional wires (5). Even without having actually resorted to the top-of-the-line mechanical wires in the

conventional approaches during the trial, it was concluded that the laser wire should remain a last choice instrument for highly specialized centers and operators in light of its narrow edge over cheaper and less dangerous techniques. Although laser energy occasionally allows successful advancement of the wire where other wires get stuck (Fig. 15.4), this aggressiveness is accompanied by an increased risk of perforations and false channels. Moreover, the cost is outrageous.

Perforations are extremely rare with conventional coronary guidewires, even those of the extra-support type (9,25). They are virtually nonexistent with the ball-tipped Magnum wire (4). Therefore, these wires should constitute the primary choice for the general attempt at chronic total coronary occlusions, reserving hydrophilic wires for failures or tough (e.g., very old) occlusions. Laser wires have no place in routine attempts.

Special Techniques

The bare wire is generally used to find and enter the stump of the occlusion. Passing the occlusion without support by a bracing catheter

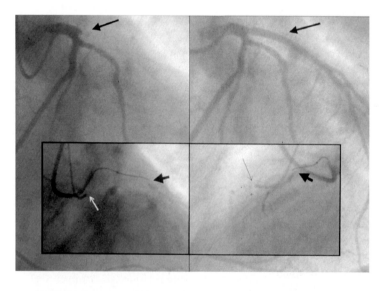

FIG. 15.4. Recanalization of a chronic total occlusion using a laser wire and simultaneous contralateral contrast medium injection. **Left panel:** proximal occlusion of the left anterior descending coronary artery (*short arrow*). **Right panel:** result after laser recanalization and implantation of a Wallstent (*short arrow*). **Insert:** Maximal advancement of the laser wire without turning on the laser (*short arrows, left:* right anterior oblique view, *right:* left lateral view). Outlining of the distal left anterior descending coronary artery, and thus the direction in which to apply laser energy, by contrast medium injection into the right coronary artery through a 4 Fr right Judkins catheter (*thin arrows*) introduced through the same femoral artery as the 7 Fr guiding catheter used for the contrast medium injection into the left coronary artery.

documents that the occlusion was very recent or extremely short. In the majority of cases, a support catheter will have to be advanced to stiffen the wire tip. Since this catheter is usually placed very distally at just a millimeter or two off the tip of the wire, the curve of the latter has to be shaped accordingly. The typical 4 to 5-mm commercial J-tip of conventional coronary guidewires will be straightened by this maneuver and steerability will be lost. Therefore, a second bend (usually into the same direction as the primary one) has to be added just 1 to 2 mm shy of the wire tip. This secondary J will afford steerability after bracing the coronary wire with the balloon catheter or after entering the occluded segment which also straightens the primary curve of the wire tip (Fig. 15.5).

The common technique for passing the occlusion is to advance the wire a few millimeters and then to follow with the balloon to reinforce it for further advancement. An alternative technique is to advance wire and balloon as a unit. In some situations, if the conventional methods fail, a safe and reliable technique is to advance the balloon head-first with the wire tip withdrawn inside the balloon.

Additional last-resort maneuvers have been advocated and used with success by especially determined operators. The first consists of the inflation of the balloon in the most distal position achievable, followed by powerful advancement of the wire, taking advantage of the excellent backup support by the wedged, inflated balloon. For this technique, the ball-tipped Magnum wire is safest as it can hardly be pushed through the vessel wall. Other wires, particularly the hydrophilic ones, portend a significant risk of false, perhaps even extravascular, pathways.

The second maneuver is only feasible with conventional over-the-wire systems. It entails advancing the coronary guidewire tail-first to conquer an exceedingly resistant, yet straight and short, occluded segment. After advancing the balloon or support catheter through the crucial segment, the wire is then used tip-first for the remainder of the intervention. This technique may be viewed as the ultimate ''poor man's'' laser technique (the hydrophilic guidewire being the common ''poor man's'' laser technique) (32). Whereas the laser wire maintains a certain directability of the advancement (Fig. 15.4), however, this approach using the stiff end of the guidewire merely affords the possibility to advance straight on.

During and after laborious endeavors to force mechanical or laser wires through resistant occlusions, it is particularly important to ascertain the proper progress of the wire as well as the correct position in the true lumen beyond the occluded segment. For this purpose, it may ex-

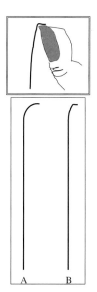

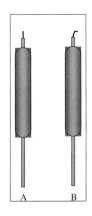

A B A B A B

FIG. 15.5. Custom shaping of guidewire tip for total occlusions. **A:** Commercial J-curve resulting in loss of steerability in action because of straightening of the curve either by the balloon advanced for support (**center panel**) or by the narrow passage in the occlusion (**right panel**). **B:** Secondary J-curve, shaped with the aid of the thumbnail 1–2 mm proximal to wire tip. This curve persists in the **center panel** and **right panel** situations and maintains steerability.

ceptionally be advisable to employ a simultaneous injection into the contralateral coronary artery in case insufficient ipsilateral collaterals are present. This method has been advocated as a routine for laser wire recanalizations and is exemplified in Figure 15.4. The second catheter can be introduced through the same femoral artery using a second puncture and for instance a tiny 4 Fr catheter without sheath. Both puncture sites can subsequently be closed using a single pressure bandage or compression device.

It makes sense to start with a balloon that is adequately sized for the final dilatation. Most modern balloons feature an excellent crossing profile. Advancing the balloon rarely causes a problem, once the wire is safely in place in the distal third of the vessel to recanalize. If exchange to a smaller balloon becomes necessary, no material is wasted because the initially selected balloon will be reused for the final dilatation. Overall, this policy saves time and money.

In terms of overall tactics, the chronic occlusion should be opened first if angioplasty for more than one lesion is planned. This provides additional collateral support in case another lesion occludes abruptly. A failure may be a reason to stop the entire procedure and perhaps recommend bypass surgery after all.

STENTING

Stenting was initially considered to be of little importance after recanalization of chronic total coronary occlusions. First, the benefit of stenting most appreciated by angioplasty operators, namely the reduction in abrupt closures, is of no immediate clinical concern with an artery that was occluded when the intervention started. Second, the reduced flow into freshly revascularized territories that is sometimes observed is considered detrimental to stent patency. Third, recanalization procedures are often time- and material-consuming. Adding more time and cost to insert stents hardly seems appealing. Fourth, the dissections and fuzzy appearances created with angioplasty are typically longer after recanalization of chronic occlusions than after dilatation of nontotal stenoses. This implies long or multiple stents and adds to the cost and the potential for restenosis and reocclusion.

Notwithstanding, randomized studies have unequivocally shown that stenting of successfully recanalized coronary segments is overall beneficial, reducing restenosis and reocclusion, which represent recognized and quite frequent problems with recanalized occlusions. Stenting also prevents other clinical events (Fig. 15.6) (33–40).

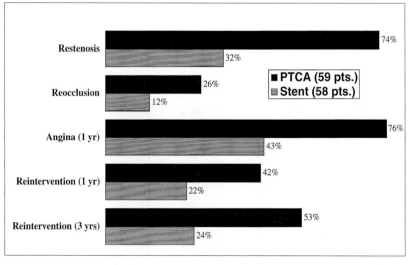

FIG. 15.6. Major results of the SICCO study (Stenting in Chronic Coronary Occlusion) randomizing patients with successfully recanalized coronary arteries to plain balloon angioplasty or stent implantation. All differences are statistically significant (33,40).

Yet, taking all the studies into consideration, only about 15% of the patients stented benefited from it. This means that roughly 6 patients have to be stented to prevent one recurrence. This amounts to additional costs of roughly $10,000 to prevent one recurrence. In addition, the stented patients with restenosis are often more difficult to treat (long in-stent restenosis) than patients with a restenosis in a nonstented segment. Side-branch occlusions are also more common with stents than without. Side branches originating just proximal to an occlusion may cause an infarction when occluded by the procedure, whereas those distal to the occluded segment may be carriers of collateral flow. Their loss may be regretted later on, when a reocclusion of the main vessel occurs or, in case of persistent patency, inverse collateral flow through such branches is solicited for disease progression in the former collateral donor.

Hence, cost-conscious operators know better than blindly follow evidence-based medicine recommendations and implant stents in all patients. They strive to narrow down the stent candidates to those with a high probability of stent benefit. If they stent about half of their patients, they stand a good chance that most of those that really need a stent get stented, and they are doing a good job at a defensible price.

SUMMARY

Chronic total coronary occlusions are a common finding in patients undergoing diagnostic coronary angiography. They constitute about 15% of targets of coronary angioplasty. In symptomatic patients, the primary goal is symptom improvement and reduction of subsequent need for coronary artery bypass surgery. In asymptomatic patients, indications for a recanalization attempt may be derived from the hope for reactivation of hibernating myocardial territories and reversed collaterals in case of disease progression in other coronary arteries.

Primary success rates have significantly improved with modern wires and more determined approaches. Theses strategies became customary when it was realized that long subintimal pathways may annihilate a recanalization at-

tempt but rarely amount to significant clinical problems and that wire perforations within the occluded segment are harmless. Laser users plainly call them ''wire exits'' to underscore their innocuousness. Primary success rates, nevertheless, remain comparably low and impose moderation in indications and investments for these types of procedures. It is clearly not worthwhile to purchase and maintain an excimer laser unit uniquely for the rare cases where only the laser wire may turn a failed attempt at recanalization into a durable success.

Recurrences after chronic occlusion angioplasty can be curtailed by judicious use of stents, just as with angioplasty of nontotal stenoses. Yet, routine stenting is not warranted, let alone cost-efficient, and overzealous stenting may bring about long and incurable in-stent restenosis, the modern nightmare of the interventional cardiologist. The role of radiation in the prevention of restenosis with this recurrence-prone indication will be defined within the next years. Again it has to be kept in mind that occlusions already consume more money than stenoses (1) and that there is little justification to expand this predicament.

Occlusion angioplasty is cherished by the experienced angioplasty operator. It represents a true technical challenge that separates the professionals from the novices. It pleases the expert to be cognizant of the fact that the inherent risk has no relationship to the intricacy of the procedure. However, even occlusion angioplasty may turn into disaster when bad luck strikes or when frustration overcomes reason and previously nonoccluded vessels are damaged while fighting with the obnoxious but harmless occlusion. Thus, the fact that the simple reocclusion of the recanalized segment will not cause ischemia, albeit true, is not very helpful because no recanalization is achieved without considerable impact on formerly healthy structures or those with dormant diseased. We may have successfully climbed the fence, but rarely without having woken up a few of the sleeping dogs. In the rare cases where problems occur, vast experience of the operating team is of essence. Hence, chronic coronary occlusion angioplasty may look like the ideal playground for the ambitious novice, but it is not.

REFERENCES

1. Bell MR, Berger PB, Menke KK, Holmes DR Jr. Balloon angioplasty of chronic total coronary artery occlusions: what does it cost in radiation exposure, time, and materials? *Cathet Cardiovasc Diagn* 1992;25:10–15.
2. Delacrétaz E, Meier B. Therapeutic strategy with total coronary artery occlusions. *Am J Cardiol* 1997;79: 185–187.
3. Meier B, Carlier M, Finci L et al. Magnum wire for balloon recanalization of chronic total coronary occlusions. *Am J Cardiol* 1989;64:148–154.
4. Allemann Y, Kaufmann U, Meyer B et al. Magnum wire for percutaneous transluminal coronary balloon angioplasty in 800 total chronic occlusions. *Am J Cardiol* 1997;80:634–637.
5. Hamburger JN, Koolen JJ, Fajadet J et al. Randomized comparison of laser guidewire and mechanical guidewires for recanalization of chronic total coronary occlusions: the TOTAL Trial. *Circulation* 1997;96[Suppl I]: I-269.
6. Freed M, Boatman JE, Siegel N, Safian RD, Grines CL, O'Neill WW. Glidewire treatment of resistant coronary occlusions. *Cathet Cardiovasc Diagn* 1993;30: 201–204.
7. Gray DF, Sivananthan UM, Verma SP, Michalis LK, Rees MR. Balloon angioplasty of totally and subtotally occluded coronary arteries: results using the Hydrophillic Terumo Radifocus Guidewire M (glidewire). *Cathet Cardiovasc Diagn* 1993;30:293–299.
8. Corcos T, Favereau X, Guerin Y et al. Recanalization of chronic coronary occlusions using a new hydrophilic guidewire. *Cathet Cardiovasc Diagn* 1998;44:83–90.
9. Reimers B, Camassa M, Di Mario C et al. Mechanical recanalization of total coronary occlusions with the use of a new guide wire. *Am Heart J* 1998;135:726–731.
10. Ivanhoe RJ, Weintraub WS, Douglas JS et al. Percutaneous transluminal coronary angioplasty of chronic total occlusions: Primary success, restenosis, and long-term clinical follow-up. *Circulation* 1992;85:106–115.
11. Puma JA, Sketch MH Jr, Tcheng JE et al. The natural history of single-vessel chronic coronary occlusion: a 25-year experience. *Am Heart J* 1997;133:393–399.
12. Finci L, Meier B, Favre J, Righetti A, Rutishauser W. Long-term results of successful and failed angioplasty for chronic total coronary arterial occlusion. *Am J Cardiol* 1990;66:660–662.
13. Bell MR, Berger PB, Bresnahan JF, Reeder GS, Bailey KR, Holmes DR Jr. Initial and long-term outcome of 354 patients after coronary balloon angioplasty of total coronary artery occlusions. *Circulation* 1992;85: 1003–1011.
14. Warren RJ, Black AJ, Valentine PA, Manolas EG, Hunt D. Coronary angioplasty for chronic total occlusion reduces the need for subsequent coronary bypass surgery. *Am Heart J* 1990;120:270–274.
15. Melchior JP, Doriot PA, Chatelain P et al. Improvement of left ventricular contraction and relaxation synchronism after recanalization of chronic total coronary occlusion by angioplasty. *J Am Coll Cardiol* 1987;4: 763–768.
16. Sirnes PA, Myreng Y, Molstad P, Bonarjee V, Golf S. Improvement in left ventricular ejection fraction and wall motion after successful recanalization of chronic coronary occlusions. *Eur Heart J* 1998;19:273–281.
17. Danchin N, Angioï M, Cador R et al. Effect of late percutaneous angioplastic recanalization of total coronary artery occlusion on left ventricular remodeling, ejection fraction, and regional wall motion. *Am J Cardiol* 1996;78:729–735.
18. Puma JA, Sketch MH Jr, Tcheng JE et al. Percutaneous revascularization of chronic coronary occlusions: an overview. *J Am Coll Cardiol* 1995;26:1-11.
19. Safian RD, McCabe CH, Sipperly ME, McKay RG, Baim DS. Initial success and long-term follow-up of percutaneous transluminal coronary angioplasty in chronic total occlusions versus conventional stenoses. *Am J Cardiol* 1998;61:23G–28G.
20. DiSciascio G, Vetrovec GW, Cowley MJ, Wolfgang TC. Early and late outcome of percutaneous transluminal coronary angioplasty for subacute and chronic total coronary occlusion. *Am Heart J* 1986;111:833–839.
21. Ellis SG, Shaw RE, Gershony G et al. Risk factors, time course and treatment effect for restenosis after successful percutaneous transluminal coronary angioplasty of chronic total occlusion. *Am J Cardiol* 1989;63: 897–901.
22. La Veau PJ, Remetz MS, Cabin HS et al. Predictors of success in percutaneous transluminal coronary angioplasty of chronic total occlusions. *Am J Cardiol* 1989; 64:1264–1269.
23. Kereiakes DJ, Selmon MR, McAuley BJ, McAuley DB, Sheehan DJ, Simpson JB. Angioplasty in total coronary artery occlusion: experience in 76 consecutive patients. *J Am Coll Cardiol* 1985;6:526–533.
24. Maiello L, Colombo A, Gianrossi R et al. Coronary angioplasty of chronic occlusions: factors predictive of procedural success. *Am Heart J* 1992;124:581–584.
25. Kinoshita I, Katoh O, Nariyama J et al. Coronary angioplasty of chronic total occlusions with bridging collateral vessels: immediate and follow-up outcome from a large single-center experience. *J Am Coll Cardiol* 1995; 26:409–415.
26. De Feyter PJ, Serruys P, Van den Brand M, Meester H, Beatt K, Suryapranata H. Percutaneous transluminal angioplasty of a totally occluded venous bypass graft: a challenge that should be resisted. *Am J Cardiol* 1989; 64:88–90.
27. Hartmann J, McKeever L, Teran J, Bufalino V et al. Prolonged infusion of urokinase for recanalization of chronically occluded aortocoronary bypass grafts. *Am J Cardiol* 1988;61:189–191.
28. Finci L, Meier B, Steffenino GD. Percutaneous angioplasty of totally occluded saphenous aortocoronary bypass graft. *Int J Cardiol* 1986;10:76–79.
29. Sievert H, Kohler KP, Kaltenbach M, Kober G. Reopening of long-segment occluded aortocoronary venous bypasses. Short- and long-term results. *Dtsch Med Wochenschr* 1988;113:637–640.
30. Finci L, Meier B, Roy P, Steffenino G, Rutishauser W. Clinical experience with the Monorail balloon catheter for coronary angioplasty. *Cathet Cardiovasc Diagn* 1988;14:206–212.
31. Wong CM, Kwong Mak GY, Chung DT. Distal coro-

nary artery perforation resulting from the use of hydrophilic coated guidewire in tortuous vessels. *Cathet Cardiovasc Diagn* 1998;44:93–96.

32. Meier B. The hydrophilic guidewire: the poor man's laser for chronic total coronary occlusions for the good and for the bad. *Cathet Cardiovasc Diagn* 1998;44: 91–92.

33. Sirnes PA, Golf S, Myreng Y et al. Stenting in chronic coronary occlusion (SICCO): a randomized, controlled trial of adding stent implantation after successful angioplasty. *J Am Coll Cardiol* 1996;28:1444–1451.

34. Anzuini A, Rosanio S, Legrand V et al. Wiktor stent for treatment of chronic total coronary artery occlusions: short- and long-term clinical and angiographic results from a large multicenter experience. *J Am Coll Cardiol* 1998;31:281–288.

35. Elezi S, Kastrati A, Wehinger A et al. Clinical and angiographic outcome after stent placement for chronic coronary occlusion. *Am J Cardiol* 1998;82:803–806, A809.

36. Moussa I, Di Mario C, Moses J, Reimers B, Di Francesco L, Blengino S, Colombo A. Comparison of angiographic and clinical outcomes of coronary stenting of chronic total occlusions versus subtotal occlusions. *Am J Cardiol* 1998;81:1–6.

37. Rubartelli P, Niccoli L, Verna E et al. Stent implantation versus balloon angioplasty in chronic coronary occlusions: results from the GISSOC trial. Gruppo Italiano di Studio sullo Stent nelle Occlusioni Coronariche. *J Am Coll Cardiol* 1998;32:90–96.

38. Suttorp MJ, Mast EG, Plokker HW, Kelder JC, Ernst SM, Bal ET. Primary coronary stenting after successful balloon angioplasty of chronic total occlusions: a single-center experience. *Am Heart J* 1998;135:318–322.

39. Hancock J, Thomas MR, Holmberg S, Wainwright RJ, Jewitt DE. Randomised trial of elective stenting after successful percutaneous transluminal coronary angioplasty of occluded coronary arteries. *Heart* 1998;79: 18–23.

40. Sirnes PA, Golf S, Myreng Y et al. Sustained benefit of stenting chronic coronary occlusion: long-term clinical follow-up of the Stenting in Chronic Coronary Occlusion (SICCO) study. *J Am Coll Cardiol* 1998;32: 305–310.

B. Treatment of Chronic Total Coronary Occlusions

Jaap N. Hamburger and *David R. Holmes, Jr.

*Department of Interventional Cardiology, Erasmus University, Heartcenter Rotterdam, 3000 Dr Rotterdam, The Netherlands; *Division of Cardiovascular Diseases and Internal Medicine, Mayo Clinic and Mayo Foundation, Department of Medicine, Mayo Medical School, Rochester, Minnesota 55905*

Percutaneous transluminal coronary angioplasty (PTCA) has established itself as an important alternative to coronary artery bypass surgery in the treatment of coronary artery disease. A continuing development of tools and techniques has led to an increase in the number and complexity of cases performed annually (1). In current angioplasty practice, the treatment of saphenous vein bypass graft disease, small diameter coronary arteries, and multivessel disease is considered as routine rather than as the exception. The recent explosive increase in the use of intracoronary stents presumably played a major role in this shift of former angioplasty boundaries (2). However, recanalization and maintenance of blood flow through a previously chronically occluded coronary artery is still a major challenge. Initially, low success rates (3–6) and high recurrence rates (7–9) hampered percutaneous attempts at recanalization of chronic occlusions. It was only after the introduction of improved guidewire technology (10–12) and the demonstration of a positive influence of intracoronary stent implantation on long-term vessel patency (13), that percutaneous treatment of chronic occlusions became an acceptable alternative for surgical treatment. In this chapter we discuss:

1. a technical approach to recanalization and adjunctive angioplasty procedures
2. currently available dedicated angioplasty hardware
3. the use of guidance for optimization of procedural results, and the
4. potential role of antithrombotic medication in sustaining long-term vessel patency.

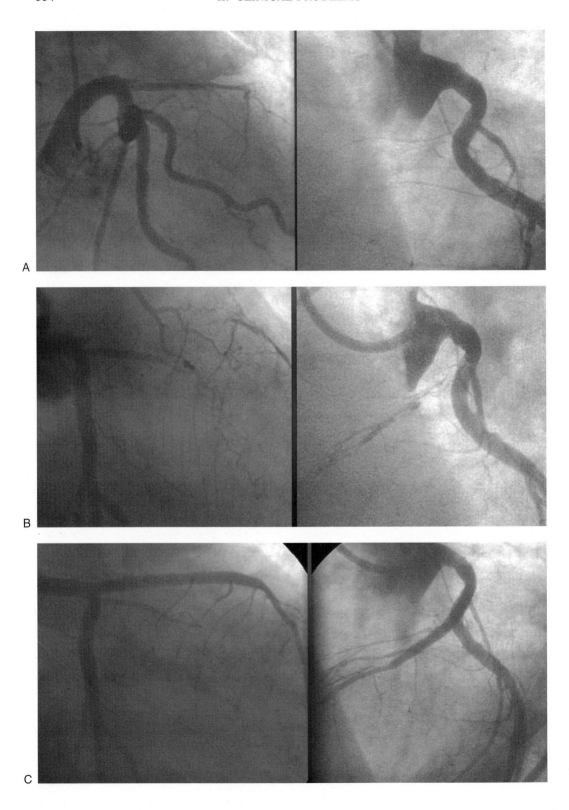

THE ACCESS

A primary condition for a successful attempt at recanalization is an optimal visualization of the local anatomy. As a rule, imaging of only the proximal part of the occlusion (i.e. the proximal stump) will not supply sufficient information to allow for reliable fluoroscopic guidance of novel, dedicated chronic occlusion guidewires. Routine puncturing of both femoral arteries allows for the insertion of a second, smaller Fr size catheter in the contra lateral coronary artery. By a combination of simultaneous bilateral injection of contrast medium into both coronary arteries, making use of the intercoronary artery collateral circulation and biplane coronary angiography, optimal information is obtained about the anatomy of the missing segment (10). A monoplane fluoroscopy system could be used, provided multiple views from different angles are made to control the alignment of the guidewire with the distal target lumen (Fig 15.7).

Of importance is the use of a guiding catheter with optimal co-axial back-up support. Typically, this could be an Amplatz left type guiding catheter for both occlusions in the left or the right coronary artery. The guiding catheter used should have a large enough lumen to accommodate the simultaneous introduction of two balloon catheters in case of presumed side-branch involvement, which potentially necessitates treatment of a bifurcation lesion using a "kissing balloon" technique.

THE GUIDEWIRES

The intrinsic capacity of a guidewire to cross a chronic total occlusion is dictated by its "steerability" (the wire tip response to subtle torque movements), pushability (or wire tip stiffness) and "crossability" (the interaction of the wire material with the occluding tissue). In the cur-rent decade we have seen the clinical introduction of various new, dedicated guidewires and guidewire systems. Within the multitude of available chronic total occlusion wires the following three major subgroups can be defined:

1. Active guidewires or guidewire systems. Examples are the laser guidewire (Spectranetics, Colorado Springs, CO) (10,14) and the activated guidewire (15), which were specially designed to cross lesions refractory to conventional guide wires. The results of several registries have suggested an advantage of the laser guidewire and the activated guidewire over conventional guide-wires (16,17). However, this advantage was not sustained in a recently performed randomized trial (18).

2. Metal tip "stiff" guidewires. A typical representative in this group is the Miracle guidewire (Asahi Intec, Japan) (11), with a short distal coil to resist wire tip entrapment in longer lesions, and supplied with a tip stiffness ranging from 3 to 12 grams.

3. Hydrophilic coated guidewires. Examples are the Choice PT or Choice Graphix guidewires (ranging from "Floppy" to "Super Support," Scimed, Minneapolis, MN), the Shinobi wire (Cordis, Miami, FL) and the Terumo Crosswire (in the U.S.: Radiofocus, or Glidewire, with a 10-gram tip stiffness) or the "Stiff wire," with a tip stiffness of 40 grams or 80 grams (Terumo, Tokyo, Japan) (12).

CROSSING THE OCCLUSION

Conventional guidewires tend to follow a path of least resistance. Unfortunately, the subendothelium is usually softer than the intraluminal, obstructing material. As a result, subintimal tracking of stiff guidewires resulting in coronary

---

FIG. 15.7. Chronic total occlusion of the left anterior descending artery. **A:** Antegrade injection, showing the proximal stump. **B:** Simultaneous bilateral injection in the left anterior descending and the right coronary artery, showing both the proximal stump and the distal lumen (right inferior oblique and left superior oblique view). **C:** Final result after implantation of a single 57-mm NIR stent (Medinol, Jerusalem, Israel). The stent was hand-crimped on a 60-mm Malvina balloon (Schneider, Bülach, Switzerland).

dissection is not uncommon. In a postmortem study, Katsuragawa et al. histologically identified approximately 200 diameter microchannels in occluded coronary segments (19). These microchannels typically would not be visible on coronary angiography, but would be large enough to carry a small-diameter, low-resistance guidewire. Assuming the potential presence of these microchannels, the tip of a balloon catheter could damage the entry point of the occlusion, thereby precluding additional attempts with different guidewires (e.g. stiffer guidewires) when needed. Thus, the importance of optimal guiding catheter support is determined by the intention to avoid using a balloon catheter for additional back-up support.

An additional, typical histologic feature is the presence of a distal, fibrotic cap. The distal cap is presumably the initial lesion, which originally gave rise to the total occlusion. Therefore, a sensible approach would be to cross the occlusion using a steerable, small-diameter (0.014 in.), low-resistance (e.g. hydrophilic coated) guidewire. In addition, the wire tip should be stiff enough to create an entry point in the stump of the occlusion and to penetrate the distal fibrotic cap.

In the presence of pre-existing microchannels, crossing of a chronic occlusion should not require any force. A ''trial and error'' approach of carefully steering and redirecting the guidewire until a channel that connects the stump with the distal parent lumen has been found, would then be the appropriate technique. In the ''microchannel scenario,'' a buckling of the guidewire means that the guidewire tip is either in the wrong microchannel, or the tip is forced in a direction at an angle with the channel lumen. Applying additional force, or using a balloon for additional support to prevent the wire from buckling, would then only increase the risk of subintimal tracking. If, despite several such attempts, there is no wire progression, a guidewire with increased tip stiffness should be chosen. When the handling of the guidewire is based on steering, rather than pushing the tip through the occlusion, while the alignment of the wire with the target lumen is continuously monitored, the risk of subintimal tracking and dissection is significantly reduced. If the tip stiffness of the guidewire is not sufficient to pierce the distal fibrotic cap, the wire tip will be deflected and again forced into a subintimal layer. Continued maneuvering of the wire could then cause the wire to perforate the adventitia, resulting in a wire exit. Although wire exits are usually benign, they have been associated with the occurrence of (late) tamponade, especially in the presence of co-medication with potent platelet aggregation blocking agents (IIb/IIIa receptor blockade, unpublished data). For this reason, the final maneuver of redirecting the guidewire tip through the distal fibrotic cap into the distal parent lumen is commonly the most critical part of the recanalization procedure. Without adequate visualization of the distal lumen, the operator will not be able to actively prevent the wire from choosing a subintimal pathway. The often very resistant nature of the distal part of an occlusion sometimes requires an exchange of the guidewire for, again, a wire with increased tip stiffness (Fig 15.8). However, it should be stressed that as long as the guidewire has not yet crossed into the distal lumen, an exchange of guidewire should never be facilitated by using a balloon or probing catheter. The reasons for this dogma are obvious: if the wire has not yet crossed the occlusion because of a subintimal position, an exchange catheter will sufficiently dissect the occluded segment as to preclude any additional guidewire attempts at recanalization. Secondly, and more urgent, in case of an undetected guidewire perforation, the introduction of an exchange catheter could alter a benign wire exit into a potentially life threatening perforation of the coronary arterial wall, requiring pericardiocentesis. Therefore, prior to advancing any device, either an antegrade or retrograde injection of contrast medium should angiographically confirm the distal, intraluminal position of the guidewire.

THE ADJUNCTIVE ANGIOPLASTY

Once the guidewire has crossed the occlusion, the operator can choose to remove, rather than push aside, the material that obstructs the original lumen. The use of various ablative tech-

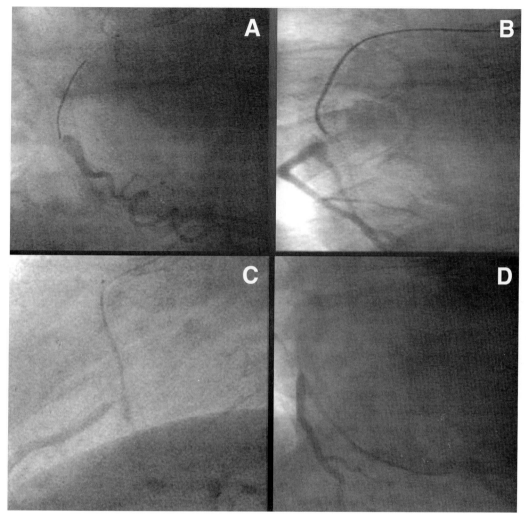

FIG. 15.8. A-C: Multiple maneuvers with the tip of a Terumo 40-gram guidewire to pierce the distal cap of a chronic total occlusion. The guidewire tip maneuvering is guided by contrast injections through the contralateral coronary artery. **D:** The tip of the guidewire has reached the true distal lumen.

niques, such as rotational atherectomy or excimer laser coronary angioplasty, has been suggested in this setting. However, a long-term clinical advantage as assessed in a prospective, randomized trial, has yet to be demonstrated (20,21). Therefore, one could argue that balloon angioplasty is still the treatment of first choice. However, a number of studies have shown a significant improvement in long-term clinical outcome following coronary stent implantation (13,22–25), the improvement typically being re-

lated to a reduction in the 6-month restenosis and/or reocclusion rates.

The often complex nature of the disease frequently dictates the need for the use of long balloons and long or multiple stents. Whether the best long-term results are achieved when stent implantation is restricted to short, suboptimally dilated segments ("spot stenting" [26]) or conversely with a full stent coverage of the entire lesion length ("full metal jacket") is still a matter of debate (Fig 15.9). Successful recanaliza-

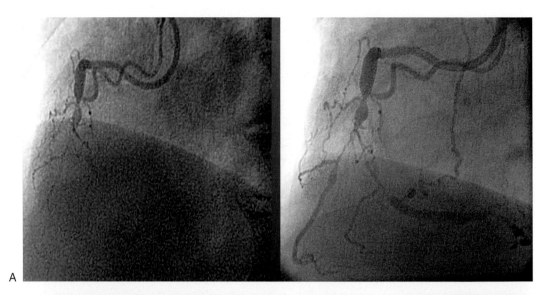

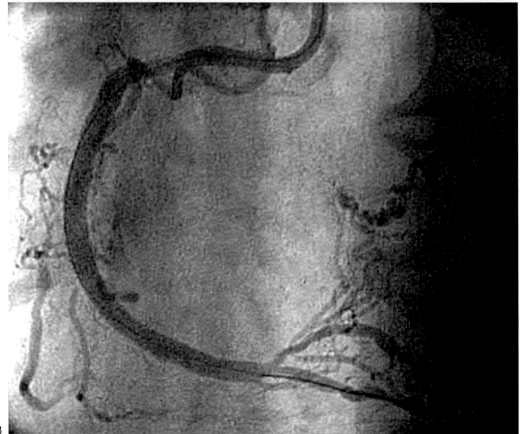

FIG. 15.9. Reconstruction of a chronically occluded right coronary artery by implantation of two 57-mm NIR stents. **A:** Initial injection. **B:** Final result.

tion of chronic total occlusions is still plagued by recurrence rates in excess of those following dilatation of coronary stenosis. Because restenosis is a function of the minimum lumen diameter, it is advisable to use a form of guidance to optimize the final result. Because stent implantation has taken such a predominant position in the recanalization procedure, intravascular ultrasound (IVUS) is probably the most useful guidance tool for optimizing stent apposition and maximizing the stent minimum lumen area relative to the media-to-media diameter at the site of stent implantation.

Finally, it has been suggested that the recurrence rate following successful recanalization of chronic occlusions is predominantly determined by the occurrence of early reocclusion (27). Therefore, the additional value of a routine use of per-procedural adjunctive medication including potent platelet aggregation blocking agents (e.g. abciximab), followed by ticlopidine or clopidogrel during the early follow-up period, needs to be assessed in a prospective study.

CONCLUSION

Percutaneous treatment of chronic total coronary occlusions has become a feasible and safe procedure. With the use of novel, dedicated guidewires, an operator technique of steering, rather than pushing the guidewire through the occlusion, and a consequent monitoring of the proper alignment of the guidewire with the distal target lumen, the procedural success rates have increased to well over 80%. Whether IVUS-guided stent implantation and periprocedural medication with platelet aggregation blocking agents will positively influence the long-term outcome needs to be evaluated.

REFERENCES

1. Windecker S, Meyer BJ, Bonzel T et al. Interventional cardiology in Europe 1994. Working Group Coronary Circulation of the European Society of Cardiology. *Eur Heart J* 1998;19(1):40–54.
2. Ruygrok PN, Serruys PW. Intracoronary stenting, from concept to custom. *Circulation* 1996;94:882–890.
3. Holmes DR, Vlietstra RE, Reeder GS et al. Angioplasty in total coronary artery occlusion. *J Am Coll Cardiol* 1984;3:845–849.
4. Meyer B, Gruentzig AR. Learning curve for percutaneous transluminal coronary angioplasty: skill, technology or patient selection. *Am J Cardiol* 1984;53:65C–66C.
5. Kereiakes DJ, Selmon MR, McAuley BJ, McAuley DB, Sheehan DJ, Simpson JB. Angioplasty in total coronary artery occlusion: experience in 76 consecutive patients. *J Am Coll Cardiol* 1985;6:526–533.
6. Stone GW, Rutherford BD, McConahay DR et al. Procedural outcome of angioplasty for total coronary artery occlusion: an analysis of 971 lesions in 905 patients. *J Am Coll Cardiol* 1990;15:849–865.
7. Serruys PW, Umans V, Heyndrickx GR et al. Elective P.T.C.A. of totally occluded coronary arteries not associated with acute myocardial infarction; short-term and long-term results. *Eur Heart J* 1985;6:2–12.
8. DiScascio G, Vetrovec GW, Cowley MJ, Wolfgang TC. Early and late outcome of percutaneous transluminal coronary angioplasty for sub acute and chronic total coronary occlusion. *Am Heart J* 1986;111:833–839.
9. Ivanhoe RJ, Weintraub WS, Douglas JS Jr et al. Percutaneous transluminal coronary angioplasty of chronic total occlusions: primary success, restenosis and long-term clinical follow-up. *Circulation* 1992;85:106–115.
10. Hamburger JN, Gijsbers GHM, Ozaki Y, Ruygrok PN, de Feyter PJ, Serruys PW. Recanalization of chronic total coronary occlusions using a laser guidewire: a pilot-study. *J Am Coll Cardiol* 1997;30:649–656.
11. Kinoshita I, Katoh O, Nariyama J et al. Coronary angioplasty of chronic total occlusions with bridging collateral vessels: immediate and follow-up outcome from a large single-center experience. *J Am Coll Cardiol* 1995; 26:409–415.
12. Lefevre T, Louvard Y, Morice MC et al. Treatment of chronic total coronary occlusion: a randomized study comparing two guidewire strategies. *Eur Heart J* 1998; (19):2674(A).
13. Sirnes PA, Golf S, Myreng Y et al. Stenting in Chronic Coronary Occlusion (SICCO): a randomized, controlled trial of adding stent implantation after successful angioplasty. *J Am Coll Cardiol* 1996;28:1444–1451.
14. Hamburger JN, Serruys PW. Laser guidewire for recanalization of chronic total occlusions. In: Beyar, Keren, Leon, Serruys, eds. *Frontiers in interventional cardiology.* London: Martin Dunitz, 1997.
15. Rees MR, Michalis LK. Activated-guidewire technique for treating chronic coronary artery occlusion. *Lancet* 1995;346:943–944.
16. Hamburger JN, Serruys PW, Gomes R et al. Recanalization of total coronary occlusions using a laser guide wire: the European TOTAL Surveillance Study. *Am J Cardiol* 1997;80:1419–1423.
17. Oesterle SN, Bittl JA, Leon MB et al., for the U.S. TOTAL investigators. Laser wire for crossing chronic total occlusions—"learning phase" results from the U.S. TOTAL Trial. *Cathet Cardiovasc Diagn* 1998;44: 235–243.
18. Serruys PW, Hamburger JN, Koolen JJ et al. Total study: randomized comparison of laser guidewire and mechanical guidewires for recanalization of chronic total coronary occlusions, the 6 month follow-up. *Eur Heart J* 1998;19:2675(A).
19. Katsuragawa M, Fujiwara H, Miyamamae M, Sasayama S. Histologic studies in percutaneous transluminal coronary angioplasty for chronic total occlusion: comparison of tapering and abrupt types of occlusion and short and

long occluded segments. *J Am Coll Cardiol* 1993;21: 604–611.

20. Appelman YEA, Koolen JJ, Piek JJ et al. Excimer laser coronary angioplasty versus balloon angioplasty in functional and total coronary occlusions. *Am J Cardiol* 1996;787:757–762.

21. Reifart N, Vandormael M, Krajcar M et al. Randomized comparison of angioplasty of complex coronary lesions at a single center. Excimer laser, rotational atherectomy and balloon angioplasty comparison (ERBAC) Study. *Circulation* 1997;96(1):91–98.

22. Goldberg SL, Colombo A, Maiello L, Borrione M, Finci L, Almagor Y. Intracoronary stent insertion after balloon angioplasty of chronic total occlusions. *J Am Coll Cardiol* 1995;26:713–719.

23. Ozaki Y, Violaris A, Hamburger JN et al. Short- and long-term clinical and quantitative angiographic results with the new, less shortening Wallstent for vessel recon-struction in chronic total occlusion: a quantitative angio-graphic study. *J Am Coll Cardiol* 1996;28:354–360.

24. Anzuini A, Rosanio S, Legrand V et al. Wiktor stent for treatment of total coronary artery occlusions: short- and long-term clinical and angiographic results from a large multicenter experience. *J Am Coll Cardiol* 1998; 31:281–288.

25. Hancock J, Thomas MR, Holmberg S, Wainwright RJ, Jewitt DE. Randomised trial of elective stenting after successful percutaneous transluminal coronary angio-plasty of occluded coronary arteries. *Heart* 79(1):18–23.

26. DeGregorio J, Kobayashi Y, Reimers B, Albiero R, Di Mario C, Colombo A. Intravascular ultrasound guided PTCA with spot stenting. *J Am Coll Cardiol* 1998;31: 387A:896–3.

27. Violaris AG, Melkert R, Serruys PW. Long-term lumi-nal renarrowing after successful elective coronary an-gioplasty of total occlusions: a quantitative angiographic analysis. *Circulation* 1995;91:2140–2150.

16

Vein Graft Lesions

A. The Focal Vein Graft Lesion

David L. Fischman and Michael P. Savage

Cardiac Catheterization Laboratory, Interventional Cardiovascular Research, Department of Cardiology, Thomas Jefferson University Hospital, Philadelphia, Pennsylvania 19107

Randomized trials of coronary artery bypass graft surgery have demonstrated significant symptom palliation as well as increased survival in certain subgroups of patients with coronary artery disease. Due to these favorable outcomes, there is a growing population of patients with prior cardiac surgery and aged bypass grafts. Management of patients with coronary artery bypass graft disease has thus become a clinical challenge of increasing magnitude.

Within the first decade of bypass surgery, most saphenous vein bypass grafts will be totally occluded or have severe atherosclerotic disease as demonstrated by angiographic studies (Fig. 16.1) (1–3). During the first year after bypass surgery, up to 15% of venous grafts are occluded. Between 1 and 6 years, the graft attrition rate is 2% per year and doubles between 6 and 10 years. By 12 years after the initial bypass surgery, approximately one-third of patients will require further revascularization (4). The clinical sequelae and mortality associated with bypass graft disease are significant. Therapy of symptomatic patients after bypass surgery is problematic, as repeat coronary bypass surgery is more technically challenging, carries increased procedural morbidity and mortality, and is less likely to provide symptomatic relief than a first operation (5,6). Thus, faced with these limitations, intensive efforts to treat the patient with bypass graft disease by transcatheter interventions have

been made. The goal of this chapter is to review the percutaneous approach to focal vein bypass graft disease and present a practical approach in the management of this growing patient population.

LIMITATIONS OF BALLOON ANGIOPLASTY

During the past two decades, extensive advances with improved early and late success rates have been demonstrated with balloon angioplasty in the native coronary circulation. The technical and clinical aspects of balloon angioplasty in saphenous vein grafts is different, however, than in the native coronary circulation. The atheromatous material, particularly in the older bypass graft, is more friable. The consequence of balloon angioplasty is thus less predictable and is hindered by high periprocedural morbidity secondary to distal embolization of atheromatous material and myocardial infarction (7–10). Risk factors for distal embolization include older graft age (3 to 5 years), presence of thrombus, and nonfocal lesions. Furthermore, long-term event-free survival remains low following balloon angioplasty due to the high incidence of restenosis, which varies with the site of angioplasty and graft age (11,12). Angiographic restenosis exceeds 50% in lesions located at the ostium or within the body of the graft. Lower restenosis rates have been reported for distal

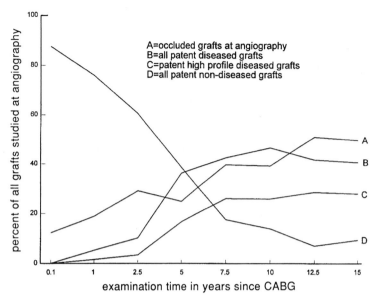

FIG. 16.1. Vein graft attrition as a function of time since coronary artery bypass surgery. CABG, coronary artery bypass graft. (From ref. 2, with permission.)

anastomotic stenoses. In addition, lesions treated less than 6 months after surgery have approximately half the incidence of restenosis than do bypass grafts older than 5 years. Plokker et al. (13) reported the long-term outcome of 454 patients treated with balloon angioplasty of saphenous vein bypass grafts (Fig. 16.2). After 5 years, only 26% of patients remained free of a major cardiac event; 26% of patients had died, and an additional 48% of patients suffered a major cardiac event (myocardial infarction, repeat bypass surgery, or repeat angioplasty). In addition to the relatively higher rates of periprocedural complications and restenosis, other

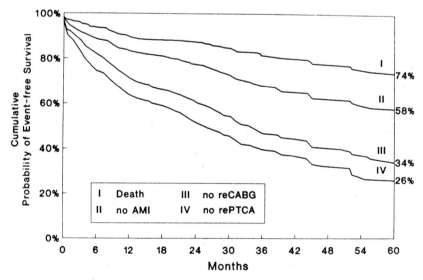

FIG. 16.2. Event-free survival after vein graft angioplasty. AMI, acute myocardial infarction; CABG, coronary artery bypass graft; PTCA, percutaneous transluminal coronary atherectomy. (From ref. 13, with permission.)

important clinical factors contribute to the unfavorable long-term outcome of patients following vein graft angioplasty. These include the relatively older age of the patients, presence of multivessel disease with frequent progression of atherosclerotic disease in sites distal to the initial lesion, and the presence of comorbid conditions.

TRANSCATHETER DEBULKING STRATEGIES

To improve on the early and late clinical outcomes following angioplasty, a variety of plaque-debulking devices have been evaluated in the treatment of vein graft disease. These include directional atherectomy, transluminal extraction, and laser angioplasty. Due to the large size and nontortuous character of saphenous vein grafts, directional atherectomy would appear to be a well-suited therapy for bypass graft stenoses. In the initial directional atherectomy registry, successful treatment without a major complication was noted in 85% of patients, although restenosis was as high as 75% in restenosis lesions versus 38% in *de novo* lesions (14). The only direct comparison of directional atherectomy versus conventional angioplasty in *de novo* vein graft stenoses was reported in the CAVEAT II trial (15). This was a randomized trial of 305 patients who were well matched with respect to graft age and target-lesion location. Directional atherectomy, as reported in this trial, resulted in an improved initial angiographic result with a larger acute gain in minimum lumen diameter as compared with balloon angioplasty (1.45 mm vs. 1.12 mm) (Fig. 16.3). Achievement of these superior angiographic results, however, was associated with a higher incidence of procedural complications, including an increased risk of distal embolization (13.4% vs. 5.1%), abrupt vessel closure (4.7% vs. 2.6%), and non–Q-wave myocardial infarction (10.1% vs. 5.8%). In addition, at 6 months, there was no difference in the restenosis rates between the two groups: 45.6% for atherectomy and 50.5% for balloon angioplasty.

An alternative device advocated for debulking atheromatous lesions in bypass grafts is the transluminal extraction-atherectomy catheter (TEC). Because of its ability to simultaneously cut and aspirate atheromatous material and clot, this device has the theoretical advantage of limiting distal embolization observed with conventional balloon angioplasty and directional atherectomy. Distal embolization has, however, been observed in greater than 10% of patients treated with this device. Safian et al. (16) reported their experience with TEC in 146 consecutive patients with saphenous vein bypass graft disease. In this series of patients, in which the average age of

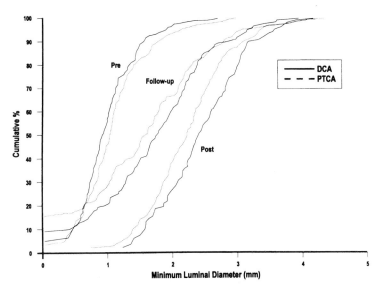

FIG. 16.3. Cumulative frequency curves showing preprocedure, postprocedure, and follow-up. The initial lumen achieved with directional coronary atherectomy (*DCA*) was greater than angioplasty (1.42 mm vs. 1.12 mm). At follow-up, late loss was greater for DCA (0.62 mm vs. 0.53 mm), leading to a slightly larger but nonsignificant net gain in the DCA group. PTCA, percutaneous transluminal coronary atherectomy. (From ref. 15, with permission.)

the treated bypass graft was 8.3 years, 21% of patients suffered an immediate angiographic complication following transluminal extraction. This included distal embolization in 11.3% of patients, no reflow in 4.4%, and abrupt closure in 5%. These angiographic complications persisted in 16% of patients despite adjunctive balloon angioplasty, which was required in 91% of lesions treated. Clinical complications included death in 2.0% of patients, myocardial infarction in 4.7% (Q-wave [2%], non–Q-wave [2.7%]), and emergent bypass surgery in 0.7%. At 6-month follow-up angiography, restenosis defined as a diameter stenosis >50% was observed in 69% of lesions, with complete occlusion in 29% of lesions. These results must be considered in light of the complex nature of bypass grafts treated, which included a high proportion of degenerated grafts with complex, ulcerated lesions containing thrombus, which clearly would not respond well to balloon angioplasty alone.

A third approach to debulking, which has been studied extensively in saphenous vein bypass grafts, has been excimer laser coronary angioplasty (ELCA). Bittl et al. (17) reported a relatively high success rate of approximately 92% in a series of 495 patients with saphenous vein graft lesions treated with excimer laser. Major complications included death in 1%, emergency bypass surgery in 0.6%, and Q-wave myocardial infarction in 2.4%. In this series of patients, a lower incidence of complications was noted in ostial lesions, discrete lesions, and smaller vein grafts. Despite the favorable initial success rate, use of laser angioplasty in vein grafts was limited by high rates of restenosis. The overall restenosis rate in this series was approximately 55%. Strauss et al. (18) reported a restenosis rate of 52%, with a 24% incidence of total occlusion at 6 months, in a multicenter study involving 106 patients with bypass graft lesions treated with excimer laser.

STENTING OF VENOUS BYPASS GRAFTS

The landmark randomized trials, STRESS and BENESTENT, demonstrated superior angio-graphic and clinical outcomes following stent placement compared with conventional angioplasty for focal lesions in native coronary arteries (19,20). These trials, however, excluded vein graft lesions. The concept of stent placement, particularly for aged bypass grafts, is appealing, given the relatively poor outcome with both balloon angioplasty and debulking strategies. A number of multicenter registries have reported relatively favorable results in saphenous vein graft lesions, with high success rates and low restenosis rates following vein graft stenting (Fig. 16.4). The multicenter Palmaz-Schatz stent registry enrolled a total of 589 patients with 624 focal vein graft lesions (21). Procedural success in this group of relatively older vein grafts (8.9 ± 4.2 years) was 98.8%, with the majority receiving a single stent (82%). Major in-hospital complications (death, myocardial infarction, or urgent coronary bypass graft surgery) occurred in only 2.9% of patients. Stent thrombosis diagnosed within the first month occurred in only 1.4% of patients. During the time period of this study, routine use of aspirin, heparin, and warfarin were employed to prevent stent thrombosis. In light of such, hemorrhagic complications associated with this intense anticoagulation regimen, requiring transfusion or vascular surgery, occurred in 14.3%. At 6-month follow-up, restenosis based on visual estimates was 30%. Coronary angiographic analysis of the first 198 patients in this registry showed an overall restenosis rate by lesion of 34%, with 22% for new lesions versus 51% in lesions treated with prior angioplasty (Fig. 16.5) (22). Restenosis was also more frequent in ostial vein graft lesions compared with nonostial lesions (61% vs. 28%, $p = .003$) (Fig. 16.6).

THE SAVED TRIAL

Based on the results of the aforementioned observational studies, the efficacy of stent placement versus angioplasty was directly compared in the prospective, randomized Saphenous Vein *De Novo* (SAVED) trial (23). In this study, 220 patients with new focal lesions in saphenous vein bypass grafts were randomly assigned to receive a Palmaz-Schatz stent (Johnson and

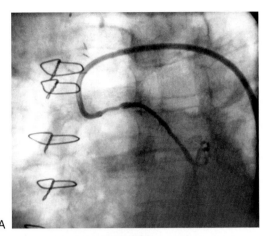

A

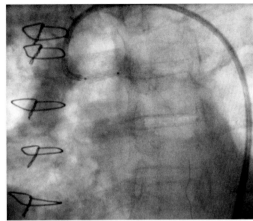

B

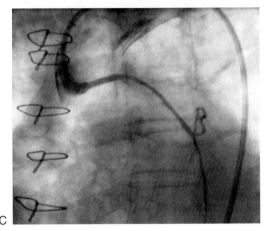

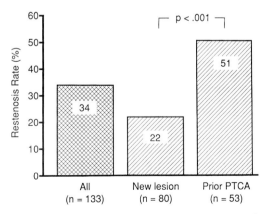

C

FIG. 16.4. Vein graft angiograms of a 68-year-old woman with unstable angina 7 years after bypass surgery. At baseline **(A)** a severe ostial lesion is noted. Use of a relatively radiopaque stent facilitates placement in the ostial location. **(B)** An excellent angiographic result is noted following placement of a 3.0 × 15.0-mm stent **(C)**.

FIG. 16.5. Restenosis of saphenous vein graft lesions after Palmaz-Schatz stent implantation. PTCA, percutaneous transluminal coronary atherectomy. (From ref. 22, with permission.)

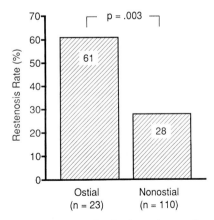

FIG. 16.6. Restenosis of vein grafts as a function of lesion location. (From ref. 22, with permission.)

Johnson International Systems, Warren, NJ) or routine angioplasty. The primary endpoint of the trial was angiographic restenosis at 6 months. The treated grafts were relatively old, approximately 10 years in both groups. Compared with balloon angioplasty, elective stent placement was associated with significantly greater angiographic procedural success (97% vs. 86%, $p <$ .01). The rate of procedural efficacy, defined as angiographic success achieved with the assigned therapy and the absence of a major in-hospital complication, was also significantly higher in the stent group than in the angioplasty group (92% vs. 69%, $p <$ .001). Thus, 31% of patients randomized to balloon angioplasty had an unsuccessful angiographic result or a major cardiac complication, or required unplanned revascularization, compared with 8% assigned to the stent group. Although there was no significant difference between the two groups in terms of major in-hospital complications, there was a trend toward fewer periprocedural non–Q-wave myocardial infarctions with stenting compared with angioplasty (2% vs. 7%). Angiographic analysis revealed an enhanced acute gain in the stent group with a larger postprocedural minimum lumen diameter (2.81 mm vs. 2.16 mm). Despite a greater late loss of luminal diameter in the stent group (1.06 mm vs. 0.66 mm), there was a significantly greater mean net gain in lumninal diameter at 6 months with stenting (0.85 mm vs. 0.54 mm). The minimum lumen diameter at 6 months was 1.73 mm in the stent group

and 1.49 mm in the angioplasty group (Fig. 16.7). Despite the relative greater benefit in luminal diameter conferred by stenting over angioplasty in saphenous vein bypass graft lesions, there was no significant benefit in the rate of angiographic restenosis. Restenosis occurred in 37% of patients in the stent group versus 46% of patients in the angioplasty group. The rate of event-free survival (freedom from death, myocardial infarction, repeat bypass surgery, and revascularization of the target lesion) at longer term follow-up was significantly greater for patients assigned to stenting than for patients assigned to angioplasty (73% vs. 58%) (Fig. 16.8). The SAVED trial thus represents the first demonstration of a transcatheter intervention that resulted in both superior angiographic and clinical outcomes compared with balloon angioplasty in saphenous vein bypass graft disease. A major limitation noted in this trial was the significant increase in bleeding and vascular complications in the stent group compared with the angioplasty group (17% vs. 5%) due to the intensive anticoagulation regimen used, which included aspirin, dipyridamole, low-molecular-weight dextran, heparin, and warfarin. Although this protocol was standard therapy when the trial was performed, subsequent studies have shown the superior safety and efficacy of aspirin and ticlopidine with stent deployment (24,25). The efficacy of this antiplatelet combination in preventing subacute thrombosis after vein graft stenting has also been demonstrated (26).

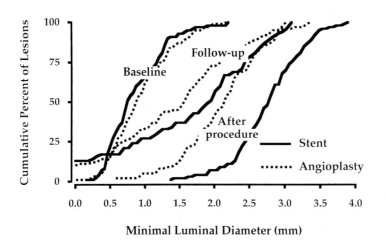

FIG. 16.7. Cumulative frequency distribution of minimum lumen diameter in the treatment groups at baseline, postprocedure, and at 6-month follow-up. (From ref. 23, with permission.)

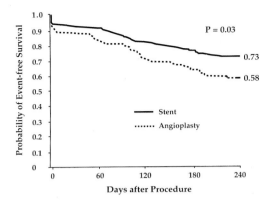

FIG. 16.8. Kaplan-Meier survival curves for freedom from major cardiac events. (From ref. 23, with permission.)

TREATMENT ALGORITHM FOR DISEASED VEIN GRAFTS

Based on the results of the various treatment modalities reviewed in this chapter, stents appear to be the treatment of choice for discrete stenoses involving the body of saphenous vein grafts. The SAVED trial demonstrated high success rates and acceptable complication and restenosis rates compared with balloon angioplasty. Although each of the atherectomy devices (directional, TEC, and laser) may be advantageous in selected patients with unfavorable lesion morphologies, a routine strategy of debulking bypass graft lesions does not appear to be warranted in light of the presented data. Whether a debulking strategy prior to stent placement will offer improved early and late results remains to be tested. Treatment of aorto-ostial lesions remains problematic. In these cases, either stenting or atherectomy with directional atherectomy or excimer laser should be considered, although restenosis is higher in this lesion subset.

FUTURE DIRECTIONS

Although stenting has been successful in selected cases, distal embolization and myocardial infarction remain significant, especially in lesions with angiographic evidence of thrombus. In these cases, adjunctive urokinase infusion has been used, with moderate success, to reduce the risk of distal immobilization. A promising technique for rapid thrombectomy without the use of thrombolytic drugs is the Possis AngioJet catheter (Possis, Minneapolis, MN) (Fig. 16.9). This device employs high-speed saline jets sprayed through an exhaust lumen to create a vacuum by means of the Bernoulli effect. As such, it is capable of evacuating thrombus. The efficacy of this device versus prolonged urokinase infusion was tested in the VeGAS (Vein Graft AngioJet Study) trial. In this randomized trial of 342 patients with intracoronary thrombus, over 50% of target lesions were in saphenous vein grafts. Rheolytic therapy proved superior to urokinase infusion, with higher procedural success, fewer bleeding complications, and a significant reduction in major adverse cardiac events (27).

Even in the absence of thrombus, distal embolization and non–Q-wave myocardial infarction are common after vein graft intervention. In the Reduced Anticoagulation Vein Graft Stent (RAVES) trial, 201 patients underwent elective stenting with contemporary techniques of high-pressure deployment and aspirin and ticlopidine therapy (28). Periprocedure myocardial infarction occurred in 28% of patients. The incidence of a myocardial infarction was directly related to lesion length: 17% for lesions less than 10 mm, 35% for lesions 10 to 20 mm, and 54% for lesions greater than 20 mm. Accordingly, efforts to prevent embolization of atheroembolic debris to the recipient native circulation are under active investigation. Promising techniques include use of PTFE-coated stents, which entrap atheroma, and distal protection devices, which combine distal graft occlusion with particulate aspiration. (29,30)

Finally, the use of platelet glycoprotein IIb/IIIa receptor antagonists have significantly reduced ischemic complications during coronary interventions. Although not formally tested in the vein graft population, a small subgroup of patients with vein graft disease were treated in the EPIC study (31). In this subgroup of 101 patients, bolus and infusion therapy resulted in a significant reduction in distal embolization compared with the placebo group (2% vs. 18%) and a trend toward a reduction in large non–Q-wave myocardial infarction (2% vs. 12%). In contrast with the results of the entire study, the early benefits achieved with abciximab was not

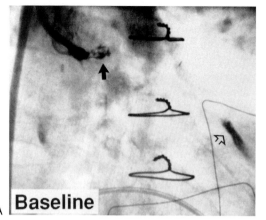

A **Baseline**

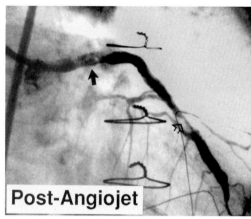

B **Post-Angiojet**

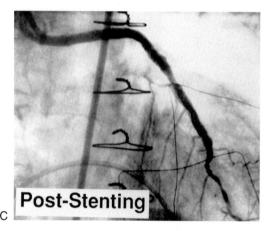

C **Post-Stenting**

FIG. 16.9. Angiograms of a 9-year-old vein graft to the left anterior descending coronary artery. At baseline **(A)** thrombotic occlusion of the proximal graft is noted (*arrow*). Restored patency of the graft is seen following thrombectomy with the An-gioJet catheter. **(B)** Subsequent treatment of severe proximal and distal graft lesions is performed with placement of coronary stents **(C)**. (From ref. 32 with permission.)

sustained over the following 6-month period. Clearly, further evaluation of this promising therapy is warranted in the treatment of saphenous vein graft disease.

REFERENCES

1. Bourassa MG, Fisher LD, Campeau L, et al. Long-term fate of bypass grafts: the Coronary Artery Surgery Study (CASS) and the Montreal Heart Institute experiences. *Circulation* 1985;72[Suppl V]:V71–V78.
2. Fitzgibbon GM, Kafka HP, Leach AJ, et al. Coronary bypass graft fate and patient outcome: angiographic follow-up of 5,065 grafts related to survival and reoperation in 1,388 patients during 25 years. *J Am Coll Cardiol* 1996;8:616–626.
3. Campeau L, Enjalbert M, Lesperance J, et al. The relation of risk factors to the development of atherosclerosis in saphenous vein bypass grafts and the progression of disease in the native circulation: a study 10 years after aortocoronary bypass surgery. *N Engl J Med* 1984;311:1329–1332.
4. Weintraub WS, Jones EL, Craver JM, Guyton RA. Fre-
quency of repeat coronary bypass or coronary angioplasty after coronary artery bypass surgery using saphenous venous grafts. *Am J Cardiol* 1994;73:103–112.
5. Cameron A, Kemp HG, Green GE. Re-operation for coronary artery disease. *Circulation* 1988;78[Suppl I]:I-158–I-162.
6. Loop FD, Cosgrove DM. Repeat coronary bypass surgery: selection of cases, surgical risks, and long-term outlook. *Mod Concepts Cardiovasc Dis* 1986;55:31–36.
7. de Feyter PJ, van Suylen R-J, DeJaegere PPT, et al. Balloon angioplasty for the treatment of lesions in saphenous vein bypass grafts. *J Am Coll Cardiol* 1993;21:1539–1549.
8. Douglas JS Jr, Gruentzig AR, King SB III, et al. Percutaneous transluminal coronary angioplasty in patients with prior coronary bypass surgery. *J Am Coll Cardiol* 1983;2:745–754.
9. Dorros G, Johnson WD, Tector AJ, et al. Percutaneous transluminal coronary angioplasty in patients with prior coronary artery bypass grafting. *J Thorac Cardiovasc Surg* 1984;87:17–26.
10. Lefkovits J, Holmes DR, Califf RM, et al. Predictors and sequelae of distal embolization during saphenous vein graft intervention for the CAVEAT-II trial: Coronary Angioplasty Versus Excisional Atherectomy Trial. *Circulation* 1995;92:734–740.

11. Platko WP, Hollman J, Whitlow PL, et al. Percutaneous transluminal coronary angioplasty of saphenous vein graft stenosis: long-term follow-up. *J Am Coll Cardiol* 1989;14:1645–1650.

12. Reeves F, Bonan R, Cote H, et al. Long-term angiographic follow-up after angioplasty of venous coronary bypass grafts. *Am Heart J* 1991;122:620–627.

13. Plokker HWT, Meester BH, Serruys PW. The Dutch experience in percutaneous transluminal angioplasty of narrowed saphenous veins used for aortocoronary arterial bypass. *Am J Cardiol* 1991;67:361–366.

14. Baim DS, Hinohara T, Holmes D, et al., for the U.S. DCA Investigator Group. Results of directional coronary atherectomy during multicenter preapproval testing. *Am J Cardiol* 1992;73:7E–11E.

15. Holmes DR Jr, Topol EJ, Califf RM, et al. A multicenter, randomized trial of coronary angioplasty versus directional atherectomy for patients with saphenous vein bypass graft lesions. *Circulation* 1995;91:1966–1974.

16. Safian RD, Grines CL, May MA, et al. Clinical and angiographic results of transluminal extraction coronary atherectomy in saphenous vein bypass grafts. *Circulation* 1994;89:302–312.

17. Bittl JA, Sanborn TA, Yardley DE, et al. Predictors of outcome of percutaneous excimer laser coronary angioplasty of saphenous vein bypass graft lesions. *Am J Cardiol* 1994;74:144–148.

18. Strauss BH, Natarajan MK, Batchelor WB, et al. Early and late quantitative angiographic results of vein graft lesions treated by excimer laser with adjunctive balloon angioplasty. *Circulation* 1995;92:348–356.

19. Serruys PW, de Jaegere P, Kiemeneij F, et al. A comparison of balloon-expandable stent implantation with balloon angioplasty in patients with coronary artery disease. *N Engl J Med* 1994;331:489–495.

20. Fischman DL, Leon MB, Baim DS, et al. A randomized comparison of coronary stent placement and balloon angioplasty in the treatment of coronary artery disease. *N Engl J Med* 1994;331:496–501.

21. Wong SC, Baim DS, Schatz RA, et al. Acute results and late outcomes after stent implantation in saphenous vein graft lesions: the multicenter USA Palmaz-Schatz stent experience. *J Am Coll Cardiol* 1995;26:704–712.

22. Fenton SH, Fischman DL, Savage MP, et al. Long-term angiographic and clinical outcome after implantation of balloon-expandable stents in aorto-coronary saphenous vein grafts. *Am J Cardiol* 1994;74:1187–1191.

23. Savage MP, Douglas J, Fischman D, et al. Coronary stents versus balloon angioplasty for aortocoronary saphenous vein bypass graft disease. *N Engl J Med* 1997; 337:740–747.

24. Schmog A, Neumann F-J, Kastrati A, et al. A randomized comparison of antiplatelet and anticoagulation therapy after the placement of coronary stents. *N Engl J Med* 1996;334:1084–1089.

25. Leon MB, Baim DS, Popma JJ, et al. A clinical trial comparing three antithrombotic-drug regimens after coronary artery stenting. *N Engl J Med* 1998;339: 1665–1671.

26. Leon MB, Ellis SG, Moses J, et al. Interim report from the Reduced Anticoagulation Vein Graft Stent (RAVES) study. *Circulation* 1996;94[Suppl]:I-683 abst).

27. Ramee SR, Baim DS, Pompa JJ, et al. A randomized, prospective, multicenter study comparing intracoronary urokinase to rheolytic thrombectomy with the POSSIS AngioJet catheter for intracoronary thrombus: final results of the VeGAS 2 Trial. *Circulation* 1998; 98[Suppl]:I-86.

28. Savage MP, Fischman DL, Ellis S, et al. Periprocedural myocardial infarction after vein graft stenting: incidence and predictive factors. *J Am Coll Cardiol* 1999;33[Suppl A]:37A.

29. Baldus S, Zeiher A, Reimers J, et al. Reduction of restenosis in venous bypass graft lesions after implantation of a covered graft stent. *J Am Coll Cardiol* 1999; 33[Suppl A]:37A.

30. Grub E, Webb J, for the SAFE Study Group. The SAFE Study. Multicenter evaluation of a protection catheter system for distal embolization in coronary venous bypass grafts (SVG's). *J Am Coll Cardiol* 1999;33[Suppl A]:37A.

31. Mak K-H, Challapalli R, Eisenberg MJ. Effect of platelet glycoprotein IIb/IIIa receptor inhibition on distal embolization during percutaneous revascularization of aortocoronary saphenous vein grafts. *Am J Cardiol* 1997; 80:985–988.

32. Savage MP, et al. *J Int Cardiol* 1997;10:145–153.

B. Diffuse Saphenous Vein Graft Disease

John S. Douglas, Jr.

Division of Cardiology, Emory University School of Medicine, Cardiac Catheterization Laboratory, Emory University Hospital, Atlanta, Georgia 30322-1104

The successful application of surgical myocardial revascularization techniques for three decades has resulted in a huge population of patients with diseased bypass grafts, the treatment of which remains one of the major challenges confronting interventional cardiologists. In no group of patients is greater wisdom required, for in these patients procedural risks are higher, long-term benefit lower, and treatment options frequently limited.

LESSONS LEARNED FROM TREATMENT OF FOCAL SAPHENOUS VEIN GRAFT DISEASE

Before extending percutaneous interventional strategies to patients with diffuse vein graft involvement, it is important to consider outcomes achieved with relatively focal disease using current technology. First, even when saphenous vein graft (SVG) narrowing involved only a short segment, intervention was associated with a substantial risk of atheroembolic MI. In a multicenter trial, during which 80% of 201 patients received a single 15-mm stent, 21% experienced an MI: CK-MB three to eight times normal in 13%, CK-MB > eight times normal in 6.5%, and Q wave 2.0% (1). Similarly, in 415 patients with single SVG interventions performed from 1995 to 1997, 84% receiving stent implantation, 32% experienced CK-MB elevation, and of those with CK-MB levels three times normal, the 30-day mortality rate was 14% (2). These reports of contemporary SVG intervention in relatively focal disease are sobering. Although a minority received IIb/IIIa inhibitors, it seems unlikely that their addition would have had major impact, given the results of vein graft intervention in EPIC and EPILOG, in which IIb/IIIa-treated patients had worse outcomes than those receiving placebo (3). Second, following successful intervention in focal SVG disease, adverse cardiac event rates related to progressive narrowing in target and nontarget SVG sites remained high during the first year and continued to occur over time. In the SAVED trial, about a third had infarction, death, or repeat revascularization within 6 months (4). Ellis et al. (5), in the careful follow-up of 103 patients after successful SVG interventions, reported event-free survival of 47% at 12 months and only 25% at 36 months (5). In this study, 82% of events occurring within the first year were attributed to progressive narrowing in the SVG that had been intervened upon. Recurring ischemic events related to the treated SVGs within the first year were due to the target lesion in two-thirds of patients, whereas events greater than 12 months after intervention were more often due to nontreated sites, which had mild (41% to 50%) narrowing

at the time of intervention. This observation that extension of disease beyond a single treatment site has important long-term implications was reinforced by recent observations that the need to treat more than one site was a strong predictor for non–target lesion disease progression (6). That is, the less focal the disease, the higher the recurrence and late-event rates. In truth, disease in aged grafts is rarely focal, and careful review of the angiogram, albeit an insensitive indicator, will often document a more generalized degenerative process than was evident at first blush.

While these observations highlight the major challenges of SVG intervention (atheroembolic infarction and recurrent ischemic events), perhaps directing one's attention to therapeutic strategies aimed at their prevention, an equally important message is a plea for caution. Given the modest benefits currently achieved with SVG intervention in the less difficult end of the disease spectrum, extending these efforts to treat diffuse disease should be undertaken only by highly experienced interventionalists in carefully selected cases in which the risk of not intervening is substantial, and, ideally, it should be done in the context of a formal investigation of one of the new strategies outlined in this chapter.

CURRENT TECHNIQUES POTENTIALLY APPLICABLE TO DIFFUSE DISEASE

Debulking prior to Stenting

Directional atherectomy has not been studied in this context in SVGs, but in CAVEAT II, MI rates for focal disease were higher with directional coronary atherectomy (DCA) than with balloon angioplasty and were associated with worse 12-month outcomes (7,8). Given these outcomes, it is highly unlikely that DCA will prove useful in preparing vein grafts for stenting. Using excimer laser angioplasty to debulk prior to stenting in 81 patients with thrombus-containing degenerated grafts, Hong et al. (9) reported favorable procedural results (9% non–Q-wave MI and 0% no reflow), but long-term outcome has not been reported. Use of a transluminal ex-

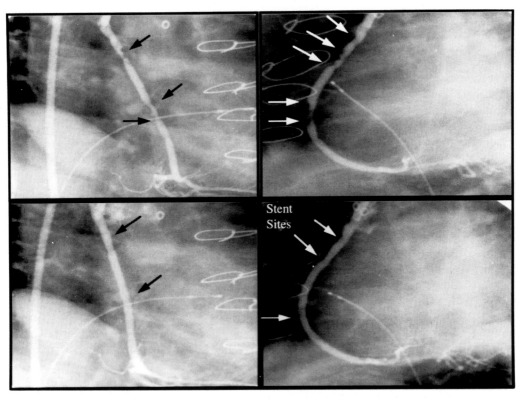

FIG. 16.10. A 60-year-old man with a history of coronary bypass surgery (12 years earlier) presented with unstable angina. He was found to have a patent LIMA graft to the left anterior descending, a patent SVG to the circumflex coronary artery, and severe diffuse disease of the SVG to the right coronary artery (**upper left,** right anterior oblique view). *Arrows* indicate sites with the most severe lesions. Because of angiographic thrombus, TEC atherectomy was performed, followed stent deployment (**lower frames**) with an excellent result and no significant creatine kinase elevation.

traction catheter (TEC) prior to stenting (Fig. 16.10) was also reported by the same group with similar outcomes (15% non–Q-wave MI, 2.2% no reflow, 2.9% abrupt closure) (9), but it should be noted that the definition of *non–Q-wave MI* was a rather high value of CK-MB: five times normal. Others have reported favorable initial outcome with TEC (10,11), but the place of these debulking strategies prior to SVG stenting is unclear, and extension of these strategies to truly diffuse disease is not justifiable.

Long Stents

Long stents are currently available in the United States, but a careful study of the use of these devices in SVGs has not be reported.

Whether benefit can be derived from long Wallstents (Sci Med-Boston Scientific) with lengths exceeding 60 mm, as has been suggested (12), seems doubtful, given the recent report of the use of Wallstents (mean lesion length < 14 mm) in 139 patients, in which 6-month outcomes were: death, 4.3%; MI, 12%; major adverse cardiac event (MACE), 24%; and restenosis, 38% (13). Intermediate-length stents (15 to 30 mm) will probably have a place in carefully selected patients without very bulky lesions, but more study is needed.

Treatment of Borderline Lesions

Because of the tendency for progression, secondary SVG sites with narrowing of ≥50% are frequently treated by interventional operators, either before or after stenting of the culprit SVG lesion. However, Ellis et al. (5) noted that ischemic events <12 months after initial treatment were most commonly related to untreated sites where some disease existed at the time of initial procedure. Not surprisingly, the frequency of nontarget, late ischemic events correlated with initial percent stenosis (initial 41% to 50%, 45% events; 31% to 40%, 18% events; ≤30%, 2% events; $p < .001$). This observation, coupled with the finding that late-event rates were low in treated lesions with narrowing <50%, raised the question of whether lesions 40% to 50% in SVGs undergoing intervention should be treated (5). This remains unanswered, and at the present time, treatment of lesions <50% is not recommended.

NEW STRATEGIES TO LIMIT EMBOLIZATION (DISTAL PROTECTION)

In view of the morbidity and mortality related to thromboatheroembolization in SVG intervention, a number of strategies are being evaluated with the goal of protecting against this complication, either by temporarily occluding graft flow and aspirating debris, by attempting to trap debris with filter-type devices or covered stents, or by using new strategies for thrombus removal.

Distal Occluder-Washout Method

Using routine percutaneous transluminal coronary atherectomy (PTCA) equipment, Shaknovich and colleagues (14) developed the distal occluder-washout (DOW) method, which involved protection of distal coronary circulation with an occlusion balloon during SVG dilation and washout steps prior to stenting implantation, as illustrated in Fig. 16.11. Using this technique in 23 grafts in 21 patients, only one non–Q-wave MI and one acute stent thrombosis were observed. No deaths, Q-wave MIs, or subacute thrombosis occurred, and, clinically significant, ''no reflow'' was avoided. Analysis of aspirate indicated an average particle size of 165 ± 44 μm, with some particles up to 600 μm in diame-

ter. Occlusion time averaged approximately 6 minutes (range, 3 to 15 minutes). We have used this strategy in a small number of patients, finding that it worked best in vein grafts to the right coronary artery, where deep seating of the guide catheter was facilitated and the ischemic burden was modest.

Emboli Containment System

The PercuSurge guidewire system (PercuSurge Inc., Sunnyvale, CA) utilizes a hollow 0.014-in. PTCA wire incorporating a compliant, inflatable, distal occlusion balloon (Fig. 16.12). During occlusion of the distal graft, PTCA and stenting can be carried out. Prior to deflation of the occlusion balloon, potentially embolic debris are aspirated from the proximal graft using a special monorail catheter. Webb et al. (15) reported that in 24 grafts aged 8.7 ± 5 years, which were stented using this protective system, creatine kinase exceeded three times normal in only one patient. No patients developed electrocardiographic evidence of MI, required surgery, or died. Of 45 aspirates, 43 (95%) had typical atherosclerotic debris, including necrotic core, foam cells, cholesterol clefts as well as fibrous caps, smooth muscle cells, and fibrin matrix (16). This system is currently undergoing multicenter FDA evaluation. In a limited experience, we have aspirated a considerable amount of atheromatous debris and found the system to be relatively easy to use. A multicenter, randomized trial is currently in progress.

Covered Stents

Stents covered with autologous venous or arterial tissue or with polytetrafluoroethylene (PTFE) have been used to seal perforations, exclude aneurysms and early results of their use in vein grafts has been reported (17–21). Covered stents offer the potential advantage of excluding, ''sequestering,'' friable atheroma and thrombotic material reducing embolic and thrombotic complications. Stedfanadis et al reconstructed an extensively diseased vein graft by use of multiple tissue-covered stents and documented excellent 6 month patency (17). PTFE covered stents

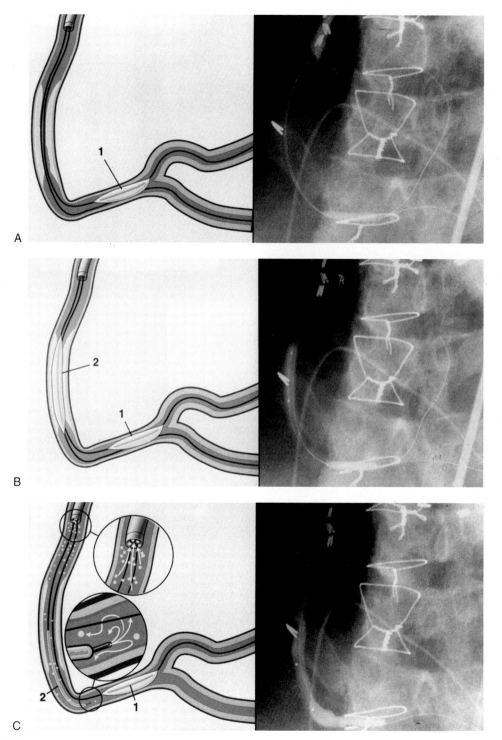

FIG. 16.11. The distal occluder-washout method. **A:** The distal occlusion step in SVG to the right coronary artery. 1, occluder balloon. **B:** Pretreatment of diseased area in the SVG. 1, occluded balloon; 2, pretreatment balloon. **C:** Washout step following pretreatment. The mixture of contrast and saline infused through the wire lumen of the deflated pretreatment balloon (*2*) is visible proximal to the inflated occluder balloon (*1*). Lack of opacification of the recipient right coronary artery is evident. (From ref. 14, courtesy of Dr. Alexander Shanknovich.)

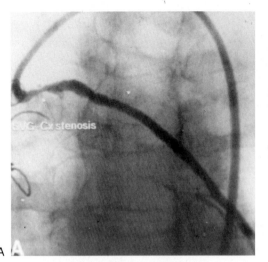

A

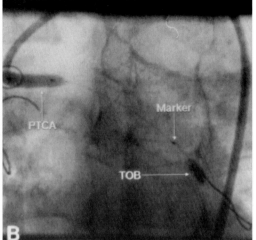

B

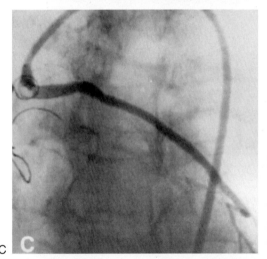

C

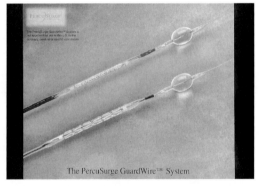

D

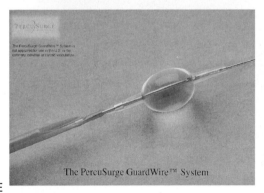

E

FIG. 16.12. Severe stenosis of proximal SVG supplying the circumflex coronary artery, left anterior oblique view **(A)**. With the total-occlusion balloon (*TOB*) inflated **(B)** the lesion is dilated and stented, and aspiration of the graft is performed with a special aspiration catheter (*arrow*). The TOB is then deflated, and angiography revealed an excellent result with a normal graft flow **(C)**. The principle illustrated can be applied to grafts with more diffuse disease. PTCA, percutaneous transluminal coronary atherectomy. (From ref. 15, courtesy of Dr. John G. Webb.) The TOB is shown inflated with stent **(D)** and aspiration catheter **(E)**.

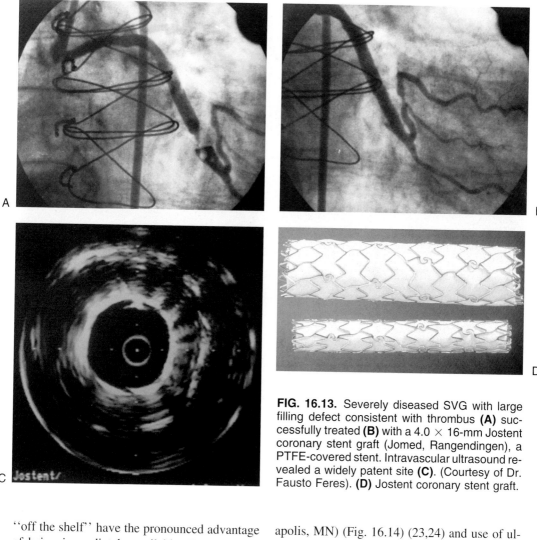

FIG. 16.13. Severely diseased SVG with large filling defect consistent with thrombus **(A)** successfully treated **(B)** with a 4.0 × 16-mm Jostent coronary stent graft (Jomed, Rangendingen), a PTFE-covered stent. Intravascular ultrasound revealed a widely patent site **(C)**. (Courtesy of Dr. Fausto Feres). **(D)** Jostent coronary stent graft.

"off the shelf" have the pronounced advantage of being immediately available. Experience is currently being accumulated (Fig. 16.13), but specific indications for their use and long-term outcome data are lacking.

Managing Graft Thrombus

In patients with unstable angina, vein graft thrombus is evident angioscopically in over 70%, and large graft thrombi are relatively common and complicate intervention by causing thromboembolic infarction and abrupt closure (22) (see Chapter 11C). Other new strategies for thrombus removal include rheolytic thrombectomy with the AngioJet (Possis Medical, Minne-

apolis, MN) (Fig. 16.14) (23,24) and use of ultrasound thrombolysis (25) (see Chapter 5H on ultrasound thrombolysis by Rosenschein). Recent reports of angioscopy following AngioJet treatment revealed effective removal of intraluminal thrombus, but some mural thrombus remained (26). However, the place of the AngioJet and ultrasound thrombolysis, both very promising strategies, has not been determined.

Several types of filters designed to trap atheromatous and thrombotic debris liberated during intervention procedures are being evaluated (Fig. 16.15), but clinical trials have not begun (27). Whether local delivery of IIb/IIIa agents will be effective in reducing thrombus burden in SVGs, as has been suggested (28), requires

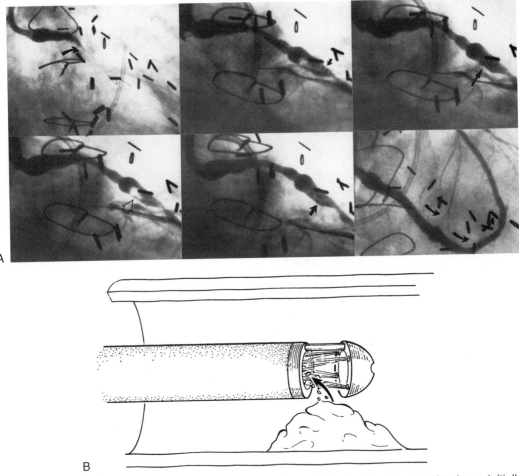

FIG. 16.14. A: Example of the use of the AngioJet to reduce the thrombus burden in an initially occluded vein graft treated with stenting, with an excellent final result **(lower right panel).** (Courtesy of Dr. Donald Baim). Diagram of the AngioJet, which has a 5 Fr working end **(B).** High-speed retrograde saline jets are directed centrally from the catheter tip into the catheter lumen, creating a vacuum that aspirates and entrains thrombus within the saline jets. The vacuum is generated according to the Bernoulli principle (24).

further study. In general, when intervention is attempted on a thrombotic graft, one or perhaps several strategies aimed at reducing the thrombus burden will be utilized in the future.

STRATEGIES TO REDUCE LATE ADVERSE EVENTS

Even if techniques are developed that permit safe and effective initial treatment of diffusely diseased vein grafts, long-term benefit will be quite modest in the majority of patients unless

effective strategies are developed that reduce restenosis and disease progression. Thus far, only a small number of patients with vein graft lesions have received catheter-based local radiation therapy. Although the initial reports have been favorable, it will be some time before the evaluation of brachytherapy in vein grafts is completed. Similarly, on-going gene therapy aimed at halting neointimal hyperplasia is focused in arterial sites, and the use of these strategies in venous grafts will follow that effort. Long-term IIb/IIIa therapy could conceivably

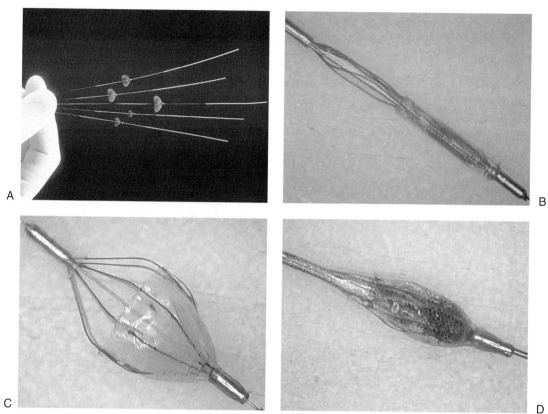

FIG. 16.15. A: A family of novel trap devices (Microvena, Inc., White Bear Lake, MN). Braided baskets of nitinol wire trap a thrombus, which is then retracted into the guide catheter (27). **B:** An umbrella-type filter utilizing 150-μm, laser-drilled holes in a polymeric shelve, which, when opened **C:** traps debris. By collapsing the umbrella, the filtered debris can be captured and removed **(D)**. (Courtesy of Angioguard, Plymouth, MN).

prove beneficial in vein graft disease by preventing thrombus formation. It is hoped that one or more of these will be effective in reducing the high event rates observed following vein graft interventions, opening the door for more aggressive intervention in diffusely diseased grafts.

REFERENCES

1. Leon MB, Ellis SG, Moses J, et al. Interim report from the reduced anticoagulation vein graft stent (RAVES) study. *Circulation* 1996;94[Suppl I]:I-683.
2. Ho KKL, Carrozza JP, Popma JJ, et al. Creatine-kinase MB isoform (CK-MB) elevations following single-vessel percutaneous revascularization of saphenous vein grafts. *Circulation* 1998;98[Suppl I]:I-353.
3. Ellis SG, Lincoff AM, Miller D, et al. Reduction in complications of angioplasty with abciximab occurs largely independently of baseline lesion morphology. *J Am Coll Cardiol* 1998;32:1619–1623.
4. Savage MP, Douglas JS Jr, Fischman DL, et al. A randomized trial of coronary stenting and balloon angioplasty in the treatment of aortocoronary saphenous vein bypass graft disease. *N Engl J Med* 1997;337:740–747.
5. Ellis SG, Brener SJ, DeLuca S, et al. Late myocardial ischemic events after saphenous vein graft intervention—importance of initially "nonsignificant" vein graft lesions. *Am J Cardiol* 1997;79:1460–1464.
6. Hong MK, Pichard AD, Wu H, et al. Predictors of long-term results after successful angioplasty in saphenous vein grafts. *Circulation* 1998;98[Suppl I]:I-353.
7. Holmes DR, Topol EJ, Califf RM, et al. A multicenter, randomized trial of coronary angioplasty versus directional atherectomy for patients with saphenous vein graft lesions. *Circulation* 1995;91:1966–1974.
8. Lefkovits J, Holmes DR, Califf RM, et al. Predictors and sequelae of distal embolization during saphenous vein graft intervention from the CAVEAT-II Trial. *Circulation* 1995;92:734–740.
9. Hong MK, Wong SC, Popma JJ, et al. Favorable results of debulking followed by immediate adjunct stent therapy for high risk saphenous vein graft lesions. *J Am Coll Cardiol* 1996;27[Suppl A]:A179.

10. Parks JM. TEC before stent implantation. *J Invas Cardiol* 1995;7[Suppl D]:10D–13D.
11. Kramer B. Optimal therapy for degenerated saphenous vein graft disease. *J Invas Cardiol* 1995;7[Suppl D]: 14D–20D.
12. Colombo, Itoh A, Hall P, et al. Implantation of the Wallstent for diffuse lesions in native coronary arteries and venous bypass grafts without subsequent anticoagulation. *J Am Coll Cardiol* 1996;53A.
13. Safian R. Transcatheter Therapeutics 1998.
14. Shaknovich A, Forman ST, Parikh MA. Novel distal occluder-wash out method of prevention of no-reflow during stenting of saphenous vein grafts. (*in press*).
15. Webb JG, Garere RG, Lo K, et al. Containment and analysis of embolic material during saphenous vein graft angioplasty. *Circulation* 1998;98[Suppl I]:I-354.
16. Webb JG. Transcatheter Therapeutics 1998.
17. Stefanadis C, Toutouzas K, Tsiamis E, et al. Total reconstruction of a diseased saphenous vein graft by means of conventional and autologous tissue-coated stents. *Cathet Cardiovasc Diagn* 1998;43:318–321.
18. Clark DA. Reconstructing diseased vein grafts—great potential raises old issues. *Cathet Cardiovasc Diagn* 1998;43:322.
19. Gerckens U, Mueller R, Cattelaens N, et al. The JoStent® stent graft: initial experience with a covered stent. *Am J Coll Cardiol* 1998;82[Suppl 7A]:615.
20. Toutouzas KP, Stefanadis CI, Tsiamis LG, et al. Stents covered by an autologous vein graft: a retrospective comparative study with conventional uncovered stents. *Circulation* 1998;98[Suppl I]:I-855.
21. Lopez A, Heuser RR, Stoeger H, et al. Coronary artery application of an endoluminal polytetrafluoroethylene stent graft: two center experience with Jomed® JoStent®. *Circulation* 1998;98[Suppl I]:I-855.
22. Silva JA, White CJ, Collins TJ, et al. Morphologic comparison of atherosclerotic lesions in native coronary arteries and saphenous vein grafts with intracoronary angioscopy in patients with unstable angina. *Am Heart J* 1998;136:156–163.
23. Ramee SR, Baim DS, Popma JJ, et al. A randomized, prospective, multi-center study comparing intracoronary urokinase to rheolytic thrombectomy with the POSSIS Angioget catheter for intracoronary thrombus: final results of the VeGAS 2 Trial. *Circulation* 1998; 98[Suppl I]:I-86.
24. Drasler WJ, Jenson ML, Wilson GJ, et al. Rheolytic catheter for percutaneous removal of thrombus. *Radiology* 1992;182:263–267.
25. Fajadet J, Calderon L, Thomas M, et al. Coronary ultrasound thrombolysis in acute coronary syndromes: the first 100 patients from the Acolysis Registry. *Circulation* 1998;98[Suppl I]:I-87.
26. Rodés J, Bilodeau L, Bonan R, et al. Angioscopic evaluation of thrombus removal by the Possis Angiojet® thrombectomy catheter. *Cathet Cardiovasc Diagn* 1998; 43:338–343.
27. Kim WH, Goldberg M, Katzer J, et al. A novel embolization trap device at the distal end of a guide wire. *Circulation* 1998;98[Suppl I]:I-354.
28. Barsness GW, Buller CE, Ohman EM, et al. Reduced thrombus burden in saphenous vein grafts with abciximab given through a local delivery catheter. *Circulation* 1998;98[Suppl I]:I-354.

C. Managing Diffuse Vein Graft Lesions: Reconstruction with Self-Expandable, Less-Shortening Wallstents

Thierry Joseph, Jean Fajadet, and Jean Marco

UCI, Clinique Pasteur, 31076 Toulouse, France

Management of patients with recurrent ischemia after coronary artery bypass graft (CABG) surgery is a difficult problem, the magnitude of which increases continuously. Angina frequently recurs after surgery, with a yearly reappearance rate of 6% to 7% after the procedure (1,2), resulting from either atherosclerosis progression in native coronary arteries or graft failure (3). The attrition rate of saphenous vein grafts (SVGs) is 10% to 20% during the first year after surgery, 1% to 2% per year between 1 and 6 years, and 4% per year between 6 and 10 years (3,4). Moreover, less than 30% of patent grafts are angiographically free of lumen stenoses at 10 years (3,4). As the number of patients who have undergone CABG continues to grow, the number of patients who need repeat revascularization increases. It has been estimated that

9% to 19% of the patients will require additional procedures within 10 years after the initial surgery (5–7).

Because repeat CABG results in increased perioperative mortality (3% to 7%), increased incidence of myocardial infarction (MI) (3% to 11%), and a less-effective symptom relief, as compared with the initial operation (4–6,8), percutaneous transluminal coronary angioplasty (PTCA) has been proposed as a reasonable alternative. However, SVG balloon angioplasty is associated with a higher rate of acute complications than observed during interventions in native coronary arteries. Distal embolization resulting from friable and ulcerated plaque is particularly frequent (from 4% to 13%) and is associated with a greater incidence of immediate and long-term adverse events (9–11). Moreover, intermediate and long-term outcomes include high rates of restenosis (up to 46%) and major adverse events (24% to 43% at 1 year and 66% to 74% at 5 years) (8,9,12–17). Either isolated implantation of Palmaz-Schatz stents (Johnson and Johnson International Systems, Warren, NJ) or stent placement after with directional coronary atherectomy or transluminal extraction catheter atherectomy has been found to improve the outcome of patients treated for focal lesions, with a restenosis rate of 13% to 37% and an event-free survival rate at 1 year of 70% to 80% (16–23). However, an optimal treatment strategy for diffuse SVG lesions is not yet determined, in particular, the need to treat 40% to 50% stenosed segments in addition to the more severe lesions. Indeed, recent data have shown that 45% of ischemic events after 1 year result from 40% to 50% of initially untreated sites (24).

We reported the immediate and intermediate clinical results of 73 patients with diffuse SVG lesions, electively treated by implantation of one or multiple self-expandable, less-shortening Wallstents, with preventive antiplatelet (aspirin, ticlopidine ± abciximab) and anticoagulant (enoxaparin) treatment.

METHODS

Between May 1, 1995, and April 30, 1997, 3,265 consecutive patients underwent PTCA in our institution, of whom 151 (4.6%) were treated for SVG lesions and 73 presented with diffuse lesions (i.e., significant lesion with length >20 mm either isolated or associated with lesions <50% stenosed). These 73 patients, considered poor candidates for repeat surgery because of advanced age, unfavorable coronary vessel anatomy, poor left ventricular function, or severe concomitant noncardiac disease, underwent SVG reconstruction with elective implantation of one or multiple Wallstents

Angioplasty Procedure

Angioplasty was performed via a transradial (41%), transfemoral (58%), and transhumeral (1%) approach, using 6 Fr (12%), 7 Fr (31%), or 8 Fr (57%) guiding catheters. The lesion was carefully crossed with a 0.014-in. guidewire and predilated with an undersized balloon inflated at 3 to 4 atm (ratio of balloon diameter to graft diameter <1) during a 30-second period, in order to prevent distal embolization. In all patients, Wallstents were used for SVG reconstruction. This stent has a self-expanding property for deployment that avoids balloon inflation and an elastic wire mesh design that allows the entrapment of friable SVG material. It is available in a large range of lengths (up to 50 mm) and sizes (up to 6.0 mm). Stents were generally chosen with a diameter 1.5 mm larger than the reference diameter and with a length 15 mm longer than lesion length. If necessary, two or more overlapped stents were implanted. If this occurred, the distal stent was deployed first and then the proximal one. Stent expansion was achieved by in-stent balloon inflation, with a ratio of balloon diameter to graft diameter <1. Intravascular ultrasound was not used during the procedure. The sheaths were removed immediately after the transradial procedure and immediately or 6 hours after the transfemoral procedure. Hemostasis was achieved by using a Perclose device or by mechanical compression (Femostop device) with 2 hours in patients treated via a transfemoral approach, and by radial compression with a tourniquet in place within 40 minutes in patients treated via a transradial approach.

After intracoronary injection of isosorbide

dinitrate (3 mg) and molsidomine (1 mg), reference vessel diameter, minimum lumen diameter, and lesion length were calculated by on-line quantitative coronary analysis (DCI Philips system). The following definitions were used for angiographic assessment:

Diffuse SVG lesion: significant lesion, with length >20 mm and either isolated or associated with lesions <50% stenosed

Thrombus: circumscribed intraluminal filling defect

Angiographic success: smooth lumen surface at the stent site, with a final diameter stenosis equal to 0

Distal embolization: new appearance of filling defects and/or abrupt cutoff of the vessel distal to the target lesion and/or decreased anterograde flow in the distal vessel previously patent, in the absence of an occlusion of the target lesion

No reflow: poor anterograde flow (thrombolysis in MI [TIMI] grade ≤ 1) not explained by dissection or high-grade residual stenosis at or adjacent to the target lesion

Abrupt closure: poor anterograde flow (TIMI grade ≤ 1) due to acute occlusion of the target lesion

Because platelet aggregation has been thought to play an important role in the ischemic complications resulting from distal embolization, all patients—at high risk for such complications—were treated at least 3 days before PTCA with aspirin (100 to 250 mg od), ticlopidine (250 mg bid), and enoxaparin (100 IU per kilogram bid). An intravenous bolus of heparin (70 IU per kilogram) was administered after arterial sheath placement, and additional heparin boluses were given to maintain the activated clotting time between 250 and 300 seconds. Fifteen (20.5%) patients were treated with abciximab therapy, with a 0.25-mg per kilogram bolus initiated just before the procedure, followed by a 10-μg per minute infusion for 12 hours. After the procedure, all patients received 1-month ticlopidine (250 qd or bid) and long-term aspirin (100 to 250 mg qd). Enoxaparin (100 IU per kilogram bid) was continued for 48 to 72 hours in 18 (24.6%) patients. Systematic serum level measurements of creatine kinase with MB fraction were not routinely performed after the procedure.

Data Analysis

Clinical, angiographic, and procedural data and postprocedural complications were prospectively entered into a computerized database (AS400, Showcase). Clinical follow-up was performed by trained personnel, who made telephone contact with the patients or their referring physicians. Information obtained included occurrence of recurrent angina, MI, subsequent cardiac catheterizations, need for repeat PTCA or additional CABG, and death (cardiac and noncardiac). Follow-up (mean length, 13 ± 8 months) was obtained in 62 (91%) of the 68 discharged, alive patients. Follow-up data were entered into the computerized database. Initial and follow-up data of the 73 studied patients were retrospectively analyzed.

RESULTS

Clinical Characteristics

Baseline characteristics are shown in Table 16.1. The study included 73 patients: 65 men and eight women; mean age, 69 ± 6 years (range, 33 to 85 years). Thirty-five of them (48%) were older than 70 years. Mean age of treated SVGs was 12 ± 2 years (range, 1 to 25 years). Thirty-two patients (45%) had a previous MI and 24 (33%) had undergone previous PTCA. At presentation, 18 patients (19%) had a recent MI and 34 (46%) presented with unstable angina.

TABLE 16.1. *Clinical characteristics*

	n (%)
Patients	73
Male	65 (89)
Age (yr)	69 ± 6
Graft age (yr)	12 ± 2
Previous MI	33 (45)
Previous PTCA	24 (33)
Unstable angina	34 (46)
Recent MI	14 (19)

MI, myocardial infarction; PTCA, percutaneous transluminal coronary angioplasty.

TABLE 16.2. *Baseline angiographic characteristics*

	%
Vessel disease	
One vessel	4
≥2 vessels	96
Ejection fraction	54 ± 15
Number of grafts	90
Target-vessel anastomosis	
LAD/diagonal branch	33
LCx/marginal branch	37
RCA	30
Graft lesion location	
Body graft	66
Proximal part	24
Distal part	10

LAD, left anterior descending artery; LCx, left circumflex artery; RCA, right coronary artery.

TABLE 16.3. *Quantitative angiographic results*

	Pre-PTCA (lesion)	Post-PTCA (stent)
RVD (mm)	3.9 ± 0.7	4.0 ± 0.6
MLD (mm)	0.2 ± 0.1	4.1 ± 0.5
Length (mm)	24.1 ± 14.0	40.0 ± 19.4
Diameter stenosis (%)	80 ± 15	4 ± 2

PTCA, percutaneous transluminal coronary angioplasty; RVD, reference vessel diameter; MLD, minimum lumen diameter.

Angiographic Characteristics

Single and multivessel disease was present in 4% and 96% of the patients, respectively (Table 16.2). Mean ejection fraction was 54% ± 15% (range, 20% to 80%).

The treated SVGs were implanted on the left anterior descending artery and/or diagonal branch (33%), the left circumflex artery and/or marginal branch (37%), and the right coronary artery (30%), respectively (see Table 16.2). One hundred six lesions were presented in 90 SVGs (1.2 lesion per graft), located on the proximal part, body graft, and distal part in 24%, 66%, and 10%, respectively. Mean length lesion was 24.1 ± 14.0 mm, and preprocedural percentage stenosis was 80% ± 15% (Table 16.3). One hundred twenty Wallstents were successfully implanted, representing 1.3 stents per graft and 1.65 stents per patient, with a mean final diameter of 4.1 ± 0.5 mm (see Table 16.3 and Fig. 16.16). No re-

Pre PTCA

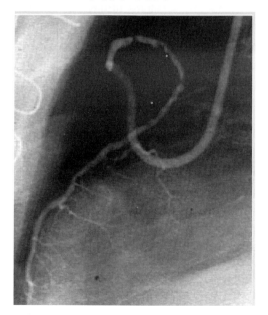

Post PTCA

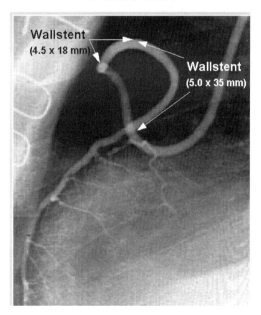

Wallstent (4.5 x 18 mm)

Wallstent (5.0 x 35 mm)

FIG. 16.16. Diffusely degenerated saphenous vein graft implanted on the left anterior descending artery before **(left panel)** and after **(right panel)** implantation of two Wallstents.

flow was observed in one patient, and distal embolization was observed in eight (11%). No abrupt closure occurred.

Other coronary lesions were treated simultaneously in 19 patients (26%). They were located on native arteries in 18 patients and on an internal mammary artery graft in one patient. Twenty-five additional stents were implanted on grafts (12) and on native arteries (13), including nine Gianturco-Roubin (Cook Inc., Bloomington, IN) stents, seven Palmaz-Schatz stents, three Wiktor (Medtronic, Minneapolis, MN) stents, three Wallstents, two Nir stents (Scimed, Maple Grove, MN), and one GFX (Medtronic AVE, Santa Rosa, CA) stent.

In-Hospital Events

In-hospital complications are reported in Table 16.4. Five patients (6.9%) died, of whom two suffered cardiac causes. The first presented with cardiogenic shock resulting from distal embolization and no reflow. The second died of ventricular fibrillation 3 days after the procedure. Noncardiac deaths included three strokes: two intracranial hemorrhages occurring 1 and 4 days after the procedure, respectively, and one subclavian dissection by guiding catheter via the transradial approach, complicated by a carotid hematoma. Among these three patients, one had received abciximab therapy during PTCA, and all were treated with enoxaparine after the procedure.

Eight other patients (11%), of whom two had received abciximab therapy, presented with non–Q-wave MIs resulting from distal embolization. One patient was electively treated with CABG 3 days after the procedure, including successful right coronary artery graft stenting but left anterior descending artery PTCA failure. One patient had transient ischemic stroke without sequela. Eight patients (11%) had vascular access complications, of whom two received blood transfusions and two required surgical repair.

Clinical Follow-Up

Clinical follow-up data (mean length, 13 ± 8 months), obtained in 62 of the 68 discharged, alive patients (91%), is presented in Table 16.5. During the follow-up period, 34% of patients presented major adverse events (death, MI, or repeat revascularization). Five patients (8.1%) died, three patients as a result of cardiac causes (4.8%). Two patients suffered fatal MIs 1 week and 3 months, respectively, after the procedure, and one presented with sudden death 6 months after PTCA. One of the noncardiac deaths resulted from stroke at 3 months. One patient (1.7%) had a nonfatal MI. Twenty-three patients (40.3%) presented with recurrent angina. A need for subsequent revascularization occurred in 16 patients (28.1%), including target-lesion revascularization in nine cases (15.8%), repeat PTCA in seven patients, and CABG in two. Angioplasty of others vessels was performed in seven patients: on native coronary arteries in four patients and on other grafts in three. No patient underwent additional revascularization for initially untreated narrowings of stented lesions.

Control angiography was performed during follow-up in 21 patients (34%), who presented clinical symptoms or a positive noninvasive ischemic test, with a delay of 2 to 15 months after stent implantation. Restenosis, defined as >50%

TABLE 16.4. *In-hospital complications*

	n (%)
Overall mortality	5 (6.9)
Cardiac death	2 (2.8)
Distal embolization	8 (11)
CABG	1 (1.4)
Subacute thrombosis	0 (0)
Vascular access	8 (11)

CABG, coronary artery bypass graft.

TABLE 16.5. *Clinical follow-up (mean, 13 ± 8 mo)*

	n (%)
Patients	62 (91)
Overall mortality	4 (6.8)
Cardiac death	3 (4.8)
Nonfatal MI	1 (1.7)
Overall revascularization	16 (28.1)
TLR	9 (15.8)
CABG	2 (3.5)
PTCA	7 (12.3)

MI, myocardial infarction; TLR, target-lesion revascularization; CABG, coronary artery bypass graft; PTCA, percutaneous transluminal coronary angioplasty.

diameter stenosis, was found in 13 patients (61.9%), of whom six had total graft occlusion.

COMMENTS

Determination of the optimal strategy for treating patients with diffuse SVG lesions remains controversial. In a pooled analysis of 16 studies, SVG balloon angioplasty is associated with a high procedural success rate (approximately 90%) and a low incidence of death (<1%), MI (<3%), distal embolization (<3%), and emergency CABG (<2%) (9–15). However, the findings of these studies should be partly relativized, because they are focused mainly on the treatment of focal lesions. It has been well established that procedural results depend in part on the diffuseness of SVG disease, age of the graft, and presence of thrombus (9,10,13,14). Intermediate and long-term outcomes include high rates of restenosis (up to 46%) and major adverse events (24% to 43% at 1 year and 66% to 74% at 5 years) (8,9,12–17). Implantation of Palmaz-Schatz stents has been shown to decrease the restenosis rate (13% to 37%) and incidence of adverse events (20% to 30% at 1 year), as compared with balloon angioplasty (16–23). But the majority of stent implantations was also performed on focal lesions. Moreover, the results of the sole randomized trial (17) are most disappointing, in particular showing a 37% restenosis rate in the stent group.

Immediate Results

In this study SAVED trial (17), successful stent implantation was achieved in all cases, in concordance with results of the previous series reporting Wallstent implantation for treating SVG disease (25–29). The frequency of in-hospital major events, including death, MI, emergency CABG, or subacute stent thrombosis, was relatively high (see Table 16.4), as compared with previous reports (0% to 11%) (16–23,25–29). Distal embolization occurred frequently; it was observed in eight patients (11%), of whom two had received abciximab during the procedure. Because serum level measurements of creatine kinase with MB fraction were not systematically performed after the pro-

cedure, some non–Q-wave MIs could have been missed, resulting in an underestimated cardiac complication rate. Our treatment strategy was initially based on an angioscopy study that found thrombi in 71% of SVGs treated by angioplasty (30), on the proved beneficial effect of the ticlopidine–aspirin association to reduce platelet aggregation and coagulation activation time during angioplasty procedures (31), and on data from the EPIC trial (32). Data from the EPIC study reported a significant reduction in distal embolization rate with abciximab therapy, as compared with placebo (2% vs. 18%). Moreover, we used Wallstents, which have a self-expanding property that avoids balloon inflation for implantation and an elastic wire mesh design that allows entrapment of friable SVG material. Nevertheless, interpretation of our results should take into account the type of lesions treated. It is well established that procedural results depend in part on the diffuseness of SVG disease, age of the graft, and presence of thrombus (9,10,13,14). Distal embolization is more frequently observed when PTCA is performed in old SVGs with diffuse disease and thrombus-containing lesions, and it is associated with a high rate of ischemic complications (9–11). The appropriate strategy for preventing or treating no reflow resulting from distal embolization is not yet established. The use of direct administration of thrombolytics remains disappointing, with a 13% occurrence of distal embolization despite preprocedural local infusion of urokinase (33,34) and only a 10% no-reflow reversal (35). The results observed after direct administration of verapamil (100 to 500 μg) are more encouraging, with a flow reestablishment in 67% to 87% of cases (35–37). More recently, intravenous administration of abciximab has been found to significantly reduced the occurrence of distal embolization in patients undergoing SVG angioplasty (2% vs. 18% in the placebo group) (32), and in some cases to rapidly restore coronary blood flow (38). Because the no-reflow phenomenon is thought to result mainly from microvascular spasm and platelet activation, an interesting pharmacologic approach might be the systematic preprocedural administration of verapamil and abciximab. Actually, new devices, such as the trap device, are also being investigated (39), but clinical trials are needed to determine the real efficacy and safety of these techniques.

Major bleeding and vascular complications significantly occurred in our study, resulting in three deaths. This probably resulted in part from the aggressive antiplatelet and anticoagulant regimen used in this study. Such complications were also frequent in the other series, despite different antiplatelet and anticoagulant treatments. They have been observed in up to 33% of patients and have been frequently related to the in-hospital deaths (16–23,25–29). De Sheerder et al. (27), who performed intra-SVG administration of thrombolytics during the procedure, reported bleeding complications in 33% of patients, including two fatal hemorrhagic strokes (27). On the other hand, no subacute stent thrombosis occurred in our study, contrasting with an incidence of 1% to 10% in other studies (16–23,25–29).

More recently, technical improvement, including the use of undersized balloons that are briefly inflated and Wallstent implantation without intrastent balloon inflation, associated with a less aggressive antiplatelet and anticoagulant regimen, resulted in an improved in-hospital outcome. Between May 1997 and January 1998, 30 other consecutive patients were been treated according to this strategy: No deaths occurred, and only two patients (6.7%) presented with distal embolization (authors' unpublished personal observation).

Intermediate Results

At a median follow-up of 13 months, 65% of patients were alive and event-free (freedom from MI and repeat revascularization). Our results were quite similar to those previously reported after SVG stent implantation, despite that our series included only patients treated for diffuse lesions. According to several studies (16,18–23, 26,29), 1-year event-free survival was 46% to 80%. It is important to note that the most disappointing results were observed in the series of De Jaegere et al. (29), in which 52% of stent implantations (mainly Wallstents) were per-

formed for treating long SVG lesions. In this study, 23% of patients presented with MI, and 50% underwent repeat revascularization at a median of 6 months after the procedure (29). Regarding these results and ours, it seems reasonable that in a patient presenting with a diffusely degenerated SVG implanted on the left anterior descending artery and without excessive surgical risk, a reoperation with implantation of the left internal mammary artery should be considered first. Adverse outcome after SVG stenting has been thought to be partly related to restenosis. Angiographic follow-up revealed a restenosis rate of 17% to 37% in the series with Palmaz-Schatz stents (16–22) and a rate of 20% to 54% in the studies with Wallstents (25–29). In our study, only symptomatic patients underwent control angiography, and the 62% restenosis rate was then probably overestimated. It is noteworthy that no patient underwent additional revascularization for initially untreated narrowings of stented lesions. This contrasted with previous studies (20,27) that reported a 27% to 34% rate of revascularization procedures in relation to SVG disease progression. This could be explained partly by our election to largely cover nonseverely diseased segments narrowing the more stenosed sites with long stents, instead of covering each severe adjacent lesion separately. Indeed, Ellis et al. (24) found that 45% of recurrent ischemic events after SVG interventions result from initially untreated 40% to 50% stenosed sites, as compared with the 19% of events related to the initially treated 40% to 50% stenosed segments. However, this strategy could have been partly the result of the high incidence of restenosis observed in our study. Regarding the choice of stent used, there are actually no data comparing different types of long stent for treating diffuse SVG disease, particularly in terms of restenosis. In our center, Wallstents are electively used in this regard, while premounted radiopaque stents, such GFX, Multilink (Guidant Inc., Santa Clara, CA), and Niroyal, are used for treating ostial SVG lesions.

CONCLUSION

This observational study suggested that reconstruction of diffusely degenerated SVGs by implantation of self-expandable, less-shortening Wallstents with preventive antiplatelet and anticoagulant treatment was associated with a significant, immediate complication rate. Intermediate clinical outcome revealed a relatively high cardiovascular morbidity and mortality rate. However, the clinical status of the studied population, at high risk for repeat CABG, should be taken into account when interpreting the results. Further studies, including new antiplatelet and anticoagulant therapy and new device technology, are needed to determine the appropriate strategy for treating such high-risk lesions, especially in order to reduce the need for repeat reinterventions.

REFERENCES

1. Campeau L, Lesperace J, Hermann J, Corbara F, Gondin CM, Bourassa MG. Loss of improvement of angina between 1 and 7 years after aortocoronary bypass surgery. *Circulation* 1979;60[Suppl I]:I1–I5.
2. Johnson WD, Kayser KL, Pedraza PM. Angina pectoris and coronary bypass surgery: patterns of prevalence and recurrence in 3105 consecutive patients followed-up to 11 years. *Am Heart J* 1984;108:1190–1196.
3. Bourassa MG, Enjalbert M, Campeau L, Lesperance J. Progression of atherosclerosis in coronary arteries and bypass grafts: ten years later. *Am J Cardiol* 1984; 53[Suppl C]:102C–107C.
4. Fitzgibbon GM, Kafaka HP, Leach AJ, Keon WJ, Hooper GD, Burton JR. Coronary bypass graft fate and patient outcome: angiographic follow-up of 5,065 grafts related to survival and reoperation in 1,388 patients during 25 years. *J Am Coll Cardiol* 1996;28:616–626.
5. Cameron A, Kemp HG, Green GE. Reoperation for coronary artery disease: 10 years of clinical follow-up. *Circulation* 1988;78[Suppl I]:I158–I162.
6. Loop FD, Lytle BW, Cosgrove DM, et al. Reoperation for coronary atherosclerosis: changing practice in 2509 consecutive patients. *Ann Surg* 1990;212:378–385.
7. Weintraub WS, Jones EL, Craver JM, Guyton RA. Frequency of repeat coronary bypass or coronary angioplasty after coronary artery bypass surgery using saphenous venous grafts. *Am J Cardiol* 1993;73:103–112.
8. Weintraub WS, Jones EL, Morris DC, King SB III, Guyton RA, Craver JM. Outcome of reoperative coronary bypass surgery versus coronary angioplasty after previous bypass surgery. *Circulation* 1997;95:868–877.
9. De Feyter PJ, Van Suylen RJ, De Jaegere PP, Topol EJ, Serruys PW. Balloon angioplasty for the treatment of lesions in saphenous vein bypass grafts. *J Am Coll Cardiol* 1993;2:1539–1549.
10. Dooris M, Hoffmann M, Glazier S, et al. Comparative results of transluminal extraction coronary atherectomy in saphenous vein graft lesions with and without thrombus. *J Am Coll Cardiol* 1995;25:1700–1705.
11. Lefkovits J, Holmes DR, Califf RM, et al, for the CAVEAT-II Investigators. Predictors and sequelae of distal

embolization from the CAVEAT-II trial. *Circulation* 1995;92:734–740.
12. Douglas JS, Gruentzig AR, King SB III, et al. Percutaneous transluminal coronary angioplasty in patients with prior coronary bypass surgery. *J Am Coll Cardiol* 1983; 2:745–754.
13. Platko WP, Hollman J, Whitlow PL, Franco I. Percutaneous transluminal angioplasty of saphenous vein graft stenosis: long-term follow-up. *J Am Coll Cardiol* 1989; 14:1645–1650.
14. Reeves F, Bonan R, Cote H, et al. Long-term angiographic follow-up after angioplasty of venous coronary bypass grafts. *Am Heart J* 1991;122:620–627.
15. Plokker TH, Meester HB, Serruys PW. The Dutch experience in percutaneous transluminal angioplasty of narrowed saphenous vein used for aortocoronary arterial bypass. *Am J Cardiol* 1991;67:361–366.
16. Brener SJ, Ellis SG, Apperson-Hansen C, Leon MB, Topol EJ. Comparison of stenting and balloon angioplasty for narrowings in aortocoronary saphenous vein conduits in place for more than five years. *Am J Cardiol* 1997;79:13–18.
17. Savage M, Douglas J, Fischman D, et al, for the Saphenous Vein De Novo Trial Investigators. Stent placement compared with balloon angioplasty for obstructed coronary bypass grafts. *N Engl J Med* 1997;337:740–747.
18. Strumpf RK, Mehta SS, Ponder R, Heuser RR. Palmaz-Schatz stent implantation in stenosed saphenous vein grafts: clinical and angiographic follow-up. *Am Heart J* 1992;123:1329–1336.
19. Pomerantz RM, Kuntz RE, Carrozza JP, et al. Acute and long-term outcome of narrowed saphenous venous grafts treated by endoluminal stenting and directional atherectomy. *Am J Cardiol* 1992;70:161–167.
20. Piana RN, Moscucci M, Cohen DJ, et al. Palmaz-Schatz stenting for treatment of focal vein graft stenosis: immediate results and long-term outcome. *J Am Coll Cardiol* 1994;23:1296–1304.
21. Fenton SH, Fishman DL, Savage MP, et al. Long-term angiographic and clinical outcome after implantation of balloon-expandable stents in aortocoronary saphenous vein grafts. *Am J Cardiol* 1994;74:1187–1191.
22. Wong SC, Baim DS, Schatz RA, et al, for the Palmaz-Schatz Stent Study Group. Immediate results and late outcome after stent implantation in saphenous vein graft lesions: the multicenter U.S. Palmaz-Schatz stent experience. *J Am Coll Cardiol* 1995; 26:704–712.
23. Braden GA, Xenopoulos NP, Young T, Utley L, Kutcher MA, Applegate RJ. Transluminal extraction catheter atherectomy followed by immediate stenting in treatment of saphenous vein grafts. *J Am Coll Cardiol* 1997; 30:657–663.
24. Ellis SG, Brener SJ, DeLuca S, et al. Late myocardial ischemic events after saphenous vein graft intervention—importance of initially ''nonsignificant'' vein graft lesions. *Am J Cardiol* 1997;79:1460–1464.
25. Urban P, Sigwart U, Kaufman U, et al. Intravascular stenting for stenosis of aortocoronary venous bypass grafts. *J Am Coll Cardiol* 1989;13:1085–1091.
26. Strauss BH, Serruys PW, Bertrand ME, et al. Quantitative angiographic follow-up of the coronary Wallstent in native vessels and bypass grafts (European experience—March 1986 to March 1990). *Am J Cardiol* 1992; 69:475–481.
27. De Scheerder IK, Strauss BH, De Feyter PJ, et al. Stent-

ing of venous bypass grafts: a new treatment modality for patients who are poor candidates for reintervention. *Am Heart J* 1992;123:1046–1054.

28. Eechout E, Goy JJ, Stauffer JC, Vogt P, Kappenberger L. Endoluminal stenting of narrowed saphenous vein grafts: long-term clinical and angiographic follow-up. *Cathet Cardiovasc Diagn* 1994;32:139–146.

29. De Jaegere PP, Van Domburg RT, De Feyter PJ, et al. Long-term clinical outcome after stent implantation in saphenous vein grafts. *J Am Coll Cardiol* 1996;28: 89–96.

30. White CJ, Ramee SR, Collins TJ, Mesa JE, Jain A. Percutaneous angioscopy of saphenous vein coronary bypass grafts. *J Am Coll Cardiol* 1993;2:1181–1185.

31. Gregorini L, Marco J, Fajadet J, et al. Ticlopidine and aspirin pretreatment reduces coagulation and platelet activation during coronary dilatation procedures. *J Am Coll Cardiol* 1997;29:13–20.

32. Mak KH, Challapella R, Eisenberg MJ, Anderson KM, Califf RM, Topol EJ. Effect of platelet glycoprotein IIb/IIIa receptor inhibition on distal embolization during percutaneous revascularization of aortocoronary saphenous vein grafts. EPIC Investigators. *Am J Cardiol* 1997;80:985–988.

33. Danardo SJ, Morris NB, Rocha-Singh KJ, Curtis GP,

Rubenson DS, Teirstein PS. Safety and efficacy of extended urokinase infusion plus stent deployment for treatment of obstructed, older saphenous vein grafts. *Am J Cardiol* 1995;76:776–780.

34. Fram DB, Primanio CA, Mitchel JF, Dougherty JE, McKay RG. Treatment of thrombotic saphenous vein bypass with the Dispatch catheter. *Cathet Cardiovasc Diagn* 1997;41:361–267.

35. Abbo KM, Dooris M, Glazier S, et al. Features and outcome of no-reflow after percutaneous coronary intervention. *Am J Cardiol* 1995;75:778–782.

36. Piana RN, Paik GY, Moscucci M, et al. Incidence and treatment of no-reflow after percutaneous coronary intervention. *Circulation* 1994;89:2514–2518.

37. Kaplan BM, Benzuly KH, Kinn JW, et al. Treatment of no-reflow in degenerated saphenous vein graft interventions: comparison of intracoronary verapamil and nitroglycerin. *Cathet Cardiovasc Diagn* 1996;39:113–118.

38. Rawitscher D, Levin TN, Cohen I, Feldman T. Rapid reversal of no-reflow using abciximab after coronary device intervention. *Cathet Cardiovasc Diagn* 1997;42: 187–190.

39. Won HK, Goldberg M, Katzentein J, et al. A novel embolization trap device at the distal end of a guidewire. *Circulation* 1998;98[Suppl I]:I354.

17

Interventional Therapy of Small Vessels

Sheldon Goldberg, Janah I. Aji, and Arun Venkat

*The Center for Cardiovascular Intervention, Cooper University Medical Center,
Camden, New Jersey 08103*

Interventional therapy in patients with smaller coronary vessels has long been recognized as problematic. Patients with smaller coronary arteries have had an historically higher risk of adverse outcomes with greater rates of periprocedural complications as well as chronic restenosis. In a retrospective review of over 5,000 cases of coronary angioplasty performed at Massachusetts General Hospital, a higher incidence of acute complications, including myocardial infarction and emergency surgery, was noted in patients with smaller vessel size. In fact, small reference diameter emerged as a strong independent predictor of adverse outcome following balloon angioplasty (1). With respect to longer term patency, small arterial diameter has been found to be associated with higher rates of restenosis. For example in the Multi Hospital Eastern Atlantic Restenosis Trial, follow-up angiography was obtained in 510 patients who underwent successful balloon angioplasty (2). Angiographic restenosis was one-third more frequent in patients with smaller vessels: By the binary definition ($\geq$50% diameter stenosis at follow-up), restenosis occurred in 34% of patients with reference diameters $\leq$2.9 mm, and the rate was significantly higher at 44% in patients with reference diameters <2.9 mm.

While coronary stent implantation has resulted in a salutary effect on angiographic and clinical restenosis compared with standard balloon angioplasty, it should be noted that studies demonstrating this clinical benefit for coronary stent placement were conducted primarily in patient populations with larger coronary arteries (i.e., those with reference vessel diameters $\geq$3 mm). Thus, the relative reduction in angiographic stenosis of 25% observed in STRESS (3) and 33% reported in Benestent (4) cannot be extrapolated to patients with smaller coronary vessels.

STUDIES OF STENT IMPLANTATION IN PATIENTS WITH SMALLER CORONARY ARTERIES

One potential problem in stenting smaller coronary arteries is the possibility of a higher incidence of stent thrombosis. This concern was raised by the data collected in the French Registry of coronary stent implantation (5). In that study, 2,900 patients who had stent implantation were treated with ticlopidine and aspirin, and 30-day follow-up was performed; 51 patients (1.8%) had stent thrombosis, and smaller balloon size was found to be a powerful predictor of this complication. Ten percent of patients in whom the procedure was performed with balloon size $\geq$2.5 mm had stent thrombosis, but only 2.3% of patients with balloon size of 3.0 mm and 1.0% of patients treated with balloons $\geq$3.5 mm in diameter developed abrupt vessel closure ($p < .001$). However, the concern over a higher incidence of abrupt closure was not observed in other trials of stent placement in smaller coronary arteries (*vida infra*).

To compare the longer term efficacy of stent implantation with balloon angioplasty in patients with smaller vessels, we analyzed the re-

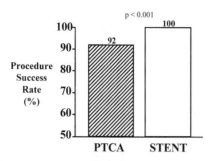

FIG. 17.1. Procedural success for stent placement versus balloon angioplasty in patients with reference vessel diameter <3.0 mm. This study was a retrospective analysis of 333 patients with smaller vessels within the overall population of 598 patients entered in the STRESS I & II trials. There is a significantly superior outcome in patients assigned to stent placement. PTCA, percutaneous transluminal coronary angioplasty.

sults from a subgroup of patients within the overall population of 598 patients entered in the STRESS I + II trial, who had reference diameters <3.0 mm by quantitative coronary angiographic analysis performed in a core angiographic laboratory (6). In that report, patients with new lesions in native coronary arteries were randomized to receive either Palmaz-Schatz stents or balloon angioplasty. The patients were treated with aspirin, postprocedure heparin, and warfarin. Follow-up angiography was performed per protocol at 6 months, and clinical follow-up was assessed after 1 year. By quantitative coronary angiographic analysis, 331 of 598

patients (56%) were determined to have reference vessel diameters <3.0 mm. Of these patients, 163 were randomly assigned to Palmaz-Schatz stent placement and 168 were assigned to balloon angioplasty. The results showed a significantly higher procedural success rate of 100% for stent placement versus 92% for standard balloon angioplasty (Fig. 17.1). This is of particular note when one considers that the stent used in this trial had a bulky delivery system and was not specifically designed for use in smaller coronary vessels. Importantly, the abrupt closure rate (3.6%) was not different for the balloon and stent groups. Compared with balloon angioplasty, stent placement resulted in a larger postprocedural lumen diameter (2.26 mm vs. 1.80 mm, $p < .001$) and a larger lumen at 6-month follow-up (1.54 vs. 1.27 mm, $p < .001$) (Fig. 17.2). Angiographic restenosis was reduced from 55% in patients treated with balloon angioplasty to 34% in patients treated with stent placement ($p < .001$) (Fig. 17.3). This superior angiographic result was accompanied by improved clinical outcome. After 1 year, event-free survival was 67% in the balloon group and 78% in the stent group (Fig. 17.4). This difference in event-free survival was due mainly to the reduced need for repeat vascularization of the target vessel. In the same report, we noted that the benefit of stenting relative to balloon angioplasty at 6 months was significant across the range of vessel sizes in terms of follow-up minimal lumen diameter (Fig. 17.5). It must be noted

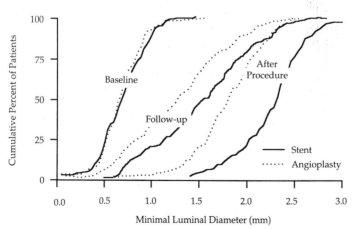

FIG. 17.2. Quantitative coronary angiographic results from the same study of patients with smaller coronary arteries. The cumulative frequency curves show that at baseline there was no difference in minimum lumen diameter between the groups assigned to stent placement or balloon angioplasty. After the procedure, a significantly larger minimum lumen diameter was observed in the stent group, and this benefit was maintained at 6-month follow-up.

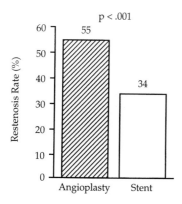

FIG. 17.3. Angiographic restenosis rates by the binary definition in the balloon and stent groups at 6 months. There was a relative reduction of 38% in restenosis rate: from 55% in the balloon group to 34% in the stent group.

that this study had several important limitations: First, it was a retrospective analysis of data gathered from a prospective, randomized trial; second, it was carried out with the use of a stent not specifically designed for smaller vessels; and finally, patients with tortuous vessels and calcified and diffuse lesions so often encountered in clinical practice were excluded from the trial.

The outcomes of coronary stent placement have also been compared for patients with large and small native coronary arteries. In one such study (7), the results of arterial scaffolding using a variety of stents were compared in 696 patients with larger (≥3 mm) coronary arteries versus 602 patients with smaller coronary arteries (reference vessel <3 mm) (Fig. 17.6). Angiographic restenosis at 6 months was 19% in patients with larger reference vessels and was significantly

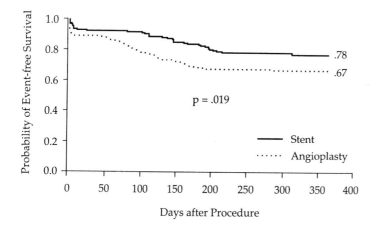

FIG. 17.4. Event-free survival (EFS) in the balloon and stent groups of patients with smaller coronary arteries. After 1 year, the EFS was only 67% in the balloon group; patients assigned to the stent group had a significantly higher EFS of 78%, mainly due to a reduced rate of repeat revascularization procedures.

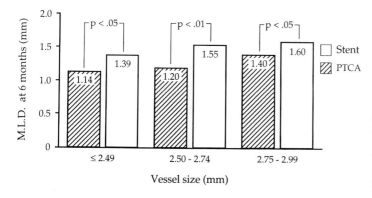

Minimal lumen diameter (*MLD*) shown as a function of vessel size in patients with smaller coronary arteries. Stent placement resulted in a larger MLD across the spectrum of reference diameters. PTCA, percutaneous transluminal coronary angioplasty.

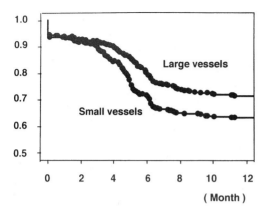

FIG. 17.6. Analyses for stenting in patients with large or small coronary arteries have [definitions as in Fig. 17.7]. The curves represent the incidence of death, myocardial infarction, surgery, or repeat intervention.

higher, at 33%, in patients with smaller coronary arteries ($p < .0001$). As expected, the absolute lumen gain was greater in patients with larger reference vessels, but absolute lumen loss was similar in the two groups; therefore, the loss index (late loss/acute gain) was less favorable in patients with smaller vessels (Fig. 17.7). An-

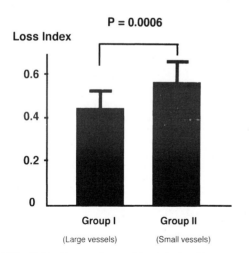

FIG. 17.7. Comparison of loss index [(postprocedure MLD—follow-up MLD)/acute gain] for patients with large reference diameters (group I: reference diameters ≥3.0 mm) versus small vessels (group II: reference diameter <3.0 mm). This indicates that the percentage of acute gain that is lost at follow-up is worse for patients with smaller vessels.

giographic predictors of freedom from restenosis included larger postprocedural stent cross-sectional area (OR 1.19, $p = .001$) and shorter lesion length (OR 1.037, $p = .01$). The event-free survival (freedom from death, myocardial infarction, coronary artery bypass graft surgery, or repeat intervention) was also more favorable in the patients with larger reference vessels (see Fig. 17.6).

The effect of vessel size on outcome after coronary stent implantation was further assessed in a study of 2,602 patients who had successful stent placement for symptomatic coronary artery disease (8). The patients were subdivided into three equal terciles of vessel size (< 2.8 to 3.2, and >3.2 mm). The event-free survival at 1 year was 69.5% in the group with the smallest vessels; it was 77.5% in the intermediate vessel size group; and it was highest, at 81%, in the tercile with the largest vessel diameters ($p < .001$) (Fig. 17.8). As noted in the previous study, the absolute late lumen loss was similar for the patients with smaller and larger vessels and the angiographic restenosis rate was highest in the patients with the smallest vessels: The restenosis rate was 38.6% in the patients with the smallest vessels; it was 28.4% in patients with intermediate vessels; and it was 20.4% for patients in the highest tercile of vessel size. Although patients with the smaller vessels had higher restenosis rates requiring more frequent repeat revascularization, within the group of patients with smaller vessels, there was a wide range of restenosis rates. Additional important independent risk factors for the development of restenosis in patients with smaller vessels included patients with a history of diabetes, prior angioplasty, the presence of lesion complexity, and multiple stent placement. As shown in Fig. 17.9, for patients with vessel size <2.8 mm, the restenosis rate was 38.6%; the presence of lesion complexity conferred a higher restenosis rate (41.6%). In patients without complex lesions, however, the restenosis rate was significantly lower (31.5%). Furthermore, restenosis ranged from 29.6% in patients without lesion complexity or diabetes mellitus to 53.5% in patients in whom both factors were present.

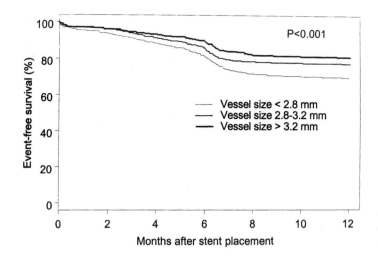

FIG. 17.8. Kaplan-Meier survival curves at 1 year for patients in three terciles of vessel size.

CASE EXAMPLE

A 62-year-old woman with insulin-dependent diabetes had bypass surgery 5 years prior to readmission with unstable angina. Angiography showed a new discrete lesion in the obtuse marginal branch of the left circumflex coronary artery (reference diameter, 2.3 mm) (Fig. 17.10A) and diffuse, complex disease of the right coronary artery, which was supplied by an occluded saphenous vein bypass graft. (Fig. 17.10B).

Stent placement was performed in the circumflex vessel with an excellent result (Fig. 17.10C) and a reasonable expectation of good long-term

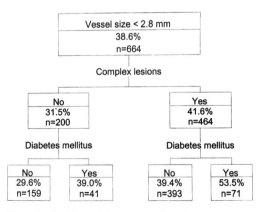

FIG. 17.9. The wide range of restenosis within the group of patients with smaller coronary arteries (reference diameter <2.8 mm). Note that restenosis can vary from about 30% in patients without complex lesions or diabetes to more than 50% in patients in whom both factors are present.

outcome. It was elected to not treat the right coronary artery because of the diffuse complex nature of the disease in the presence of diabetes. The restenosis risk could be estimated to be over 50% for this type of vessel (see Fig. 17.9).

CLINICAL IMPLICATIONS

To date, studies have shown that small vessel size is an important risk factor for the development of restenosis and the need for repeat revascularization when either balloon angioplasty or stent implantation is performed. Preliminary evidence suggests that stenting may be superior to balloon angioplasty for the therapy of patients with smaller coronary arteries, but at present we are awaiting the results of randomized trials to assess the long-term efficacy of stent placement in this important cohort of patients. We have also learned that other factors, including the presence of lesion complexity, more diffuse disease requiring multiple stents, and diabetes, adversely effect outcome. Future studies will need to address the following key issues in an attempt to further enhance long-term patency.

Optimization of Stent Placement Technique

In this regard, second- and third-generation coronary stents specifically designed for use in smaller vessels need to be studied in terms of long-term outcome. The use of intravascular ultrasound in order to properly size and oppose

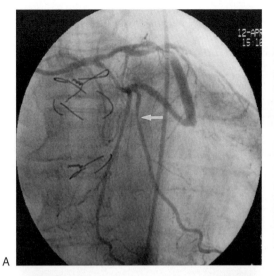

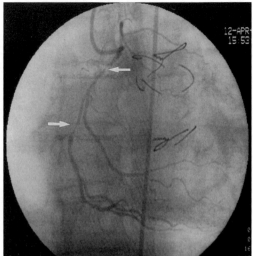

A

B

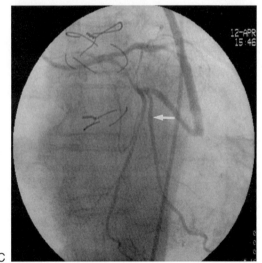

C

FIG. 17.10. A: Angiogram showing a discrete, noncomplex lesion in the obtuse marginal branch of the left circumflex coronary artery in a patient with diabetes. The reference vessel diameter was 2.3 mm. The risk of restenosis can be estimated to be approximately 40%. **B:** The same patient after placement of a 2.5 × 8.0-mm ACS Multilink Duet stent (Guidant Inc., Santa Clara, CA). Note that the stented area is the largest segment of the treated vessel. **C:** The right coronary angiogram from the same patient. There is diffuse disease and the reference diameter is 2.25 mm. The risk of restenosis was estimated to be >50%. This lesion was not revascularized because of the potential for poor long-term outcome.

stents needs further consideration. The role of debulking to reduce plaque burden as an adjunct to stent placement also needs further study. Since the results of plaque excision prior to stent placement have shown promising results in pilot studies in patients with larger coronary arteries (9,10), the role of debulking lesions with rotational atherectomy prior to stent placement needs formal evaluation in patients with smaller vessels.

Adjunctive Pharmacologic Agents

The results from the Epistent trial (11) suggest an important role for IIb/IIIa receptor antago-

nists not only in terms of reducing myocardial infarction, but also for reducing clinical restenosis in certain patient subgroups (i.e., those with diabetes). The adjunctive use of this class of compounds, therefore, may play a particularly important role in the therapy of patients with small vessels.

Local Radiation

This investigational therapy appears promising in patients in whom intimal proliferation plays a critical role in the restenosis process (12). The efficacy of this approach will require the development of user-friendly, cost-effective devices for this substantial population of patients.

REFERENCES

1. Palacios et al. Outcomes of coronary intervention in patients with small vessels. J Am Coll Cardiol 1999 (*in press*).
2. Hirshfeld JW, Schwartz JS, Jugo R, et al. Restenosis after coronary angioplasty: a multivariate statistical model to relate lesion and procedure variables to restenosis. *J Am Coll Cardiol* 1991;18:647–656.
3. Fischman DL, Leon MB, Baim DS, et al. A randomized comparison of coronary-stent placement and balloon angioplasty in the treatment of coronary artery disease. *N Engl J Med* 1994;331:496–501.
4. Serruys PW, Dejaegere P, Kiemeneij F, et al. A comparison of balloon-expandable-stent implantation with balloon angioplasty in patients with coronary artery disease. *N Engl J Med* 1994;331:489–495.
5. Karrillon GJ, Morice MC, Benveniste E, et al. Intracoronary stent implantation without ultrasound guidance and with replacement of conventional anticoagulation by antiplatelet therapy: 30-day clinical outcome of the French Multicenter Registry. *Circulation* 1996;94:1519–1527.
6. Savage MP, Fischman DL, Rake R, et al. Efficacy of coronary stenting versus balloon angioplasty in small coronary arteries. *J Am Coll Cardiol* 1998;31:307–311.
7. Akiyama T, Moussa I, Reimers B, et al. Angiographic and clinical outcome following coronary stenting of small vessels. *J Am Coll Cardiol* 1998;32:1610–1618.
8. Elezi S, Kastrati A, Neumann F, Hadamitzky M, Dirschinger J, Schomig A. Vessel size and long-term outcome after coronary stent placement. *Circulation* 1998;98:1875–1880.
9. Moussa I, Moses J, DiMario C, et al. Stenting after optimal lesion debulking (SOLD registry). *Circulation* 1998;98:1604–1609.
10. Goldberg S, Aji J. Plaque excision combined with stent placement: can a poor "finisher" become a good "starter"? *Circulation* 1998;98:1591–1593.
11. EPISTENT Investigators. Evaluation of platelet IIb/IIIa inhibitor for stenting. Randomised placebo-controlled and balloon-angioplasty-controlled trial to assess safety of coronary stenting with use of platelet glycoprotein-IIb/IIIa blockade. *Lancet* 1998;352(9122):87–92.
12. Teirstein PS, Massullo V, Jani S, et al. Catheter-based radiotherapy to inhibit restenosis after coronary stenting. *N Engl J Med* 1997;336:1697–1703.

18

Complete Versus Incomplete Revascularization

David P. Faxon and Christakis Christodoulou

*University of Southern California School of Medicine, Division of Cardiology,
Los Angeles, California 90033*

BACKGROUND

Fundamental to the large-scale growth and success of angioplasty as a popular and effective mode of coronary artery revascularization has been the use of angioplasty for the treatment of patients with multivessel coronary disease. Studies show that multivessel disease patients constitute the majority of patients now undergoing the procedure. Nearly all studies also show that the majority of patients with multivessel disease treated with angioplasty are incompletely revascularized (1). Incomplete revascularization is most commonly defined as the presence of a residual stenosis of more than 50% in an artery of greater than 1.5 mm diameter. Incomplete revascularization can occur intentionally, when the operator dilates only those lesions or arteries that are thought by the operator to be the cause of the patient's symptoms, or unintentionally, when one or more lesions cannot be dilated or fails to be effectively treated.

FUNDAMENTALS OF INCOMPLETE REVASCULARIZATION

Understanding the significance of coronary obstructions and their treatment has come a long way over the past 10 years. When coronary angioplasty first began, the large profile and stiffness of the balloon catheters made it difficult to reach and dilate distal lesions and lesions in small arteries. As technology advanced, it became possible to dilate many more stenoses or lesions within the epicardial coronaries. How-

ever, with the widespread use of angioplasty in multivessel disease patients, incomplete revascularization became more common, largely due to the inability to dilate chronic total occlusions. The widespread practice of incomplete revascularization in multivessel disease was contrary to surgical data that suggested that incompletely revascularized patients have higher event rates in future years (2). In fact, complete surgical revascularization is still defined as the successful bypass or revascularization of all large epicardial coronaries. This definition does not take into account the lesion location, degree of stenosis, or the degree of myocardial ischemia. The advent of minimally invasive cardiac surgery direct coronary artery bypass (MIDCAB), with only left internal mammary artery (LIMA) to the LAD insertion, has impacted the approach taken by surgeons and interventionalists. More attention is now paid to the importance of the size of the vessel and the degree of myocardial ischemia, with incomplete revascularization as a strategy in certain patients with multivessel coronary artery disease.

One of the most important considerations in incomplete revascularization is identifying and selecting the lesion or lesions that are contributing to the patient symptoms or prognosis. In 1986, Wohlgelernter and colleagues (3) first defined such a lesion as a "culprit lesion." They described the efficacy of single-vessel percutaneous transluminal coronary angioplasty (PTCA) in 27 patients with unstable angina. In 75% of patients, they were able to identify a

TABLE 18.1. *Studies identifying culprit lesions*

Study	Year	% of Culprit Lesions	Criteria to identify a culprit lesion
Wohlgelernter (3)	1986	75%	ECG distribution of ischemia
Ambrose (5)	1988	58%	Angiographic characteristics
Breisblatt (6)	1995	21%	Operator-defined, using a combination of the above

culprit lesion by distribution on EKG (of ischemia) or anatomic features of the lesions. All patients were successfully treated by angioplasty and showed an excellent medium-term outcome. Unfortunately, subsequent studies have shown that identifying a culprit lesion is difficult, even in the setting of unstable angina (Table 18.1) (4–6). A culprit lesion is a concept originally used in the setting of unstable angina and it may not be reasonable to expand this definition to lesions found during elective cardiac catheterization, because in this setting, identifying a culprit lesion is often more difficult and treating all lesions may be necessary to improve symptoms. Of note is that in the BARI trial (4), only 21% of lesions were identified as culprit, using angiographic appearance.

If a culprit lesion can be identified, then incomplete revascularization has several advantages. First, it makes the angioplasty technically easier, particularly when only a single lesion is dilated. It might also result in a lower risk of complications, as well as subsequent restenosis. Bourassa et al. followed 757 patients, of whom only 132 had been completely revascularized, and found that repeat PTCA within the first year was more common in the completely revascularized group (40% versus 30%, $p < .05$) (1).

While identification of a culprit lesion can be difficult, it is facilitated by the distribution of EKG changes, as demonstrated by Wohlgelernter (3), and/or by angiographic criteria, as described by Ambrose et al. (5). Unfortunately, estimating the degree of luminal stenosis and morphology of a lesion is an unreliable predictor of outcome and has significant interobserver variability. Other approaches include imaging techniques, such as exercise thallium-201. Breisblatt et al. (6) evaluated 85 patients with multivessel disease and performed preangioplasty exercise thallium testing to help identify the ischemic area. This approach helped

identify the primary stenosis in 93% of patients. A follow-up thallium was then performed 2 weeks to 1 month later. At that time, 38 (47%) patients showed evidence of ischemia in another territory and underwent a second angioplasty. At 1-year follow-up, in the group that had no ischemia after the first angioplasty, only 13% required angioplasty of a second vessel. In the other group, 79% required multivessel angioplasty. Thus, thallium can be used preangioplasty as an adjunct to identifying the culprit lesion. The use of IVUS and Doppler flow wires have further helped define culprit lesions in the setting of routine angioplasty and some operators now rely on these to identify significant stenoses in a patient that may not have undergone any preprocedural noninvasive evaluation.

Finally, in a study by Faxon et al. (7), incompletely revascularized patients were characterized as functionally adequate or inadequate. Functionally adequate revascularization was done when all the stenoses in bypassable vessels supporting viable myocardium were successfully dilated. Not surprisingly, functionally adequate revascularization resulted in significantly fewer adverse events (death MI or CABG) at 1 year and showed no difference from those patients who were completely revascularized.

OUTCOMES OF INCOMPLETE REVASCULARIZATION

Studies looking at the long-term outcome of a strategy of incomplete revascularization have been mixed (Table 18.2). In general, clinical trials have not demonstrated any difference in overall mortality between the two strategies. While four studies showed no difference in outcome with complete revascularization (8–10,13), six studies showed significant and important differences (1,7,11,12,14,15). In the largest published study to date on this subject,

TABLE 18.2. *Long-term outcomes of incomplete revascularization strategy*

Author	R	>	FU (y)	Death	MI	% CABG	PTCA	Asymptomatic
Bell (10)	C	356	2	NS	NS	NS	NS	NS
	IR	511						
Faxon (7)	C	72	1	3	7	15	30	76
	IR	67		6	13	18	19	67
Reeder (8)	O	127	2	3	7	33	20	69
	IR	159		5	9.4	35	8	67
Thomas (9)	C	19	2	0	0	5	11	63
	IR	73		0	1	1	12	63
Deligonul (13)	C	118	2	5	2.5	7	14	80
	IR	225		5.4	3.5	16	13	78
Vandormael (15)	C	35		0	3	3	3	63
	IR	31		0	0	16	16	63
Mabin (14)	C	31	1	0	3	13	6	87
	IR	35		0	3	23	6	63
O'Keefe (12)	C	445	4.5	1				67
	IR	201		12				67
Bourassa (1)	C	132	9	2.6	22	32	30	—
	IR	625		22	17	14	40	—
Cowley (11)	C	91	3					92
	IR	248						74

R, degree of revascularization; C, complete; IR, incomplete revascularization; FU(y), follow-up (in years).

Bourassa and colleagues studied 757 patients with multivessel disease from the 1985–86 NHLBI PTCA registry and followed them for 9 years (1). Of these patients, only 132 were completely revascularized. Compared to patients with incomplete revascularization, these patients were older ($p < .05$), more likely to be female ($p < .05$), and more likely to have had recent myocardial infarction ($p < .05$), or unstable angina ($p < .001$). They also were much more likely to be patients who had urgent or emergent PTCAs ($p < .001$), which is not surprising given that the objective in these procedures is primarily to deal with the lesion involved in the acute coronary syndrome. Early death, Q-wave myocardial infarction, and CABG rates were higher in those with incomplete revascularization ($p < .05$); however, at 9 years, follow-up rates of repeat PTCA, death, Q-wave MI, and recurrent angina, were not different (Table 18.2).

Most reported studies do demonstrate a higher incidence of recurrent angina and the need for bypass surgery in patients with incomplete revascularization. Cowley and colleagues evaluated 370 patients, who were followed for 27 months after angioplasty (11). The 3-year, event-free survival for the entire group was 76.5%. Complete revascularization was strongly and negatively associated with long-term cardiac events. Using a Cox proportional hazard regression analysis, better left ventricular ejection fraction, lower Canadian Cardiovascular Society anginal class, less severe complex disease, and complete revascularization were associated with better event-free survival. Interestingly enough, when incomplete revascularization was defined as no stenosis of greater than 60% in large vessels, an improved prediction occurred. Other studies have also emphasized that the degree of incomplete revascularization is most important. In a study mentioned above by Faxon et al. (7), it was shown that if adequate revascularization was realized (defined as revascularization of all stenoses greater than 50% in vessels greater than 1.5 mm in diameter and serving viable territory), then no difference was found when compared with completely revascularized patients. However, when lesions were left in bypassable vessels that served viable territory, the outcome was much poorer, principally because of the need for repeat bypass surgery. The location of the lesion is also important and this has not been clearly defined in previous

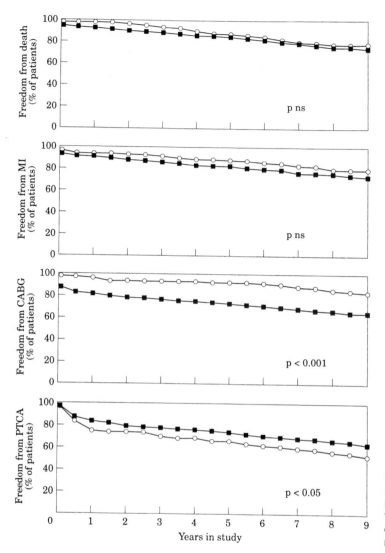

FIG. 18.1. Life table analysis plots showing the cumulative 9-year event-free rates in patients with complete (○) versus patients with incomplete (■) revascularization. Used by permission.

studies. In a study from the NHLBI PTCA Registry (1), a favorable 1-year outcome (defined as no clinical events and minimal or no angina), was highly predicted by the absence of a significant proximal stenosis of more than 50%. The importance of proximal versus distal disease is probably a surrogate for the size of the ischemic myocardium. As pointed out in the study by Cowley (11), other factors such as LV function, age, and comorbidity need to be taken into consideration in determining long-term outcome and therefore, the appropriateness of incomplete revascularization in any individual patient.

The surgical studies have also addressed the outcome of incomplete revascularization following bypass surgery. Importantly, incomplete revascularization is rarely a deliberate strategy following surgery. By and large, the surgical studies show that incompletely revascularized patients fare worse. The most recent study on this subject was by Jones et al. (2). They followed a total of 2,860 patients over a period of 12 years. These patients had all undergone CABG. All had multivessel disease and 803 patients were deemed to have undergone incomplete revascularization. However, in this group, the patients had more prior MI's, worse left ventricular function, and more three-vessel disease. Not surprisingly, these patients fared worse, with more MIs and poorer survival rates, except at 12 years, when the two subgroups appear to equalize. Of note was the analysis of the vessels left unrevascularized. The investigators found that incomplete revascularization of the LAD territory or multiple unrevascularized zones fared worst, followed by RCA and left circumflex. This is consistent with the importance of the location and the size of the ischemic territory. To date, the surgical studies lack randomization and the majority of patients with incomplete revascularization are those with diffuse disease, poor LV function, distal disease, and disease that is otherwise not amenable to bypass.

The only randomized comparisons of complete versus incomplete revascularization are from the randomized trials of PTCA versus bypass surgery. In particular, the BARI Trial did not require complete revascularization by either technique (17–18). As expected, the surgical patients had significantly more vessels bypassed than the PTCA patients had dilated. Thus, the outcome can be viewed as a comparison of complete (surgery) versus incomplete (PTCA) revascularization. In this study, in-hospital and 5-year death and nonfatal MI rates were equal. Only the need for repeat revascularization was different (8% for surgery and 54% for PTCA). In a multivariate analysis, incomplete revascularization was not associated with death or MI, but was associated with the need for bypass surgery during follow-up. These findings have been supported by other major randomized trials (19).

PRACTICAL APPROACH

There are a number of important factors to consider when deciding if incomplete revascularization is appropriate in a patient with multivessel disease. Careful attention should be given to the severity of angina symptoms, the presence of heart failure, and whether or not the patient has diabetes. If bypass surgery is a possibility, an estimate of surgical risk is also important. The results of exercise testing, stress thal-

lium, or stress echo, in combination with the angiogram, should be reviewed to help determine if one or more culprit lesions can be identified.

Lesion morphology, particularly irregular lesions suggesting plaque rupture and filling defects that may indicate thrombi (particularly in patients with unstable angina or recent MI), should be looked for carefully. If all significant lesions can be dilated, complete revascularization should be done, as long as it can be obtained with reasonable safety. If not, the significant lesions that are left behind should probably not serve more than 10% of the viable myocardium. If this cannot be achieved, patients with low surgical risk should be referred for surgical revascularization. In treated diabetic patients who have three-vessel disease (particularly if diffuse), even if complete revascularization is possible, bypass surgery with a LIMA graft is preferable, as demonstrated by the BARI Trial (17).

The optimal management of patients with multivessel disease is to do complete revascularization if at all possible (Fig. 18.2). Incomplete revascularization should be considered if the patient is at high risk for surgery or has steno-

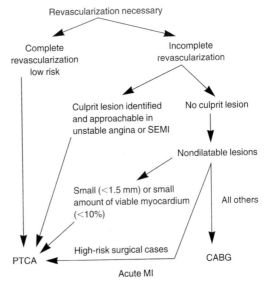

FIG. 18.2. Decision analysis in incomplete revascularization.

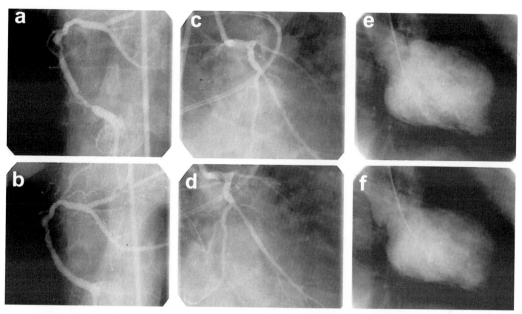

FIG. 18.3. An example of incomplete but adequate revascularization (**panels A–F**). The mid and distal right coronary artery were successfully dilated (**panels A and B**), as well as the first obtuse marginal (**panels C and D**). The LAD lesion was not dilated (**panels C and D**), since it served nonviable myocardium, as shown on the left ventriculogram (**panels E and F**).

ses that cannot be dilated and are not functionally important, because they serve nonviable territory or less than 10% of the viable myocardium (Fig. 18.3). In addition, stenoses in small vessels (e.g., <1.5 mm diameter) that are not suitable for bypass or angioplasty can also be left untreated. The successful dilation of the culprit lesion is critical for a favorable long-term outcome. The culprit lesion should always be the first lesion attempted and if successfully dilated, all other stenoses should be attempted in order of their significance. In some circumstances, the procedure can be staged with the culprit lesion dilated first and the remaining lesions dilated at another setting.

If a lesion is of questionable significance (e.g., ≤50% stenosis) and therefore it is not clear whether it contributes to the patient's symptoms, several approaches are possible. First, the procedure can be staged with the culprit or most important lesion dilated. Subsequently, the patient undergoes an exercise test to determine the functional significance of the remaining lesion(s). If the test is negative, then no further angioplasty is necessary. Alternatively, measurement of coronary flow reserve using a Doppler flow wire at the time of initial angioplasty can also distinguish the functional significance to the stenoses (Fig. 18.4).

An alternative approach to incomplete revascularization in patients in whom complete revascularization is not possible is the use of "hybrid" revascularization. Reports from several groups have shown that combining minimally invasive coronary artery bypass surgery with angioplasty can result in complete revascularization without the need for open heart surgery or incomplete revascularization by angioplasty. A recent study suggests that this approach is most attractive for patients with relative contraindications for cardiopulmonary bypass and in whom minimal surgery is possible, but not all vessels can be bypassed (20). "Hybrid" revascularization in all patients needing complete revascularization with LAD involvement might offer the advantages of a LIMA to the LAD and angio-

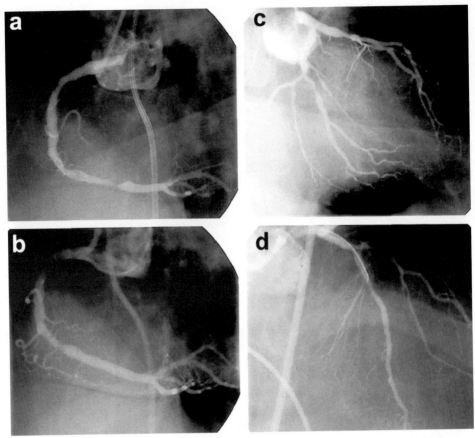

FIG. 18.4. An example of complete revascularization. The RCA lesion was successfully stented (**panels A and B**), but the LAD and OMB lesions were shown to have normal coronary flow reserve using Doppler flow (**panels C and D**) and these were not dilated.

plasty to other vessels without cardiopulmonary bypass or a midsternotomy scar. Clearly more studies are necessary to evaluate this approach.

SUMMARY

Angioplasty should be viewed as a palliative procedure for the treatment of coronary artery disease, a chronic, progressive disease. Revascularization remains the mainstay of therapy, since it is so effective in reducing symptoms. However, the only effective way to stem the course of coronary artery disease is to modify risk factors, with the goals of preventing new stenoses and stabilizing vulnerable plaques that can lead to acute coronary artery syndrome.

Since the goals of revascularization in the absence of left main disease or three-vessel disease are to relieve symptoms rather than impact survival, it makes sense that incomplete revascularization, with a functionally adequate result that leaves the patient symptom-free and is achieved with the lowest risk, is a reasonable approach for many patients. Future advances in angioplasty techniques are likely to reduce the number patients with incomplete revascularization.

Minimal bypass surgery combined with angioplasty or a "hybrid" strategy has already received some attention and may be a viable solution for patients who would otherwise be incompletely and inadequately revascularized.

REFERENCES

1. Bourassa MG, Yeh W, Holubkov R, Sopko G, Detre KM, for the Investigators of the NHLBI PTCA Registry. Long-term outcome of patients with incomplete versus complete revascularization after multivessel PTCA. *Eur Heart J* 1998;19:103–111.
2. Jones EL, Weintraub WS. The importance of completeness of revascularization during long-term follow-up after coronary artery operations. *J Thorac Cardiovasc Surg* 1996;112:227–237.
3. Wohlgelernter D, Cleman M, Highman HA, Zaret BL. Percutaneous transluminal coronary angioplasty of the "culprit lesion" for management of unstable angina pectoris in patients with multivessel coronary artery disease. *Am J Cardiol* 1986;58:400–464.
4. Williams DO, Baim DS, Bates E et al. Coronary anatomic and procedural characteristics of patients randomized to coronary angioplasty in the Bypass Angioplasty Revascularization Investigation (BARI). *Am J Cardiol* 1995;75:27–33.
5. Ambrose JA, Hjemdahl-Monsen CE, Borrico S, Gorlin R, Fuster V. Angiographic demonstration of a common link between unstable angina pectoris and non–Q-wave acute myocardial infarction. *Am J Cardiol* 1988;61: 244–247.
6. Breisblatt WM, Barnes JV, Weiland F, Spaccavento LJ. Incomplete revascularization in multivessel percutaneous transluminal coronary angioplasty: the role for stress thallium-201 imaging. *J Am Coll Cardiol* 1998;11: 1183–1190.
7. Faxon DP, Ghalilli K, Jacobs AK et al. The degree of revascularization and outcome after multivessel coronary angioplasty. *Am Heart J* 1992;123:854–859.
8. Reeder GS, Holmes DR, Detre K et al. Degree of revascularization in patients with multivessel coronary disease: a report from the NHLBI PTCA Registry. *Circulation* 1988;77:638–644.
9. Thomas ES, Most AS, Williams DO. Coronary angioplasty for patients with multivessel coronary artery disease: follow-up clinical status. *Am Heart J* 1988;115: 8–13.
10. Bell MR, Bailey KR, Reeder GS et al. Percutaneous transluminal angioplasty in patients with multivessel coronary disease: how important is complete revascularization for cardiac event-free survival? *J Am Coll Cardiol* 1990;16:553–562.
11. Cowley MJ, Vandermael M, Topol EJ et al. Is traditionally defined complete revascularization needed for patients with multivessel disease treated by elective coronary angioplasty? *J Am Coll Cardiol* 1993;22: 1289–1297.
12. O'Keefe JH, Rutherford BD, McConahay DR et al. Multivessel coronary angioplasty from 1980 to 1989: procedural results and long-term outcome. *J Am Coll Cardiol* 1990;16:1097–1102.
13. Deligonul U, Vandormael MG, Kern MJ et al. Coronary angioplasty: a therapeutic option for symptomatic patients with two and three vessel coronary disease. *J Am Coll Cardiol* 1988;11:1173–1179.
14. Mabin TA, Holmes DR, Smith HC et al. Follow-up clinical results in patients undergoing percutaneous transluminal coronary angioplasty. *Circulation* 1985;71: 754–760.
15. Vandormael MG, Chaitman BR, Ischinger T et al. Immediate and short-term benefit of multilesion coronary angioplasty: influence of degree of revascularization. *J Am Coll Cardiol* 1985;6:983–991.
16. Shaw RE, Anwar A, Myler RK et al. Incomplete revascularization and complex lesion morphology: relationship to early and late results in multivessel coronary angioplasty. *J Invest Cardiol* 1990;2:93–101.
17. The Bypass Angioplasty Revascularization Investigation (BARI) Investigators. Comparison of coronary bypass surgery with angioplasty in patients with multivessel disease. *N Engl J Med* 1996;335:217–225.
18. Botas J, Stadius ML, Bourassa MG et al. Angiographic correlates of lesion relevance and suitability for percutaneous transluminal coronary angioplasty and coronary artery bypass grafting in the Bypass Angioplasty Revascularization Investigation Study (BARI). *Am J Cardiol* 1996;77:805–814.
19. King SB, Lembo NJ, Weintraub WS et al. Emory Angioplasty Versus Surgery Trial (EAST): design, recruitment, and baseline description of patients. *Am J Cardiol* 1995;75:42–59.
20. Friedrich GJ, Bonatti J, Dapunt OE. Preliminary experience with minimally invasive coronary artery bypass surgery combined with coronary angioplasty. *N Engl J Med* 1997;336:1454–1455.

19

The Patient with Very Poor Left Ventricular Function

A. Managing the Patient with Severe Left Ventricular Dysfunction

Gregory W. Barsness and *David R. Holmes, Jr.

Department of Cardiology, °Department of Medicine, Mayo Medical School, Division of Cardiovascular Diseases and Internal Medicine, Mayo Clinic and Mayo Foundation, Rochester, Minnesota 55905

Anatomy and symptomatic status shape the clinical management of patients with severe left ventricular dysfunction. In patients with suitable coronary anatomy and evidence of ischemia, the decision to proceed with revascularization requires evaluation and understanding of symptom status, comorbid conditions, availability of revascularization options, overall risk, and patient preferences. There is a significant relationship between poor left ventricular function and poor outcome after coronary revascularization (1,2). Moreover, a clinical history of heart failure, irrespective of ejection fraction, is also independently associated with increased mortality (3). Although surgical revascularization may afford prognostic benefit among patients with moderately depressed ejection fraction, (4,5) it is increasingly the patient with debilitating angina and an ischemic cardiomyopathy with an ejection fraction of less than 25% who presents for palliation.

Because of associated high procedural morbidity and mortality, these patients with severe ventricular dysfunction may not be considered viable candidates for surgical intervention. Often, these patients have undergone previous surgical revascularization, as well, further complicating the issue of repeat revascularization. In these cases, percutaneous revascularization is an appropriate option and may provide the patient with both symptom relief and improved prognosis. Despite the emergence of alternative medical and invasive revascularization techniques, such as growth factor therapy, myocardial laser revascularization, and external counterpulsation, percutaneous coronary intervention remains the preferred mechanical revascularization technique in the vast majority of patients with dilatable lesions. This chapter reviews our approach to percutaneous revascularization in the high-risk patient with severe left ventricular dysfunction.

PATIENT SELECTION— CHARACTERISTICS AND PREPARATION

The importance of sufficient preparation prior to high-risk coronary interventions cannot be overstated. This includes preparing the patient, as well as adequately addressing the procedural and technical concerns as an operator. Initial attention should be directed at determining the potential benefits and risks of any planned procedure. Prior to undertaking the procedure, discussion with the patient and family should include risks of the procedure and potential options. Due to the demonstrated prognostic benefits of complete revascularization with coronary bypass surgery in patients with depressed ventricular function, patients without significant comorbidity who are acceptable surgical candidates should generally be referred for bypass surgery unless all lesions can be treated percutaneously. Most patients with severe left ventricular dysfunction, however, are not candidates for surgical intervention, and percutaneous intervention is the mechanical revascularization procedure of choice.

Due to the inherent risk of intervention in patients with severe ventricular dysfunction, every effort should be made to identify areas of myocardial viability to assure that a successful intervention will provide the anticipated benefits of amelioration of ischemia and improvement in regional myocardial function (6). This is particularly true in the case of patients who are unable to undergo complete revascularization via the percutaneous approach. Identification of areas of ischemic burden may help to target specific ischemia-producing lesions among a host of potential candidates.

Although identification of ischemia is helpful in developing a revascularization strategy, the absence of ischemia or viability by noninvasive assessment does not exclude the potential benefit of revascularization. The extent of viable but ischemic myocardium has been shown to determine the degree of improvement in left ventricular function after surgical revascularization (7), but even positron emission tomography (PET), the gold standard for viability assessment, may underestimate the degree of myocardial recovery after revascularization. Between 10% and 20% of segments identified as nonviable by noninvasive imaging techniques demonstrate improved function after either CABG or percutaneous revascularization (8). Given this caveat, we use dobutamine echocardiography or thallium redistribution perfusion imaging in the assessment of ischemia and viability, as these methods have reasonable sensitivity and specificity in identifying areas of viability and predicting subsequent improvement in regional wall motion after revascularization (9).

Risk Assessment

Procedural risk may be increased due to poor left ventricular function alone, or as a result of underlying complicated, multivessel coronary disease. The latter risk profile is of particular concern. For many such patients, percutaneous revascularization is one of the only choices for palliation of medically refractory angina, because mortality with coronary bypass surgery may approach 20%, whereas the initial results of percutaneous intervention in these patients may be more favorable (Tables 19.1 and 19.2) (10–37).

The same characteristics that put a patient at patient high-risk for coronary bypass also predispose to poor outcome after percutaneous intervention. Preliminary registry data in high-risk patients with ejection fraction <25%, multivessel coronary disease, and objective ischemia highlight a high periprocedural event rate and suggest similar early attrition rates with percutaneous coronary intervention or coronary bypass grafting (16). The risk of hemodynamic collapse due to abrupt closure associated with failed percutaneous coronary intervention is related to the presence of multivessel disease, diffuse disease, a large myocardial territory at risk, and preprocedural stenosis (7). Various methods of predicting risk for poor outcome after percutaneous coronary intervention have included the jeopardy score, originally developed by Califf and colleagues (38) and modified by Ellis (39). As modified by Ellis, the total jeopardy score is defined as the net ventricular dysfunction anticipated following abrupt closure. This is calculated by allowing one point for each of the six myocardial regions (Table 19.3) in the distribution of a significant (70%) stenosis, and 0.5 points for each area of baseline hypokinesis not supplied through a significant stenosis. In this study, a jeopardy score of more than 2.5 was a univariate predictor of mortality. The extent of myocardium at risk is of particular concern in the case of collateral circulation, when total jeopardized myocardial territory may be quite extensive. Although the incidence and, possibly, the importance of abrupt closure has been modified somewhat with advent of the platelet glycoprotein IIb/

TABLE 19.1. *Outcome of coronary bypass grafting in patients with severe LV dysfunction: contemporary series*

Study (Reference)	Period	N	EF (%)	Primary indication	Number of grafts	30-Day mortality (%)	1-Year mortality (%)	Long-Term mortality (%, period)
Pagano(27)	1994–96	39	23[a]	Elective	3.0	5.7	14 (6-mo)	—
Baumgartner(28)	1990–96	61	≤25	(Semi)elective	4.0	8	—	—
Salati(29)	1992–95	31	25[a]	Elective	2.6	0	—	—
Dietl(30)	1991–95	163	22[a]	Mix	3.4	10	—	—
Calhoun(31)	1992–94	12	21[a]	Elective/CHF	—	17	—	—
Christenson(32)	1990–93	91	21[a]	Mix/angina	4.6	14.3	—	—
Krucoff(10)	1990–93	21	<25	Elective	—	14	33	—
Lee(33)	1986–93	35	25[a]	Elective/ICD[b]	2.7	3.7	—	29 (3-year)
He(34)	1986–93	52	<30	Repeat CABG	—	33	—	—
Langenburg(35)	1983–93	96	20[a]	Elective	3.0	8	—	—
Mickleborough(36)	1982–93	79	18[a]	Mix	3.6	3.8	6	32 (5-year)
Townend(37)	1991–92	15	20[a]	Elective/CHF	2.7	13	40[c]	—
Dreyfus(38)	1990–92	46	23[a]	Elective	3.8	10.9	13	—
Lindelow(39)	1988–92	7	24[a]	Elective/ischemia[c] MR	2-5	—	—	40 (3-year)[d]
Kaul(40)	1987–92	210	≤20	Mix	—	8	18	27 (5-year)
Elefteriades(41)	1986–92	83	25[a]	(Semi)elective	2.7	8.4	13	20 (3-year)
Hausmann(42)	1986–92	265	24[a]	Elective/Angina	2.9	7.6	10.9	13.1 (3-year)
Herlitz(43)	1988–91	7	≤20	—	—	—	—	29 (2-year)
Milano(44)	1981–91	118	21[a]	Mix	3.7	11	22.8	42.5 (5-year)
Lansman(45)	1986–90	42	16[a]	Mix	3.5	4.8	12	66 (6-year)
Luciani(46)	1985–90	20	22[a]	Mix/angina	2.2	20	—	20 (5-year)

[a] Mean
[b] Patients received implantable cardiac defibrillator (ICD) implantation at the time of CABG
[c] Includes one patient who underwent successful heart transplantation 8 months after CABG
[d] Includes 5 patients who did not undergo combined valvular procedure
EF, ejection fraction; MR, mitral regurgitation; CHF, congestive heart failure.

TABLE 19.2. *Results of percutaneous coronary intervention in patients with severe LV dysfunction: contemporary series*

Study (Reference)	Period	N	EF (%)	Lesions successful/ attempted	Major complications (%)	In-Hospital MACE (%)	30-Day mortality (%)	Late mortality (%)
Unselected:								
Mayo(unpublished)	1994–97	392	29[a]	1.4/1.6	—	17	—	15 (1yr)
Krucoff(10)	1990–93	29	<25	—	—	—	10	45 (1yr)
Maiello(47)	1987–91	100	30[a]	1.5/1.8	12	13	—	23[c] (19mo[a])
CPS support:								
Shawl(20)	1988–91	107	19[a]	1.8/1.9	0	4.7	—	23 (2yr)
Teirstein(48)	1989–90	126	≤20	1.6/1.8	41	8	—	—
Pavlides(22)	1987–90	15	21[a]	—	13	0	0	—
IABP support:								
Kreidieh(49)	1987–91	16	<30	—/1.6	6	12	—	6 (1 yr)
Stent support:								
Saucedo(26)	–1997[b]	85	<25	—	—	2.35	—	6.1 (1yr)
Supported:								
Ferrari(50)	1990–93	35	30[a]	1.7/2.0	5.7	2.8	8.6	29.6 (2yr)

[a] Mean
[b] Abstract published 1998
[c] Includes 9% in-hospital mortality plus follow-up mortality in 75 patients with clinically successful initial procedures
EF, ejection fraction; MACE, major adverse cardiac events, including death, myocardial infarction, and repeat revascularization.

TABLE 19.3. *Six coronary segments used to determine the myocardial jeopardy score (39)*

Coronary segment
Left anterior descending artery(LAD)
1. LAD (body)
2. First major septal perforator
3. First major diagonal branch
Left circumflex coronary artery
4. Left circumflex (body)
5. Major marginal branch
6a. Left posterior descending (PDA)
Right coronary artery
6b. Right PDA

IIIa inhibitors and stent use (10–12), the underlying principles and predictors of poor outcome remain unchanged.

Timing

Developing an interventional plan in patients with severe ventricular dysfunction requires evaluation of viable revascularization options and proper counseling of the patient. For this reason, sequential angiography followed by intervention in the same setting is often inadvisable in these cases. It is obvious that the patient must fully understand the potential risks and benefits of any planned procedure, and simultaneous counseling of family members is often beneficial. While it requires an additional procedure for the patient, delaying the intervention allows for optimization of medical management, surgical consultation regarding potential backup or hybrid procedures, and consultation with colleagues regarding optimal approaches for the intervention. In the case of patients who are critically ill, of course, delaying the procedure may not be possible.

Because of the observed association between a history of congestive heart failure and poor outcome, particularly in patients with a low ejection fraction, the timing of percutaneous intervention should be carefully considered in patients with recent symptoms of heart failure (3). Patients who are decompensated are at increased risk and may benefit from aggressive medical management of left ventricular dysfunction prior to a planned intervention.

Finally, whereas most of the patients with severely depressed ventricular function undergoing percutaneous revascularization will not be candidates for surgical backup support in the event of procedural failure, preprocedural planning for insertion of a left ventricular assist device as a bridge to transplantation is a potential option. At the very least, terms of discontinuation of support need to be addressed with the patient and family prior to initiation of the procedure.

GENERAL CONSIDERATIONS

Access Site

We have not generally found it necessary to use any other than a femoral access site. Advantages of this approach include the ability to increase sheath size as needed and switch out for support devices, should this be necessary. We place an 8 Fr arterial sheath and use 8 Fr guiding catheters in most instances to allow adequate coronary visualization and support. Right-heart catheterization is also performed to assess and optimize filling pressures. When relying on standby support, we place 4 Fr sheaths in the contralateral artery to provide ready access. A contrast injection of 20 to 40 cc through a pigtail catheter placed in the abdominal aorta may be used to perform peripheral arteriographic assessment of the adequacy of the femoro-iliac system and descending aorta for the introduction of support devices.

Anticoagulation

The appropriate level of procedural anticoagulation depends on the type of intervention performed, concomitant medication use, and type of mechanical support. In general, anticoagulation requirements in high-risk percutaneous interventions are similar to that described elsewhere in this text for routine procedures. The major difference is in the case of nonheparin coated systems for cardiopulmonary support (CPS), when the activated clotting time must be maintained in the range of greater than 400 seconds. The routine use of aspirin is necessary as is additional anticoagulation with ticlopidine or clopidogrel, in the cases of stenting.

Sedation

The extensive vascular manipulation required in initiating high-risk interventional procedures necessitates adequate sedation. Because proper visualization of the coronary tree and lesions of interest is a fundamental concern for the interventionalist, patients who are not fully able to cooperate may be best served by induction of general anesthesia. In this way, extraneous patient movements can be minimized and attention can be devoted to performance of the procedure. Although not required, general anesthesia may be instituted electively prior to initiation of cardiopulmonary support (CPS) due to the large catheters required for this procedure and potential for discomfort to the patient.

Contrast

Contrast agent selection can be important in reducing adverse events in high-risk interventional procedures. While first-generation ionic agents may be well tolerated in low-risk procedures, the high osmolality and calcium chelating effects of these agents can compound difficulties with hypotension and dysrhythmia in poorly compensated patients. Beyond this, however, there is considerable debate regarding the optimal contrast agent. The second-generation, low-osmolality agents, both ionic and nonionic, induce less adverse hemodynamic effects and are better tolerated in the high-risk setting. Although nonionic agents appear to have somewhat less anticoagulant effect than ionic agents, the beneficial impact of ionic agents in high-risk interventions continues to be controversial. Contrast-related adverse events are infrequent with these second-generation agents, and either group of agents can likely be used without significant detrimental effects. Iodixanol, an isosmolar, nonionic agent, may be better tolerated than previously available agents, and randomized trials are ongoing to evaluate the potential benefit in high-risk interventions.

Multivessel Interventions

For patients with multivessel disease and severe ventricular dysfunction, complete functional revascularization may provide significant improvement in symptoms and outcome, even if complete anatomic revascularization is not possible. The strategy of revascularization must be individualized according to clinical and anatomic criteria, as the order and number of lesions attempted has a direct impact on the safety and potential benefit of the procedure. As discussed above, the identification of segments supplying ischemic and viable myocardium is important in recognizing appropriate targets for intervention.

Once identified, revascularization targets can be approached in a systematic fashion based on the amount of jeopardized myocardium and the presence of collateral circulation. In the presence of a total occlusion supplying a large territory of jeopardized myocardium, failed intervention on the vessel supplying collaterals may be catastrophic. For this reason, the occluded vessel should be attempted first to provide adequate antegrade flow to this territory. After successful intervention on the occluded vessel, one may approach the lesion in the vessel that supplies collaterals with relative safety. Other lesions can be approached based on the size of myocardium at risk, with those lesions affecting the greatest territory approached first. Because of diminishing return, revascularization of lesions supplying small areas of myocardium should generally not be attempted. In the case of vein graft disease, due to the high rate of restenosis, it is preferable to attempt revascularization via the native system whenever possible to provide the highest chance of a durable result.

In addition, whereas a 2-day, staged procedure may be entertained when intervention is planned on two or more lesions affecting large areas of myocardium, in many cases, particularly those involving mechanical support, all revascularization is performed in the same setting. When only a suboptimal result can be achieved or when further attempts at intervention would compromise the safety of the patient, staging may also be appropriate. In this case, the patient can be transferred to a monitored bed, generally with the arterial sheath in place, and maintained on a heparin infusion. Intraaortic balloon pump support may be initiated or continued as discussed below. Many of these patients will also be continued on a glycoprotein IIb/IIIa inhibitor overnight with appropriate reduction in the heparin dosing. Repeat angiography the following day can be used to assess the status of the initial lesion, with a decision made at that time regarding the need for additional intervention on the original or additional lesions.

SUPPORTED INTERVENTIONS

Not all patients with severe ventricular dysfunction require mechanically supported interventions. Patients who are well compensated, without clinical evidence of heart failure, and who require treatment of a vessel supplying only a modest myocardial territory, can undergo revascularization at experienced centers with only standby support. As lesion complexity and the amount of myocardium at risk increases, however, the anticipated risk of serious adverse results increases as well. In such cases, particularly in patients with unstable symptoms recalcitrant to medical therapy, percutaneous support devices are essential to the interventional plan.

THE INTRAAORTIC BALLOON PUMP

Use of the intraaortic balloon pump (IABP) decreases oxygen demand by reducing the myocardial workload, providing pulsatile flow support with an augmentation of cardiac output by 0.5 to 0.8 L/minute, reduced left ventricular end diastolic pressure (10%–20%), and a similar reduction in the pulmonary capillary wedge pressure (Table 19.4). Although markedly improving diastolic perfusion pressure (40), aortic counterpulsation has not been demonstrated to

improve coronary blood flow past a hemodynamically significant stenosis. In coronary segments without obstructive lesions, however, aortic counterpulsation increases oxygen delivery through a 25% increase in coronary blood flow (41). For this reason, the benefit of IABP use may be more pronounced after intervention, when obstructing lesions have been successfully modified and the increased perfusion pressure is translated into improved coronary flow. Prior to intervention or after unsuccessful intervention, IABP use provides benefit primarily through afterload reduction and decreased myocardial oxygen consumption.

Early reports of elective IABP support in high-risk interventions demonstrated a high procedural success rate and low short-term cardiovascular event rates. However, this success came at the price of a vascular complication rate of up to 11% (42,43). Subsequent trials in acute ischemic syndromes have suggested variable efficacy depending on the underlying condition. A randomized trial of IABP use for 48 hours after rescue angioplasty demonstrated a beneficial effect on sustained patency, with decreased in-hospital infarct-related artery occlusion and recurrent ischemia (44); however, the PAMI II trial failed to show a significant benefit of early IABP support after primary angioplasty in high-risk patients. There was a significant increase in local vascular access-site complications (45).

Despite the lack of adequate randomized studies, the hemodynamic support and coronary perfusion properties associated with IABP support may contribute to a successful procedural outcome and provide additional benefit in the vulnerable period immediately following the procedure (Fig. 19.1). Although the IABP may be inserted quickly in the event of hemodynamic instability during a procedure, we choose to introduce prophylactic aortic counterpulsation in the majority of very high-risk percutaneous coronary intervention cases. Advantages of IABP use include ready availability, quick, easy insertion, and the availability of routine support. The device is contraindicated in cases of severe aortoiliac disease or severe aortic valvular regurgitation. With newer catheter designs, serious complications are rare, but may include gas leak

TABLE 19.4. *Intraaortic balloon pump hemodynamic effects*

Peak systolic arterial pressure	−
End-diastolic aortic pressure	− −
Diastolic aortic pressure	+ + + +
Mean aortic pressure	0
LVEDP/PCWP	−
Heart rate	−
Cardiac output	+ +

LVEDP, left ventricular end diastolic pressure; PCWP, pulmonary capillary wedge pressure.

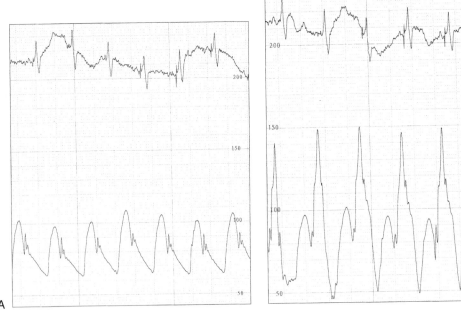

FIG. 19.1. Blood pressure before **A:** and after **B:** initiation of aortic counterpulsation in a 53-year-old man with unstable angina, an ejection fraction <15%, and systemic hypotension. Note the diastolic pressure augmentation with initiation of IABP support prior to intervention on a lone patent saphenous vein graft.

into the arterial space, vascular injury, infection, bleeding, thrombocytopenia, and embolic events (Table 19.5).

PERCUTANEOUS CARDIOPULMONARY SUPPORT

Percutaneous cardiopulmonary support (CPS) is used in the extremely high-risk patient when hemodynamic collapse during intervention is strongly anticipated or when the result of such collapse, even if temporary, would be catastrophic. Successful insertion and use of CPS depends on team members trained in the initiation of CPS. The National Registry of Elective Cardiopulmonary Bypass Supported Angioplasty evaluated cardiopulmonary bypass support in patients with an ejection fraction of less than 25%, a target vessel supplying more than half of the viable myocardial territory, or both (46). This multicenter registry demonstrated the feasibility of supported high-risk angioplasty, and demonstrated this technique to be equally

effective as a prophylactic or a standby device (21). Although complications were significantly increased in the prophylactic group, mortality was significantly less in patients with an ejection fraction of less than 20% who were treated in this group. Importantly, CPS was required in only 8% of the patients in the standby group. Additional evaluation of 109 consecutive patients demonstrated the feasibility of CPS-supported angioplasty in high-risk patients with unstable angina and severely reduced left ventricular function (32).

Because of the difficulty in predicting which patients will need CPS initiation, CPS is usually used as a standby procedure in the event of complete hemodynamic collapse. While CPS initiation is a relatively rare occurrence for most operators, performing high-risk interventions may result in situations requiring cardiopulmonary support, and it is therefore useful to be familiar with the technique. CPS is also helpful as a planned procedure in very high-risk patients, such as those undergoing intervention on a lone

TABLE 19.5. *IABP versus CPS*

	IABP	CPS
Percutaneous insertion	Yes, rapid	Yes, difficult
Prophylactic use	Yes	Usually not
Pulsatile flow	Yes	No
Ventricular support	Left	Right and Left
Hemodynamic support	Minor (0.5–0.8L/min)	Complete (3.5–5.0L/min)
Oxygenation support	No	Yes
Support independent of rhythm	No	Yes
Provides afterload reduction	Yes	Some
Augments distal coronary flow:		
Past stenosis	No	No
Without stenosis	Yes	Minimal
Hemolysis	Mild	Significant
Heparinization requirements	Low	High[a]
Maximal duration of therapy	>48 hours	6–8 hours[a]
Indications	High risk PCI	High risk PCI[a]
	Bridge to surgery	
	Refractory angina	
	Cardiogenic shock	
	Failure to wean CPS	
	Bridge to transplant or LVAD	
Contraindications	Significant AR	Lack of familiarity or technical support
	Significant AA	PVD
	Severe PVD	
	Significant arrhythmia	
Complications	Vascular	Vascular
	Nerve injury	Nerve injury
	Infection	Infection
	Hemolysis	DIC, hemolysis
	Bleeding	Bleeding
	Thrombocytopenia	Anemia
	Systemic embolism	Anaerobic metabolism
	Limb ischemia	Poor CNS perfusion
		Fluid third-spacing
		Hypokalemia
		Hypomagnesemia
		May require surgical vascular closure or prolonged vessel compression
		Arterial and/or venous thrombosis
		Limb ischemia

[a] See text

IABP, intraaortic balloon pump; CPS, cardiopulmonary support; PCI, percutaneous coronary intervention; LVAD, left ventricular assist device; AR, aortic regurgitation; AA, aortic aneurysm; PVD, peripheral vascular disease; DIC, disseminated intravascular hemolysis; CNS, central nervous system.

patent vessel, as standby use may not be reliable, particularly in centers unaccustomed to performing the procedure. If started within 10 minutes of sustained cardiac arrest, however, CPS may improve the chance of survival (47). True bail-out hemodynamic support with CPS is usually not indicated, as patients who lack an organized rhythm and those without significant cardiac function after intervention typically have no clearly defined endpoint, unless imminent car-

diac transplantation is entertained. In this case, CPS is an appropriate bridge to early insertion of a left ventricular assist device, but termination of support must be considered early in these cases.

The attractiveness of CPS lies in the fact that, unlike IABP support, it provides complete circulatory support, regardless of underlying rhythm or left ventricular function. This system can maintain a cardiac output of up to 5L/min while unloading the left ventricle and reducing the pulmonary wedge pressure to less than 5 mm Hg. This may reduce left ventricular workload and oxygen requirements. Additionally, coronary perfusion may be secondarily improved due to the reduced left ventricular end-diastolic pressure and slightly increased diastolic perfusion pressure. However, CPS offers poor myocardial protection from prolonged ischemia (34) and is not appropriate for prolonged use in all patients. Although patients may adapt over time to the nonpulsatile flow provided by CPS (48), the acute processes of "coronary steal," involving segments with significant stenoses and impaired microvascular perfusion, in such a setting may predispose to progressive myocardial dysfunction.

In general, total bypass times of 6 to 8 hours may be tolerated, but hemolysis, disseminated intravascular coagulation, and extracellular fluid shifts prevent longer support with older systems (See Table 19.5). The consumptive coagulopathy accompanying platelet and clotting cascade activation have been reduced with newer heparin-coated systems, which permit prolonged operation without the use of high-dose systemic heparin. However, these new systems do not obviate the need for changing system components periodically, nor do they seem to significantly reduce the potential for intracardiac thrombus or vascular complications (34,49,50). The perfusion problems and poor myocardial protection related to nonpulsatile flow have yet to be over-

come with prolonged support. In patients with a stable rhythm, IABP support and early weaning of CPS remains the preferred strategy.

CPS TECHNIQUE

Percutaneous cardiopulmonary support requires the insertion of large-bore cannulae into the femoral artery and vein. Blood is withdrawn via a cannula placed at the level of the right atrium and circulated through a membrane oxygenator and heat exchanger to be reintroduced into the arterial circulation via the femoral artery (Fig. 19.2). To institute CPS, right femoral arterial and venous access is obtained via the modified Seldinger technique. An 8 Fr arterial and 7 Fr venous sheath are placed. It is important to obtain arterial access at the level of the common femoral artery below the inguinal ligament, because placement of the cannula in the superficial or profunda femoral artery can result in significant vascular trauma. Contrast injection into the aorto-iliac system is necessary to document patency and degree of tortuosity. Significant tortuosity or stenoses preclude the placement of the large 18 to 20 Fr cannulae on the affected side.

If unaffected by significant peripheral vascular disease, left common femoral arterial access is obtained using the same technique as on the right. A pulmonary artery catheter is inserted through the right venous sheath to measure cardiac output and pulmonary pressures. After systemic anticoagulation to an ACT of >400 sec-

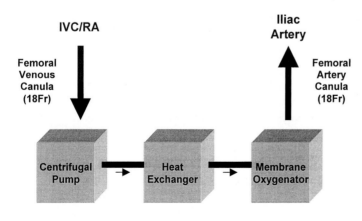

FIG. 19.2. Schematic drawing of percutaneous cardiopulmonary support (*CPS*) circuitry. Blood is withdrawn via an 18 Fr femoral venous catheter placed to the level of the junction of the inferior vena cava (*IVC*) and the right atrium (*RA*) and is propelled by a centrifugal pump through a membrane oxygenator and heat exchanger. The warmed and oxygenated blood is then reintroduced to the patient via an 18 Fr catheter residing in the femoral artery, providing complete cardiopulmonary support.

onds, which generally requires 200–300 units of heparin/kg, sequential dilatation of the arteriotomy site to 14 Fr is performed over the 0.038-in. guidewire. This requires a large skin nick. The 18 Fr arterial cannula and dilator are then carefully advanced as a unit with a twisting, forward motion. The dilator is then removed and the cannula clamped. Blood loss can be significant with this step if not performed quickly. A similar technique is used to insert the venous sheath into the left femoral vein and, under fluoroscopic guidance, advanced to the caudal margin of the right atrium, and both cannulae are sutured in place at the groin.

The CPS circuit is primed, and with the help of an assistant, the venous cannula and venous connection tubing from the CPS console are "topped off" with saline and quickly mated to avoid air trapping in the tubing. The clamp is then removed. The same steps are performed to connect the arterial cannula, making certain that no air is trapped in the arterial circuit. It is helpful to perform these connections under a flow of saline from a syringe, which can help replace the volume lost when the tubing is rotated to make the ends meet. Once initiated, CPS is continued for the duration of the intervention and during transfer to the intensive care unit. Pulmonary capillary wedge pressure should be maintained at greater than 5 mm Hg with a mean blood pressure of 60–80 mm Hg during the procedure. Once initiated, CPS is continued for the duration of the intervention and during transfer to the intensive care unit. CPS is gradually weaned in the ICU by decreasing the flow rate. The use of IABP may be required during this process, and in these instances should often be continued for a period of 24–48 hours in the intensive care setting.

STENT

While not generally considered a support device, the development of improved coronary stents and simplified antiplatelet regimens has revolutionized all aspects of percutaneous intervention. Procedural ischemia is one of the primary limiting factors in the setting of a severely impaired ventricle, because this can lead to rapid, progressive worsening of cardiac function and sudden hemodynamic collapse. By reducing the need for prolonged balloon inflations, stents decrease procedural ischemic time and lead to a more predictable result and improved acute outcome. A recent study reported a favorable 1-year mortality of 6.1% among patients with a left ventricular ejection fraction of less than 25% after coronary stenting (36). Additionally, a decrease in the incidence of subacute closure to <1% with the use of stents in routine cases also translates into improved results in high-risk patients.

Recent advances in stent design may further improve these results. The availability of low-profile, trackable stents permits primary delivery of stents to the site of stenosis without predilation. This technique has the potential to dramatically decrease procedural ischemia, and in certain instances is the preferred method of delivery. In most instances, however, a gentle, primary dilation prior to stent placement is preferred, because this improves visualization of the lesion and distal coronary bed during stent positioning. Imprudent advancement of a stent to the site of a tight stenosis without adequate visualization often paradoxically increases contrast requirements and ischemic time, thereby increasing the likelihood of major complications.

ANTIPLATELET AGENTS

While controversial, the use of platelet glycoprotein IIb/IIIa inhibitors in the setting of high-risk percutaneous intervention is gaining favor. Without adequate clinical studies to guide practice in this situation, we nevertheless generally administer these agents to improve the likelihood of procedural success and possibly to improved long-term outcome. Theoretical advantages of platelet inhibition include the amelioration of intravascular thrombotic complications and the prevention of periprocedural non-Q-wave myocardial infarction, which is discussed in greater detail elsewhere in this text. A caveat to this recommendation is in patients who may require CPS, because the high activated clotting time required with this procedure could predispose patients to severe hemorrhagic and vascular complications with concomitant platelet inhibition.

POSTPROCEDURAL MANAGEMENT

A vital part of immediate postprocedural care involves providing adequate monitoring and ready access to emergency support services. While many patients with depressed ventricular function will require intensive care monitoring after high-risk percutaneous coronary intervention, certain patients may be followed on monitored "stepdown" beds (Table 19.6), provided there are adequate trained staff and monitoring capabilities to respond to potentially catastrophic events. Potential ischemic complications may include chest pain, dysrhythmia, or significant hypotension in the postprocedural period. For these and other indications suggestive of ischemia, it is recommended that early repeat catheterization be performed to evaluate the anatomic result. In addition, monitoring of the vascular access sites for bleeding and maintenance of pulses is imperative, particularly in the cases involving IAPB or CPS. In an intensive care setting, hemodynamic and electrocardiographic monitoring, as well as intake and output measurements, are helpful to guide further therapy in fluid management.

As discussed above, prolonged aortic counterpulsation may be of value in patients left with a suboptimal result and poor antegrade flow or significant residual stenosis. In these patients, intensive care unit monitoring with intraaortic balloon pumping for 24 to 48 hours may lessen the incidence of vessel reocclusion (44). Continued heparinization is required with activated partial thromboplastin times in the range of 50–60.

TABLE 19.6. *Patients suitable for non-ICU management after high-risk percutaneous coronary intervention*

Indications of suitability
No episodes of distal embolization or no-reflow
Stented or "stentlike" angiographic result
Normotensive without mechanical or inotropic support
Stable rhythm

SUMMARY

Although percutaneous intervention in patients with severe left ventricular dysfunction entails increased risk, revascularization can reduce the ischemic burden in these patients and improve long-term prognosis. Risk assessment and appropriate planning and patient preparation are of utmost importance and can help improve the likelihood of a successful outcome. Patients with demonstrable ischemia in the distribution of an approachable coronary lesion or lesions are suitable candidates for percutaneous revascularization. Clinical assessment and optimization of hemodynamic and volume status prior to intervention is essential, as is proper medical management of heart failure and ischemic symptoms. Surgical consultation is also helpful prior to initiation of the procedure to discuss the possibility of surgical backup or availability and appropriateness of ventricular assist device support (Fig. 19.3).

Specific procedural approaches will necessarily vary depending on the underlying patient characteristics. Procedural outcome has become somewhat more predictable with the development of improved coronary stents and simplified antiplatelet regimens, largely due to the ability to decrease the duration of myocardial ischemia. Judicious use of adjunctive medications and mechanical devices, such as glycoprotein IIb/IIIa antagonists and stents, can decrease procedure time, myocardial ischemia, and contrast load, resulting in improved procedural outcome. In select cases, primary stenting without predilation of the lesion can also be helpful in minimizing ischemic time, although impaired lesion visualization can paradoxically increase the duration of ischemia and contrast requirements.

The decision to proceed with mechanical support is also based on underlying patient characteristics. Many patients with well-compensated left ventricular dysfunction can undergo intervention at experienced centers with only standby IABP support. However, in unstable patients or those at high risk due to complex anatomy or a large territory of jeopardized myocardium, prophylactic IABP placement is recommended. For patients at very high risk, such as those undergoing intervention on a lone patent vessel, prophy-

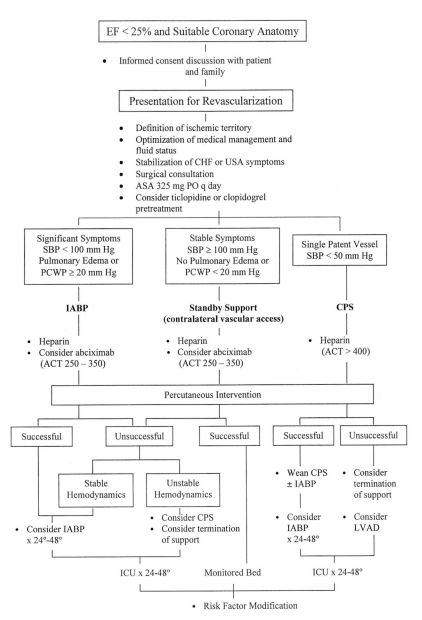

FIG. 19.3. Management algorithm for high-risk percutaneous coronary intervention in patients with severe left ventricular dysfunction.

lactic CPS may be used to support the patient in whom hemodynamic instability would be catastrophic.

REFERENCES

1. Hartzler GO, Rutherford BD, McConahay DR, Johnson WJ, Giorgi LV. "High-risk" percutaneous transluminal coronary angioplasty. *Am J Cardiol* 1988;61:33–37G.

2. Alderman EL, Fisher LD, Litwin P et al. Results of coronary artery surgery in patients with poor left ventricular function (CASS). *Circulation* 1983;68:785–795.

3. Anderson RD, Ohman EM, Holmes DR et al. The prognostic value of congestive heart failure in patients undergoing percutaneous coronary interventions. *J American Coll Cardiol* 1998;32:936–941.

4. Bounous EP, Mark DB, Pollock BG et al. Surgical survival benefits for coronary disease patients with left ventricular dysfunction. *Circulation* 1988;78:I151–I157.

5. Mark DB, Nelson CL, Califf RM et al. Continuing evo-

lution of therapy for coronary artery disease: initial results from the era of coronary angioplasty. *Circulation* 1994;89:2015–2025.

6. Ryan TJ, Bauman WB, Kennedy JW et al. Guidelines for percutaneous transluminal coronary angioplasty. A report of the American Heart Association/American College of Cardiology Task Force on Assessment of Diagnostic and Therapeutic Cardiovascular Procedures (Committee on Percutaneous Transluminal Coronary Angioplasty). *Circulation* 1993;88:2987–3007.

7. Bergelson BA, Jacobs AK, Cupples LA et al. Prediction of risk for hemodynamic compromise during percutaneous transluminal coronary angioplasty. *Am J Cardio* 1992;70:1540–1545.

8. Bonow RO. The hibernating myocardium: implications for management of congestive heart failure. *Am J Cardiol* 1995;75:17A–25A.

9. Castro PF, Bourge RC, Foster RE. Evaluation of hibernating myocardium in patients with ischemic heart disease. *Am J Med* 1998;104:69–77.

10. Pagano D, Townend JN, Littler WA, Horton R, Camici PG, Bonser RS. Coronary artery bypass surgery as treatment for ischemic heart failure: the predictive value of viability assessment with quantitative positron emission tomography for symptomatic and functional outcome. *J Thorac Cardiovasc Surg* 1998;115:791–799.

11. Baumgartner FJ, Omari BO, Goldberg S et al. Coronary artery bypass grafting in patients with profound ventricular dysfunction. *Tex Heart Inst J* 1998;25:125–129.

12. Salati M, Lemma M, Di Mattia DG et al. Myocardial revascularization in patients with ischemic cardiomyopathy: functional observations. *Ann Thorac Surg* 1997; 64:1728–1734.

13. Dietl CA, Berkheimer MD, Woods EL, Gilbert CL, Pharr WF, Benoit CH. Efficacy and cost-effectiveness of preoperative IABP in patients with ejection fraction of 0.25 or less. *Ann Thorac Surg* 1996;62:401–408.

14. Calhoun WB, Mills RM Jr., Drane WE. Clinical importance of viability assessment in chronic ischemic heart failure. *Clin Cardiol* 1996;19:367–369.

15. Christenson JT, Maurice J, Simonet F et al. Effect of low left ventricular ejection fractions on the outcome of primary coronary bypass grafting in end-stage coronary artery disease. *J Cardiovasc Surg* 1995;36:45–51.

16. Krucoff MW, Jones RH, O'Connor CM et al. The high-risk myocardial ischemia trial (HIRMIT) randomized pilot and registry: 6 day, 6 week, 6 month & 1 year mortality. *Circulation* 1994;90:I-334.

17. Lee JH, Konstantakos AK, Murrell HK et al. Late results with concomitant coronary artery bypass grafting and ICD implantation. *J Cardiac Surg* 1996;11:165–171.

18. He GW, Acuff TE, Ryan WH, He YH, Mack MJ. Determinants of operative mortality in reoperative coronary artery bypass grafting. *J Thorac Cardiovasc Surg* 1995; 110:971–978.

19. Langenburg SE, Buchanan SA, Blackbourne LH et al. Predicting survival after coronary revascularization for ischemic cardiomyopathy. *Ann Thorac Surg* 1995;60: 1193–1196, 1196–1197(discussion).

20. Mickleborough LL, Maruyama H, Takagi Y, Mohamed S, Sun Z, Ebisuzaki L. Results of revascularization in patients with severe left ventricular dysfunction. *Circulation* 1995;92:II73–II79.

21. Townend JN, Pagano D, Allen SM et al. Results of surgical revascularization in ischaemic heart failure without angina. *Eur J Cardiothorac Surg* 1995;9: 507–513,513–514(discussion).

22. Dreyfus GD, Duboc D, Blasco A et al. Myocardial viability assessment in ischemic cardiomyopathy: benefits of coronary revascularization. *Ann Thorac Surg* 1994; 57:1402–1407.

23. Lindelow B, Andersson B, Waagstein F, Bergh CH. Prognosis of alternative therapies in patients with heart failure not accepted for heart transplantation. *J Heart Lung Transplant* 1995;14:1204–1211.

24. Kaul TK, Agnihotri AK, Fields BL, Riggins LS, Wyatt DA, Jones CR. Coronary artery bypass grafting in patients with an ejection fraction of twenty percent or less. *J Thorac Cardiovasc Surg* 1996;111:1001–1012.

25. Elefteriades JA, Tolis G Jr., Levi E, Mills LK, Zaret BL. Coronary artery bypass grafting in severe left ventricular dysfunction: excellent survival with improved ejection fraction and functional state. *J Am Coll Cardiol* 1993; 22:1411–1417.

26. Hausmann H, Ennker J, Topp H et al. Coronary artery bypass grafting and heart transplantation in end-stage coronary artery disease: a comparison of hemodynamic improvement and ventricular function. *J Cardiac Surg* 1994;9:77–84.

27. Herlitz J, Brandrup G, Caidahl K et al. Death, mode of death, morbidity and requirement for rehospitalization during 2 years after coronary artery bypass grafting in relation to preoperative ejection fraction. *Coron Artery Dis* 1996;7:807–812.

28. Milano CA, White WD, Smith LR et al. Coronary artery bypass in patients with severely depressed ventricular function. *Ann Thorac Surg* 1993;56:487–493.

29. Lansman SL, Cohen M, Galla JD et al. Coronary bypass with ejection fraction of 0.20 or less using centigrade cardioplegia: long-term follow-up. *Ann Thorac Surg* 1993;56:480–485.

30. Luciani GB, Faggian G, Razzolini R, Livi U, Bortolotti U, Mazzucco A. Severe ischemic left ventricular failure: coronary operation or heart transplantation? *Ann Thorac Surg* 1993;55:719–723.

31. Maiello L, Colombo A, Gianrossi R, Almagor Y, Finci L. Survival after percutaneous transluminal coronary angioplasty in patients with severe left ventricular dysfunction. *Chest* 1994;105:733–740.

32. Shawl FA, Quyyumi AA, Bajaj S, Hoff SB, Dougherty KG. Percutaneous cardiopulmonary bypass-supported coronary angioplasty in patients with unstable angina pectoris or myocardial infarction and a left ventricular ejection fraction ≤25%. *Am J Cardiol* 1996;77:14–19.

33. Teirstein PS, Vogel RA, Dorros G et al. Prophylactic versus standby cardiopulmonary support for high risk percutaneous transluminal coronary angioplasty. *J Am Coll Cardiol* 1993;21:590–596.

34. Pavlides GS, Hauser AM, Stack RK et al. Effect of peripheral cardiopulmonary bypass on left ventricular size, afterload and myocardial function during elective supported coronary angioplasty. *J Am Coll Cardiol* 1991; 18:499–505.

35. Kreidieh I, Davies DW, Lim R, Nathan AW, Dymond DS, Banim SO. High-risk coronary angioplasty with elective intra-aortic balloon pump support. *Int J Cardiol* 1992;35:147–152.

36. Saucedo JF, Popma JJ, Mehran R et al. Clinical outcomes of patients with low left ventricular ejection frac-

tion undergoing intracoronary stenting. *J Am Coll Cardiol* 1998;31:235A.

37. Ferrari M, Scholz KH, Figulla HR. PTCA with the use of cardiac assist devices: risk stratification, short- and long-term results. *Cathet Cardiovasc Diagn* 1996;38: 242–248.

38. Califf RM, Phillips HR, Hindman MC et al. Prognostic value of a coronary artery jeopardy score. *J Am Coll Cardiol* 1985;5:1055–1063.

39. Ellis SG, Myler RK, King III SB et al. Causes and correlates of death after unsupported coronary angioplasty: implications for use of angioplasty and advanced support techniques in high-risk settings. *Am J Cardiol* 1991; 68:1447–1451.

40. Gurbel PA, Anderson RD, MacCord CS et al. Arterial diastolic pressure augmentation by intra-aortic balloon counterpulsation enhances the onset of coronary artery reperfusion by thrombolytic therapy. *Circulation* 1994; 89:361–365.

41. Kern MJ, Aguirre F, Bach R, Donohue T, Siegel R, Segal J. Augmentation of coronary blood flow by intra-aortic balloon pumping in patients after coronary angioplasty. *Circulation* 1993;87:500–511.

42. Kahn JK, Rutherford BD, McConahay DR, Johnson WL, Giorgi LV, Hartzler GO. Supported "high risk" coronary angioplasty using intraaortic balloon pump counterpulsation. *J Am Coll Cardiol* 1990;15: 1151–1155.

43. Voudris V, Marco J, Morice MC, Fajadet J, Royer T. "High-risk" percutaneous transluminal coronary angioplasty with preventive intraaortic balloon counterpulsation. *Cathet Cardiovasc Diagn* 1990;19:160–164.

44. Ohman EM, George BS, White CJ et al. The use of aortic counterpulsation to improve sustained coronary artery patency during acute myocardial infarction: results of a randomized trial. *Circulation* 1994;90: 792–799.

45. Stone GW, Marsalese D, Brodie BR et al. A prospective, randomized evaluation of prophylactic intraaortic balloon counterpulsation in high risk patients with acute myocardial infarction treated with primary angioplasty. *J Am Coll Cardiol* 1997;29:1459–1467.

46. Vogel RA, Shawl F, Tommaso C et al. Initial report of the national registry of elective cardiopulmonary bypass supported coronary angioplasty. *J Am Coll Cardiol* 1990;15:23–29.

47. Overtie PA. Emergency use of portable cardiopulmonary bypass. *Cathet Cardiovasc Diagn* 1990;20:27–31.

48. Monties JR. The living organism and artificial organs. *Artif Organs* 1998;22:358–361.

49. Muehrcke DD, McCarthy PM, Stewart RW et al. Complications of extracorporeal life support systems using heparin-bound surfaces. The risk of intracardiac clot formation. *J Thorac Cardiovasc Surg* 1995;110:843–851.

50. Ihno T, Nakagawa T, Furukawa H et al. Various problems during long-term percutaneous cardiopulmonary support. *Artif Organs* 1997;21:766–771.

B. Shock in the Setting of Acute Myocardial Infarction

David Hasdai and *David R. Holmes, Jr.

*Department of Cardiology, Rabin Medical Center, Beilinson Campus, 49100 Petah Tikva, Israel;
*Division of Cardiovascular Diseases and Internal Medicine, Mayo Clinic and Mayo Foundation,
Department of Medicine, Mayo Medical School, Rochester, Minnesota 55905*

INCIDENCE OF CARDIOGENIC SHOCK

Cardiogenic shock (CS) is a well-known complication of acute myocardial infarction (AMI). As early as 1912, Herrick reported one of the first series of patients developing CS after obstruction of major coronary arteries (1). Herrick described the development of a weak, rapid pulse, feeble cardiac tones, dyspnea, and cyanosis in patients with angina. Outcome was very poor in that series of patients.

In the modern era, CS occurs in 5% to 15% of patients with AMI (2–6). CS in the setting of AMI remains a harbinger of extremely poor prognosis, being the most common cause of in-hospital mortality complicating AMI. Indeed, patients with CS account for a large proportion of the morbidity and mortality of AMI (2,3,6–8). For example, although shock occurred in only 7.2% of patients in the large, multicenter Global Utilization of Streptokinase and Tissue-Plasminogen Activator for Occluded Coronary Arteries (GUSTO-I) trial, this patient group accounted for 58% of all mortality in the entire trial (6). While outcome of AMI has improved for most patients, data from the Worcester Heart Attack Study have demonstrated that in-hospital mortality of shock patients did not improve between 1975 and 1988 (3). Thus, CS remains a major therapeutic challenge for cardiologists.

Cardiogenic shock may develop in the early stages of AMI, or more commonly after the first few hours. Indeed, in the GUSTO-I trial, almost 90% of the patients with CS developed shock after enrollment (6). This may reflect a selection bias in enrollment of patients; clinicians may have been reluctant to enroll CS patients to a trial of thrombolytic therapy when other options were available. Obtaining written informed consent for participation in a randomized trial from a patient in CS may also be difficult. Thus, in the broader patient population with AMI, a larger proportion of patients may present with CS.

This chapter reviews the current status of treatment for CS with emphasis on percutaneous interventions and assist devices.

PATHOPHYSIOLOGY

Alonso et al. (9) compared the pathological findings of 22 patients who died after CS developed in the setting of AMI with ten patients who died from AMI without CS. Total left ventricular damage averaged 51% (range 35%–68%) in the CS patients and 23% (range 14%–31%) in the non-CS patients. These findings are in accord with other autopsy studies reporting a loss of more than 40% of the left ventricular myocardium among patients with CS (2). However, CS may also develop in cases of less severe myocardial damage related to associated complications such as right ventricular infarction, acute mitral regurgitation, or ventricular-septal defect. In addition, in patients with regional abnormalities in cardiac function due to prior infarcts, but a well-compensated global function owing to hypercontractility of the uninvolved region, a small infarct in the normal region of the heart may result in CS. In all of the above cases, systemic perfusion of vital organs is compromised due to reduced cardiac function. This results in a downward spiral with increasing organ hypoperfusion, reduced renal and cerebral function, altered metabolism, and worsening coronary blood flow. Current supportive therapy for CS is thus aimed toward restoring and then stabilizing systemic perfusion by increasing cardiac contractility and/or reducing the systemic resistance to blood flow.

CLINICAL AND PHYSICAL FEATURES

As described by Herrick (1) almost 90 years ago, the physical findings generally detected during CS include hypotension, a weak, rapid pulse, pulmonary rales, cyanosis, altered sensorium, and cold, clammy skin. Despite the advent of modern-technology diagnostic devices such as echocardiography used to assess cardiac function among patients with AMI and CS, the physical examination remains a valuable tool both for the diagnosis of CS as well as for prognostic purposes. We have recently demonstrated (10) that findings derived from physical examination, such as altered sensorium and cold, clammy skin, were important independent predictors of 30-day mortality among patients with CS (odds of dying 1.68 times higher in the presence of each of these conditions). In addition, the prognostic value of a simple parameter such as reduced urine output was similar to the prognostic value of the pulmonary capillary wedge pressure, the former parameter being much more readily available and risk-free. Invasive monitoring, therefore, does not supplant a thorough physical examination.

RIGHT-HEART CATHETERIZATION

There is a great deal of controversy regarding the role of right-heart catheterization in the management of CS. Holmes et al. (11) recently reported that among patients in the GUSTO-I trial, outcome was better in those who received a more aggressive therapeutic approach, including right-heart catheterization. Another report, in contrast, asserted that the use of right-heart catheterization for hemodynamic monitoring in critically ill patients, including those with CS, was associated with increased mortality (12). It is not clear if the increased mortality in that study reflected (a) a wider group of patients in whom the risk benefit may not have been favorable,

(b) procedural complications associated with the insertion of the catheter, (c) complications of prolonged monitoring, or (d) suboptimal interpretation of the derived data or ineffective guidance of pharmacological therapy based on these data. In our recent report from GUSTO-I (10), patients with CS who underwent right-heart catheterization had better prognoses than those who did not. There results may be biased in that the patients with the more favorable outcomes were more likely to receive aggressive treatment including right-heart catheterization.

Our prior report (10) also demonstrated that data derived from right-heart catheterization were of prognostic significance. The most significant predictor of 30-day mortality was the value of the cardiac output; a decrease in cardiac output of 1 liter/minute for values below 5.1 liters/minute was associated with reduced survival (1.75 times greater risk of dying at 30 days). Pulmonary capillary wedge pressure measurements were also of prognostic value, with both an increase in pulmonary capillary wedge pressure for values above 20 mm Hg and a decrease in pulmonary capillary wedge pressure for values under 20 mm Hg associated with greater odds of 30-day mortality.

The measurement of hemodynamic parameters from right-heart catheterization in shock patients is not only of prognostic significance but may also be of therapeutic benefit. For example, our data indicated that patients with cardiac output >5.1 liters per minute and CS had a bad prognosis similar to that of shock patients with cardiac output <5.1 liters per minute, yet the former group likely would not require positive inotropic support, whereas the latter group might benefit from such therapy.

Our data also provided possible therapeutic targets for patients with shock. Cardiac output and pulmonary capillary wedge pressure measurements of 5.1 liters per minute and 20 mm Hg, respectively, were associated with lower mortality, whereas values above or below were associated with increased mortality. Although there is much information that can be derived from invasive monitoring, there are few widely-accepted guidelines for tailoring the management of shock patients based on the derived data.

THE INTRAAORTIC BALLOON PUMP

The intraaortic balloon pump (IABP) is a valuable assist device used to stabilize patients with CS. The device is inserted percutaneously through 9 or 10 Fr sheaths, although sheathless devices have recently been introduced. IABP use increases diastolic coronary arterial perfusion and reduces systemic afterload without increasing myocardial oxygen demand. Use of the IABP may also enhance the efficacy of thrombolytic therapy in states of low coronary perfusion pressure (13,14). It is worth emphasizing, however, that despite the widespread use of the IABP for CS, we have seen little firm evidence in the data that IABP use improves outcome. Nevertheless, preliminary data supports that IABP in conjunction with revascularization may favorably affect outcome. For example, Anderson et al. (15) reported that the use of IABP in the GUSTO-I trial was associated with a trend toward lower 30-day and 1-year mortality rates. Kovack et al. (16) also reported that the use of IABP significantly improved in-hospital outcome of CS patients receiving thrombolytic therapy for AMI. Two important points were emphasized in the latter study:

1. IABP may be used in the community-hospital setting in the CS patient until transfer of the patient to a facility where percutaneous or surgical revascularization procedures can be performed.
2. IABP in itself does not alter outcome. Rather, IABP should be used to stabilize the CS patient until revascularization is completed.

REPERFUSION AND REVASCULARIZATION

Given that the patency of the infarct-related artery is most strongly associated with acute and long-term survival among patients with CS (8), current therapy is primarily aimed toward reperfusion of the infarct-related artery. Reperfusion may be achieved pharmacologically or through percutaneous or surgical revascularization.

There have been no trials in which patients with AMI presenting with CS have been specifically randomized to thrombolytic therapy or placebo. However, the Gruppo Italiano per lo Studio della Streptochinasi nell' Infarto Miocardico (GISSI) study, comparing streptokinase with control, included patients with CS (17): 69.9% of the 146 patients presenting with CS and receiving streptokinase died within 21 days, as compared with 70.1% of the 134 control CS patients. In contrast, an analysis of large trials comparing thrombolytic therapy for AMI with control demonstrated that among patients presenting with a systolic blood pressure <100 mm Hg, mortality was reduced from 35.1% in the control group to 28.9% in patients receiving thrombolytic therapy (18). The proportion of patients with hypotension who were in CS was not defined (18). A retrospective analysis of patients admitted to Duke University Medical Center in the years 1987 through 1988 also demonstrated high mortality rates in CS patients receiving thrombolytic therapy; among patients treated with thrombolytic therapy alone, the in-hospital mortality rate was 58% (8). The lack of benefit of thrombolytic agents in CS may be attributed to reduced coronary thrombolysis in states of the low perfusion pressure (13,14,16.)

Given the discouraging results attained with thrombolytic therapy for patients with CS, there is an emerging interest in the use of mechanical revascularization in CS patients. Although the reported results with mechanical revascularization seem slightly better than those attained with thrombolytic therapy, there may be a selection bias in clinical practice regarding the use of mechanical revascularization (19–21); the clinical and angiographic profile of patients undergoing angioplasty is often more favorable than patients receiving medical therapy alone.

A recent prospective randomized trial of 55 patients with CS following AMI compared revascularization (surgical or percutaneous) with medical therapy (22). The study was stopped prematurely due to low enrollment. However, in this small cohort emergent angioplasty did not improve outcome. In contrast, both Holmes et al. (6,11) and Berger et al. (21) reported from the GUSTO-I trial that revascularization was associated improved survival. Moreover, Berger et al. (21) demonstrated that CS patients who underwent successful angioplasty had better outcomes than those who had unsuccessful angioplasty. Thus, there are currently no prospective, randomized data that mechanical revascularization improves the outcome of CS patients, but there are several compelling reports indicating that the use of angioplasty among CS patients was associated with improved outcome.

The concerns regarding the selection bias of CS patients treated with angioplasty pertain to surgical revascularization. Series of surgical patients with CS have been reported, showing relatively good outcome (approximately 40% mortality) (23–26). By and large, these reports were from the preangioplasty era. In addition, as explained above, in most of these reports, IABP was used to stabilize the CS patient until surgical revascularization was achieved. Bypass surgery has one major advantage over percutaneous revascularization, in that more complete revascularization may be more commonly attained with bypass surgery, thereby enabling restoration of normal blood flow and better cardiac function to a greater proportion of the heart. However, given the lag period between the acute event and attainment of revascularization during surgery (27), angioplasty of the culprit lesion should be performed promptly, if possible. Thereafter, bypass surgery should be contemplated if indicated.

CONCLUSION

Cardiogenic shock remains a common and ominous complication of AMI. Although there are no prospective, randomized data that the use of percutaneous assist devices and mechanical revascularization are associated with improved outcome, based on the encouraging results reported in the literature regarding the use of an aggressive approach for CS patients, we currently recommend that patients with CS complicating AMI undergo coronary angiography as soon as possible followed by percutaneous or surgical revascularization. IABP should be contemplated, especially if the patient is refractory to supportive pharmacological therapy.

The mortality rates of CS complicating AMI remain unacceptably high. For example, even among CS patients who received an aggressive therapeutic approach in the GUSTO-I trial, over 50% died at 30 days. Therefore, other pharmacological and mechanical therapeutic approaches are exigent if outcome of CS is to be substantially improved.

REFERENCES

1. Herrick JB. Clinical features of sudden obstruction of the coronary arteries. *JAMA* 1912;39:2015–2020.
2. Califf RM, Bengtson JR. Cardiogenic shock. *N Engl J Med* 1994;330:1724–1731.
3. Goldberg RJ, Gore JM, Alpert JS et al. Cardiogenic shock after acute myocardial infarction—incidence and mortality from a community wide perspective 1975–1988. *N Engl J Med* 1991;325:1117–1122.
4. Scheidt S, Ascheim R, Killip T. Shock after acute myocardial infarction: a clinical and hemodynamic profile. *Am J Cardiol* 1970;26:556–564.
5. Gheorghiade M, Anderson J, Rosman H et al. Risk identification at the time of admission to coronary care unit in patients with suspected myocardial infarction. *Am Heart J* 1988;116:1212–1217.
6. Holmes DR Jr, Bates ER, Kleiman NS et al. Contemporary reperfusion therapy for cardiogenic shock: The GUSTO-I Trial experience. *J Am Coll Cardiol* 1995; 26:668–674.
7. Bates ER, Topol EJ. Limitations of thrombolytic therapy for acute myocardial infarction complicated by congestive heart failure and cardiogenic shock. *J Am Coll Cardiol* 1991;18:1077–1084.
8. Bengtson JR, Kaplan AJ, Pieper KS et al. Prognosis in cardiogenic shock after acute myocardial infarction in the interventional era. *J Am Coll Cardiol* 1992;20: 1482–1489.
9. Alonso DR, Scheidt S, Post M, Killip T. Pathophysiology of cardiogenic shock. Quantification of myocardial necrosis, clinical, pathologic and electrocardiographic correlations. *Circulation* 1973;48:588–596.
10. Hasdai D, Holmes DR Jr, Califf RM et al. Cardiogenic shock complicating acute myocardial infarction: predictors of mortality. *Am Heart J* 1999;138:21–31.
11. Holmes DR Jr, Califf RM, Van de Werf F et al. Differences in countries' use of resources and clinical outcome for patients with cardiogenic shock after myocardial infarction: results from the GUSTO trial. *Lancet* 1997; 349:75–78.
12. Connors AF Jr, Speroff T, Dawson NV et al. The effectiveness of right heart catheterization in the initial care of critically ill patients. SUPPORT Investigators. *JAMA* 1996;276:889–897.
13. Prewitt RM, Gu S, Garber PJ, Ducas J. Marked systemic hypotension depresses coronary thrombolysis induced by intracoronary administration of recombinant tissue-type plasminogen activator. *J Am Coll Cardiol* 1992; 20:1626–1633.
14. Prewitt RM, Gu S, Schick U, Ducas J. Intraaortic balloon counterpulsation enhances coronary thrombolysis induced by intravenous administration of a thrombolytic agent. *J Am Coll Cardiol* 1994;23:794–798.
15. Anderson RD, Ohman EM, Holmes DR Jr. et al. Use of intraaortic balloon counterpulsation in patients presenting with cardiogenic shock: observations from the GUSTO-I Study. *J Am Coll Cardiol* 1997;30:708–715.
16. Kovack PJ, Rasak MA, Bates ER, Ohman EM, Stomel RJ. Thrombolysis plus aortic counterpulsation: improved survival in patients who present to community hospitals with cardiogenic shock. *J Am Coll Cardiol* 1997;29:1454–1458.
17. Gruppo Italiano per lo Studio della Streptochinasi nell' Infarto Miocardico. Effectiveness of intravenous thrombolytic therapy in acute myocardial infarction. *Lancet* 1986;1:397–401.
18. Fibrinolytic Therapy Trialists' (FTT) Collaborative Group. Indications for fibrinolytic therapy in suspected acute myocardial infarction: collaborative overview of early mortality and major morbidity results from all randomised trials of more than 1000 patients. *Lancet* 1994; 343:311–322.
19. Hochman JS, Boland J, Sleeper LA et al. Current spectrum of cardiogenic shock and effect of early revascularization on mortality. *Circulation* 1995;91:873–881.
20. Eltchaninoff H, Simpfendorfer C, Franco I, Raymond RE, Casale PN, Whitlow PL. Early and 1-year survival rates in acute myocardial infarction complicated by cardiogenic shock: a retrospective study comparing coronary angioplasty with medical treatment. *Am Heart J* 1995;130:459–464.
21. Berger PB, Holmes DR Jr, Stebbins AL, Bates ER, Califf RM, Topol EJ. Impact of an aggressive invasive catheterization and revascularization strategy on mortality in patients with cardiogenic shock in the Global Utilization of Streptokinase and Tissue Plasminogen Activator for Occluded Coronary Arteries (GUSTO-I) Trial: An observational study. *Circulation* 1997;96:122–127.
22. Stauffer JC, Urban P, Bleed D et al. Results of the "Swiss" multicenter evaluation of early angioplasty for shock following myocardial infarction. *Circulation* 1997;96:I-206.
23. Dunkman WB, Leinbach RC, Buckley MJ et al. Clinical and hemodynamic results of intraaortic balloon pumping and surgery for cardiogenic shock. *Circulation* 1972; 46:465–477.
24. Bardet J, Masquet C, Khan JC et al. Clinical and hemodynamic results of intraaortic balloon counterpulsation and surgery for cardiogenic shock. *Am Heart J* 1977; 93:280–288.
25. DeWood MA, Notske RN, Hensley GR et al. Intraaortic balloon counterpulsation with and without reperfusion of myocardial infarction shock. *Circulation* 1980;61: 1105–1112.
26. Subramanian VA, Roberts AJ, Zema MJ et al. Cardiogenic shock following acute myocardial infarction: late functional results after emergency cardiac surgery. *N Y State J Med* 1980;80:947–952.
27. Berger PB, Stensrud PE, Daly RC et al. Time to reperfusion and other procedural characteristics of emergency coronary artery bypass surgery after unsuccessful coronary angioplasty. *Am J Cardiol* 1995;76:565–569.

20

Proximal Left Anterior Descending Disease

A. The Role of PTCR in Proximal Left Anterior Descending Disease

Corrado Vassanelli, *Giuliana Menegatti, and *Jonata Molinari

Department of Medical Sciences, University "A. Avogadro," Division of Cardiology, 28100 Novara, Italy; °Division of Cardiology, University Hospital, University of Verona, 37126 Verona, Italy

BACKGROUND

Stenoses in the proximal left anterior descending (LAD) coronary artery are considered a life-threatening disease (1–3), because of the large amount of myocardium at risk in these cases, and because these cases are associated with lower immediate and long-term success rate after balloon angioplasty (4–6). Despite considerable incidence of this disease in patients without acute myocardial infarction (7,8) (8.5% in our experience in single-vessel coronary artery disease), the published reports on percutaneous interventions in proximal LAD stenoses are few, the definitions conflicting, the techniques different, the long-term results scarce, and the optimal strategy of treatment still controversial.

Following the American Heart Association definition (9), the proximal LAD is the segment starting at the takeoff of the circumflex coronary artery and ending before the origin of first septal perforator, without taking into account the takeoff of the first diagonal. This definition, given before the advent of interventional cardiology, contrasts with that of other authors who included the origin of the first septal perforator (6). More appropriate seems the definition of Ten Berg (7), who classified as proximal LAD the segment ending before the takeoff of the first side branch (either the first septal perforator or the first diagonal branch). A proximal lesion can be classified as ostial if the origin of the LAD is truly involved.

Most authors consider a proximal LAD lesion significant if the narrowing is greater than 70% of the vessel diameter (the 70% diameter stenosis definition); however, in some series, especially of very proximal location, narrowing greater than or equal to 50% was considered significant (the 50% diameter stenosis definition) (6,8).

The choice of the best treatment in symptomatic patients with isolated proximal LAD lesion and good left ventricular function is still debated. However, there is agreement that in these patients a more aggressive strategy, mainly to improve long-term outcome, is warranted.

THE SURGICAL APPROACH

Although three randomized trials (the Coronary Artery Surgery Study, the VA Coronary Artery Bypass Surgery Cooperative Study and the European Coronary Surgery Study) (10–12) failed to demonstrate that surgical revascularization improves the survival rate or decreases the rate of myocardial infarction in the subgroup of patients with single-vessel disease, the poor prognosis associated with proximal LAD lesion and the excellent long-term patency rate of left internal mammary artery (LIMA) grafting seemed to warrant a surgical revascularization even in single-vessel disease.

The first randomized prospective trial comparing PTCA and LIMA grafting in patients with proximal LAD disease and good left ventricular function (the SALAD trial) (13), did not demonstrate a significant difference in the rate of composite endpoint of death and myocardial infarction at a 24-month follow-up. However, the CABG-treated patients were more frequently free from adverse events than PTCA-treated patients (86% versus 43%), mainly because of a higher risk of restenosis, of a more frequent need for antianginal treatment, and subsequent revascularization procedures.

In a randomized prospective study on medical therapy, balloon angioplasty or bypass surgery (the Medicine, Angioplasty or Surgery Study [MASS]) (14), the use of left internal mammary artery grafting for the treatment of patients with stable angina, isolated severe stenosis of proximal LAD, and normal left ventricular function, was associated with a higher event-free survival rate due to a lower reintervention rate than PTCA or medical treatment alone during an average follow-up of 3 years.

However, there was a significant progression of coronary atherosclerosis in untreated vessels in all groups, and the three therapeutic options resulted in a similar success rate in terms of abolishing limiting angina and in an equally low incidence of death or myocardial infarction during the follow-up period. These results were confirmed after 5 years of follow-up (15).

Coronary revascularization without cardiopulmonary bypass and cardioplegic arrest through a small anterior thoracotomy has been introduced as an alternative to the conventional approach (16,17). This approach, called minimally invasive direct coronary artery bypass (MIDCAB) is presently performed almost exclusively to treat single-vessel LAD disease not amenable to PTCR, through LIMA grafting. Although this technique has raised a great enthusiasm among cardiac surgeons and cardiologists, many issues have yet to be defined (18).

THE INTERVENTIONAL APPROACH

In general, prevention of acute complications and restenosis after percutaneous interventions may be accomplished by judicious choice of technique (or combination of techniques) and by the optimization of the results. This is of particular importance in proximal LAD lesions, which, because of the great amount of elastic fiber in the vessel wall (19), frequently have a substantial elastic recoil (20) and a high restenosis rate at follow-up after balloon dilatation (21,22).

For the interventional cardiologist, two major strategies are emerging for the treatment of these lesions, mainly intended to reduce the restenosis rate: elective stenting and the combination of stenting with a debulking technique.

The BENESTENT I and STRESS I trials (23,24) have consistently shown the advantage of stenting over standard PTCA in reducing the risk of angiographic and clinical restenosis in the treatment of *de novo*, short lesions in large arteries (lumen diameter ≥3.0 mm). In the subgroup analysis of the BENESTENT trial (23), the restenosis rate in patients with proximal LAD disease randomized to stent was reduced to the same extent as in the other patients. In the LAD subgroup of the STRESS I study, (25) the net gain was greater after stenting, and this resulted in a much lower restenosis rate compared to PTCA (32.9% versus 52.6%, $p < .01$). This translated into an improved event-free survival rate in the LAD stent population, whereas there was no difference in survival rates in the non-LAD stent and PTCA group. The advantage of elective stenting is confirmed by the BENESTENT II trial (26). In patients with LAD lesions assigned angiographic follow-up, the minimum lumen diameter (MLD) was significantly higher (1.78 mm versus 1.56 mm, $p = .004$) and the event-free survival rate was significantly better (83.8% versus 73.4%, $p = .005$) in the group treated with stents as compared to those randomized to PTCA (Macaya C. Data presented at the BENESTENT II Symposium, ESC Stockholm, 1997).

Phillips et al. (27) reported a single-center experience in 65 consecutive patients who received a stent for treatment of LAD lesions proximal to the first septal branch and compared them with 56 patients matched for clinical and anatomical characteristics treated with standard PTCA during the same time period. Late loss was similar between the two groups, and patients who received a coronary stent had a higher net gain (1.41 ± 0.89 versus 0.85 ± 0.83, $p < .001$) and a lower angiographic restenosis rate (20% versus 52%, $p < .001$).

The advantage of primary stenting over standard PTCA has been confirmed by Versaci et al. (8) in 120 symptomatic patients with isolated stenosis of proximal LAD. In a highly select population with reasonably good left ventricular function (ejection fraction ≥0.40) and short lesions located in vessels >3.0 mm in diameter, the patients randomized to implantation of a slotted tubular stent had a 12-month restenosis rate (by the 50% diameter stenosis definition) significantly lower (19% versus 40%) and event-free survival better (87% versus 70%) than those in patients randomized to standard PTCA.

Cost-effectiveness analyses (using a decision-analytic model) suggest that the strategy of elective stent implantation in proximal LAD stenoses in vessels ≥3.0 mm in diameter is less expensive at medium term than so-called "provisional stenting" (defined as a narrowing <25% after conventional balloon dilatation) (28). The advantage is attributed to reduced probabilities of death, myocardial infarction, and repeat revascularization. Due to the higher effectiveness of stenting compared to aggressive PTCA (94% versus 84%), the resultant net benefit was in favor of stent implantation (cost-effectiveness ratio of $9.708/patient for stent implantation versus $13.674/patient for conventional PTCA).

In vessels with an angiographic diameter <3.0 mm, the decision of whether to stent should be a balance between the amount of acute elastic recoil and the risk of occurrence of in-stent restenosis at follow-up.

An alternative emerging strategy to improve immediate and long-term results of percutaneous treatment of lesions in proximal LAD is to reduce the plaque burden with a debulking technique, like directional or rotational atherectomy, prior to stent implantation.

Although it is difficult to separate the effects of procedural variables from those of lesion subsets, it has been suggested that balloon-to-artery ratio and higher inflation pressures have an impact on restenosis only if optimal stent dimensions are not achieved (29). In a recent study (30) on 382 lesions treated with 476 Palmaz-Schatz stents (Johnson and Johnson International Systems, Warren, NJ) with angiographic and intravascular ultrasound follow-up available, the three strongest predictors of in-stent restenosis were the ostial lesion location, the intravascular ultrasound (IVUS) preinterventional plaque burden at the lesion site (plaque/total arterial area), and the postinterventional lumen dimensions.

The rationale for device synergy comes from a combination of the effects of atherectomy and of stenting. Atherectomy, reducing the plaque burden, decreases the resistance of the vessel wall, allowing complete stent expansion, and also possibly removes the source of cells promoting the intimal hyperplasia. Stent implantation, improving the inner surface of the vessel by tackling the dissections and preventing the early and late recoil, optimizes the postinterventional lumen dimensions.

Recent reports have shown that the combination of stent placement with high-speed rotational or directional atherectomy have better immediate and long-term results than stent implantation alone.

In most cases, calcifications are responsible for incomplete stent expansion, according to Mintz et al. (31), thus increasing the risk of restenosis. Although not specifically addressed in proximal LAD lesions, the experiences reported by Hoffman et al. (32) and Moussa et al. (33) suggest that rotational atherectomy and stent placement are complementary in large, calcified vessels. In these studies of complex lesions, the acute gain after rotational atherectomy and stent placement was high (2.17 ± 0.60 mm and 2.10 ± 0.61 mm respectively) and the target lesion revascularization rate at follow-up reasonably low (12.2% and 17% respectively).

In a retrospective study, Kobayashi et al. (34) compared the results of stenting alone to those of DCA followed by stenting in 200 lesions located in large (≥3.0 mm) LAD coronary arteries. Compared to stenting alone, debulking plus stenting obtained a significantly larger acute lumen gain (2.85 ± 0.66 mm versus 2.25 ±

0.60 mm), lower late loss index (0.26 ± 0.23 versus 0.47 ± 0.39) and a lower restenosis rate (6.5% versus 23.5%).

Bramucci (personal communication during Endovascular Therapy Course, Paris, May 1998) evaluated the effect of DCA and of subsequent stent application in a series of 42 very proximal LAD lesions. The MLD after DCA increased from 2.48 ± 0.51 mm to 3.45 ± 0.49 mm after adjunctive stent, with a decrease of percent diameter stenosis from 28% ± 14% to 4% ± 10%. At angiographic follow-up, MLD was 2.35 ± 1.50 mm and the percent diameter stenosis was 29% ± 30%. Three patients (7.1%) needed repeat revascularization (two by CABG and one by repeat DCA).

In the pilot phase of the prospective SOLD trial (35), 90 lesions underwent DCA followed by implant of slotted tubular stents. Clinical success was 97.2%. Stenting after plaque removal optimized the MLD, which increased significantly from 2.32 ± 0.59 mm to 3.45 ± 0.53 mm. At angiographic follow-up, the loss index was 0.29 and restenosis rate (by the 50% diameter stenosis definition) was 7.4%.

TECHNICAL CONSIDERATIONS

Some specific technical considerations have to be made for the treatment of proximal LAD lesions. In patients with chest pain, equivocal proximal LAD stenosis (i.e. a diameter stenosis ranging from 30% to 50%), and ambiguous results from noninvasive tests, we evaluate the physiologic significance of the lesion at the diagnostic catheterization, by intracoronary pressure measurement using a pressure guidewire. The calculation of myocardial fractional flow reserve during maximal hyperemia by adenosine is safe and useful in clinical decision making (36).

Although the use of IVUS is not routine in our institution, the information obtained by IVUS is particularly useful for planning the procedure, especially in cases with suspected involvement of the origin of the left circumflex coronary artery.

An important technical aspect is to find the angiographic projection which best visualizes the entire lesion and the left main bifurcation (in very proximal lesions) and the separation with the first diagonal branch (for the more distal lesions).

The femoral approach is still our preferred strategy in high risk patients in whom a circulatory support by intraaortic balloon pumping is planned via the contralateral femoral access; however, if elective stenting is planned, a radial approach is chosen. Presently, a prophylactic balloon pump is inserted before dilation of proximal LAD lesion only in patients presenting with cardiogenic shock.

When choosing the guiding catheter we look for one that provides good support; we prefer an Amplatz left or an extra back-up configuration. In elective procedures in noncomplex lesions, a 6 Fr size is used, while in emergency cases or when a complex procedure is anticipated, a larger size is used because it gives a good support and allows the use of all types and sizes of stents and of additional devices such as catheters for high-speed or directional atherectomy.

In all cases, we presently use as a first choice a radiotransparent guidewire with high support characteristics. The use of a guidewire with multiple markers to obtain a proper positioning might be of some help in very proximal lesions, but it is not routinely used.

In very proximal severe lesions of large vessels, (especially in chronic total occlusions) a frequent problem to overcome is the prolapse of the guidewire in the left circumflex coronary artery while trying to cross the lesion. In these cases, especially when the left main is short or absent, we use nitinol wires with hydrophilic coating, gently advance the dilating balloon or, preferably, use a multifunctional catheter to maintain the position and the direction of the wire and increase the support of the system. In some cases, with disease at the origin of the left circumflex, there is some concern about the need to protect the left circumflex coronary artery with a wire. The wire positioned in the left circumflex may also be used as a marker of the vessel takeoff for a proper deployment of the stent in the LAD.

It has to be noted that predilation with balloons of standard length often involves the left main. In these cases, it is necessary to check the flow in the left circumflex, and to keep the duration of the balloon inflation short (25–30 seconds).

Considering of the difficulty of the deployment of a self-expandable stent, we prefer a balloon-expandable stent with high radial force of slotted tubular or cell design. These include the Palmaz-Schatz Crown, NIR (Scimed, Maple Grove, MN), ACS Multi-Link Rx Duet (Guidant Inc. Santa Clara, CA), and beStent (Medtronic Inc., Minneapolis, MN) stents. The new generation AVE GFX (Arterial Vascular Engineering, Division of Medtronic, Santa Rosa CA) stent my well be a very reasonable alternative. In order to ensure proper stent position without prolapse in the distal left main or in the circumflex, it is particularly useful to use a radiopaque stent or a stent with radiopaque markers at margins. In most cases, stent position has to be checked with multiple injection and stent deployment must be made under fluoroscopic control to avoid allowing the stent to move or embolize. Particular attention has to be paid to the presence of a disease of the distal left main stem.

To reduce the risk of edge dissections, the length of the balloon has to closely match that of the stent, minimizing the amount of bare balloon expanded outside the stent. We select high-pressure, minimally compliant delivery balloon, potentially obviating the need for an additional postdilation balloon. With the latest generation, very low-profile, premounted stents, the target lesion can be crossed primarily with the stent-balloon assembly and the stent can be delivered without predilatation, deployed, and fully expanded with the same balloon (stent-assisted angioplasty).

Stenting of *de novo* lesions was usually accomplished with full coverage of the lesion (normal to normal vessel). This strategy is sometimes difficult in proximal lesions, because the stent itself might protrude into the left main or jeopardize the origin of side branches. For this reason and because of the evidence that long stenting is associated with higher restenosis rate, recently we adopt the "spot-stenting" technique, trying to cover the lesion with the shortest possible stent, especially in small vessels.

Since the introduction of stents, the use of perfusion balloons, either in high risk patients or in bail-out settings, has been abandoned.

Surgery could be considered if the invasive cardiology team does not have sufficient experience in stenting, especially for ostial lesions or obstructions involving major side branches (large first diagonal branch), which require special skills.

Directional coronary atherectomy is suitable for large (>3 mm) left anterior vessels with or without plaques extending to the left main stem. To obtain better results of DCA, whenever possible, we do not fully predilate the lesion, in order to have maximum plaque removal and to better localize the site of atherectomy. If complementary stenting is planned, a less aggressive atherectomy may be adequate to improve vessel compliance at the lesion site, facilitating stent delivery and allowing its optimal expansion.

In lesions strictly located to the proximal LAD, rotational atherectomy is a good choice for removing part of the plaque before balloon dilation and stent implantation, preventing plaque shift in the left circumflex, and reducing elastic recoil. However, rotational atherectomy is applied only if calcifications are visible on fluoroscopy; otherwise, rotablation is not routinely used because the procedure is too long, difficult, and expensive.

REFERENCES

1. Mock MB, Ringquist I, Fisher LD et al. Survival of medically treated patients in the Coronary Artery Surgery Study (CASS) registry. *Circulation* 1982;66: 652–658.
2. Califf RM, Tomabechi Y, Lee KL et al. Outcome in one-vessel coronary artery disease. *Circulation* 1983; 67:283–290.
3. Klein LW, Weintraub WS, Agarwal JB et al. Prognostic significance of severe narrowing of the proximal portion of the left anterior descending coronary artery. *Am J Cardiol* 1986;58:42–46.
4. Topol EJ, Ellis SG, Fishman J et al. Multicenter study of percutaneous transluminal angioplasty for right coronary artery ostial stenosis. *J Am Coll Cardiol* 1987;9: 1214–1218.
5. Hirschfeld JW, Schwartz JS, Jugo R et al., and the M-Heart Investigators. Restenosis after coronary angioplasty: a multivariate statistical model to relate lesion and procedure variables to restenosis. *J Am Coll Cardiol* 1991;18:647–656.

6. Frieson JH, Dimas AP, Whitlow PL et al. Angioplasty of the proximal left anterior descending coronary artery: initial success and long-term follow-up. *J Am Coll Cardiol* 1992;19:745–751.

7. Ten Berg JM, Gin MTJ, Ernst SMPG et al. Ten-year follow up of percutaneous transluminal coronary angioplasty for proximal left anterior descending coronary artery stenosis in 351 patients. *J Am Coll Cardiol* 1996; 28:82–88.

8. Versaci F, Gaspardone A, Tomai F, Crea F, Chiariello L, Gioffrè PA. A comparison of coronary artery stenting with angioplasty for isolated stenosis of the proximal left anterior descending coronary artery. *N Engl J Med* 1997;336:817–822.

9. Austin WG, Edwards JE, Freye RL et al. A reporting system on patients evaluated for coronary artery disease: report of the Ad Hoc Committee for Grading of Coronary Artery Disease, Council on Cardiovascular Surgery. American Heart Association. *Circulation* 1975;51: 7–40.

10. Coronary Artery Surgery Study Group. Coronary Artery Surgery Study (CASS): a randomized trial of coronary artery bypass surgery: survival data. *Circulation* 1983; 68:939–950.

11. VA Coronary Artery Bypass Surgery Cooperative Study Group. Eighteen-year follow-up in the Veterans Affairs cooperative study of coronary artery bypass surgery for stable angina. *Circulation* 1992;86:121–130.

12. European Coronary Surgery Study Group. Long-term results of prospective randomized study of coronary artery bypass surgery in stable angina pectoris. *Lancet* 1982;1173–1180.

13. Goy JJ, Eeckhout E, Vogt P et al. Coronary angioplasty versus left mammary artery grafting for isolated proximal left anterior descending artery stenosis. *Lancet* ,3: 1449–1453.

14. Hueb WA, Bellotti G, De Oliveira SA et al. The Medicine, Angioplasty or Surgery Study (MASS): a prospective, randomized trial of medical therapy, balloon angioplasty or bypass surgery for single proximal left anterior descending artery stenoses. *J Am Coll Cardiol* 1995;26: 1600–1605.

15. Hueb W, Cardoso RH, Soares PR et al. The Medicine, Angioplasty and Surgery Study (MASS): a prospective randomized trial of medical therapy, balloon angioplasty or bypass surgery for single proximal left anterior descending artery stenoses. *J Am Coll Cardiol* 1998; 31[Suppl C]:386C(abst).

16. Calafiore AM, Angelini GD, Bergsland J et al. Minimally invasive coronary artery bypass grafting. *Ann Thorac Surg* 1996;62:1545–1548.

17. Calafiore AM, DiGiammarco G, Teodori G et al. Left anterior descending coronary artery grafting via left anterior small thoracotomy without cardiopulmonary bypass. *Ann Thorac Surg.* 1996;61:1658–1665.

18. Fann JI, Stevens JH, Pompili MF, Burdon TA, Reitz BA. Minimally invasive coronary artery bypass grafting. *Curr Opin Cardiol* 1997;12:482–487.

19. Boucek RJ, Morales AR, Romanelli R et al. *Coronary artery disease: pathologic and clinical assessment.* Baltimore: Williams & Wilkins, 1984:66–85.

20. Rozenman Y, Gilon D, Welber S, Sapoznikov D, Gots-man MS. Clinical and angiographic predictors of immediate recoil after successful coronary angioplasty and relation to late restenosis. *Am J Cardiol* 1993;72: 1020–1025.

21. Topol EJ, Leya F, Pinkerton CA et al. A comparison of directional atherectomy with coronary angioplasty in patients with coronary artery disease. *N Engl J Med* 1993;329:221–227.

22. Adelman AG, Cohen EA, Kimball BP et al. A comparison of directional atherectomy with balloon angioplasty for lesions of the left anterior descending coronary artery. *N Engl J Med* 1993;329:228–233.

23. Serruys PW, DeJaegere P, Kiemeneij F et al., for the BENESTENT study group. A comparison of balloon-expandable-stent implantation with balloon angioplasty in patients with coronary artery disease. *N Engl J Med* 1994;331:489–495.

24. Fischman DL, Leon MB, Baim DS et al., for the Stent Restenosis Study Investigators. A randomized comparison of coronary-stent placement and balloon angioplasty in the treatment of coronary artery disease. *N Engl J Med* 1994;331:496–501.

25. Heuser RR, Wong SC, Chuang YC et al. The LAD subgroup in the stent restenosis study (STRESS): the most pronounced antirestenosis effect of stenting. *Eur Heart J* 1995;16:291(abst).

26. Serruys PW, van Hout B, Bonnier H et al., for the BENESTENT Study Group. Randomized comparison of implantation of heparin-coated stents with balloon angioplasty in selected patients with coronary artery disease (BENESTENT II). *Lancet* 1998;352:673–681.

27. Phillips PS, Segovia J, Alfonso F et al. Advantage of stents in the proximal left anterior descending coronary. *Am Heart J* 1998;135:719–725.

28. Iñiguez A, Navarro F, Valdesuso R, Córdoba M, Ayala R, Almeida P. Cost-effectiveness of stent implantation versus "stent-like" result after balloon dilation of lesions located in the proximal segment of the left anterior descending artery. *Eur Heart J* 1997;18[Suppl]: 2773(abst).

29. Mintz GS, Hoffmann R, Mehran R et al. In-stent restenosis: the Washington Hospital Center Experience. *Am J Cardiol* 1998;81(7A):7E–13E.

30. Hoffmann R, Mintz GS, Mehran R et al. Intravascular ultrasound predictors of angiographic restenosis in lesions treated with Palmaz-Schatz stents. *J Am Coll Cardiol* 1998;31:43–49.

31. Mintz GS, Popma JJ, Pichard AD et al. Patterns of calcification ion coronary artery disease: a statistical angiography in 1155 lesions. *Circulation* 1995;91: 1959(abst).

32. Hoffman R, Mintz GS, Kent KM et al. Is there an optimal therapy for calcified lesions in large vessels? Comparative acute and follow-up results of rotational atherectomy, stents, or the combination. *J Am Coll Cardiol* 1997;29[Suppl A]:68A(abst).

33. Moussa I, Di Mario C, Moses J et al. Coronary stenting after rotational atherectomy in calcified and complex lesions. Angiographic and clinical follow-up results. *Circulation* 1997;96:128–136.

34. Kobayashi Y, Moussa I, De Gregorio J et al. Low restenosis rate in lesions of the left anterior descending coro-

nary artery with stenting following directional coronary atherectomy. *J Am Coll Cardiol* 1998;31[Suppl A]: 378A(abst).

35. Moussa J, Moses J, Di Mario C, King T, Reimers B, Colombo A. Immediate and short-term results of the pilot phase of stenting after optimal lesion debulking:

"the SOLD Trial." *J Am Coll Cardiol* 1997;29[Suppl A]:415A(abst).

36. Pijls NHJ, De Bruyne B, Peels K et al. Measurement of fractional flow reserve to assess the functional severity of coronary-artery stenoses. *N Engl J Med* 1996;334: 1703–1708.

B. The Role of Bypass Surgery in Proximal Left Anterior Descending Coronary Artery Disease

J-J Goy and Eric Eeckhout

Division of Cardiology, University Hospital, 1011 Lausanne, Switzerland

BACKGROUND

Historical data about the natural history and the clinical significance of isolated proximal left anterior descending coronary artery (LAD) are still confusing. Many trials have been published, but suffered from major bias of selection or are simply retrospective (1–3). Moreover most of them include and analyze together patients who have had myocardial infarction, with or without a normal left ventricular function. However, in spite of these limitations, we can find some consistency in the prognosis of patients with such lesions when only medical treatment is applied. Data from the early 1980s suggest that at 6 years the incidence of death is around 25%, compared to only 14% for patients with isolated right coronary stenosis. The same conclusions arise from other nonrandomized studies or registries (3–5). This poorer prognosis seems to be even worse when left ventricular dysfunction is present. Nowadays, the use of new antianginal drugs in addition to aggressive lipid lowering therapy may seriously modify these historical data. In spite of the limitations in evaluating the value of medical therapy, it is generally accepted in daily practice that patients with a 70% or greater stenosis of the proximal LAD should be revascularized, provided that silent or clinical ischemia has been documented. In fact, most patients will remain symptomatic despite optimal medical

treatment. When an intermediate stenosis is present, between 50% to 70%, the use of intracoronary Doppler flow or pressure measurements is helpful in making a decision (6–7). This data has led us to adopt a particular attitude regarding patients with proximal LAD stenosis.

REVASCULARISATION PROCEDURES

The management of patients with proximal LAD stenosis is of critical importance and remains controversial. Apart from medical therapy, the clinician has a choice between four interventional strategies:

1. percutaneous transluminal coronary angioplasty (PTCA),
2. stent implantation in addition to PTCA,
3. surgery with implantation of the left internal mammary artery, and
4. surgery with implantation of the left internal mammary artery by a minimal invasive surgical approach.

The last option is still in clinical evaluation and long-term data are required to fully define the role of this new surgical approach.

There is still some debate regarding patients with proximal LAD stenosis, and surgeons often advocate a surgical approach. On the other hand, cardiologists define an isolated proximal LAD stenosis as one of the best indications for coronary angioplasty. The survival rate of patients with multivessel coronary artery disease and proximal LAD lesion is 92% at 5 years and 75% at 10 years after cardiac surgery (8). When the left internal mammary artery is used, the in-hospital mortality (<30 days) is very low (<2%) and the relief of angina is excellent, with 92% of the patients free of symptoms at 5 years (9). In a similar group of patients with proximal LAD stenosis and multiple-vessel disease, medical treatment carries a significantly worse prognosis, with a survival rate of 83% and 64% at 5 and 10 years, respectively, as shown by the European Coronary Surgery study (10). Thus, the benefit of surgery over medical therapy in the specific group of patients with proximal LAD stenosis and multiple-vessel disease is widely accepted.

However, coronary angioplasty has to be considered as a possible option for coronary revascularization. Angioplasty is usually performed in patients with single-vessel disease and offers a slight benefit over medical therapy at 6 months in terms of exercise tolerance and relief of angina, as demonstrated by Parisi et al. (11). That study, however, involved a heterogeneous group of patients with a single coronary artery stenosis of any vessel. The number of patients with LAD stenosis is unknown, and the conclusions drawn by Parisi and et al. might be slightly different for the particular group of patients with proximal LAD stenosis. Based on retrospective data, the survival rate after angioplasty for single coronary stenosis compares favorably with surgery in heterogeneous group of patients (12). Another retrospective evaluation of a group of proximal LAD stenosis treated with angioplasty shows the 5-year actuarial freedom from cardiac death to be 97% and from death and myocardial infarction to be 94%. Adding surgical or percutaneous revascularization to cardiac death and myocardial infarction, the proportion of patients free from events decreases to 71% (13). The initial success rate of angioplasty is high (<95%), but 25% to 30% of the patients experience a recurrence of symptoms caused by a restenosis within the first 6 months after the initial intervention, making additional investigations, angiography,

and angioplasty necessary, thereby increasing the final cost and the morbidity. Although the in-hospital outcome is similar in patients treated with surgery or angioplasty, the length of the in-hospital stay and the cost and morbidity of the procedure are lower for the latter. These advantages are counterbalanced by the need for further reintervention to achieve a good clinical result, which penalizes patients treated with angioplasty. Several ongoing studies have compared surgery and angioplasty in patients with ischemic heart disease (14–17). In most of them, except for the RITA trial (15), patients with single coronary stenosis are excluded. In the RITA trial, the results of the subgroup of patients with proximal LAD lesion have not yet been reported. The major problem with the RITA trial is that its patients represent a "melting pot" of many different coronary situations (such as various ejection fractions, proximal or distal stenosis, one or more stenoses on a vessel, various sizes of vessel, and presence of collaterals), making extrapolation of their conclusions to any individual patient difficult.

The use of stents will certainly decrease the need for additional revascularization and the occurrence of acute complications as reported in previous trials comparing PTCA alone with PTCA followed by stent implantation (18–20). This is particularly true for the proximal LAD (21,22). Versaci et al. demonstrated a 40% restenosis rate following conventional angioplasty, versus 19% with stenting in this particular setting. Similar results were reported in the large multicenter BENESTENT II trial with 38% and 16%, respectively. As a corollary, the incidence of cardiac related events in the BENESTENT II LAD subgroup was 13.1% versus 23.9%, whereas repeat intervention rates were 8.6% and 18% respectively. Because the long-term outcome after coronary stenting seems particularly favorable (23), the technique will likely be used more and more often. There is a scarcity of data comparing coronary artery bypass grafting (CABG) to PTCA in patients with single-vessel disease. We designed two prospective randomized trials. In the first trial, conventional PTCA was compared to CABG (left internal mammary artery grafting) and in the second, one PTCA followed by stent implantation was also compared to CABG.

CONVENTIONAL PERCUTANEOUS TRANSLUMINAL CORONARY ANGIOPLASTY VERSUS CORONARY ARTERY BYPASS GRAFTING

In a first trial, surgery using left internal mammary artery grafting was compared with conventional angioplasty in a group of patients with isolated proximal LAD stenosis, documented clinical or silent ischemia, and normal left ventricular ejection fraction. Previous Q-wave myocardial infarction, unstable angina pectoris, or left ventricular ejection fraction below 0.50 were exclusion criteria.

Study design made provision for clinical and functional assessments at 6 months and 1, 2, 3, 4 and 5 years after treatment. Clinical parameters prospectively collected were cardiac death, myocardial infarction (Q- and non–Q-wave), repeat revascularization, angina functional class, exercise tolerance, clinical need for repeat angiography, and postprocedural antianginal drug regimen. Functional status was estimated by means of the functional class and stress test. The interim analysis at 2 years did not show a significant difference for death or myocardial infarction (24). Additional revascularization was sig-

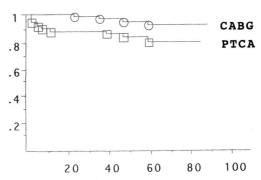

FIG. 20.1. Kaplan-Meier curve of the population free from death and myocardial infarction (months).

nificantly more frequent after PTCA than after CABG. At 5 years, the incidence of death was similar but myocardial infarction occurred more frequently in the PTCA group, mainly because of a higher incidence of non–Q-wave myocardial infarction related to subacute or acute closure during PTCA (Table 20.1). However, the incidence of Q-wave myocardial infarction was not different between CABG and PTCA. Non–Q-wave myocardial infarction was defined as a CK rise ≥ 2 the normal values with a CK MB fraction of $\geq 10\%$ of the total CK for both treatment groups. The survival curve for death and myocardial infarction show a significant difference between CABG and PTCA, but again only

TABLE 20.1. *Primary endpoints at 5 years*

Endpoint	PTCA ($n = 68$)	CABG ($n = 66$)	Relative risk	p value
Death:				
Cardiac death	1 (1.5)	1 (1.5)		.8
Noncardiac death	5 (7.5)	1 (1.5)		
MI:				
<6 months	8 (11)	2 (3)		
>6 months	2 (4)	1 (1)		
Total	10 (15)	3 (4)		.0001
MI and cardiac death:	11 (16)	4 (6)	2.6 (1.1–5.4)	.0004
Revascularization:				
PTCA	13 (19)	6 (9)		
CABG	3 (5)	0		
PTCA + CABG	10 (15)	0		
Any	26 (38)	6 (9)	4.2 (2.8–5.6)	.0001
Any endpoint:	30 (44)	9 (14)	4.2 (2.8–5.6)	.0001

MI, myocardial infarction; PTCA, percutaneous transluminal coronary angioplasty; CABG, coronary artery bypass grafting.

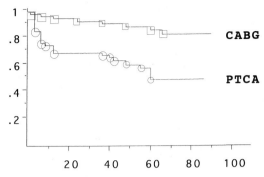

FIG. 20.2. Kaplan-Meier curve of the event free population (month) ($p < .05$).

TABLE 20.3. *Functional class at follow-up*

	PTCA ($n = 68$)	CABG ($n = 66$)
I	50 (74%)	47 (71%)
II	14 (21%)	17 (26%)
III	3 (4.5%)	2 (3 %)
IV	1 (1.5%)	0

PTCA, percutaneous transluminal coronary angioplasty; CABG, coronary artery bypass grafting.

due to an excess of non–Q-wave myocardial infarction in the PTCA group (Figs. 20.1, 20.2). As at 2 years, additional revascularization was significantly more frequent after PTCA (Table 20.2) and, finally, 73% of the patients randomized to PTCA did not require LAD revascularization, compared to 92% in the CABG group. Interestingly, in the PTCA group more non-LAD revascularizations were performed. A higher incidence of repeat angiography in these patients may lead to PTCA because of the "oculostenotic" reflex. The symptomatic assessment showed a dramatic and similar improvement, in that more than 70% of patients in both group were asymptomatic (Table 20.3). We concluded that both surgery and angioplasty improve the clinical status of patients with isolated proximal LAD stenosis with a very low mortality at 5 years. The higher incidence of myocardial infarction with PTCA is due to periprocedural

TABLE 20.2. *Incidence and localization of the revascularization procedures*

	PTCA ($n = 68$)	CABG ($n = 66$)
Patients with revascularization	26 (36%)	6 (9%)
Number of procedures	37	6
LAD revascularization	18 (26%)	3 (4.5%)
Non-LAD revascularization	8 (12%)	3 (4.5%)
No revascularization of the LAD	50 (73%)	63 (95%)

LAD, left anterior descending coronary artery; PTCA, percutaneous transluminal coronary angioplasty; CABG, coronary artery bypass grafting.

complications. The risk of additional revascularization is also higher after PTCA.

Very similar conclusions arise from the MASS trial (25). Indeed, the incidence of any adverse events was significantly lower in the surgical group compared to medical or percutaneous approaches, although the incidence of death and myocardial infarction did not. The differences are mainly due to a higher need for reintervention in the medical and percutaneous treatment.

PERCUTANEOUS TRANSLUMINAL CORONARY ANGIOPLASTY WITH STENT IMPLANTATION VERSUS COMPARE CORONARY ARTERY BYPASS GRAFTING

As discussed previously the use of stents should decrease both the incidence of acute complications and of restenosis. Therefore, we design a new trial (the SIMA trial) comparing stent implantation versus left internal mammary grafting in patients with isolated proximal LAD stenosis with a left ventricular ejection fraction >0.45. Randomization started in 6 European centers in October 1994 and ended in March 1998. A total of 123 patients were included: 63 in the stent group and 60 in the CABG group. Ultimately, two patients had to be excluded and 121 patients were finally analyzed. Lesion type was similar in both groups, with about 60% of B1 and B2 lesions. The mean reference diameter of the vessel was 3.1 mm in the stent group and 3.2 mm in the CABG group, and the percentage stenosis was 76% and 77% respectively. In the stent group, more than 50% of the patients received a Palmaz-Schatz stent (Johnson and Johnson International Systems, Warren, NJ) but the Micro-Stent (Arterial Vascular Engineering,

TABLE 20.4. *Immediate outcome of the patients randomized in the SIMA trial*

	Stent ($n = 62$)	CABG ($n = 59$)	p value
Immediate outcome	1–3 stents 98%	LIMA 98% (min. surg. $n = 6$)	N.S.
Protocol deviation	No stent (1 pt)	SVG (1 pt) 1 LIMA +1 SVG (1 pt)	
Reference diameter	3.1 (2.9–3.39		
MLD post-stenting	3.0 (2.7–3.2)		
% stenosis poststenting	7 (5–12)		
CK (baseline)	121 (81–165)	109 (68–151)	N.S.
CK-MB (baseline)	14 (10–16)	11 (8–14)	
CK (postprocedure)	130 (66–196)	1106 (454–1758)	<.05
CK-MB (postprocedure)	18 (8–28)	64 (25–104)	<.05

PTCA, percutaneous transluminal coronary angioplasty; CABG, coronary artery bypass grafting; MLD, minimum lumen diameter; SVG, saphenous vein graft; LIMA, left internal mammary artery; min. surg., minimal invasive surgery.

Division of Medtronic, Santa Rosa CA), the NIR stent (Scimed, Maple Grove, MN), the Multi-Link stent (Guidant Inc. Santa Clara, CA), the beStent (Medtronic Inc., Minneapolis, MN) and the Jostent (Jomed International AB, Drottning-gatan, Sweden) were also implanted. In the stent group, the final in-stent residual stenosis was 7%. Stent implantation was not possible in one patient and in the surgical group one patient received a saphenous vein graft and one patient received a saphenous vein graft in addition to the mammary artery graft (Table 20.4). The incidence of acute events was similar. One patient in the stent group died and three had non–Q-wave myocardial infarctions. In the CABG group, one patient had a Q-wave myocardial infarction and one a non–Q-wave myocardial infarction. Finally, 93% of the patients in the stent group were free of acute events compared to 96% in the CABG group (Table 20.5). The incidence of minor events such as arrhythmias or bleeding was significantly higher in the CABG

group (See Table 20.5). The mean length of the in-hospital stay was 13 days in the CABG group compared to 2.6 days in the stent group (Table 20.6). An interim analysis will be made at 2 years and a quality of life assessment will also be available. At present, we conclude that both CABG and PTCA followed by stent implantation are safe and efficient with a low and comparable incidence of acute complications. However, long-term results are required before definitive conclusions can be drawn.

LIMITATIONS

The major limitation of trials comparing CABG to PTCA is the definition of non–Q-wave myocardial infarction, especially in the surgical group. It is usually based on the importance of CK rise, but the line between ischemia and necrosis is still unclear and controversial. Thus, in all the trials described here, the incidence of non–Q-wave myocardial infarction may be underestimated, depending on the definition. From trials comparing CABG to PTCA, we have learned that survival and incidence of myocardial infarction are comparable between the two therapies (26). Thus, quality of life should be, in upcoming trials, a primary endpoint.

In view of these results, both surgery and angioplasty are acceptable treatments for an isolated proximal LAD stenosis. Indication for angioplasty in the treatment of single LAD stenosis should be considered in the light of these results. After surgery, some patients will develop other

TABLE 20.5. *In-hospital complications*

	Stent ($n = 62$)	CAGB ($n = 59$)	p value
Death	1 (2%)	0	
Q-wave MI	0	1 (2%)	
Non-Q-wave MI	3 (5%)	1 (2%)	
CVS	0	0	N.S.
Re-PTCA	0	0	
Urgent CAGB	0	0	
Any event	4 (7%)	2 (4%)	

PTCA, percutaneous transluminal coronary angioplasty; CABG, coronary artery bypass grafting; N.S., not significant.

TABLE 20.6. *Length of the in-hospital stay (days)*

	Stent (n = 62)	CABG (n = 59)	p value
Total number in-hospital	2.6 (1.7–3.5)	13 (9–18)	<.0001
Intensive care unit	1.2 (0.6–1.7)	2.3 (1.8–2.7)	<.0001
Ward	1.3 (0.9–1.6)	11 (6–15)	<.0001

lesions of the right or circumflex artery; in those, angioplasty can certainly be used. Moreover, adequate control risk factors can probably slow the progression of the atherosclerotic process. The possible need for future reintervention should not influence the choice of treatment when proximal LAD stenosis is documented.

CONCLUSIONS

Isolated proximal LAD stenosis and normal left ventricular function comprise a particular subset of coronary disease patients. When an aggressive approach is required, PTCA and CABG can both be safely recommended. CABG still has a place in the treatment of these lesions but only if the left internal mammary artery is used. Clearly, the final choice between CABG, PTCA, and PTCA with stent implantation should be based on the angiographic aspect of the lesion, the estimated rate of complications, and a careful discussion with the patient, who must be fully informed of both the advantages and possible complications of each treatment option. Physicians should consider CABG and PTCA with stent implantation as complementary therapeutic options in patients with ischemic heart disease and isolated proximal LAD stenosis, knowing that for some patients CABG is the best choice and for others PTCA is better. However, based on the data of the literature, if PTCA is planned, additional stenting should be performed in patients with single proximal LAD stenosis.

REFERENCES

1. Brooks N, Cattell M, Jennings K, Balcon R., Honey M, Layton C. Isolated disease of left anterior descending coronary artery. Angiographic and clinical study of 218 patients. *Br Heart* 1982;47:71–77.
2. RITA Participants. Coronary angioplasty versus coronary artery bypass surgery: the Randomized Intervention Treatment of Angina (RITA) trial. *Lancet* 1993; 341:573–580.
3. King S, Lembo N, Weintraub W et al., for the Emory Angioplasty Versus Surgery (EAST). A randomized trial comparing coronary angioplasty with coronary bypass surgery. *N Engl J Med* 1994;331:1044–1050.
4. Hamm C, Reimers J, Ischinger T, Rupprecht H-J, Berger J, Bleifeld W, for the German angioplasty bypass surgery investigation. A randomized study of coronary angioplasty compared with bypass surgery in patients with symptomatic multivessel coronary disease. *N Engl J Med* 1994;331:1037–1043.
5. Califf R, Tomabechi Y, Lee K et al. Outcome in one-vessel coronary artery disease. *Circulation* 1983;67: 283–290.
6. Klein L, Weintraub W, Agarwal J et al. Prognostic significance of severe narrowing of the proximal portion of the left anterior descending coronary artery. *Am J Cardiol* 1986;58:42–46.
7. Pijls N, De Bruyne B, Peels K et al. Measurement of fractional flow reserve to assess the functional severity of coronary artery stenoses. *N Engl J Med* 1996;334: 1703–1708.
8. De Bruyne B, Bartunek J, Sys S, Pijls N, Heyndrickx G, Wijns W. Simultaneous coronary pressure and flow velocity measurements in humans. Feasibility, reproducibility, and hemodynamic dependence of coronary flow velocity reserve, hyperemic flow versus pressure slope index, and fractional flow reserve. *Circulation* 1996;94:1842–1849.
9. Varnauskas E, and the European Coronary Surgery Study Group. Twelve-year follow-up of survival in the randomized European Coronary Surgery Study. *N Engl J Med* 1988;319:332–337.
10. Mark DB. Assessment of prognosis in patients with coronary artery disease. In: Rougin GS, Califf RM, O'Neil WW, Philips HR III, Stach RS, eds. *Interventional cardiovascular medicine: principles and practice.* New York: Churchill Livingstone, 1994.
11. Webster J, Moberg C, Zincon G. Natural History of severe proximal coronary artery diseases as documented by coronary cineangiography. *Am J Cardiol* 1974;33: 195–200.
12. Sergeant P, Lesaffre E, Flameng W, Ruy R. Internal mammary artery: methods of use and their effect on survival. *Eur J Cardiothorac Surg* 1990;4:72–78.
13. Parisi A, Folland E, Hartigan P. A comparison of angioplasty with medical therapy in the treatment of single vessel coronary artery disease. *N Engl J Med* 1992;326: 10–16.
14. Akins C, Block P, Palacios I, Gold H, Carroll D, Grunkemeier G. Comparison of coronary artery bypass grafting and percutaneous transluminal coronary angioplasty as initial treatment strategies. *Ann Thorac Surg* 1989; 47:507–516.

15. Frierson J, Dimas A, Whitlow P et al. Angioplasty of the proximal left anterior descending coronary artery: initial success and long-term follow-up. *J Am Cardiol* 1992;19:745–751.

16. BARI, CABRI, EAST, GABI and RITA: coronary angioplasty on trial. *Lancet* 1990;335:1315–1316 (editorial).

17. Kramer J, Proudfit W, Loop F et al. Late follow-up of 781 patients undergoing percutaneous transluminal coronary angioplasty or coronary artery bypass grafting for an isolated obstruction in the left anterior descending coronary artery. *Am Heart J* 1989;118:1144–1153.

18. Fischman D, Savage M, Leon M et al., for the STRESS investigators. Acute and late angiographic results of the STent REStenosis Study (STRESS). *J Am Coll Cardiol* 1994;23:60A(abst).

19. Serruys P, de Jaegere P, Kiemeneij F et al. A comparison of balloon expandable stent implantation with angiography in patients with coronary disease. *N Engl J Med* 1994;331:489–495

20. Serruys P, van Hout B, Bonnier H et al., for the BENESTENT Study Group. Randomised comparison of implantation oh heparin-coated stents with balloon angioplasty in selected patients with coronary artery disease (BENESTENT II). *Lancet* 1998;352:673–681.

21. Versaci F, Gaspardone A, Phil M et al. A comparison of coronary-artery stenting with angioplasty for isolated stenosis of the proximal left anterior descending coronary artery. *N Engl J Med* 1997;336:817–822.

22. Goy J-J., Eeckhout E. Intracoronary stenting. *Lancet* 1998;351:1943–1949.

23. Pocock S, Henderson R, Richards A et al. Meta-analysis of randomised trials comparing coronary angioplasty with bypass surgery. *Lancet* 1995;346:1184–1189.

24. Goy J-J, Eeckhout E, Burnand B et al. Coronary angioplasty versus left internal mammary artery grafting for isolated proximal left anterior descending artery stenosis. *Lancet* 1994;343:1449–1453.

25. Hueb W, Bellotti G, Almeida de Olivera S et al. The medicine angioplasty or surgery study (MASS): a prospective, randomized trial of medical therapy, balloon angioplasty or bypass surgery for single proximal left anterior descending artery stenoses. *JACC* 1995;26:1600–1605.

26. Goy J-J, Eeckhout E, Burnand B et al. Coronary angioplasty versus left internal mammary artery grafting for isolated proximal left anterior descending artery stenosis. *Lancet* 1994;343:1449–1453.

21

Overview of Treatment Selection for Multivessel Disease

A. Multivessel Disease: Medical and Revascularization Options

James G. Jollis and *Daniel B. Mark

*Division of Cardiology, *Department of Medicine, Duke University Medical Center, Durham, North Carolina 27708-3485*

Coronary artery disease (CAD) is a chronic disorder that many patients must endure for decades. The course of the disease for an individual patient is typically characterized by long periods of clinical stability punctuated by acute exacerbation, often taking the form of unstable angina or acute myocardial infarction (MI). Management of the patient with multivessel coronary artery disease requires an understanding of the natural history of CAD along with the potential short- and long-term effects of the different treatment options available. Multivessel CAD may either be diagnosed at cardiac catheterization or suspected from the result of a stress test. For this chapter, we assume the patient has already undergone cardiac catheterization and that the clinician is now faced with the problem of deciding which treatment option to pursue. The major management options in this setting involve choices of medication and coronary revascularization techniques. Other portions of this text review the technical aspects of revascularization. In this chapter, we briefly examine the key concepts involved in the prognostic stratification of the patient with multivessel disease. We then show how the prognosis of the patient relates to treatment selection.

PROGNOSIS IN THE MEDICALLY TREATED PATIENT

CAD Risk Continuum

It is important to understand that multivessel coronary artery disease is not a homogeneous anatomic or prognostic entity and includes both very low risk and very high risk individuals (1). Consequently, merely establishing the presence of multivessel disease is not sufficient to define proper management. Rather, the efficient estimation of the patient's short- and long-term risk of adverse cardiac events (especially death and MI) is the principal foundation on which treatment decisions are made. It is conceptually helpful in thinking about the risks of coronary disease to view the patient's prognosis as the sum of the risks attributable to the patient's current disease state and the risk that the patient's disease will progress to a higher or lower risk state.

The risks associated with the patient's current disease state can be understood with reference to four major types of prognostic measures (Table 21.1). The strongest individual prognostic indicator in coronary disease is the extent of left ventricular damage present. Typically, the ejection fraction is the variable most often used to summarize the state of left ventricular function

TABLE 21.1. *Major prognostic factors in coronary disease relating to current risk state*

Left ventricular function/damage
   History or prior MI
   Congestive heart failure symptoms
   Cardiomegaly on chest radiography
   Ejection fraction
   Regional left ventricular wall-motion abnormalities
   Left ventricular diastolic function
   Mitral regurgitation
   Atrial fibrillation
   Conduction disturbances on ECG
Coronary disease severity
   Anatomic extent of CAD
   Transient ischemia
   Collaterol vessels
Ongoing coronary plaque event
   Symptom course (unstable, progressive, stable)
   Transient ischemia
   Hematologic milieu
Electrical instability
   Ventricular arrhythmias
   Late potentials
   Decreased heart rate variability

From ref. 1, with permission.

(2). However, because it is a ratio (stroke volume over left ventricular end-diastolic volume), compensatory responses to left ventricular damage that serve to maintain cardiac output (e.g., Frank Starling mechanism) may make the ejection fraction an optimistic measure of true left ventricular contractile abilities (3). More recent studies have therefore focused directly on ventricular volumes as indicators of myocardial systolic dysfunction and decompensation (4). Even the observation at left ventricular angiography of a dilated left ventricle (an informal ventricular volume assessment) indicates a higher risk state for any given ejection fraction value than that same ejection fraction with a nondilated ventricle. Cardiomegaly on the plain chest radiograph is a similar measure that has been shown repeatedly to have independent prognostic value (5–7). Another such measure is the presence and severity of congestive heart failure symptoms. (6,8) For any given ejection fraction value, symptomatic heart failure indicates a patient at substantially higher risk than a similar patient without congestive heart failure symptoms (9).

Ischemic mitral regurgitation is now recognized as an important and often underdiagnosed problem in multivessel coronary disease patients (6,10,11). Overall, about 20% of CAD patients presenting for diagnostic cardiac catheterization have some degree of mitral regurgitation, and 3% have severe regurgitation. Pathophysiologically, there are three major forms of this disorder, each with somewhat different prognostic implications. The most common form is papillary muscle dysfunction, which is typically due to posterior wall infarction caused by occlusion of the circumflex or right coronary arteries. Such infarcts result in posteromedial papillary muscle dysfunction and restriction of the posterior mitral valve leaflet. Mitral regurgitation resulting from papillary muscle dysfunction may be associated with a good long-term prognosis if it is caused by a culprit lesion in the arterial supply to the papillary muscle that can be revascularized, and if the overall state of the left ventricle is good. The second type of mitral regurgitation seen in ischemic heart disease is that resulting from global left ventricular dilation with secondary disruption of the function of the mitral valve apparatus. Dilation of the left ventricle caused by ischemic damage will move the papillary muscles out of proper alignment, with resulting incomplete systolic coaptation of the mitral leaflets and varying degrees of regurgitation. In addition, long-standing left ventricular dilation may result in secondary dilation of the mitral annulus, also disrupting proper valvular function. This form of mitral regurgitation is associated with a poor prognosis, largely because of the severity of underlying left ventricular dysfunction. The final and least common type of ischemic mitral regurgitation is papillary muscle rupture, which typically occurs as a consequence of acute MI and is seen in less than 1% of such patients. The picture here is one of abrupt hemodynamic deterioration with acute pulmonary edema and a rapid downhill course unless the disorder is promptly recognized and aggressively treated. In studies in the Duke Database for Cardiovascular Diseases, we have found that mitral regurgitation of 1 + or greater severity is a significant adverse prognostic factor, and severe regurgitation is a major independent determinant of survival in coronary disease (11–13). Because mitral regurgitation provides a form of afterload reduction to the left ventricle, the combination of a significantly depressed left ventricular ejection fraction and moderate or severe mitral regurgitation is a worrisome one, because it indicates that the true systolic performance of the ventricle is probably significantly worse than the ejection fraction would suggest.

There is an ongoing debate about whether ventricular arrhythmias and late potentials are merely markers of a significantly damaged myocardium or are actually independent indicators of a separate dimension of risk for the patient with coronary disease (14). A similar debate exists about the prognostic significance of atrial arrhythmias and interventricular conduction defects. Atrial fibrillation is an uncommon arrhythmia in coronary disease, with an estimated prevalence 0.6% in the Coronary Artery Surgery Study (CASS) registry (15). The CASS investigators reported that atrial fibrillation in coronary disease correlated particularly with the presence of ischemic mitral regurgitation and with symptomatic heart failure. Even after accounting for these factors, however, atrial fibrillation was associated with approximately a doubling of the patient's risk of dying, compared with sinus rhythm. Similar observations have been made about interventricular conduction disturbances, particularly left bundle branch block or incomplete conduction defects that did not meet full criteria for left bundle branch block (16).

After left ventricular function, the most important prognostic characteristics of the coronary disease patient relate to the anatomic extent and severity of coronary atherosclerosis. Traditionally, the extent of disease is measured as "the number of diseased vessels." In this system, the coronary tree is divided into three distributions: the left anterior descending (including diagonal branches), the left circumflex (including marginal branches), and the posterior descending artery. If a 70% (visual assessment) or greater diameter stenosis is present in any large segment of the distribution, it is considered "significant." Conceptually, the number of diseased vessels is intended to convey a sense of the magnitude of jeopardy faced by the corresponding three major segments of the left ventricle. While this classification is very widely used,

it is insufficiently informative for either clinical decision making or for prognostic studies. For example, a patient with a 75% distal right coronary lesion and a 75% second circumflex marginal lesion has two-vessel disease, as does a patient with a 99% proximal left anterior descending lesion and a proximal 99% right coronary lesion (assuming right dominance), but they clearly have significantly different prognoses and may require different therapeutic strategies.

Over the last two decades, many investigators have tried to improve the "number of diseased vessels" classification system. Although some innovations may provide a more informative and prognostically rich classification, no such effort to date has met with general clinical acceptance. The one system that has achieved some use in research studies is the coronary artery jeopardy score derived by Johnson and colleagues at the Massachusetts General Hospital and validated independently by Califf and colleagues at Duke (17). The score divides a stereotypic coronary tree into six major segments and assigns two points to each segment with a 70% or greater stenosis. The score values thus range from 0 (no significant CAD) to 12 (significant left main and right CAD) and stratify prognosis significantly better than a simple, number of diseased vessels classification. However, the score has several important limitations that are characteristic of most attempts in this area. First, all lesions of 70% or greater are treated as prognostically equivalent without taking into account the true amount of myocardium at risk or the varying risk associated with different degrees of "significant" coronary stenosis. Second, the score does not take into account the presence of serial lesions or collateral vessels, and the variable branching pattern of the coronary tree in different patients cannot be accounted for. Third, the score does not consider morphologic and pathophysiologic characteristics of the atherosclerotic plaques, such as the presence of attached thrombus. Finally, the viability of myocardium downstream from each lesion is not considered in assessing whether that lesion truly "jeopardizes" myocardium.

New approaches in this area involve taking

advantage of powerful new computerized coronary tree programs that allow for processing of much more detailed information than the typical clinician is capable of assimilating. Our group proposed an intermediate strategy that took advantage of more detailed information available from the typical clinician interpretation of the coronary angiogram, but did not require quantitative analysis of the coronary tree or computer processing to create the score (1,18,19). The Duke Index (Table 21.2), which is hierarchical and assigns each patient to the worst category applicable to them, takes into account prognostically important information about lesion severity (e.g., a 95% lesion represents a higher risk than a 75% stenosis) and location (e.g., a proximal lesion represents a higher risk than a nonproximal lesion, especially in the left anterior descending artery). To keep this system relatively simple, categories with similar prognoses were collapsed together to reduce the total number of categories in the final index. Prognostic weights have been assigned using Cox regression analyses and a linear transformation so that the score ranges from 0 (no CAD) to 100 ($\geq$95% left main disease). This new index can identify important anatomic subsets of patients with multivessel disease who derive particular benefit from percutaneous transluminal coronary angioplasty (PTCA) or from coronary artery bypass

TABLE 21.2. *Duke prognostic CAD index*

Extent of CAD	Prognostic weight (0–100)
No CAD $\geq$ 50%	0
1 VD 50%–74%	19
>1 VD 50%–74%	23
1 VD 75%	23
1 VD $\geq$ 95%	32
2 VD	37
2 VD, both $\geq$ 95%	42
1 VD, $\geq$ 95% proximal LAD	48
2 VD, 95% LAD	48
2 VD, $\geq$ 95% proximal LAD	56
3 VD	56
3 VD, $\geq$ 95% in at least one	63
3 VD, proximal LAD	67
3 VD, $\geq$ 95% proximal LAD	74
Left main 75%	82
Left main $\geq$ 95%	100

VD, ventricular damage; LAD, left anterior descending.

graft (CABG) that were not evident using the overall number of diseased vessels classification (20–22).

Work in quantitative coronary angiography has challenged the primacy of the long-accepted, visually determined, "significant" coronary stenosis (23). While the percent diameter stenosis assessed by quantitative coronary angiography is undoubtedly both more accurate and more consistent than the visual determination, it is as yet unclear that use of these measurements improves clinical decision making or prognostic risk stratification. Investigators in the Angioplasty Compared to Medicine (ACME) study found that visual stenosis measurement actually correlated better with exercise capacity on the treadmill than did stenosis measurements with quantitative angiography or hand-held calipers (24).

The occurrence of transient ischemia provides another marker of the severity of CAD. Although many investigators refer to this phenomenon as "silent ischemia," the use of this term emphasizes an artificial dichotomy among ischemic episodes that is probably no longer relevant. The original reason for making such a distinction was based on Cohn's hypothesis that silent ischemia reflected a "defective anginal warning system" that would place patients who manifested this phenomenon at a particularly increased risk of adverse prognostic events relative to their symptomatic counterparts (25). For the most part, the defective anginal warning system theory has not been borne out by the evidence. It is now well established that many CAD patients have a majority of their ischemic events without symptoms (26,27). Growing evidence now suggests that ischemia occurs on a continuum and that the frequency and extent of transient ischemic episodes (both symptomatic and silent) correlate strongly with the severity of underlying coronary disease. What remains unsettled is the extent to which transient ischemia provides independent prognostic information about the patient's disease beyond that available from an examination of the coronary arteriogram. It is possible, and many clinicians believe, that transient ischemia during exercise testing or ambulatory monitoring helps to differentiate otherwise similar-looking coronary lesions with differing "functional" importance (26)

The third major group of prognostic variables related to risks of the current disease state in CAD consists of indicators of whether a recent coronary plaque event has occurred. Current thinking, supported by a growing body of pathologic, angioscopic, and ultrasound data, is that atherosclerotic plaque rupture is the initiating event for most of the adverse clinical consequences of coronary disease (28–30). Coronary plaque rupture appears to occur most commonly in high-risk plaques, which are those with a cholesterol-rich core and a thin, fibrous cap (30,31). Rupture appears to take place most often at the shoulder of the plaque in an area where the plaque cap is particularly thin. The proximate cause is still a matter of active investigation and is believed related to transient hemodynamic changes, as well as to changes in the composition of the plaque itself (32). In particular, the presence of inflammatory cells and metalloproteinases released by these cells may be responsible for creating the predisposition to rupture (33). The inflammatory reaction in the plaque may be infectious in etiology, although proof of this is still lacking (34). The extent of disruption of the plaque cap caused by rupture varies considerably. In less severe cases, there is minimal associated thrombus formation; the plaque may enlarge during the healing process, but otherwise such cases are usually asymptomatic. At the other end of the spectrum, severe disruption of the plaque cap may lead to a large, obstructive coronary thrombus and acute MI. Interestingly, while most of the focus in the treatment of coronary disease has been on plaques judged to be "significant" by coronary angiography (i.e., at least 75% stenosis), these are not the only plaques that are now believed to be associated with risk for rupture and associated thrombosis. The "insignificant" plaques that are noted with varying frequency on coronary angiography and that are not suitable for treatment with either PTCA or CABG are now believed to be a significant source of plaque events for many coronary disease patients (28,29).

Clinically, the principal marker of an unstable coronary plaque is a change in the patient's symptom pattern, typically manifesting as a sudden increase in the frequency, severity, or ease with which ischemic attacks are provoked. In a detailed evaluation of the prognostic information available from the patient's routine anginal history, we found that the presence of increasingly progressive symptoms over the preceding 6 weeks and a greater frequency of symptoms were both strong predictors of prognosis, even when information on left ventricular ejection fraction and coronary disease severity from cardiac catheterization was taken into account (35). Conversely, a stable symptom pattern suggests the absence of a recent plaque event of clinical consequence, although there are clearly some situations in which a crescendo pattern of ischemia develops without the patient's awareness of symptoms.

Despite the substantial limitation of symptom status as a measure of disease activity, as yet there is not a more efficient objective method for identifying CAD patients experiencing a significant plaque event. Neither exercise testing nor ambulatory monitoring is practical for screening for plaque events, as they cannot be repeated frequently enough to provide adequate surveillance. It is quite clear from recent work (and our own experience bears this out) that plaque events can develop and progress quite rapidly, so that it is possible for a patient to have a negative adequate exercise study and shortly after to develop a large anterior MI.

The fourth major domain of CAD risk relates to the electrical stability (or lack thereof) of the myocardium. A large number of studies have evaluated the relationship between various forms of ventricular arrhythmias and prognosis in coronary disease. In general, the findings from these studies are that malignant ventricular arrhythmias (e.g., sustained ventricular tachycardia, ventricular fibrillation) are significant adverse prognostic markers except when they occur in the earliest phase (e.g., first 48 hours) of acute MI. The significance of lesser degrees of ventricular arrhythmias, such as frequent premature ventricular contractions or nonsustained ventricular tachycardia, remains more controversial. There are two points of view represented in current literature. One suggests that these lesser ventricular arrhythmias are markers for myocardial electrical instability. The other point of view is that such arrhythmias are a consequence of left ventricular dysfunction and scarring and do not convey independent prognostic information. This debate has been complicated by the findings of the Cardiac Arrhythmia Suppression Trial (CAST), showing that antiarrhythmic drugs that were quite effective in suppressing ventricular arrhythmias actually increased mortality in a cohort of post-MI patients (36). In contrast, beta blockers and coronary bypass surgery, two therapies whose primary impact is on ischemia rather than on arrhythmias, have both been reported to diminish sudden cardiac death (37,38).

The measurement of late potentials on the signal-averaged ECG has been used to identify patients at risk for sudden cardiac death. Late potentials are believed to indicate the electrophysiologic substrate for reentrant ventricular tachycardia, and numerous studies have reported that late potentials are powerful adverse prognostic findings that are independent of the results of ambulatory monitoring for ventricular arrhythmias and left ventricular ejection fraction (39). The clinical utility of this measure continues to be debated. Investigations into heart rate variability have yielded another marker for high risk that is of uncertain pathophysiologic or therapeutic significance (40–42). Heart rate variability is presumed to reflect the net effects of the parasympathetic and sympathetic nervous systems, both of which have been shown to be important in affecting the threshold for ventricular fibrillation. Neither late potentials nor heart rate variability has yet been accepted as part of the standard risk assessment for CAD.

Along with these measures of risk from the current disease state, prognosis in coronary disease depends importantly on the probability that the disease process will move to a higher or lower risk state. For the most part, we now believe that shifts in risk state are related to changes in coronary plaques, as described earlier. Because detection of plaque events is still very indirect and imprecise, our understanding of their pathophysiology remains poor. It is believed that high-risk atherosclerotic plaques, that

is, those plaques that have a large liquid cholesterol core and a thin, fibrous cap (as discussed), cycle through phases of particular vulnerability to rupture because of inflammation and healing responses due to factors that are incompletely defined. A vulnerable, high-risk plaque is one in which a plaque event can be initiated by normal physiologic stresses on the circulatory system. In the setting of a vulnerable plaque, a fortuitous triggering event (such as a surge in blood pressure that might be caused by a sudden change in physical activity or emotional state) might then initiate an active plaque event (43). At present, the best we can do to identify the major risks of progression of disease is to target those factors that predict the occurrence of the disease, namely, the standard cardiovascular risk factors such as smoking, diabetes, hypertension, and hypercholesterolemia.

EFFECTS OF MEDICAL THERAPY ON PROGNOSIS

As fundamental as the question is, surprisingly little of the literature on the prognosis of CAD deals with the issue of whether medical therapy itself affects the natural history of the disease. Most prognostic studies of CAD have passively assumed that medical therapy does not affect outcome and that all forms of medical therapy perform equivalently in this regard. It is now clear, however, that these are pragmatic rather than scientific decisions. Given the profusion of individual therapeutic agents available for treatment of CAD and the lack of consensus about the optimal medical regimen for any given type of patient, analysis of the effects of medical therapy can become prohibitively complex outside the realm of a carefully controlled, randomized trial. The complexity of the problem notwithstanding, there is now strong evidence that many agents do in fact affect survival in CAD.

Some of the most convincing evidence available to date about the benefits of medical therapy in CAD relate to aspirin (44). Because platelets are one of the principal participants in the thrombotic consequences of a coronary plaque event, platelet inhibition is now viewed as a key therapeutic strategy in controlling the acute manifestations of the disease. Evidence about the survival benefits of aspirin come from several, large-scale trials (44,45). In the asymptomatic population (subjects with preclinical CAD), the evidence is still inconclusive, although aspirin has been shown to reduce the risk of first nonfatal MI by 33%. In chronic stable angina, the Physician's Health Study (46) reported an 87% statistically significant reduction in the risk of first nonfatal MI and a 49% nonstatistically significant reduction in mortality. In unstable angina, aspirin has been shown in four randomized trials to improve prognosis relative to placebo, producing reduction in mortality and MI rates of near 50% (45). In acute MI, the ISIS II trial showed that low-dose aspirin given immediately reduced the 30-day mortality by a magnitude equivalent to and additive with that of thrombolytic therapy. At least eight separate trials have evaluated the role of aspirin after acute MI. While individually these trials have arrived at conflicting conclusions, when pooled, they suggest a 10% to 15% reduction in long-term mortality and a 20% to 30% reduction in reinfarction (44).

Glycoprotein IIb/IIIa receptor antagonists are a newer, more powerful class of antiplatelet agents. To date, only intravenous forms of these drugs have been approved for use in the United States. Abciximab is approved for use as an adjunct to percutaneous coronary intervention procedures, while eptifibatide and tirofiban are approved for use in acute coronary syndrome patients (47–51). Several oral glycoprotein IIb/IIIa blockers are being studied in ongoing clinical trials for secondary prevention (52).

Beta-adrenergic blocking agents are another class of pharmacologic agents for which there is strong evidence of prognostic benefit in CAD. Most of the data available so far, however, relate to the acute MI and post-MI phases of the disease. There are no data supporting the use of prophylactic beta-blockers in asymptomatic subjects, and there are no adequate controlled data about the survival effects of beta-blockers in stable angina. Three double-blind, randomized trials have compared beta-blockers with placebo in unstable angina (45). A metaanalysis of the available trials indicates a 13% reduction

in the risk of progression of acute MI (46). However, no clear effect on mortality has yet been demonstrated. In acute MI patients not receiving thrombolytic therapy, beta-blockers lower mortality by approximately 15% when given acutely (53). They also lower mortality by around 20% and reduce the risk of reinfarction by approximately 25% when started in the predischarge phase and continued for the first several years after MI. Whether beta-blockers also provide prognostic benefits in patients who are given reperfusion therapy is at present less clear-cut. The mechanism of benefit of beta-blockers in preventing cardiac death is uncertain, may be multifactorial, and is believed to be a class effect rather than the property of one or more of the individual agents in this class of drugs.

Nitrates are the oldest class of pharmacologic agents used for treatment of ischemic heart disease. There are no controlled trials that have tested the prognostic effects of these drugs on asymptomatic subjects or on patients with stable angina. There are also no randomized, placebo-controlled trials in unstable angina dealing with the effects on cardiac events. The GISSI 3 (transdermal glyceryl trinitrates) (54) and the ISIS 4 (isosorbide mononitrate) (55) trials showed that routine nitrate use for 6 weeks after acute MI in a population receiving thrombolytic therapy does not produce a clinically relevant benefit. In addition, the long-term prognostic effects of nitrates after MI remain undefined, although one retrospective study has suggested benefit. The potential mechanism of prognostic benefit with nitrates is assumed to relate to their hemodynamic effects (decreased preload and afterload) or their direct dilating effects on epicardial coronary vessels and collateral vessels. In addition, an antiplatelet effect of nitrates has been suggested (56).

The role of calcium channel blocking agents as antianginal drugs remains controversial (57). Five trials of nifedipine in acute MI have all shown better survival in the placebo-treated patients. A randomized trial on amlodipine, a second-generation dihydroperidine with a longer duration of action than nifedipine, showed no difference in mortality for patients with ischemic cardiomyopathy (58). One large trial of diltiazem in acute MI showed no overall mortality effect but an increased mortality in patients with impaired left ventricular function and a decreased mortality in the subgroup of patients with well-preserved left ventricular function (59). Two trials of verapamil in acute MI have reported beneficial trends for the treatment group. Diltiazem has also been shown to reduce early nonfatal reinfarction in patients with non–Q-wave MI (60). Calcium blockers have vasodilatory properties that make them potent antianginal agents, and they also reduce cardiac preload and afterload. In addition, some work has suggested that these drugs may inhibit the progression of atherosclerosis. However, the potential for adverse prognostic effects, particularly in patients with left ventricular dysfunction, is disturbing and remains incompletely defined at present. Therefore, many have advised using these drugs as second- or third-line agents in CAD patients (45).

Angiotensin-converting enzyme (ACE) inhibitor use has substantially increased over the last few years following the demonstration in several clinical trials of an improved survival for patients with left ventricular dysfunction and acute MI (54,55,61–65). Two trials have also suggested that these agents may produce a reduction in nonfatal MI, although the mechanism for this has yet to be defined (61).

Cholesterol-lowering agents, specifically drugs that inhibit HMG-CoA reductase, have most recently been shown to reduce cardiac events and mortality. Such benefits have been seen for asymptomatic patients with elevated lipid panels (66,67) and for symptomatic patients with known coronary disease (68,69).

In summary, there is much evidence that medical therapy importantly affects the prognosis of CAD, although not necessarily always in a beneficial fashion. In addition, it seems reasonable to assume that medical therapy has improved in its efficacy over the past 20 years, although few direct empirical data are available to support this contention. The relationship between the prognostic effects of medial therapy and the angiographic extent of CAD has gone largely unexplored.

EFFECTS OF REVASCULARIZATION THERAPY ON CAD PROGNOSIS

Much of our understanding of the prognostic effects of coronary revascularization come from the earlier work comparing coronary bypass surgery with medical therapy (12,70). Investigations by our group and others using statistical models have shown that coronary bypass surgery acts specifically to reduce long-term mortality risk attributable to coronary disease by an amount proportional to the extent of the coronary disease present. In other words, an effective coronary bypass surgery procedure substantially mitigates or even neutralizes the risk of dying attributable to the coronary disease present. Bypass surgery, however, does not alter the risk from noncoronary prognostic factors, such as older age or low ejection fraction. It also does not prevent the subsequent occurrence of MI (71). What coronary bypass surgery does do is to make any subsequent MI likely to be significantly smaller than it otherwise would have been, and consequently more survivable for the patient (72).

The prognostic benefits of coronary bypass surgery can be summarized in terms of its relative effect (e.g., a 50% reduction in the risk of dying relative to medical therapy) or its absolute effect (e.g., an increase in the 5-year survival rate from 75% to 95%), or both. The relative scale tells us about the magnitude of efficacy of the procedure. Thus, bypass surgery in a patient with critical left main disease produces a substantially greater relative reduction in mortality risk than does a procedure performed on a patient with two-vessel disease, even though both patients may have a significant improvement in their life expectancy from the procedure. On the other hand, the absolute difference in survival rates with surgery versus medicine provides information reflecting both the relative efficacy of the procedure and the degree of risk associated with continued conservative (i.e., medical) therapy. Thus, a group of patients with three-vessel disease who are 55 years old and have good left ventricular function and no major comorbidity will have the same relative benefit from bypass surgery as a group of patients with same coronary anatomy who are all 75 years old and have an ejection fraction of 35%, but the latter group will have a substantially greater absolute increment in their survival from the procedure. In other words, while bypass surgery does not work any better in high-risk patients, the relative benefits of the procedure are magnified by the noncoronary factors that increase the patient's medical risk of cardiovascular death. The largest survival benefits of bypass surgery in absolute terms are thus observed in patients with the most severe CAD and the highest absolute medical risk.

The prognostic effects of coronary angioplasty and other percutaneous interventions relative to medicine and bypass surgery have been addressed by a number of studies. We examined our experience with over 9,000 patients with symptomatic CAD treated with medicine, coronary angioplasty, or coronary bypass surgery at Duke Medical Center over a 7-year period (18,73). Our major findings can be summarized

as follows (Figs. 21.1 through 21.7). In patients with the most severe coronary disease (i.e., three-vessel disease, and two-vessel disease with a 95% proximal left anterior descending lesion), bypass surgery significantly improved survival relative to both medical therapy and angioplasty. In intermediate levels of CAD (i.e., other forms of two-vessel disease), revascularization appeared to offer a modest survival benefit, with coronary angioplasty having a slight advantage over bypass surgery because of its lower procedural mortality rate. In single-vessel disease patients, revascularization did not offer any prognostic advantage up to 5 years over initial medical therapy.

A number of randomized trials have compared angioplasty and bypass surgery for multivessel coronary disease, including BARI, CABRI, EAST, RITA, GABI, and ERACI (74–82). To date, these studies have shown similar survival to 5 years, with a slight advantage for bypass surgery (75). Angioplasty involves lower costs with the initial procedure, while the

1 Vessel Disease

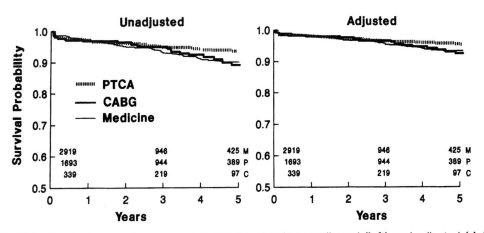

FIG. 21.1. Survival curves for one-vessel disease showing unadjusted **(left)** and adjusted **(right)** comparisons of the three treatment groups to demonstrate absolute survival differences. The x-axis shows follow-up time out to 5 years. The y-axis shows cardiovascular survival probability from 1.0 to .5. Numbers at the bottom of the plots show number of patients in each treatment group remaining to be followed at 0, 3, and 5 years of follow-up. PTCA, percutaneous transluminal coronary angioplasty (*P*); CABG, coronary artery bypass graft surgery (*C*); *M,* medically treated. (From ref. 18, with permission.)

2 Vessel Disease

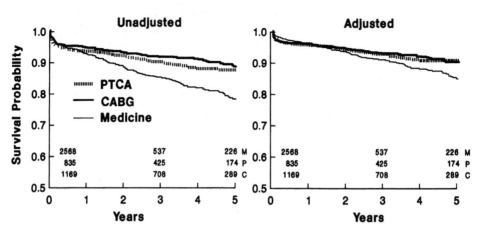

FIG. 21.2. Survival curves for two-vessel disease. See Fig. 21.1 for orientation. PTCA, percutaneous transluminal coronary angioplasty (*P*); CABG, coronary artery bypass graft surgery (*C*); *M*, medically treated. (From ref. 18, with permission.)

3 Vessel Disease

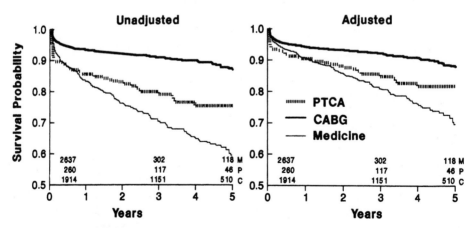

FIG. 21.3. Survival curves for three-vessel disease. See Fig. 21.1 for orientation. PTCA, percutaneous transluminal angioplasty (*P*); CABG, coronary artery bypass graft surgery (*C*); *M,* medically treated. (From ref. 18, with permission.)

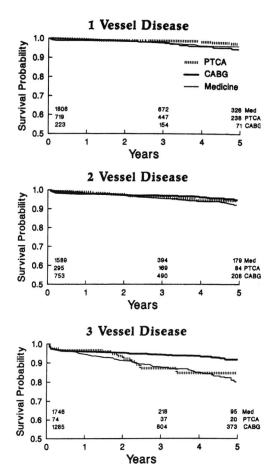

FIG. 21.4. Adjusted survival curves for one-, two-, and three-vessel disease, excluding patients with acute MI within 2 weeks. Patterns seen in Figs. 21.1 through 21.3 are clearly preserved in the nonacute MI portion of the study population. PTCA, percutaneous transluminal coronary angioplasty; CABG, coronary artery bypass graft surgery; Med, medically treated. (From ref. 18, with permission.)

need for repeat procedures following angioplasty results in similar costs over the long term (83). Both surgery and angioplasty have undergone significant improvement since these trials were completed, and the relative superiority of either technique as currently practiced is still uncertain. Coronary stents, now used in approximately 50% or more percutaneous coronary interventions, have significantly reduced early complications and the need for repeat proce-

dures relative to balloon angioplasty (84). Use of adjunctive abciximab and coronary stenting together appears to provide the lowest early complication rate and best long-term outcomes of any of the percutaneous strategies (85). Bypass surgery has also been associated with declining procedural mortality.

OVERVIEW OF THE THERAPEUTIC APPROACH TO THE PATIENT WITH MULTIVESSEL CAD

Despite the enormous number of revascularization procedures done in the United States each year, there is surprisingly still no consensus about their appropriate use. There are six main factors that we take into account when assessing treatment options for multivessel disease patients: (a) their overall risk of cardiac events with continued medical therapy, considering the factors described earlier in this chapter; (b) the projected prognostic benefits of revascularization as described in the last section of this chapter; (c) the severity of ischemic symptoms and associated impairment of functional status; (d) the technical feasibility of percutaneous interventions and of CABG; (e) the presence and extent of major comorbidity; and (f) the patient's preferences. The first two considerations generally dictate that for significant left main disease or high-risk multivessel disease (e.g., with a proximal high-grade left anterior descending stenosis and depressed left ventricular function, or an acute coronary syndrome), bypass surgery remains the preferred option. Limitations in physical activities and functional status caused by ischemic symptoms are another indication for revascularization. Coronary angioplasty demonstrated a modest advantage over medical therapy in improving exercise performance and symptom relief in single-vessel disease in the ACME trial (86). For multivessel disease patients, both angioplasty and surgery improve functional status relative to medicine (87). In addition, results from the EAST and BARI trials suggest that bypass surgery is associated with somewhat better symptom relief in such patients than is angioplasty (83,88). Whether an individual patient is having enough ischemic symptoms to make revascularization the preferred approach depends

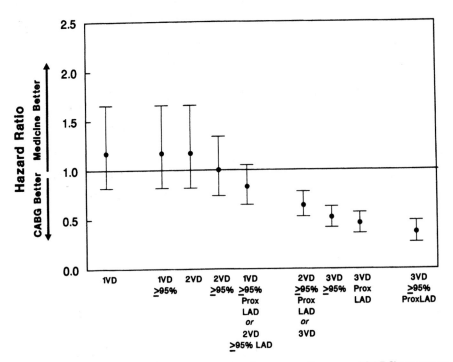

FIG. 21.5. Hazard (mortality) ratios for coronary artery bypass graft surgery (*CABG*) versus medicine calculated from the Cox regression model to evaluate relative survival differences. *Points* indicate hazard ratios for each level of the CAD index; *bars* indicate 99% confidence intervals. *Horizontal line* at ratio of 1.0 indicates point of prognostic equivalence between treatments. Hazard ratios below the line favor CABG; those above the line favor medicine. VD, vessel disease; Prox LAD, proximal left anterior descending artery. (From ref. 18, with permission.)

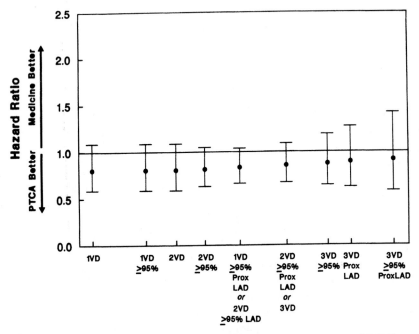

FIG. 21.6. Hazard ratios for percutaneous transluminal coronary angioplasty (*PTCA*) versus medicine. See Fig. 21.5 for orientation. *Points* below 1.0 favor PTCA. VD, vessel disease; Prox LAD, proximal left anterior descending coronary artery. (From ref. 18, with permission.)

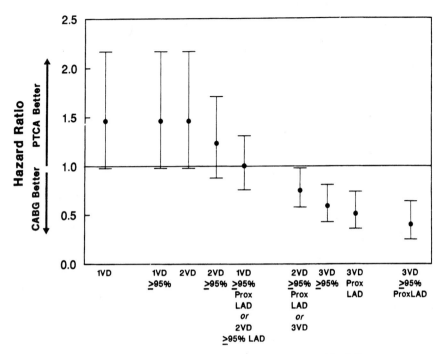

FIG. 21.7. Hazard ratios for coronary artery bypass graft surgery (*CABG*) versus percutaneous transluminal coronary angioplasty (*PTCA*). See Figure 21.5 for orientation. *Points* below 1.0 favor CABG. VD, vessel disease; Prox LAD, proximal left anterior descending coronary artery. (From ref. 18, with permission.)

on both the initial success of medical therapy in controlling such symptoms and the willingness of the patient to accept the procedural risks of revascularization to achieve better symptom control and higher functional status.

A number of anatomic considerations guide selection of coronary revascularization techniques. Morphologic lesion characteristics that favor percutaneous interventions include short length, lack of calcification, location in a large-caliber vessel, and lack of involvement of a branching vessel. Characteristics that make percutaneous intervention less likely to be successful include tortuous vessels, long-standing total occlusions, and eccentric or ostial plaques. Significant left main lesions (e.g., ≥50% diameter stenosis) generally preclude percutaneous intervention in the left coronary system unless the system is "protected" by a previously placed bypass graft. The availability of and experience with percutaneous techniques such as coronary stents, directional and rotational atherectomy,

and laser have broadened the range and complexity of lesions that may be successfully approached. The presence of anatomic characteristics unfavorable to percutaneous intervention will often lead us to recommend bypass surgery in patients for whom revascularization is deemed desirable.

Anatomic and morphologic considerations may also weigh against selection of bypass surgery as the preferred therapeutic option. Diffuse distal vessel disease or small vessel diameter may preclude satisfactory placement of grafts. Lack of adequate bypass conduit because of previous vein stripping, bypass surgery, or subclavian artery disease (limiting internal mammary artery flow) may also limit the therapeutic choices. Similarly, previous inflammatory pericardial processes or severely impaired left ventricular function are factors that may weigh against selection of bypass surgery. The availability of and experience with newer surgical techniques, such as use of the radial artery conduit, may broaden the range of complex patients that can be considered for surgery.

Major comorbidity, such as advanced chronic obstructive lung disease or dialysis-dependent renal failure, substantially alters the risk:benefit ratio for invasive therapies. Unfortunately, these patients often present with high-risk multivessel disease and thus pose the dilemma of having the most to gain from invasive therapy but also the highest risk of major complications and a prolonged postprocedural recovery. The literature in this area is still inadequate to define when, in these patients, the risks associated with their comorbidity exceed the projected benefits of revascularization. Thus, each clinician tends to approach such patients with a level of aggressiveness dictated by their recent experience with other similar patients (e.g., ''The last patient like this I did an angioplasty on did great'' or '' ... spent months in the ICU after the procedure.'') Clearly, more work is needed in this area to put therapeutic decision making on a firmer footing.

We listed patient preferences last in the factors we consider when making treatment recommendations for our patients, not because they are least important but because it is least clear how best to assess and incorporate them. Some patients come to the hospital expressing strong preferences for a particular therapy or strong aversions to a particular therapy, often based on experiences of family members, friends, or colleagues. Such opinions may reflect an inadequate information base rather than carefully reasoned preferences. Of course, deciding whether to undergo a high-risk angioplasty or bypass operation is not like deciding which automobile or television to buy. Consumers usually have a much better understanding of what such purchases will provide in the way of benefits. In addition, consumers do not usually face an overt risk of immediate death or major comorbidity from their nonmedical purchasing decision.

In contrast, selecting medical therapy or one of several revascularization options is usually done without a full understanding of the choices or their downstream consequences and does involve some immediate personal risk of death or major disability. We have investigated better ways of incorporating personal patient prefer-

ences into the therapeutic decision-making process as part of the Ischemic Heart Disease Patient Outcome Research Team (PORT) project. One such method involves the use of an interactive video disk that presents to the patient an individualized risk profile and a thorough description of treatment options (89). Work in this project has shown that patients vary greatly in the degree to which they are bothered by anginal symptoms and diminished functional status. The also vary greatly in their willingness to accept short-term risk in exchange for long-term gains. With the growth of the electronic media, we anticipate that bedside tools will become readily available to help better educate the patient on treatment options and to allow therapeutic decisions to better reflect the preferences of the patient along with the objective risk:benefit considerations.

REFERENCES

1. Mark DB. Assessment of prognosis in patients with coronary artery disease. In: Roubin GS, Califf RM, O'Neill WW, Phillips HR III, Stack RS, eds. *Interventional cardiovascular medicine: principles and practice.* New York: Churchill Livingstone, 1994:165–185.
2. Pryor DB, Bruce RA, Chaitman BR, et al. Task force I: determination of prognosis in patients with ischemic heart disease. *J Am Coll Cardiol* 1989;14(4): 1016–1025.
3. Konstam MA, Kronenberg MW, Udelson JE, et al. Effectiveness of preload reserve as a determinant of clinical status in patients with left ventricular systolic dysfunction. *Am J Cardiol* 1992;69:1591–1595.
4. Eng C. Enlargement of the heart. *Heart Failure* 1991; 15–24.
5. Harrell FE Jr, Lee KL, Califf RM, Pryor DB, Rosati RA. Regression modeling strategies for improved prognostic prediction. *Stat Med* 1984;3:143–152.
6. Harris PJ, Harrell FE Jr, Lee KL, Behar VS, Rosati RA. Survival in medically treated coronary artery disease. *Circulation* 1979;60:1259–1269.
7. Hammermeister KE, DeRouen TA, Dodge . Variables predictive of survival in patients with coronary disease: selection by univariate and multivariate analyses from the clinical, electrocardiographic, exercise, arteriographic, and quantitative angiographic evaluations. *Circulation* 1979;59:421–430.
8. Bounous EP Jr, Mark DB, Pollock BG, et al. Surgical survival benefits for coronary disease patients with left ventricular dysfunction. *Circulation* 1988;78[Suppl I]:I151–I157.
9. Clements IP, Brown ML, Zinsmeister AR, Gibbons RJ. Influence of left ventricular diastolic filling on symptoms and survival in patients with decreased left ventricular systolic function. *Am J Cardiol* 1991;67: 1245–1250.

10. Tcheng JE, Jackman JD, Nelson CL, et al. Outcome of patients sustaining acute ischemic mitral regurgitation during myocardial infarction. *Ann Intern Med* 1992;117: 18–24.

11. Hickey MS, Smith LR, Muhlbaier LH, et al. Current prognosis of ischemic mitral regurgitation: implications for future management. *Circulation* 1988;78[Suppl I]:I51–I59.

12. Califf RM, Harrell FE Jr, Lee KL, et al. The evolution of medical and surgical therapy for coronary artery disease: a 15-year perspective. *JAMA* 1989;261: 2077–2086.

13. Rankin JS, Livesey SA, Smith LR, et al. Trends in the surgical treatment of ischemic mitral regurgitation: effects of mitral valve repair on hospital mortality. *Semin Thorac Cadiovasc Surg* 1989;1:149–163.

14. Califf RM, McKinnis RA, Burks J, et al. Prognostic implications of ventricular arrhythmias during 24 hour ambulatory monitoring in patients undergoing cardiac catheterization for coronary artery disease. *Am J Cardiol* 1982;50:23–31.

15. Cameron A, Schwartz MJ, Kronmal RA, Kosinski AS. Prevalence and significance of atrial fibrillation in coronary artery disease (CASS Registry). *Am J Cardiol* 1988;61:714–717.

16. Bateman TM, Weiss MH, Czer LSC, et al. Fascicular conduction disturbances and ischemic heart disease: adverse prognosis despite coronary revascularization. *J Am Coll Cardiol* 1985;5:632–639.

17. Califf RM, Phillips HR, Hindman MC, et al. Prognostic value of a coronary artery jeopardy score. *J Am Coll Cardiol* 1985;5:1055–1063.

18. Mark DB, Nelson CL, Califf RM, et al. The continuing evolution of therapy for coronary artery disease: initial results from the era of coronary angioplasty. *Circulation* 1994;89(5):2015–2025.

19. Smith LR, Harrell FE Jr, Rankin JS, et al. Determinants of early versus late cardiac death in patients undergoing coronary artery bypass graft surgery. *Circulation* 1991; 84[Suppl III]:245–253.

20. Mark DB, Nelson CL, Harrell FE Jr, et al. Improved survival benefits with coronary angioplasty and coronary bypass surgery: assessment using a new coronary prognostic index. *Circulation* 1992;86:I-536(abst).

21. Hammond HK, Kelly TL, Froelicher VF, Pewen W. Use of clinical data in predicting improvement in exercise capacity after cardiac rehabilitation. *J Am Coll Cardiol* 1985;6:19–26.

22. Jones RH, Hannan EL, Hammermeister KE, et al. Identification of preoperative variables needed for risk adjustment of short-term mortality after coronary artery bypass graft surgery. *J Am Coll Cardiol* 1996;28: 1478–1487.

23. Uren NG, Melin JA, De Bruyne B, Wijns W, Baudhuin T, Camici PG. Relation between myocardial blood flow and the severity of coronary-artery stenosis. *N Engl J Med* 1994;330:1782–1788.

24. Folland ED, Vogel RA, Hartigan P, et al., and the Veterans Affairs ACME Investigators. Relation between coronary artery stenosis assessed by visual, caliper, and computer methods and exercise capacity in patients with single-vessel coronary artery disease. *Circulation* 1994; 89:2005–2014.

25. Cohn PF. Silent myocardial ischemia in patients with a defective anginal warning system. *Am J Cardiol* 1980; 45:697–702.

26. Rocco MB, Nabel EG, Campbell S, et al. Prognostic importance of myocardial ischemia detected by ambulatory monitoring in patients with stable coronary artery disease. *Circulation* 1988;78:877–884.

27. Pepine CJ. Is silent ischemia a treatable risk factor in patients with angina pectoris? *Circulation* 1990;82: II135–II142.

28. Davies MJ, Thomas AC. Plaque fissuring: the cause of acute myocardial infarction, sudden ischemic death, and crescendo angina. *Br Heart J* 1985;53:363–373.

29. Davies MJ, Thomas A. Thrombosis and acute coronary-artery lesions in sudden cardiac ischemic death. *N Engl J Med* 1984;310(18):1137–1140.

30. Falk E. Morphologic features of unstable atherothrombotic plaques underlying acute coronary syndromes. *Am J Cardiol* 1989;63:114E–120E.

31. Fernandez-Ortiz A, Badimon JJ, Falk E, et al. Characterization of the relative thrombogenicity of atherosclerotic plaque components: implications for consequences of plaque rupture. *J Am Coll Cardiol* 1994;23(7): 1562–1569.

32. Rasheed Q, Nair R, Sheehan H, Hodgson JM. Correlation of intracoronary ultrasound plaque characteristics in atherosclerotic coronary artery disease patients with clinical variables. *Am J Cardiol* 1994;73:753–758.

33. Davies MJ. Reactive oxygen species, metalloproteinases, and plaque stability. *Circulation* 1998;97: 2382–2383.

34. Mehta JL, Saldeen TG, Rand K. Interactive role of infection, inflammation and traditional risk factors in atherosclerosis and coronary artery disease. *J Am Coll Cardiol* 1998;31:1217–1225.

35. Califf RM, Mark DB, Harrell FE Jr, et al. Importance of clinical measures of ischemia in the prognosis of patients with documented coronary artery disease. *J Am Coll Cardiol* 1988;11:20–26.

36. Echt DS, Liebson PR, Mitchell LB, et al., and the CAST Investigators. Mortality and morbidity in patients receiving encainide, flecainide, or placebo. The Cardiac Arrhythmia Suppression Trial. *N Engl J Med* 1991; 324(12):781–788.

37. Holmes DR, Davis KB, Mock MB, et al., Participants in the Coronary Artery Surgery Study. The effect of medical and surgical treatment on subsequent sudden cardiac death in patients with coronary artery disease: a report from the coronary artery surgery study. *Circulation* 1986;73:1254–1263.

38. Furberg CD, Hawkins CM, Lichstein E. Effect of propranolol in postinfarction patients with mechanical or electrical complications. *Circulation* 1984;69:761–765.

39. Steinberg JS, Regan A, Sciacca RR, Bigger JT, Fleiss JL. Predicting arrhythmic events after acute myocardial infarction using the signal-averaged electrocardiogram. *Am J Cardiol* 1992;69:13–21.

40. Kleiger RE, Miller JP, Bigger JT, Moss AJ. Decreased heart rate variability and its association with increased mortality after acute myocardial infarction. *Am J Cardiol* 1987;59:256–262.

41. Bigger JT Jr, Fleiss JL, Steinman RC, Rolnitzky LM, Kleiger RE, Rottman JN. Correlations among time and frequency domain measures of heart period variability two weeks after acute myocardial infarction. *Am J Cardiol* 1992;69:891–898.

42. Tung CY, Lam LC, Waugh RA, et al. Clinical, pharmacologic health status, and socioeconomic correlates of heart rate variability in coronary disease. *Circulation* 1995;92:145A.

43. Muller JE, Abela GS, Nesto RW, Tofler GH. Triggers, acute risk factors and vulnerable plaques: the lexicon of a new frontier. *J Am Coll Cardiol* 1994;23(3):809–813.

44. Antiplatelet Trialist's Collaboration. Collaborative overview of randomized trials of antiplatelet therapy. I. Prevention of death, myocardial infarction, and stroke by prolonged antiplatelet therapy in various categories of patients. *BMJ* 1994;308:81–106.

45. Braunwald E, Mark DB, Jones RH, et al. Unstable angina: diagnosis and management. *AHCPR* 1994;94:0682.

46. Yusuf S, Wittes J, Friedman L. Overview of results of randomized clinical trials in heart disease: II. Unstable angina, heart failure, primary prevention with aspirin, and risk factor modification. *JAMA* 1988;260:2259–2263.

47. The PRISM Plus Study Investigators. Inhibition of the platelet glycoprotein IIb/IIIa receptor with tirofiban in unstable angina and non-Q-wave myocardial infarction. *N Engl J Med* 1998;338:1488–1497.

48. The PRISM Study Investigators. A comparison of aspirin plus tirofiban with aspirin plus heparin for unstable angina. *N Engl J Med* 1998;338:1498–1505.

49. The EPIC Investigators. Use of a monoclonal antibody directed against the platelet glycorprotein IIb/IIIa receptor in high-risk coronary angioplasty. The EPIC Investigation. *N Engl J Med* 1994;330:956–961.

50. The EPILOG Investigators. Platelet glyocprotein IIb/IIIa receptor blockade and low-dose heparin during percutaneous coronary revascularization. *N Engl J Med* 1997;336:1689–1696.

51. The PURSUIT Investigators. Inhibition of platelet glycoprotein IIb/IIIa with eptifibatide in patients with acute coronary syndromes without persistent ST-segment elevation. *N Engl J Med* 1998;339:436–443.

52. Cannon CP, McCabe CH, Borzak S, et al., for the TIMI 12 Investigators. Randomized trial of an oral platelet glycoprotein IIb/IIIa antagonist, sibrafiban, in patients after an acute coronary syndrome: results of the TIMI 12 Trial. *Circulation* 1998;97:340–349.

53. Yusuf S, Wittes J, Friedman L. Overview of results of randomized clinical trials in heart disease. I. Treatments following myocardial infarction. *JAMA* 1988;260:2088–2093.

54. Gruppo Italiano per lo Studio della Sopravvivenza nell'Infarto Miocardico. GISSI-3: effects of lisinopril and transdermal glyceryl trinitrate singly and together on 6-week mortality and ventricular function after acute myocardial infarction. *Lancet* 1994;343:1115–1122.

55. ISIS-4 Collaborative Group. ISIS-4: a randomised factorial trial assessing early oral captopril, oral mononitrate, and intravenous magnesium sulphate in 58,050 patients with suspected acute myocardial infarction. *Lancet* 1995;345:669–685.

56. Diodati J, Theroux P, Latour JG, Lacoste L, Lam JYT, Waters D. Effects of nitroglycerin at therapeutic doses on platelet aggregation in unstable angina pectoris and acute myocardial infarction. *Am J Cardiol* 1990;66:683–688.

57. Held PH, Yusuf S, Furberg CD. Calcium channel blockers in acute myocardial infarction and unstable angina: an overview. *BMJ* 1989;299:1187–1192.

58. Packer M, O'Connor CM, Ghali JK, et al. Effect of amlodipine on morbidity and mortality in severe chronic heart failure. *N Engl J Med* 1996;335:1107–1114.

59. The Multicenter Diltiazem Postinfarction Trial Research Group. The effect of diltiazem on mortality and reinfarction after myocardial infarction. *N Engl J Med* 1988;319:385–392.

60. Gibson RS, Boden WE, Theroux P, et al., the Diltiazem Reinfarction Study Group. Diltiazem and reinfarction in patients with non-Q-wave myocardial infarction. *N Engl J Med* 1986;315:423–429.

61. Yusuf S, Pepine CJ, Garces C, et al. Effect of enalapril on myocardial infarction and unstable angina in patients with low ejection fractions. *Lancet* 1992;340:1173–1178.

62. SOLVD Investigators. Effect of enalapril on survival in patients with reduced left ventricular ejection fractions and congestive heart failure. *N Engl J Med* 1991;325:293–302.

63. Kjekshus J, Swedberg K, Snapinn S. Effects of enalapril on long-term mortality in severe congestive heart failure. *Am J Cardiol* 1992;69:103–117.

64. Pfeffer MA, Braunwald E, Moye LA, et al., for the SAVE Investigators. Effect of captopril on mortality and morbidity in patients with left ventricular dysfunction after myocardial infarction. Results of the survival and ventricular enlargement trial. *N Engl J Med* 1992;327:669–677.

65. The ACE Inhibitor Myocardial Infarction Collaborative Group. Indications for ACE inhibitors in the early treatment of acute myocardial infarction. *Circulation* 1998;97:2202–2212.

66. Shepherd J, Cobbe SM, Ford I, et al., for the West of Scotland Coronary Prevention Study Group. Prevention of coronary heart disease with pravastatin in men with hypercholesterolemia. *N Engl J Med* 1995;333:1301–1307.

67. Downs JR, Clearfield M, Weis S, et al., for the AFCAPS/TexCAPS Research Group. Primary prevention of acute coronary events with lovastatin in men and women with average cholesterol levels. *JAMA* 1998;279:1615–1622.

68. Scandinavian Simvastatin Survival Study Group. Randomised trial of cholesterol lowering in 4444 patients with coronary heart disease: the Scandinavian Simvastatin Survival Study (4S). *Lancet* 1994;344:1383–1389.

69. Sacks FM, Pfeffer MA, Moye LA, et al., for the CARE Investigators. Cholesterol And Recurrent Events (CARE). *N Engl J Med* 1996;335:1001–1009.

70. Yusuf S, Zucker D, Peduzzi P, et al. Effect of coronary artery bypass graft surgery on survival: overview of 10-year results from randomised trials by the Coronary Artery Bypass Graft Surgery Trialists Collaboration. *Lancet* 1994;344:563–570.

71. Davis KB, Alderman EL, Kosinski AS, Passamani E, Kennedy JW. Early mortality of acute myocardial infarction in patients with and without prior coronary revascularization surgery. *Circulation* 1992;85:2100–2109.

72. Wiseman A, Waters DD, Walling A, Pelletier GB, Roy D, Theroux P. Long-term prognosis after myocardial infarction in patients with previous coronary artery bypass surgery. *J Am Coll Cardiol* 1988;12:873–880.

73. Jones RH, Kesler K, Phillips HR, et al. Long-term survival benefit of CABG and PTCA in patients with coronary artery disease. *J Thorac Cardiovasc Surg* 1996; 111:1013–1023.
74. BARI Investigators. Comparison of coronary bypass surgery with angioplasty in patients with multivessel disease. *N Engl J Med* 1996;335:217–225.
75. The Writing Group for the Bypass Angioplasty Revascularization Investigation (BARI) Investigators. Five-year clinical and functional outcome comparing bypass surgery and angioplasty in patients with multivessel coronary disease: a multicenter randomized trial. *JAMA* 1997;277:715–721.
76. Pocock SJ, Henderson RA, Rickards AF, et al. Meta-analysis of randomised trials comparing conronary angioplasty with bypass surgery. *Lancet* 1995;346:1184–1189.
77. RITA Trial Participants. Coronary angioplasty versus coronary artery bypass surgery: the Randomised Intervention Treatment of Angina (RITA) trial. *Lancet* 1993; 341:573–580.
78. King SB III, Lembo NJ, Weintraub WS, et al., for the Emory Angioplasty versus Surgery Trial. A randomized trial comparing coronary angioplasty with coronary bypass surgery. *N Engl J Med* 1994;331:1044–1050.
79. Hamm CW, Reimers J, Ischinger T, Rupprecht HJ, Berger J, Bleifeld W, for the German Angioplasty Bypass Surgery Investigation. A randomized study of coronary angioplasty compared with bypass surgery in patients with symptomatic multivessel coronary disease. *N Engl J Med* 1994;331:1037–1043.
80. Sim I, Gupta M, McDonald K, Bourassa MG, Hlatky MA. A meta-analysis of randomized trials comparing coronary artery bypass grafting with percutaneous transluminal coronary angioplasty in multivessel coronary artery disease. *Am J Cardiol* 1995;76:1025–1029.
81. Rodriguez A, Mele E, Peyregne E, et al., for the ERACI Investigators. Three-year follow-up of the Argentine Randomized Trial of Percutaneous Transluminal Coronary Angioplasty Versus Coronary Artery Bypass Surgery in Multivessel Disease (ERACI). *J Am Coll Cardiol* 1996;27:1178–1184.
82. CABRI Trial Participants. First-year results of CABRI (coronary angioplasty versus bypass revascularization investigation). *Lancet* 1995;346:1179–1184.
83. Hlatky MA, Rogers WJ, Johnstone I, et al., for the BARI Investigators. Medical care costs and quality of life after randomization to coronary angioplasty or coronary bypass surgery. *N Engl J Med* 1997;336:92–99.
84. Goy JJ, Eeckhout E. Intracoronary stenting. *Lancet* 1998;351:1943–1949.
85. The EPISTENT Investigators. Randomised placebo-controlled and balloon-angioplasty-controlled trial to assess safety of coronary stenting with use of platelet glycoprotein IIb/IIIa blockade. *Lancet* 1998;352:87–92.
86. Parisi AF, Folland ED, Hartigan P. A comparison of angioplasty with medical therapy in the treatment of single-vessel coronary artery disease. *N Engl J Med* 1992;326:10–16.
87. Mark DB, Nelson C, Delong E, et al. Comparison of quality of life outcomes following coronary angioplasty, coronary bypass surgery and medicine. *J Am Coll Cardiol* 1993;21(2):216A(abst).
88. Weintraub WS, Mauldin PD, Becker E, Kosinski AS, King SB. A comparison of the costs of and quality of life after coronary angioplasty or coronary surgery for multivessel coronary disease: results from the Emory Angioplasty Versus Surgery Trial (EAST). *Circulation* 1995;92:2831–2840.
89. Liao L, Jollis JG, Delong ER, Peterson ED, Morris KG, Mark DB. Impact of an interactive video on ischemic heart disease patient decision making. *J Gen Int Med* 1996;11:373–376.

B. Approaching Multivessel Coronary Artery Disease

Daniel L. Dries and Bernard J. Gersh

Division of Cardiology, Georgetown University Medical Center, Washington, DC 20007-2197

Current approaches for the treatment of coronary artery disease include medical management, risk factor reduction, percutaneous coronary revascularization, and surgical revascularization. The available data supporting which option to choose for a given situation have evolved over the last three decades and highlight the important role that randomized, prospective clinical trials have played in advancing clinical cardiology, in particular the management of coronary artery disease. In the early 1970s, the treatment options included medical therapy or consideration of surgical revascularization. Three historic trials from the late 1970s improved our understanding of which patients might benefit from surgical revascularization. With the introduction of percutaneous revascularization in the 1980s, a technology that continues to evolve in rapid fashion, the therapeutic options available to the cardiologist managing a patient with coronary artery disease have expanded further.

This chapter discusses the available data related to an evidence-based approach to the patient with multivessel coronary artery disease, in addition to addressing the art of medicine in applying the published data to the individual patient in whom factors including lifestyle, occupation, socioeconomic status, and compliance are integral components of the therapeutic strategy.

SURGICAL REVASCULARIZATION COMPARED WITH MEDICAL MANAGEMENT

Three landmark prospective, randomized clinical trials provide the majority of data on which to base the decision to treat the patient with multivessel coronary artery disease with surgical revascularization as opposed to medical management. These trials were the European Coronary Surgery Study (ECSS), the Veterans Administration Coronary Artery Bypass Surgery Cooperative Study (VACS) group, and the Coronary Artery Surgery Study (CASS) (1–4). In the VACS, 68 male patients who had stable angina for 6 months were randomly assigned to treatment. In the ECSS, 768 men with multivessel disease who had angina for more than 3 months were randomly assigned to treatment. Finally, the CASS enrolled 780 patients with single-vessel or multivessel coronary artery disease. The characteristics of the patients enrolled in these trials are shown in Table 21.3.

In each trial, the most consistent and important conclusions were that patients with left main coronary artery disease or three-vessel coronary artery disease and impaired left ventricular systolic function had the greatest benefit from coronary artery bypass graft (CABG) surgery compared with medical management. A greater ischemic burden, as indirectly quantified by the severity of angina, also identified patients with

TABLE 21.3. *Clinical and angiographic characteristics of 2,649 patients enrolled in seven randomized trials of coronary artery bypass grafting versus initial medical therapy for chronic coronary artery disease*

Characteristic	Patients (%)
Age distribution (yr)	
≤40	8.5
41–50	38.2
51–60	46.0
>60	7.3
Ejection fraction (%) (n = 2,474)	
<40	7.2
40–49	12.5
50–59	28.0
≥60	52.3
Male	96.8
Severity of angina (CCS classification)	
None	11.2
Class I or II	53.8
Class III or IV	35.0
History	
Myocardial infarction	59.6
Hypertension	26.0
Heart failure	4.0
Diabetes mellitus	9.6
Smoking (n = 1,949)	83.5
Current smokers (n = 2,298)	45.5
ST segment depression >1 mm	
Resting (n = 2,423)	9.9
Exercise (n = 1,985)	70.5
Drugs at baseline	
Beta-blockers (n = 2,308)	47.4
Antiplatelet agents (n = 1,195)	3.2
Digitalis (n = 2,319)	12.9
Diuretics (n = 1,940)	12.6
No. of vessels diseased	
Left main artery	6.6
One vessel[a]	10.2
Two vessels[a]	32.4
Three vessels[a]	50.6
Location of disease	
Proximal left anterior descending	59.4
Left anterior descending diagonal	60.4
Circumflex	73.8
Right coronary	81.6

Data on some characteristics are not available for all patients: When data are available in less than 90% of the patients, numbers of patients with available data are shown in parentheses. Abnormal ejection fraction was defined as ≤50% and significant coronary stenosis as >50% diameter reduction.

[a] Without left main artery.

From ref. 5,. with permission.

three-vessel disease who had a large benefit from surgical revascularization, as demonstrated by large absolute and relative reductions in the risk for all-cause mortality compared with comparable patients treated medically.

The conclusions from the individual trials were confirmed and expanded in an important metaanalysis of seven randomized trials of CABG versus an initial strategy of medical therapy for chronic coronary artery disease (5). The seven trials in the metaanalysis included the three already mentioned as well as four other small trials (50 patients per treatment arm). In total, 2,649 patients were randomized to medical therapy or CABG primarily for stable angina pectoris. For this metaanalysis, original clinical and angiographic data were collected and analyzed using uniform definitions: abnormal ejection fraction (EF) was defined as an EF ≤50%, and a significant coronary artery stenosis was defined as >50% diameter reduction, as assessed angiographically. Patients were overwhelmingly men between the ages of 40 and 60 years. Of major importance to the extrapolation of these data to the present era is the recognition that only about one-half of the patients were tak-

ing beta-adrenergic receptor blockers and only 3% were receiving antiplatelet drugs at baseline.

The metaanalysis confirmed that the survival advantage of CABG over medical therapy was proportional to the number of diseased coronary arteries: significant for three vessels (RR, 0.58; $p < .001$) and left main coronary artery (RR, 0.32; $p = .004$) and, in particular, to involvement of the left anterior descending coronary artery (RR, 0.58, even if only one- or two-vessel disease) (Table 21.4). Thus, the greatest absolute mortality benefit for CABG was demonstrated in the patients with the highest preoperative risk. These subgroups included patients with left main coronary disease (4,6), left main "equivalent" disease (7), and three-vessel disease and impaired left ventricular function (8).

Although the relative benefits were similar regardless of left ventricular function, the absolute benefit was greater among patients with a lower EF as a result of the higher mortality rates in

TABLE 21.4. *Outcomes[a] of various subgroups receiving medical therapy (MT) versus coronary artery bypass grafting (CABG) trials at 5 years*

Subgroup	Overall numbers deaths	MT mortality patients	Odds ratio rate (%)	p for CABG vs. MT (95% CI)	p for vs. MT	Interaction
Vessel disease						
One vessel	21	271	9.9	0.54 (0.22–1.33)	0.18	0.19
Two vessels	92	859	11.7	0.84 (0.54–1.32)	0.45	
Three vessels	189	1341	17.6	0.58 (0.42–0.80)	<0.001	
Left main artery	39	150	36.5	0.32 (0.15–0.70)	0.004	
No LAD disease						
One or two vessels	50	606	8.3	1.05 (0.58–1.90)	0.88	0.06
Three vessels	46	410	14.5	0.47 (0.25–0.89)	0.02	
Left main artery	16	51	45.8	0.27 (0.08–0.90)	0.03	
Overall	112	1067	12.3	0.66 (0.44–1.00)	0.05	
LAD disease present						
One or two vessels	63	524	14.6	0.58 (0.34–1.01)	0.05	0.44
Three vessels	143	929	19.1	0.61 (0.42–0.88)	0.009	
Left main artery	22	96	32.7	0.30 (0.11–0.84)	0.02	
Overall	228	1549	18.3	0.58 (0.43–0.77)	0.001	
LV function						
Normal	228	2095	13.3	0.61 (0.46–0.81)	<0.001	0.90
Abnormal	115	549	25.2	0.59 (0.39–0.91)	0.02	
Exercise test status						
Missing	102	664	17.4	0.69 (0.45–1.07)	0.10	0.37
Normal	60	585	11.6	0.78 (0.45–1.35)	0.38	
Abnormal	183	1400	16.8	0.52 (0.37–0.72)	<0.001	
Severity of angina (CCS)						
Class 0, I, II	178	1716	12.5	0.63 (0.46–0.87)	0.005	0.69
Class III, IV	167	924	22.4	0.57 (0.40–0.81)	0.001	

LAD, left anterior descending coronary artery; LV, left ventricle.
[a] Note significant heterogeneity of treatment effect among angiographic and clinical subgroups.
From ref. 5, with permission.

the patients with lower EF. Additionally, it was demonstrated that absolute and relative mortality benefits were greater for patients with evidence of myocardial ischemia, as demonstrated by severe angina or an abnormal result of an exercise test. An additional finding of the metaanalysis, related to the greater statistical power of combining the patients from seven randomized trials, was that patients with three-vessel coronary disease and normal left ventricular function and patients with significant stenosis in the proximal left anterior descending artery also experienced a survival benefit with surgical revascularization. In general, however, the greatest absolute benefit for CABG was demonstrated in the patients with evidence of the most severe ischemic extent of coronary artery disease or left ventricular dysfunction. Patients with severe left ventricular dysfunction were excluded from the three major trials comparing CABG with medical therapy. In addition, several nonrandomized registry studies emphasized the benefit of surgery over medical therapy in patients with multivessel disease and severe angina pectoris, regardless of left ventricular function (9).

In attempting to apply the results of the randomized trials to current clinical practice, we must appreciate some of the limitations of these data. These trials did not include patients older than age 65 years and included mostly men. Currently, more than 50% of CABG procedures are performed in patients older than age 65 years (10). The only trial to include internal mammary artery grafts was CASS, in which only 14% of patients received an internal thoracic conduit. Aspirin and lipid-lowering agents, in particular the 3-hydroxy-3-methylglutaryl-coenzyme A reductase inhibitors, were not widely used in the patients allocated to medical or surgical therapy. Clearly, the use of the internal mammary conduit has improved long-term graft patency (11), and the importance of lipid-lowering and antiplatelet therapy in improving long-term saphenous vein graft patency was not recognized until after the completion of these studies (12,13). Finally, there have been substantial improvements in preoperative evaluation, cardioplegia, intraoper-

ative anesthesia, and postoperative care since the 1970s.

SURGICAL OR PERCUTANEOUS REVASCULARIZATION?

The available data, despite the limitations, have clearly demonstrated that revascularization is the optimal strategy for most patients with multivessel coronary artery disease, especially if they have evidence of moderate-to-severe inducible ischemia and left ventricular systolic impairment or severe ischemia irrespective of left ventricular function. The area of controversy remains which method of revascularization, surgical or percutaneous, is preferred. We next consider the available data regarding the relative benefits of percutaneous versus surgical revascularization for patients with multivessel coronary artery disease and a clinical profile that indicates that revascularization is the preferred treatment strategy.

There have been several trials comparing elective percutaneous transluminal coronary angioplasty (PTCA) with CABG as methods of revascularization in patients with multivessel coronary disease (14–19). What is most important to emphasize about each of these six trials is the highly selective nature of the enrolled patients. The characteristics of the patients are presented in Table 21.5. Overall, of 91,730 screened patients, only 5.2% were randomly assigned to a study group. It is also important to appreciate that most of the patients in these trials had well-preserved EFs that ranged from 56% to 63%. Close to two-thirds of patients were excluded for left main coronary disease, diffuse disease, chronic total occlusion, or presumed inability to achieve complete "functional" revascularization (20). Therefore, many subsets of patients previously demonstrated to achieve the greatest absolute benefit from surgical revascularization were excluded from these studies.

What each of the six trials demonstrated was no difference in mortality or the combined endpoint of death and nonfatal myocardial infarction between patients randomized to percutaneous angioplasty or surgical revascularization

TABLE 21.5. *Characteristics of patients from six randomized trials of coronary artery bypass surgery compared with percutaneous transluminal coronary angiography*

Characteristic	RITA (14)	ERACI (15)	GABI (16)	EAST (17)	CABRI (18)	BARI (19)
Patients enrolled (no.)	1011	127	359	392	1054	1829
Patients screened (no.)	27,975	1409	8981	5118	23,047	25,200
Median age (yr)	57	58	59	62	61	62
Men (%)	81	85	89	74	78	73
Diseased vessels (no.)	≥1	≥2	≥2	≥2	≥2	≥2
Mean ejection fraction	—	0.61	—	0.61	0.63	0.57
Class III–IV angina, %	59	—	65	80	62	—

BARI, Bypass Angioplasty Revascularization Investigation; CABRI, Coronary Angioplasty Bypass Revascularization Investigation; EAST, Emory Angioplasty versus Surgery Trial; ERACI, Argentine Trial of PTCA versus CABG; GABI, German Angioplasty Bypass Surgery Investigation; RITA, Randomised Intervention Treatment of Angina Trial.
From ref. 20, with permission.

(Figs. 21.8 through 21.10). Although there were differences between the trials in endpoints and follow-up time, they were sufficiently similar to lend themselves to a metaanalysis. Two metaanalyses have been completed, including each of the previously mentioned trials except for BARI (21,22).

The metaanalysis by Pocock et al. (21) included 3,371 patients, of whom 1,661 were randomized to CABG and 1,710 to PTCA. The mean follow-up time was 2.7 years. The incidence of all-cause mortality was similar for those assigned to CABG (4.4%) and those as-

signed to PTCA (4.6%) (RR, 1.08; 95% CI: 0.79, 1.50). The incidence of the composite endpoint of death or nonfatal myocardial infarction was also similar for those assigned to CABG (7.6%) and those assigned to PTCA (7.9%) (RR, 1.10; 95% CI: 0.89, 1.37). The incidence of repeat revascularization within 1 year was 33.7% in patients allocated to PTCA and 3.3% in those assigned to CABG ($p < .001$). Revascularization rates over a 7-year period are illustrated in Fig. 21.9, with the majority of repeat PTCAs performed within the first year (23). Within the patients allocated to an initial strategy of PTCA

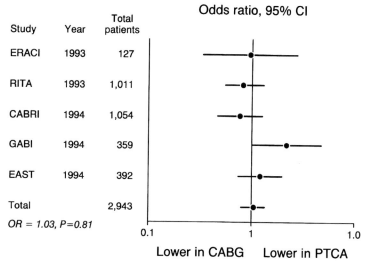

FIG. 21.8. Overall combined risk for death and nonfatal myocardial infarction in five randomized trials comparing percutaneous transluminal coronary angioplasty (*PTCA*) with coronary artery bypass graft (*CABG*) surgery. CABRI, Coronary Angioplasty Bypass Revascularization Investigation; EAST, Emory Angioplasty versus Surgery Trial; ERACI, Estudio Randomizado Argentino de Angioplastia vs Cirugia (Argentine Trial of PTCA versus CABG); GABI, German Angioplasty Bypass Surgery Investigation; OR, odds ratio; RITA, Randomised Intervention Treatment of Angina. (From ref. 22, with permission.)

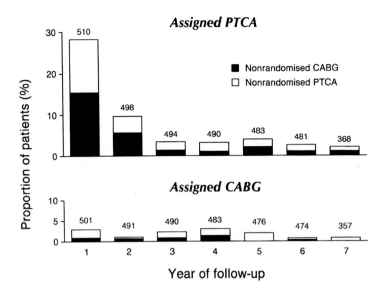

Assigned PTCA

Assigned CABG

Year of follow-up

FIG. 21.9. Reintervention rates by year of follow-up for each treatment group. Numbers at top of blocks indicate number of patients at the start of each year. CABG, coronary artery bypass grafting; PTCA, percutaneous transluminal coronary angioplasty. (From ref. 23, with permission.)

who underwent a subsequent revascularization procedure, these consisted of almost equal numbers of repeat PTCA and CABG procedures. The prevalence of class II angina was greater in the group treated with PTCA at 1 year than in those treated with CABG, but this difference had diminished by 3 years.

The BARI trial deserves individual emphasis because it was the largest of the PTCA versus CABG trials, and it has provided some additional and important insights into the best approach to the patients with multivessel coronary artery disease. It was designed originally as an "equivalence" trial. Close to 30% of eligible patients were randomized, and of these, 40% had three-vessel disease and 22% had an EF <50%. The 5-year mortality rate was 10.7% in those assigned to CABG and 13.7% in those randomized to PTCA, corresponding to a 22% relative risk reduction in favor of CABG that did not achieve statistical significance. The incidence of death or Q-wave myocardial infarction by 5

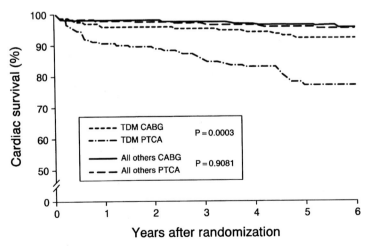

FIG. 21.10. Cardiac survival after assignment to percutaneous transluminal coronary angioplasty (*PTCA*) and coronary artery bypass grafting (*CABG*) in 353 patients with treated diabetes mellitus (*TDM*) and in 1,476 patients without diabetes or with diabetes not receiving treatment. (From The BARI Investigators. Influence of diabetes on 5-year mortality and morbidity in a randomized trial comparing CABG and PTCA in patients with multivessel disease: the Bypass Angiography Revascularization Investigation [BARI]. *Circulation* 1997;96:1761–1769. By permission of the American Heart Association.)

years was 19.4% in those randomized to CABG and 21.3% for those assigned to PTCA.

An interesting result from a predefined subgroup analysis was that in patients with diabetes ($n = 353$) receiving treatment (either with insulin or an oral hypoglycemic agent), there was a significant mortality benefit associated with CABG compared with PTCA (see Fig. 21.10). The 5-year mortality rate in treated diabetic patients assigned to CABG was 19.4% compared with 34.5% in those assigned to PTCA ($p = .003$). These data are supported by a subgroup analysis from CABRI that showed 2-year mortality rates of 15.6% in the treated diabetic patients who had PTCA and 3.5% in the treated diabetic patients who had CABG (Bertrand M. Long-term follow-up of European revascularization trials, read at 68th Scientific Sessions, American Heart Association, Anaheim, California, November 16, 1995).

The diabetic patients did tend to have a greater extent of coronary disease and a greater prevalence of left ventricular dysfunction. Whether these data suggest that CABG is preferred to PTCA in the higher risk patient with multivessel coronary disease or rather relate to a unique interaction between diabetes and percutaneous coronary intervention cannot be answered from these data. These data await further confirmation and mechanistic elucidation in prospective studies. Nonetheless, at the present time, the BARI data as well as other observational and subgroup studies suggest that in treated diabetic patients with multivessel coronary artery disease, regardless of the presence or absence of left ventricular systolic dysfunction, it is important to revascularize the patient as completely as possible and that strong consideration should be given to surgical revascularization.

It is important to consider whether PTCA and CABG are indeed equivalent modes of coronary revascularization in all patients with multivessel coronary artery disease. Certainly, multivessel coronary artery disease affects a heterogeneous population. For example, the patient with a discrete lesion in the right coronary and circumflex artery with preserved systolic ventricular dysfunction is not comparable in terms of prognosis to the patient with three-vessel coronary disease and an EF of 35%.

The results of the CABG versus medical therapy trials suggested that the greatest absolute benefit of surgical revascularization was demonstrated in the highest-risk patients, in particular, those with both multivessel coronary disease and left ventricular dysfunction as well as those with multivessel coronary disease and a large ischemic burden, as evidenced by exercise treadmill testing or the severity of angina. Of course, anginal severity per se is not equivalent to ischemic burden as assessed by nuclear imaging, because a single stenosis can cause considerable angina. However, in general, it is reasonable to conclude from the CABG versus medical therapy trials that in addition to left ventricular dysfunction, the presence of a large ischemic burden in conjunction with multivessel disease, especially if the proximal left anterior descending coronary artery is involved, identifies a subset of patients that appear to benefit most in terms of absolute and relative mortality risk from surgical revascularization.

The patients enrolled in the recent PTCA versus CABG trials were relatively low risk, and this deserves emphasis for the clinician extrapolating these data to an individual patient. For example, 70% of the participants in these trials had either one- or two-vessel coronary artery disease. Perhaps most importantly, fewer than 20% had left ventricular dysfunction. In BARI, close to 60% of patients had two-vessel coronary artery disease. In comparison, in the prior trials comparing CABG to medical therapy, 60% of patients had left main or three-vessel coronary artery disease and 20% of patients had significant left ventricular dysfunction. Thus, the present trials of PTCA versus CABG included a significant proportion of patients in whom, based on the data from the trials comparing surgical with medical management, surgical revascularization did not offer a mortality benefit compared with medical therapy. Also, in terms of statistical power, these trials cannot eliminate the possibility of a mortality benefit in favor of CABG. Moreover, most of the patients enrolled in these studies had anatomy that was amenable to complete revascularization if the approach were percutaneous.

Many patients have multivessel disease that is so diffuse and severe that complete revascularization is not possible using percutaneous approaches. In these patients, complete surgical revascularization is always preferred to incomplete revascularization using a percutaneous approach unless there are mitigating circumstances, such as an unacceptably high surgical risk. Thus, the present trials comparing PTCA with CABG are applicable to low-risk patients with multivessel coronary disease in which percutaneous or surgical revascularization approaches would offer *similar* completeness of revascularization. However, the ratio of screened to enrolled participants in these trials illustrates that the majority of patients with multivessel coronary artery disease are not in this category.

MULTIVESSEL CORONARY ARTERY DISEASE: A PRACTICAL APPROACH BASED ON THE EVIDENCE

Importance of a Comprehensive Approach

The importance of carefully assessing each patient's risk profile is based on the surgical versus medical therapy trials (VACS, ECSS, and CASS) in which the greatest absolute benefit for CABG was seen in the patients with the highest preoperative risk. Specifically, patients with the most severe symptoms, ischemia, extent of coronary artery disease, and left ventricular dysfunction had the greatest comparative benefit. In the majority of patients with multivessel coronary artery disease and a moderate-to-large ischemic burden, revascularization is usually the preferred treatment approach. We emphasize that in addition to revascularization, an aggressive approach to risk factor modification and the judicious use of adjunctive pharmacologic approaches are equally important. For example, lipids should be lowered according to target goals for secondary prevention (i.e., low-density lipoprotein cholesterol ≤ 100 mg/dL) using dietary modification and treatment with a 3-hydroxy-3-methylglutaryl-coenzyme A reductase inhibitor if neces-

sary. Aspirin and beta-adrenergic receptor blockers both have demonstrated an ability to reduce the risk for subsequent cardiac events in patients with established coronary artery disease. Weight loss in overweight individuals, smoking cessation, and control of hypertension are of equal importance.

Defining Individual Risk Profiles

For the patient with multivessel coronary disease, determination of the need for revascularization depends on defining the patient's overall risk. Patients at high risk include those with three-vessel coronary artery disease and left ventricular dysfunction and those with left main coronary artery disease. These patients should always be considered candidates for revascularization. The metaanalysis of the CABG versus medical therapy data also demonstrated a survival advantage from surgical revascularization in patients with two-vessel coronary artery disease if one of the vessels was the proximal left anterior descending artery, as well as in patients with three-vessel coronary artery disease and normal left ventricular dysfunction. However, we emphasize that the decision has to be individualized. We advocate a surgical revascularization approach to the patient with significant (>50%) left main stenosis or significant three-vessel coronary artery disease in association with a large ischemic burden, severe symptoms, or impaired left ventricular dysfunction.

In patients at moderate risk, two-vessel coronary artery disease not involving the proximal left anterior descending coronary artery and preserved left ventricular dysfunction, both PTCA and CABG are reasonable options, given suitable anatomy for either approach. Such patients can expect similar outcomes with regard to survival and freedom from nonfatal myocardial infarction, but they should be aware that the PTCA approach is associated with a substantially greater risk for repeat revascularization within the next 1 to 3 years.

Once a decision is made to proceed with revascularization, either to alleviate medically refractory symptoms or to obtain a survival benefit, the selection of PTCA or CABG as the preferred method of revascularization depends on several factors. Some of the important considerations include patient preferences, specific coronary anatomy, status of left ventricular function, total ischemic burden, and ability of a percutaneous approach to offer a degree of revascularization comparable to a surgical approach.

The clinician confronted with the patient with multivessel coronary disease that is amenable to either a percutaneous or a surgical approach should be well aware of the highly select group of patients included in the recent clinical trials that compared PTCA with CABG. For the patient with multivessel coronary disease and moderate-to-severe left ventricular dysfunction, the current data do not support the contention that PTCA offers outcomes comparable to those of CABG. Likewise, in the patient with a large ischemic burden, regardless of the left ventricular dysfunction, it is extremely important to revascularize the patient as completely as possible (24). In many instances, this is best achieved by a surgical approach. Finally, the diabetic patient with multivessel coronary disease did better with surgical revascularization in the recent BARI experience. The reasons for this are unclear, and these data need to be confirmed.

At the present time, it appears reasonable to have a low threshold to proceed with a surgical approach to achieve the most complete degree of revascularization possible in the diabetic patient with multivessel coronary artery disease. In each instance, the decision must be individualized and based on an understanding of the available data and an assessment of the individual patient's risk profile, as evidenced by the presence or absence of important comorbidities, such as diabetes, the total ischemic burden, and the status of left ventricular function.

MULTIVESSEL CORONARY ARTERY DISEASE AND SEVERELY IMPAIRED LEFT VENTRICULAR FUNCTION

The approach to patients with significantly impaired left ventricular function and multivessel coronary artery disease continues to evolve. These patients, broadly defined as those with an EF $\leq$ 20% to 30%, were excluded from the trials

that compared medical therapy with surgical revascularization. Advances have been made in our understanding of the pathophysiology and prognostic import of hibernating myocardium, and improvements in the surgical approach to these patients have resulted in observational data suggesting a low operative mortality in these patients previously considered to be at prohibitively high surgical risk.

The CASS Registry demonstrated that patients with lower EFs derived the greatest absolute and relative benefits from surgery compared with medical therapy (25,26). The 5-year survival rates in the medical and surgical groups were 54% and 68%, respectively, in patients with an EF $<$ 35% (p = .0007). In patients with an EF $<$ 25%, the 5-year survival rates in the surgical and medical groups were 63% and 43%, respectively (25). The CASS investigators found that for the patients without angina who presented with preoperative symptoms of heart failure, the mortality rates were 23% for both the medical and surgical groups. The patients with preoperative angina, however, had mortality rates of 39% in the surgical group compared with 62% in the medical group (p = .0006).

The results of CASS, which suggested a benefit of revascularization in patients with angina and left ventricular dysfunction, are perhaps the expression of the more recent experience with the use of preoperative viability testing to identify hibernating myocardium in patients with multivessel coronary disease and moderate-to-severe left ventricular dysfunction (27–30). In other words, the presence of angina pectoris was an indirect marker for the presence of myocardial viability. Recent data suggested that in patients with moderate-to-severe left ventricular dysfunction, the presence of viable myocardium, identified either by the use of positron emission tomography or nuclear scanning, identifies patients who can expect improvement in ventricular function after surgery and improvement in symptoms of heart failure (31).

There is evidence that, in patients with multivessel coronary disease and significant left ventricular dysfunction, survival with surgical revascularization is superior to medical therapy in a patient population with various degrees of preoperative angina and heart failure. The experience from Duke University reported on the results of CABG in 118 patients with an EF of 25% or less (32). In this series, the operative mortality was 11%. The survival at 1 and 5 years in these patients was 77.2% and 57.5%, respectively, which is better than the estimated survival from medical therapy alone.

In most series (33–38), the operative mortality rate has been reduced to less than 10% as a result of improvements in preoperative, operative, and postoperative management, including, in particular, the preoperative use of a pulmonary artery catheter to optimize hemodynamic status preoperatively and improvements in cardioplegia. Many patients with multivessel coronary artery disease and evidence of myocardial viability present with only symptoms of heart failure. Therefore, the clinician should be aware that the *absence of angina* or a history of infarction does not exclude the possibility that the patient presenting with heart failure due to systolic dysfunction has an ischemic etiology and, possibly, hibernating myocardium.

It is recommended that all patients with newly diagnosed left ventricular systolic dysfunction undergo either an invasive or a noninvasive test to define the etiology of left ventricular dysfunction. If an ischemic etiology is suggested by a large ischemic burden on a noninvasive nuclear study, then cardiac catheterization to assess coronary anatomy and the potential for revascularization is warranted, provided the patient is otherwise a candidate for CABG. If an ischemic etiology is suggested by large, fixed perfusion defects, then an evaluation for the presence of viable, hibernating myocardium is also appropriate. Given the extreme limitation of donor hearts for cardiac transplantation, it is extremely important to be aggressive in considering these options in patients with a severe ischemic cardiomyopathy. More prospective data are required to better define the important variables that identify patients with ischemic cardiomyopathy likely to benefit and, equally importantly, those likely not to benefit from surgical revascularization.

FUTURE DIRECTIONS

Because of logistic and ethical concerns, the trials comparing medical therapy with CABG done in the 1970s are unlikely to be repeated despite substantial improvements in medical therapy and surgical techniques. The role for surgical revascularization in the patient at high risk, such as the patient with left main disease or triple-vessel disease and left ventricular dysfunction, has been established. Clinical trials have convincingly demonstrated that PTCA and CABG offer similar results in terms of survival and freedom from nonfatal cardiac events in the patient with moderate risk (mostly two-vessel coronary artery disease with normal left ventricular function). Randomized trials comparing PTCA with medical therapy have been limited to patients with single-vessel coronary disease. Given the remarkable, demonstrated efficacy of the statin drugs to prevent recurrent ischemic events, it would be reasonable to consider a clinical trial comparing PTCA with medical therapy in patients with moderate-risk multivessel coronary disease. Another unanswered question remains the relative efficacies of PTCA or CABG in patients at higher risk (i.e., those demonstrated to benefit more from surgical revascularization than from medical therapy). With the improved technology and medical therapy for percutaneous interventions, such as coronary stenting and the use of the glycoprotein IIb/IIIa inhibitor agents, allowing interventional cardiologists to approach chronic coronary occlusions, it seems reasonable to consider future trials of PTCA versus CABG in these higher risk populations. Finally, the BARI results that suggested that patients with diabetes receiving treatment with oral hypoglycemic agents or insulin benefited more from CABG than from PTCA need further validation.

CONCLUSIONS

The data available from clinical trials over the last 20 years have demonstrated that the majority of patients with multivessel coronary artery disease benefit from revascularization. CABG is associated with an approximately 50% risk reduction in moderate- to high-risk groups compared with medical therapy. These patients include those with three-vessel disease and depressed left ventricular function, left main disease, and left main "equivalent" disease. In these patients, surgical revascularization is preferred. In patients at moderate risk, mostly including those patients with two-vessel coronary artery disease and normal left ventricular function, the major clinical dilemma in the 1990s is which modality of revascularization to use: PTCA or CABG. The available clinical data suggest that in these patients at moderate risk, comprising the overwhelming majority of patients included in the PTCA versus CABG trials, PTCA and CABG are both acceptable and associated with a similar 3-year risk for mortality or the combined endpoint of death or nonfatal myocardial infarction. However, patients initially treated with PTCA can expect a substantially increased risk for repeat revascularization procedures during the initial 3 years. Finally, in patients with severely depressed left ventricular dysfunction, multivessel coronary artery disease, and evidence of myocardial viability, surgical revascularization can be offered at a reasonable mortality rate and, based on observational data, may improve survival and symptoms of heart failure.

REFERENCES

1. European Coronary Surgery Study Group. Long-term results of prospective randomised study of coronary artery bypass surgery in stable angina pectoris. *Lancet* 1982;2:1173–1180.
2. The VA Coronary Artery Bypass Surgery Cooperative Study Group. Eighteen-year follow-up in the Veterans Affairs Cooperative Study of Coronary Artery Bypass Surgery for stable angina. *Circulation* 1992;86: 121–130.
3. Alderman EL, Bourassa MG, Cohen LS, et al. Ten-year follow-up of survival and myocardial infarction in the randomized Coronary Artery Surgery Study. *Circulation* 1990;82:1629–1646.
4. Caracciolo EA, Davis KB, Sopko G, et al. Comparison of surgical and medical group survival in patients with left main coronary artery disease. Long-term CASS experience. *Circulation* 1995;91:2325–2334.
5. Yusuf S, Zucker D, Peduzzi P, et al. Effect of coronary artery bypass graft surgery on survival: overview of 10-year results from randomised trials by the Coronary Artery Bypass Graft Surgery Trialists Collaboration. *Lancet* 1994;344:563–570.
6. Second Interim Report by the European Coronary Surgery Study Group. Prospective randomised study of coronary artery bypass surgery in stable angina pectoris. *Lancet* 1980;2:491–495.
7. Caracciolo EA, Davis KB, Sopko G, et al. Comparison of surgical and medical group survival in patients with left main equivalent coronary artery disease. Long-term CASS experience. *Circulation* 1995;91:2335–2344.

8. Passamani E, Davis KB, Gillespie MJ, Killip T. A randomized trial of coronary artery bypass surgery. Survival of patients with a low ejection fraction. *N Engl J Med* 1985;312:1665–1671.
9. Kaiser GC, Davis KB, Fisher LD, et al. Survival following coronary artery bypass grafting in patients with severe angina pectoris (CASS). An observational study. *J Thorac Cardiovasc Surg* 1985;89:513–524.
10. Loop FD, Lytle BW, Cosgrove DM, et al. Influence of the internal-mammary-artery graft on 10-year survival and other cardiac events. *N Engl J Med* 1986;314:1–6.
11. Graves EJ, Gillum BS. 1994 summary: National Hospital Discharge Survey. Hyattsville, Maryland: U.S. Department of Health and Human Services, Public Health Service, Centers for Disease Control and Prevention, National Center for Health Statistics, 1996.
12. Pearson T, Rapaport E, Criqui M, et al. Optimal risk factor management in the patient after coronary revascularization. A statement for healthcare professionals from an American Heart Association Writing Group. *Circulation* 1994;90:3125–3133.
13. Goldman S, Copeland J, Moritz T, et al., and the Department of Veterans Affairs Cooperative Study Group. Starting aspirin therapy after operation. Effects on early graft patency. *Circulation* 1991;84:520–526.
14. RITA Trial Participants. Coronary angioplasty versus coronary artery bypass surgery: the Randomized Intervention Treatment of Angina (RITA) trial. *Lancet* 1993; 341:573–580.
15. Rodriguez A, Boullon F, Perez-Balino N, Paviotti C, Liprandi MI, Palacios IF. Argentine randomized trial of percutaneous transluminal coronary angioplasty versus coronary artery bypass surgery in multivessel disease (ERACI): in-hospital results and 1-year follow-up. ERACI Group. *J Am Coll Cardiol* 1993;22:1060–1067.
16. Hamm CW, Reimers J, Ischinger T, Rupprecht HJ, Berger J, Bleifeld W. A randomized study of coronary angioplasty compared with bypass surgery in patients with symptomatic multivessel coronary disease. German Angioplasty Bypass Surgery Investigation. *N Engl J Med* 1994;331:1037–1043.
17. King SB III, Lembo NJ, Weintraub WS, et al. A randomized trial comparing coronary angioplasty with coronary bypass surgery. Emory Angioplasty versus Surgery Trial. *N Engl J Med* 1994;331:1044–1050.
18. CABRI Trial Participants. First-year results of CABRI (Coronary Angioplasty versus Bypass Revascularisation Investigation). *Lancet* 1995;346:1179–1184.
19. The Bypass Angioplasty Revascularization Investigation (BARI) Investigators. Comparison of coronary bypass surgery with angioplasty in patients with multivessel disease. *N Engl J Med* 1996;335:217–225.
20. Solomon AJ, Gersh BJ. Management of chronic stable angina: medical therapy, percutaneous transluminal coronary angioplasty, and coronary artery bypass graft surgery. Lessons from the randomized trials. *Ann Intern Med* 1998;128:216–223.
21. Pocock SJ, Henderson RA, Rickards AF, et al. Meta-analysis of randomised trials comparing coronary angioplasty with bypass surgery. *Lancet* 1995;346: 1184–1189.
22. Sim I, Gupta M, McDonald K, Bourassa MG, Hlatky MA. A meta-analysis of randomized trials comparing coronary artery bypass grafting with percutaneous transluminal coronary angioplasty in multivessel coronary artery disease. *Am J Cardiol* 1995;76:1025–1029.

23. Henderson RA, Pocock SJ, Sharp SJ, et al., for the Randomised Intervention Treatment of Angina (RITA-1) trial participants. Long-term results of RITA-1 trial: clinical and cost comparisons of coronary angioplasty and coronary-artery bypass grafting. *Lancet* 1998;352: 1419–1425.

24. Bell MR, Gersh BJ, Schaff HV, et al. Effect of completeness of revascularization on long-term outcome of patients with three-vessel disease undergoing coronary artery bypass surgery. A report from the Coronary Artery Surgery Study (CASS) Registry. *Circulation* 1992;86: 446–457.

25. Alderman EL, Fisher LD, Litwin P, et al. Results of coronary artery surgery in patients with poor left ventricular function (CASS). *Circulation* 1983;68:785–795.

26. Killip T, Passamani E, Davis K. Coronary Artery Surgery Study (CASS): a randomized trial of coronary bypass surgery. Eight years follow-up and survival in patients with reduced ejection fraction. *Circulation* 1985; 72:V102–V109.

27. Arnese M, Cornel JH, Salustri A, et al. Prediction of improvement of regional left ventricular function after surgical revascularization. A comparison of low-dose dobutamine echocardiography with ^{201}Tl single-photon emission computed tomography. *Circulation* 1995;91: 2748–2752.

28. Pagley PR, Beller GA, Watson DD, Gimple LW, Ragosta M. Improved outcome after coronary bypass surgery in patients with ischemic cardiomyopathy and residual myocardial viability. *Circulation* 1997;96: 793–800.

29. Haas F, Haehnel CJ, Picker W, et al. Preoperative positron emission tomographic viability assessment and perioperative and postoperative risk in patients with advanced ischemic heart disease. *J Am Coll Cardiol* 1997; 30:1693–1700.

30. Bonow RO. Identification of viable myocardium (Editorial). *Circulation* 1996;94:2674–2680.

31. Di Carli MF, Asgarzadie F, Schelbert HR, et al. Quantitative relation between myocardial viability and improvement in heart failure symptoms after revascularization in patients with ischemic cardiomyopathy. *Circulation* 1995;92:3436–3444.

32. Milano CA, White WD, Smith LR, et al. Coronary artery bypass in patients with severely depressed ventricular function. *Ann Thorac Surg* 1993;56:487–493.

33. Pigott JD, Kouchoukos NT, Oberman A, Cutter GR. Late results of surgical and medical therapy for patients with coronary artery disease and depressed left ventricular function. *J Am Coll Cardiol* 1985;5:1036–1045.

34. Dreyfus G, Duboc D, Blasco A, et al. Coronary surgery can be an alternative to heart transplantation in selected patients with end-stage ischemic heart disease. *Eur J Cardiothorac Surg* 1993;7:482–487.

35. Christakis GT, Weisel RD, Fremes SE, et al. Coronary artery bypass grafting in patients with poor ventricular function. Cardiovascular Surgeons of the University of Toronto. *J Thorac Cardiovasc Surg* 1992;103: 1083–1091.

36. Kron IL, Flanagan TL, Blackbourne LH, Schroeder RA, Nolan SP. Coronary revascularization rather than cardiac transplantation for chronic ischemic cardiomyopathy. *Ann Surg* 1989;210:348–352.

37. Van Trigt P. Ischemic cardiomyopathy: the role of coronary artery bypass. *Coron Artery Dis* 1993;4:707–712.

38. Bounous EP, Mark DB, Pollock BG, et al. Surgical survival benefits for coronary disease patients with left ventricular dysfunction. *Circulation* 1988;78:I151–I157.

22

Coronary Stent Retrieval: Devices and Techniques

Kirk N. Garratt

Mayo Graduate School of Medicine and Cardiovascular Diseases and Internal Medicine, Adult Cardiac Catheterization Laboratory, St. Mary's Hospital, Mayo Clinic and Foundation, Department of Medicine, Rochester, Minnesota 55905

The benefit of coronary stent use has been established, and accordingly stent utilization continues to increase. In 1998 an estimated 450,000 coronary stents were placed in the United States and it is estimated that this number may approach 850,000 within 3 years. With the development and use of coronary stents, a new set of technical problems and potential complications has arisen.

During the earliest period of stent use, new systems for the conduct of angioplasty had to be invented. New equipment and techniques were needed to accommodate the bulky first-generation stents. Since coronary stents were unavailable for an extended period during which operators were keenly interested in using them, many interventionalists obtained stents approved for noncoronary uses (biliary and peripheral vascular applications chiefly) and mounted them manually onto coronary angioplasty balloons. Since little was known about optimal properties of stent delivery balloons, stents slipped free of their delivery balloons with regularity. Furthermore, under many circumstances, the safety of stent insertion was uncertain. Since only one first-generation stent was available with a protective sheath integrated into the delivery system, some operators developed *ad hoc* systems for protecting and delivering stents into tough spots. Although clever, these systems were often unreliable. Combining with a steep initial learning curve for stent procedures in general, this early period offered ample opportunity to experience stent delivery failures.

Stent failures can be categorized into three types:

1. inability to deploy, successful stent retraction,
2. inability to deploy, unsuccessful stent retraction, stent loss, and
3. inability to deploy, unsuccessful stent retraction, stent loss with retrieval.

The first category requires little commentary, since successful stent retraction usually results in no significant additional patient risk. The second category includes stents lost through embolization and those left behind when deployed in a vascular segment other than the target segment. The third category is perhaps the most interesting, since it entails several novel techniques and the use of equipment that was previously unfamiliar to cardiac interventionalists (although very familiar to vascular radiologists).

In this chapter, the methods for avoiding the need for coronary stent retrieval, the clinical consequences of stent loss, and the techniques useful for retrieving lost stents will be reviewed.

INCIDENCE OF STENT LOSS

The actual frequency of stent loss and retrieval is very hard to determine, because this event has not been tabulated in most large interventional databanks, and it is almost certain to be widely under-reported. Furthermore, it is virtually certain that some stents pose a greater risk of dislodgment from their delivery balloons than others. Although not documented, there is a prevailing belief (probably founded) that unprotected, flexible coil stents pose the greatest risk of damage or dislodgment owing to the relatively delicate nature of these devices. The most delicate design is the free-helical design Medtronic Wiktor stent (Medtronic, Inc., Minneapolis, MN) (1). In the North American Medtronic Wiktor stent study, mechanical delivery problems resulted in stent delivery failure in 17 of 355 patients (4.8%), but irretrievable stent loss occurred in only two patients (0.6%) (2).

Most operators claim that their rate of stent loss is quite low. Alfonso and colleagues described a stent embolization rate of less than 2% for a consecutive series of 500 patients treated with a variety of stent designs (3). More recently, Cantor and colleagues described their experience with 1,303 stent placement attempts occurring between March 1994 and June 1996 (4). They observed stent delivery failure (defined as inability to deliver the stent to the target lesion or inability to deploy it accurately and adequately) in 108 cases (8.3%). An attempt to withdraw the stent was made in almost all cases, and they were successful in retrieving the stent in 45% of these attempts. In 38% of these cases (3.1% of the total population) the stent embolized peripherally. A stent was dislodged in the left main artery in 4% of cases. In about one-third of initially unsuccessful stent placement attempts, a subsequent stent was placed successfully.

CLINICAL CONSEQUENCES OF STENT LOSS

The consequences of a stent loss episode are presumed to hinge on a few factors:

1. the clinical setting in which the stent procedure is undertaken,
2. the ultimate location of a lost or embolized stent, and
3. the likelihood of blood flow impediment resulting from a misplaced stent.

Almost all high-volume stent operators have experienced stent embolization into the peripheral arterial bed, and almost all believe that the event is benign under almost all conditions. Clearly, embolization into the cranial circulation should be avoided to minimize risk of cerebral complications. Otherwise, peripheral stent embolization *per se* rarely causes an overt clinical problem.

However, there may be an association between a stent loss episode and adverse clinical events. Cantor (4) reported that stent deployment failure was associated with an in-hospital adverse event rate of 19%, including three deaths, a 5% incidence of nonfatal myocardial infarction, and a 16% rate of urgent coronary artery bypass surgery. Furthermore, 39% of these patients had experienced death, myocardial infarction, or the need for additional target lesion revascularization within 6 months of their stent loss episode. These data suggest that stent loss may identify a population of patients at increased risk of adverse clinical events, which themselves may or may not be the consequence of the stent loss event.

AVOIDING STENT LOSS EPISODES

Colombo has described stent detachment as a "problem solved by preventing its occurrence" (5). This would seem unarguable, but the harsh truth is that there is little confirmed information regarding factors contributing to an increased risk of stent loss. For the most part, interventionalists are dependent on the anecdotal reports of high-volume operators about their perceptions and impressions regarding risk.

In Cantor's large published experience in 1,303 consecutive patients (4), 40% were undergoing stent implantation as a planned elective procedure, 18% were treated for an abrupt closure or threatened abrupt closure event, and 43% were treated for a nonischemic, suboptimal angioplasty event. By 1999 standards, this distribution of stent indications seems skewed toward less elective and more urgent stent procedures: in our laboratory at Mayo Clinic, stents are used in more than 70% of patients and the significant majority are placed for elective indications. Indeed, our "preemptive" use of coronary stents has led to a significant decline in the frequency of abrupt vascular closure events (6). It seems reasonable to anticipate that the more challenging clinical and angiographic circumstances surrounding the stent event would have an impact on the risk of stent loss, but there are insufficient data to analyze this issue fully.

Most experienced operators identify arterial calcification (as a marker of reduced coronary compliance), proximal vessel tortuosity, and poor guide catheter support as important elements contributing to stent loss risk. Although insufficient data are available to be certain of this, experience and reason support these claims. There is also a widespread belief that newer stent designs are less prone to stent loss. Some stent systems have been designed with the explicit intent to reduce this risk (NIR stent with SOX [Scimed, Maple Grove, MN], sheathed ACS Multi-Link stent [Guidant Inc. Santa Clara, CA]) but there does appear to be a lower reported incidence of stent loss with newer generation stents, even those stents without special protective mechanisms. Since newer stents are typically mounted on lower profile delivery balloons, it does not necessarily follow that they would be less likely to slip from their delivery catheters. For example, the Medtronic beStent (Medtronic Inc., Minneapolis, MN) experienced a higher rate of stent dislodgment than had been predicted, prompting a suspension of the beStent clinical trial in late 1997. A problem with insufficient crimping of the larger beStent iteration (BEL design) was identified and corrected, and the trial was resumed. Despite this, it does appear that stent engineers have, in general, created improved production systems resulting in better stent adherence for balloon-mounted stents.

A few technical innovations have been proposed to reduce the risk of stent loss. "Homemade" stent sheaths made of 6 Fr or larger multipurpose catheters have been used to protect stents, but they are almost never needed with contemporary stents. Colombo and coworkers have advocated an altered balloon surface structure meant to improve the reliability of stent adherence to the balloon (7). Rokas and colleagues have described an innovative technique for using a guidewire to strap a stent onto the high-pressure-tolerant ACS Flowtrack autoperfusion balloon catheter (Guidant Corp) (8). In this imaginative approach, a guidewire is advanced through the central catheter lumen, out of a proximal perfusion port, over the outer surface of the balloon, then back into the central lumen through a distal perfusion port. If a stent is mounted onto the balloon before the wire is threaded through the catheter in this fashion, then the wire essentially straps the stent onto the balloon between the proximal and distal perfusion ports, making loss of the stent during advancement very unlikely. The guidewire is retracted once the balloon is in position to permit stent placement.

STENT RETRIEVAL DEVICES

Several techniques have been derived empirically for the recovery of damaged or misplaced stents. A discussion of the various devices that have been found useful for this purpose follows. (Table 22.1)

Loop Snare

Figure 22.1A, these are closed-loop snare devices that can be used to grasp a stent (9,10). Such devices have been used widely in vascular radiology and cardiology procedures for retrieval of retained components, such as fractured guidewires or retained components. These devices consist of a movable wire contained within an outer plastic catheter. The wire passes through the catheter, exits the distal tip, then is folded over and re-enters the distal catheter tip. Movement of one or both ends of the wire allows the snare to be opened or closed. The loop snare can be passed over the distal end of a damaged

TABLE 22.1. *Equipment for removal of deployed stents*

Loop snares
Basket retrieval devices
Biliary stent forceps
Biopsy or alligator forceps
Cook retained fragment retrieval tool
Miscellaneous retrieval tools

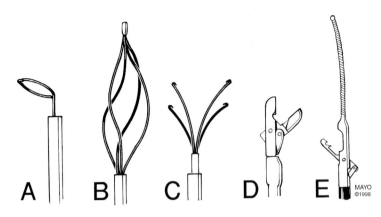

FIG. 22.1. Devices useful for recovering damaged coronary stents. **A:** Loop snare. **B:** Basket retrieval device. **C:** Biliary stone forceps. **D:** Biopsy forceps. **E:** Cook retained fragment retriever.

stent and cinched tightly; the snare and the stent system can then be withdrawn safely.

Snares can be fashioned in the laboratory from a 300-cm coronary wire and a 5 Fr diagnostic catheter. The loops of these "homemade" snares exit the catheter tip in the same axis as the catheter, though, and can be difficult to negotiate over a damaged stent. Commercial loop snares are available with loops that extend either in the direction of the long axis of the delivery catheter, or folded to open at a 90 degree angle from the delivery catheter (like a halo); these are generally of greater utility in recovery damaged stents. Loop snares are available with loop diameters ranging from 0.5 cm to 5 cm, and have catheter bodies that are 4 or 5 Fr in diameter. Commercial catheters are available in up to 150-cm lengths. Most loop snares have only moderate radiopacity.

The loop can be advanced over the distal end of the guidewire to seize a stent, but under these circumstances the coronary position of the guidewire must be sacrificed. Alternatively, the loop can be passed over the proximal end of the delivery catheter first (outside the body) advanced through the hemostatic sheath, and along the balloon shaft until it reaches the stent. In this fashion the loop snare can be used to recover a damaged stent without loss of the coronary guidewire position.

Basket Retrieval Device

As shown in Figure 22.1B, the basket retrieval device consists of a set of helically-arranged loops that can be expanded or collapsed. Originally designed to remove ureteral and biliary stones, this device can be used to trap lost or retained components within its loops (9). It can be used to catch a stent from the side and pull it free of a deployment balloon. This device works best if the stent has been damaged and misshapen such that a portion of the stent projects laterally away from the deployment balloon. Under some circumstances, it may be possible to recover the stent without sacrificing the position of the coronary guidewire across the target lesion. Basket retrieval devices are available commercially from several companies and are available in a variety of expanded sizes and catheter lengths.

Biliary Stone Forceps Device

As shown in Figure 22.1C, the biliary stone forceps device consists of a set of curved, finger-like projections that can be expanded/extended or contracted/retracted. This device was designed for percutaneous removal of obstructive stones in the biliary tree. Manipulating the "fingers" of this device, an operator can grab hold of lost or retained components. This device is most useful in recovering partially expanded stents, or in situations in which a portion of a stent has become separated from the deployment balloon catheter. Under these circumstances, it is often possible to remove a damaged stent without having to lose the guidewire position. Biliary forceps are available with catheter bodies of 4 or 5 Fr, and in lengths of 130 cm. The retracted device has fair visibility under fluoroscopy, but the extended finger-like projections have poor radiopacity. It is possible to damage vascular structures with the sharp fingers of this device and it must be handled cautiously.

Biopsy or Alligator Forceps

As shown in Figure 22.1D, the biopsy or alligator forceps devices have distal tip modifications that allow grasping of structures through a "biting jaws" action. Myocardial bioptomes are the most familiar example of such a tool. Although a variety of forceps devices are available, most are not suitable for vascular use, because (a) the shaft diameter is too large, (b) the device is too rigid to passed safely in the arterial system, and/or (c) the catheter length (often 80–90 cm) may be inadequate. Myocardial bioptomes and long alligator forceps have both been used to recover stents successfully (11,12). The thinner, softer, and longer disposable bioptomes may offer advantages. Although bioptome jaws are not meant for cutting through metal, it is possible that aggressive gripping with such a device could sever a thin metal stent.

Cook Retained Fragment Retrieval Tool

As shown in Figure 22.1E, the retained fragment retrieval tool catheter, manufactured by Cook, Inc. (Bloomington, IN) has a guidewire attached to its distal end, resembling a fixed-wire angioplasty balloon catheter. An articulating arm operable from the proximal hub permits grasping and retrieving of retained equipment fragments. This catheter was developed for use by vascular radiologists aiming to retrieve retained components. The device is available in 80-cm and 145-cm lengths. Its bulk and rigidity make it unattractive for use within coronary arteries, but it has been used in our laboratory to recover damaged stents from within the aorta.

CORONARY STENT RETRIEVAL TECHNIQUE

Stents Within the Coronary Artery

Management of a misplaced or embolized stent that is within the coronary artery will typi-

cally involve minimizing the consequences of the event rather than retrieving the stent. Occasionally, a relatively intact stent that has slipped free of its deployment balloon catheter may be retrieved by advancing a 2.0-mm balloon through it, inflating the balloon distally, and retracting (9,13,14). For 3.0-mm vessels and larger this is a reasonably safe thing to do: remember, 6 Fr directional coronary atherectomy devices have a profile as large as an inflated 2.0 mm balloon, so these vessels should accommodate this maneuver. Even more rarely, it may be possible to insert one of the retrieval devices described above into the vessel to grasp the stent. This requires clearance to have the devices work properly, and should only be considered in large vessels such as saphenous vein grafts. There is certainly the potential for vascular injury through scraping from an edge of the stent when an attempt is made to drag it from the vessel. For this reason, most stents embolized into the coronary system are best managed by full complete deployment: advance an appropriately sized angioplasty balloon over the position of the stent and inflate it to fix the position of the stent and minimize its effects on blood flow (9,15). It is ideal to advance the balloon through the center of the stent and expand it in the usual fashion, but if this is not possible, it is better to push the stent out of the lumen than to leave it unexpanded within the lumen. At least one case report has detailed the consequences of an unrecognized stent embolization into a left anterior descending artery which led to recurrent ischemic symptoms and repeat catheterization (15). In this case, the embolized stent was expanded successfully several weeks after its initial placement attempt.

Stents Outside the Coronary Artery

The approach to recovery of a damaged, misplaced or embolized stent will depend on the type of stent involved. The following sections describe the approach used in our laboratory for flexible coil-type stents and the more rigid slotted-tube–designed stents. To date, there is insufficient experience in recovery of self-expanding stents to comment on best approaches for retrieval of them.

Flexible Coil Stents

Small, unsheathed flexible coil stents with relatively low mass, mounted on a factory-issued deployment balloon catheter, have been very popular but are currently being outpaced by the rapid development of slotted-tube variants with increased flexibility and trackability. These stents are susceptible to damage during attempted placement.

If stent placement is interrupted or fails, and the stent is still intact and attached to the deployment balloon catheter, then the delivery catheter should be withdrawn. Although manufacturers warn operators not to attempt to pull stents back into a guide catheter once they have exited, stents can usually be withdrawn safely if the guide catheter distal tip has an excellent coaxial relationship to the proximal arterial segment being approached. If this is not the case, then the guide catheter should be retracted until a favorable alignment between guide and stent delivery catheter can be achieved. This can usually be achieved in the ascending aorta, but if any doubt exists the system should be retracted to the descending aorta to below the level of the renal arteries. This not only minimizes the risk should the stent be stripped free of the delivery balloon, but it also simplifies approaching the stent with a retrieval device if withdrawal fails. On occasion, removal may require retracting the guiding catheter to the distal end of the intraarterial sheath, which results in tip straightening (Fig. 22.2). It is usually possible to retain the guidewire position with these maneuvers. Using high-resolution fluoroscopy, it is usually possible to determine if the stent is being displaced from the deployment balloon as the system is retracted; some stents are easily seen making this maneuver is somewhat safer.

Retraction of the stent into the guide catheter may fail if a proper alignment cannot be achieved. In this circumstance, the edge of the

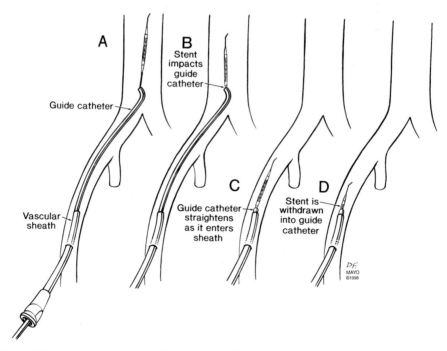

FIG. 22.2. Withdrawing an undeployed stent from the coronary artery into the guide requires that there be an excellent coaxial relationship; otherwise, the stent may be stripped off of the balloon. Achieving this coaxial relationship is dependent upon the specific guide catheter configuration and its relationship to the coronary ostium. In some patients, the guide catheter may require withdrawal part of the way into the sheath to straighten it out.

catheter tip may deform the stent or strip it free of the delivery catheter. If the stent cannot be withdrawn into the guide catheter, then the guide and stent catheters should be withdrawn simultaneously and removed from the body. Stent manufacturers usually suggest removal of the vascular sheath as well, but this can result in the stent becoming dislodged in the skin and it complicates vascular access, even if a guidewire is left in place. If the stent fails to come out with the other gear, it has been dislodged at the distal tip of the hemostatic sheath and can be retrieved using one of the retrieval devices described above. Alternatively, the guide catheter can be removed and a retrieval device can be advanced alongside the deployment catheter. The devices described above will pass alongside most stent delivery catheters as long as an 8 Fr or larger sheath has been used, and those available with 4 Fr shafts will pass through 6 Fr sheaths if the stent delivery catheter has been taken out.

An important caveat is to leave the stent on the wire, even if the coronary position has been lost. The wire provides a "lifeline" to the stent; once the wire is removed, the stent becomes subject to embolization and can place the operator in a situation in which stent retrieval is extraordinarily difficult.

If a stent is in a large vascular space it may be retrieved using one of the retrieval devices discussed above. Whenever possible the stent should be retracted to below the level of the renal arteries. The easiest device to use is the loop snare (Fig. 22.3). The guide catheter may be withdrawn to ease passage of the retrieval device, but the stent delivery catheter may be left in place to buttress the stent and help identify its location. The loop snare is inserted through the hemostatic valve alongside the stent delivery catheter, and advanced until it is superior to the damaged stent. The guidewire is retracted until it is below the level of the snare. The loop snare is opened and passed over the guidewire tip, then retracted until the stent is within the hold of the loop. Both the loop snare and the delivery catheter are removed as a single unit. As mentioned in the device section above, it may be possible to advance the loop snare from the proximal end of the system and approach the damaged stent

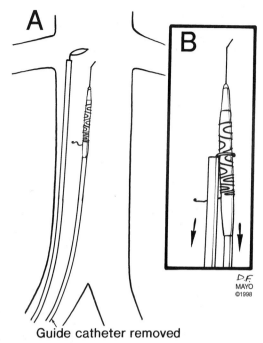

Guide catheter removed

FIG. 22.3. Loop snare to retrieve damaged flexible-coil type stent. **A:** The loop is advanced alongside the damaged stent then passed over the guidewire and stent delivery catheter from above (i.e., from distally). **B:** The loop is placed over the damaged stent. The stent catheter and loop snare are then retracted together. It is also possible to place the loop over the delivery catheter shaft outside the body, before advancing it through the vascular sheath, thereby approaching the damaged stent from below (i.e., from the proximally).

from below, thereby allowing recovery of the stent without necessarily sacrificing guidewire position. This maneuver is easier if the delivery balloon has been removed and the loop snare is advanced over the proximal end of the guidewire.

Flexible coil stents can usually be retrieved without loss of the guidewire position using biliary forceps (Fig. 22.4). For example, if a stent is damaged at the coronary ostium, the delivery balloon catheter can be removed and a long biliary forceps catheter inserted through the guide catheter. With the tip of the guide catheter approximated to the damaged stent, the "fingers" of the biliary forceps are opened and advanced

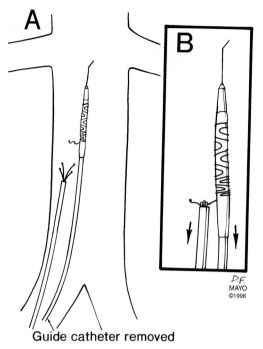

Guide catheter removed

FIG. 22.4. Biliary forceps for grasping flexible-coil type stent. **A:** The forceps are advanced alongside the stent. **B:** The damaged portion of the stent is grasped with the forceps. The stent delivery catheter and forceps are removed together.

out of the guide catheter. The "fingers" are closed around the stent and it is pulled into the guide catheter. With care, this can be done without trapping the guidewire.

The basket retrieval device may also be used, but it is more difficult to control and can easily trap the guidewire along with the damaged stent (Fig. 22.5). This device is generally of most use when a flexible coil stent has a portion of stent material projecting away from the delivery catheter at an angle approaching 90 degrees.

Slotted-Tube Stents

Unlike the flexible coil stents, the rigid slotted-tube stents are generally constructed of sheets of metal that are cut or stamped in such a fashion as to make windows in the sheet of material which enlarge upon stent expansion. These stents typically are more rigid and cannot

be unraveled or otherwise streamlined for removal. Newer stent designs that mimic loops or coils bonded to one another in a series of repeating elements tend to behave more like classic slotted tube designs, and are included in this category for the purposes of this discussion.

In general, older slotted-tube stents, such as the Johnson and Johnson JJIS stent (Johnson and Johnson International Systems, Warren, NJ), should be deployed rather than extracted if malposition occurs. Attempts to remove damaged or partially expanded high-mass slotted tube stents have been successful (16–18), but can result in substantial vascular injury at the arterial exit site. This is especially true of Johnson and Johnson peripheral or biliary stents. These are still used widely for treatment of very large conduits such as saphenous vein graft lesions. A fully or partially expanded peripheral or biliary stent might be recoverable using the snare balloon technique

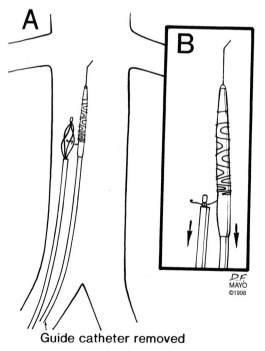

Guide catheter removed

FIG. 22.5. Basket retrieval device for removing damaged flexible-coil stent. **A:** The device is advanced alongside the damaged stent. **B:** The damaged portion of the stent is grasped with the forceps. The stent delivery catheter and forceps are removed together.

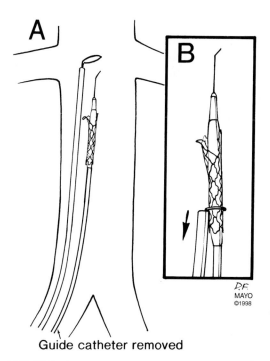

Guide catheter removed

FIG. 22.6. Loop snare device for retrieving rigid, slotted-tube stents. **A:** Loop is advanced over the distal end of stent and balloon catheter. **B:** Grasping the stent near its proximal limit will ease passage through the vascular sheath.

(Fig. 22.6). The snare can be used to collapse the stent as much as possible, near the proximal end of the stent. It may then be retracted into the vascular sheath. However, be advised that this can be a difficult and fruitless endeavor. Despite attempts with large sheaths—up to 14 Fr—it can be very difficult to appropriately position a crushed stent into the opening of the vascular sheath and retract it. Typically the stent becomes hung up at the mouth of the sheath, causing the sheath to collapse and making further retraction impossible. It has been recommended that the entire apparatus (stent, recovery tool, and hemostatic sheath) then be removed as a unit, hopefully while maintaining a vascular access wire. Unfortunately, the stent can become lodged in the subcutaneous tissues as you try to extract it, and it may necessitate a common femoral arteriotomy to complete removal. For this reason, and in view of the essentially universal benignity of lower extremity stent emboliza-

tion, it may be wiser to simply allow the stent to embolize distally at this point. If an appropriately sized peripheral vessel can be identified, the stent can be positioned there.

The Cook retrieval device is also useful for removing slotted tube design stents, especially those with low mass (Fig. 22.7). As with the loop snare, the goal is to grasp the damaged stent at the proximal end to ease its passage through the vascular sheath. The same cautions apply as discussed above.

Happily, the newer, low-mass slotted tube-type stents are not as problematic in this regard. They usually can be retrieved by entrapment with a loop snare and retraction through the hemostatic sheath; even if the edge of the stent catches the sheath, the low-mass stents will usually collapse enough to come out. Replacement of the vascular sheath is then recommended.

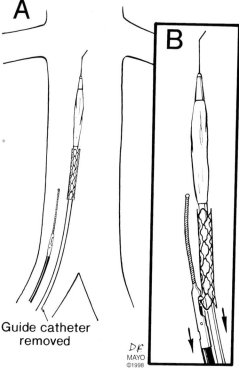

Guide catheter removed

FIG. 22.7. Use of the Cook retained fragment retrieval tool for removal of slotted-tube–design stent. **A:** Tool is advanced along side-stent delivery catheter. **B:** The stent is grasped at its proximal end and retracted through vascular sheath.

MANAGING DELIVERY BALLOON LEAKAGE AND RUPTURE

An additional area that can be problematic involves balloon dysfunction during stent expansion. Delivery balloon rupture may cause the balloon to become trapped in a partially deployed stent. Happily, this problem is uncommon and is most likely to occur when a fibrocalcific lesion has been inadequately predilated and the delivery balloon has been inflated to a pressure beyond its tolerance limit. The initial impulse is to pull firmly on the trapped balloon, but this can displace the stent without freeing the balloon, and create a situation in which the stent can be neither deployed successfully nor retrieved.

In vein grafts or large right coronary arteries, it may be possible to advance the guide catheter into the vessel until it abuts the damaged balloon. At this point, pulling the balloon toward the guide will cinch the guide into the stent which will often cause the balloon to come free. Another option is to advance a fixed-wire balloon catheter ("balloon-on-a-wire system") alongside the trapped balloon and into the stent. Although somewhat more difficult to manipulate, fixed-wire balloons enjoy a very low profile which is critical in this application. Inflation of the fixed-wire balloon may allow enough expansion of the stent so that the trapped balloon can be removed.

Stent leakage is somewhat more common, and occurs most often when a hand-mounted stent has pinched the delivery balloon and created a pinhole leak. If the deployment balloon is leaking but not ruptured, the situation can be remedied using a brief, rapid, high-pressure inflation designed to force the balloon to expand fully before it can rupture (9). Attaching the inflation port of a leaking balloon to a power injector and providing a brief, high-pressure, low-volume power inflation has been successful in expanding such stents further, permitting withdrawal of the damaged balloon. The best settings to use will vary according to the situation, but we have been successful using injections of 20–30 cc/sec over 0.5–1.0 sec, setting pressure maximums at 400–600 mm Hg (27–41 bars). Higher pressure limits may exceed the tolerance of the catheter body, thereby involving the risk of catheter (rather than balloon) rupture. Newer balloon technologies may reduce the risk of pinhole leaks (7).

It should be noted that occasionally a balloon rupture can be a useful thing. Baggy ruptured balloons easily snag undeployed stents, and have been used to extract unexpanded stents (19).

CONCLUSION

Stent retrieval is best avoided, but since the criteria identifying high-risk patients have not been defined, it is likely that all stent operators will have an opportunity to retrieve some stents. In the absence of definitive data, vascular noncompliance (evidenced by angiographic calcification or difficulty advancing other equipment into the target vessel), tortuosity, pre-existing vascular disruption, and poor guide support are likely correlates of stent placement failure.

Specific stent retrieval techniques are varied and a number of approaches have been successful. The best retrieval technique to use will depend primarily on the location of the damaged stent and the type of stent used. The loop snare is probably the most consistently helpful retrieval device. With all retrieval systems and strategies it is important to maintain a guidewire through the stent whenever possible to stabilize the position of the stent until it can be recovered. Distal embolization into the peripheral circulation below the level of the renal arteries, or deployment in a small peripheral vessel, are alternatives to management of a damaged stent, but a reasonable effort should be made to recover damaged stents in most cases.

Stent loss events correlate with an increased risk of adverse clinical events. It is not clear whether stent loss is causal with respect to these clinical events (some data suggest this is not the case) or if patients with high-risk circumstances are more likely to experience trouble with stent placement. In either case, stent mishaps should be considered serious events and heightened clinical vigilance is warranted for these patients.

REFERENCES

1. White C. The Wiktor and Wiktor-i stents. In: Serruys PW , Kutryk MJB, eds. *Handbook Of Coronary Stents*, 2nd ed. St Louis: Mosby, 1998:31–44.
2. Garratt KN, White CJ, Buchbinder M et al. Wiktor stent placement for unsuccessful coronary angioplasty: the American experience. *J Inv Cardiol* 1995;7[Suppl C]: 35C.
3. Alfonso F, Martinez D, Hernandez R et al. Stent embolization during intracoronary stenting. *Am J Cardiol* 1996; 78:833–835.
4. Cantor WJ, Lazzam C, Cohen EA et al. Failed coronary stent deployment. *Am Heart J* 1998;136(6):1088–1095.
5. Colombo A. Stent retrieval. In: Serruys PW, Kutryk MJB, eds. *Handbook Of Coronary Stents*, 2nd ed. St Louis: Mosby, 1998:275–282.
6. Suh WW, Grill DE, Rihal CS, Bell MR, Holmes DR Jr, Garratt KN. Availability of intracoronary stents is associated with decreased abrupt vascular closure rates and improved early clinical outcomes. Submitted to *Circulation*.
7. di Mario C, Reimers B, Reinhardt R, Ferraro M, Moussa I, Colombo A. New stent delivery balloon: a technical note. *Cathet Cardiovasc Diagn* 1997;42:452–456.
8. Rokas SG, Antonellis IP, Patsilinakos SP et al. New method for placement of intracoronary stents in order to avoid their embolization in the intravascular space. *Cathet Cardiovasc Diagn* 1998;45(2):183–187.
9. Foster-Smith KW, Garratt KN, Higano ST, Holmes DR Jr. Retrieval techniques for managing flexible intracoronary stent misplacement. *Cathet Cardiovasc Diagn* 1993;30:63–68.
10. Elsner M, Peifer A, Kasper W. Intracoronary loss of balloon-mounted stents: successful retrieval with a 2 mm—''Microsnare''—device. *Cathet Cardiovasc Diagn* 1996;39:271–276.
11. Berder V, Bedossa M, Gras D, Paillard F, Le Breton H, Pony JC. Retrieval of a lost coronary stent from the descending aorta using a PTCA balloon and biopsy forceps. *Cathet Cardiovasc Diagn* 1993;28:351–353.
12. Eeckhout E, Stauffer JC, Goy JJ. Retrieval of a migrated coronary stent by means of an alligator forceps catheter. *Cathet Cardiovasc Diagn* 1993;30:166–168.
13. Wong PH. Retrieval of undeployed intracoronary Palmaz-Schatz stents. *Cathet Cardiovasc Diagn* 1995;35: 218–223.
14. Cishek MB, Laslett L, Gershony G. Balloon catheter retrieval of dislodged coronary artery stents: a novel technique. *Cathet Cardiovasc Diagn* 19995;34(4): 350–352.
15. Kirk MM, Herzog WR. Deployment of a previously embolized, unexpanded, and disarticulated Palmaz-Schatz stent. *Cathet Cardiovasc Diagn* 1997;42: 331–334.
16. Kobayashi Y, Nonogi H, Miyazaki S, Daikoku S, Yamamoto Y, Takamiya M. Successful retrieval of unexpanded Palmaz-Schatz stent from left main coronary artery. *Cathet Cardiovasc Diagn* 1996;38(4):402–404.
17. Rozenman Y, Burstein M, Hasin Y, Gotsman MS. Retrieval of occluding unexpanded Palmaz-Schatz stent from a saphenous aorto-coronary vein graft. *Cathet Cardiovasc Diagn* 1995;34(2):159–161.
18. Veldhuijzen FL, Bonnier HJ, Michels HR, el Gamal MI, van Gelder BM. Retrieval of undeployed stents from the right coronary artery: report of two cases. *Cathet Cardiovasc Diagn* 1993;30:245–248.
19. Bersin RM, Gold RS Jr. Balloon rupture during peripheral stent implantation: a new technique for balloon retrieval. *Cathet Cardiovasc Diagn* 1993;29(4):292–295.

23

Management of Vascular Sheath Following PTCA

A. Vascular Closure Devices for Immediate Sheath Removal after Coronary Interventions: Luxury or Necessity?

Sigmund Silber

Department of Cardiology, University of Munich, Dr. Mueller Hospital, 81379 Munich, Germany

Coronary interventions are usually performed by the femoral approach; the brachial approach is showing a continuously declining trend (1). Patients undergoing the femoral approach, however, are usually immobilized overnight, which may result in significant discomfort with increased back pain and need for analgesics (2). Noncompliance of the patients regarding strict bedrest after the procedure has been reported to be a substantial factor for femoral complications after PTCA, increasing the risk of hematoma formation and of rebleeding (3). Sandbags do not reduce vascular complications and even increase patients' discomfort (4). Mechanical compression devices could not effect clinically relevant advantages (3,5).

Reducing the sheath size was presumed to result in fewer local vascular complications (6). Although newer, 6 Fr guiding catheters even allow safe stenting in 3.5 mm-vessels, there was no reduction in bleeding complications related to the reduction in sheath size (1,7,8). This miniaturization of equipment also led to a revival of the transradial approach, which was initially suggested for diagnostic angiography (9). Although the transradial approach for PTCA is more time-consuming and has a considerable learning curve, it remarkably increases patients' comfort and decreases bleeding complications (10).

With the current standard stent regimen using aspirin and ticlopidine (or clopidogrel), major local bleeding complications may still occur in approximately 2.5% (11,12). It has been estimated that major access site complications increase the hospital length of stay by approximately 2 days, adding roughly $2,000 to the overall procedural costs (13,14). Furthermore, glycoprotein-IIb/IIIa inhibitors (GP-IIb/IIIa inhibitors) are increasingly used in high- and low-risk patients; although the increased rate of bleeding complications in the EPIC study could be significantly reduced by decreasing the concomitant heparin dosage, the EPILOG and RESTORE trials still revealed a rate of major bleeding of 1.8% and 2.5% respectively in the patients treated with GP-IIb/IIIa inhibitors and of 2.3% to 3.1% in the placebo groups (15,16). The use of low molecular weight heparin in patients at high risk for stent thrombosis may also be associated with a higher bleeding risk (17).

The clinical use of vascular closure devices for rapid hemostasis after femoral access was first reported in 1991 (18). Ever since, these devices undoubtedly have proven to increase patients' comfort and decrease burden for the medical staff; they may also reduce hospital costs by shortening the length of stay. Patients may be ambulated almost immediately after diagnostic coronary angiography. They may also be discharged many hours earlier than the 6-hour supine restriction period enforced by most centers after diagnostic catheterization (14). After coronary interventions, patient comfort is additionally increased by immediate sheath removal (19–21).

The purpose of this chapter is to summarize the basic concepts and the clinical results of the four prevailing vascular closure devices after transfemoral coronary interventions and immediate sheath removal.

THE VASOSEAL DEVICE

Concept

VasoSeal, the "Vascular Hemostatic Device" (VHD, Datascope Corp., Montvale, NJ, USA) works predominantly by collagen-induced thrombus generation. It consists of purified collagen plugs that induce the formation of a hemostatic cap directly over the arterial puncture site. Biodegradable collagen induces platelet activation and aggregation, releasing coagulation factors and resulting in the formation of fibrin and the subsequent generation of a thrombus (22). Collagen is ultimately degraded and resorbed by granulocytes and macrophages. Antigenicity of purified collagen is considerably reduced and, although allergies to collagen are described (23), allergic reactions to collagen used for hemostasis have not been a clinical problem (24–26).

VasoSeal is the oldest of the clinically used sealing devices (18). It is comprised of four parts: a blunt-tipped, 11 Fr dilator, one of seven differently sized 11.5 Fr sheaths selected by length using a preprocedure needle-depth measurement technique, and two 90 mg collagen cartridges. (Details of these four parts are described elsewhere [25,26].) When the sheath is pulled, a short guidewire is inserted and the existing sheath is removed while maintaining manual compression. Then the blunt-tipped, 11 Fr dilator is inserted via the guidewire just down to the site of the arterial puncture. The 11.5 Fr sheath is advanced over the dilator down to the arterial surface. While still holding pressure, the dilator and the guidewire are removed and the collagen cartridge is deployed with a "push-and-pull" movement. We usually use only one cartridge of collagen, since we know from previous studies that one collagen plug is as effective as two plugs but is better tolerated (27–29). Recently, VasoSeal "ES" was released, introducing an enhanced guidance using a removable J-segment wire.

Clinical Results

Over 500,000 VasoSeal devices have been deployed worldwide. Reported deployment success rates vary from 88% (30) to 100% (20,24,31) (Table 23.1). Time to hemostasis for sheath removal immediately after the intervention varies from 5 to 8 minutes (20,25,26). A recently published study reported a mean time to hemostasis of 13.1 ± 6.1 minutes for VasoSeal deployment immediately after PTCA in 95 patients (32). Time to ambulation was not the primary endpoint in most controlled studies. The lower range time to ambulation after immediate sheath removal is 6 to 9 hours (20) with a mean

TABLE 23.1. *Relevant characteristics of the four prevailing vascular closure devices*

	VasoSeal	Angio-Seal	Duett	Perclose, Inc.
Deployment success rate	88%–100%	91%–100%	98%–100%	90%–100%
Time to hemostasis	5min–13min	2min–4min	4min–6min	11min–19min
Time to ambulation	6h–9h	6h–8h	2h–6h	4h–7h
Minor complications	8%	5.9%	2.1%	5.3%
Major complications	up to 5.3%	up to 1.3%	up to 1%	up to 4%

Data are based on immediate sheath removal after coronary intervention value of 8.7 ± 5.3 hours (32). In that "early" mobilization study, 52% of the patients receiving VasoSeal immediately after PTCA were mobilized after 6 hours and 82% after 10 hours (32). None of these patients was mobilized earlier than 6 hours.

Minor local complications have been reported in 8% and major complications in 5.3% of the 2,073 PTCA patients analyzed in 15 studies (20) (Table 23.1). This figure is comparable to a recently published single-center experience with major local complications in 5% of the 204 anticoagulated patients (33). Intraarterial insertions of VasoSeal with resultant leg ischemia have been reported in 0.3% to 2% (15/2,229) of the patients (20).

In our study addressing an identical sheath dwell time, and therefore an identical level of anticoagulation in the VasoSeal and the manual groups, there was no statistical difference regarding local complications. Although the incidence of medium or large hematoma was low, the trend toward decreasing smaller hematomas was counterbalanced by an increased risk of larger hematomas or a major complication, and may in part explain some of the published controversial findings (29).

THE ANGIO-SEAL DEVICE

Concept

Angio-Seal, the "Hemostatic Puncture Closing Device" (HPCD), was originally developed by the Kensey Nash Corporation, Exton, PA, USA, then distributed by Quinton Instruments and Sherwood, followed by Tyco, and now by St. Jude Medical Devices (Minneapolis, MN). It works predominantly by mechanical forces ("sandwich technique") and also by a collagen-induced thrombus formation.

Angio-Seal provides a mechanical block of the arterial puncture site with an anchor from inside the artery, guiding and holding the collagen in the tract (34). It consists of four components within a single delivery device ("carrier") requiring an 8 Fr sheath: an anchor, a collagen plug, a connecting suture, and a tamper. All three components deployed into the patient are completely resorbable; the anchor is made from polyglycolic and polylactic acids. The small plug contains only about 15 mg collagen. The technique of its deployment has been described in detail elsewhere (35,36). In brief, a short guidewire is inserted and the existing sheath removed while hemostasis is maintained with manual compression. The location of the end of the 8 Fr sheath is determined by the presence of blood flow through the modified dilator. The sheath–dilator combination is then advanced 1 cm further down the puncture site inside the artery lumen. The dilator is then removed and the carrier device introduced into the 8 Fr sheath. After the collagen is deployed, a tamper is pushed downwards to compress the collagen against the outer arterial wall; and a spring is attached between the tamper and a metal tag fixed to the positioning suture, thus applying continuous pressure on the tamper.

In our study, the reduction of the spring deployment time from 30 minutes to 5 minutes was not related to an increased risk of bleeding or other vascular complications (19). This technique makes handling of Angio-Seal easier, because the suture may be cut while the patients are still on the table in the catheterization laboratory. Furthermore, patients can be transferred much faster to the intermediate care unit, thereby reducing the burden on the personnel in the catheterization laboratory.

Clinical Results

Angio-Seal has been used in over 400,000 patients. Deployment success rates are in the range from 91% (37) to 100% (19,20). Data on time to hemostasis for sheath removal immediately after the intervention are sparse and in the range of 2 to 4 minutes (20), reflecting our own experience in over 2,000 applications. Regarding time to ambulation, no study specifically investigating early ambulation has been fully published. The shortest time interval between deployment and ambulation in a U.S. multicenter trial was 8 hours (36) (Table 23.1). For diagnostic patients, a time to ambulation of 1 hour (38), and even 20 minutes (39) was considered to be safe.

Minor local complications have been reported

in 5.9% (254 patients) and major complications in 0.4% of the 254 PTCA patients (20) (Table 23.1). A recently published report on 411 consecutive patients revealed a major complication rate of 1.3% (40). An inadvertent complete intraarterial deployment of Angio-Seal with resultant leg ischemia requiring surgical removal of the entire system was not published until recently (41).

Interestingly, the 8 Fr Angio-Seal is also safe and effective for 9 Fr sheaths (42). A newly developed 6 Fr device has been tested in France and is now available in Europe.

THE DUETT DEVICE

Concept

The Duett is a novel vascular sealing device (Vascular Solutions, Minneapolis, MN) which incorporates a unique low-profile balloon-positioning catheter in combination with a biological procoagulant mixture containing collagen and thrombin. It works purely by generating a thrombus.

The low-profile catheter (3 Fr) incorporates a moveable core wire that allows *in vivo* modifications of the balloon dimensions. When the device is inflated, the balloon assumes an elliptical shape with a significantly larger diameter (6 mm) and a relatively short length. This configuration provides optimal temporary sealing of the arterial puncture from the luminal side by ensuring a large surface area of balloon in apposition to the puncture site and at the same time minimizing obstruction to flow through the lumen of the vessel. The procoagulant is a suspension comprised of 250 mg bovine microfibrillar collagen (Avitene, Davol Inc., Woburn, MA) and 10,000 units bovine thrombin (Jones Medical Inc., St. Louis, MO). This combination may be optimal for achieving rapid hemostasis at the arterial puncture site. The suspension incorporating both of these hemostatic agents is designed to have a suitable viscosity for injecting through the side arm of most vascular sheaths, yet have a consistency that would be likely to maintain the procoagulant material at the desired location in the periarterial space at the puncture site.

These aspects of the device may partially explain the remarkable absence of any delayed oozing from the arterial access site, of the sort that frequently plagues other sealing approaches, causing significant nursing and patient concerns. Detailed descriptions of the device appear elsewhere (43,44). In previously reported preclinical studies, the Duett was able to achieve rapid and reliable hemostasis in a canine model, regardless of sheath size or degree of anticoagulation (43).

Clinical Results

After the first clinical investigational protocol was approved by the International Ethics Committee in Freiburg, Germany, we applied this novel device for the first time in humans. A total of 24 patients were enrolled (44). For the PTCA patients, mean time to hemostasis, including deployment time and compression time, was 11.4 ± 2.9 minutes with a compression time ("time to hemostasis" in the old sense) of 6.0 ± 2.2 (44) minutes and a time to ambulation of 16.3 ± 4.9 hours (44) (Table 23.1). The most important concern related to the use of this device was the risk of inadvertent intravascular injection. Including measurements of several coagulation parameters, there was no evidence of intraarterial injection or leakage (44). No other major complication occurred (44). Our study was followed by the first U.S. feasibility trial of the device. The preliminary results in 43 patients were recently presented. The 11 interventional patients with immediate sheath removal showed a mean time to hemostasis of 4.6 ± 2.1 minutes with a mean time to ambulation of 5.4 ± 2.0 hours (45). All 40 patients with ultrasound follow-up showed no major complications. Considering the relatively low number of patients, deployment success rates are in the range from 98% to 100% (44,45). In a large, single-center study (46) as well as in the multicenter European registry with a total of 1,587 patients enrolled, patients were ambulated 2 to 6 hours after the intervention. Minor complications have been reported in 2.1% and major complications in 1%. An inadvertent intraarterial injection of the procoagulant occurred in four patients (0.3%) and was successfully treated by intraarterial infusion of urokinase in three cases and surgical repair in one. Overall, the Duett has been applied in over 3,500 cases worldwide. Enrollment into the US/European multicenter SEAL trial has just been completed, with 630 patients randomized (5:3) to Duett or manual compression. With 391 Duett applications, the results are pending.

THE PERCLOSE, INC. DEVICES

Concept

The series of Perclose, Inc. devices (Redwood City, CA) does not use collagen or thrombin; it is based solely on nonabsorbable sutures (47). The Prostar devices use four needles (two sutures); the Techstar devices two needles (one suture). The 11 Fr and 9 Fr Prostar devices have been discontinued; 8 Fr and 10 Fr Prostar are available for use with 8 Fr to 10 Fr sheaths; the 6 Fr and 7 Fr Techstar devices are for use with 5 Fr to 7 Fr sheaths.

The Perclose, Inc. devices include a number of components, including a 0.035-in. guidewire, a knot-pushing tool, a predilator for the subcutaneous tissue, and the suture-containing device itself (48). The needles exiting the device just inside the artery are drawn through the arterial wall and reenter the device outside the artery. As the ends of the sutures are pulled out, the suture loop is pulled against the arterial wall. Once it is apparent that hemostasis will be achieved, the guidewire is removed with further sequential tightening of the suture pairs (48).

Recently, the use of Perclose, Inc. devices in the brachial artery after coronary intervention was suggested (49). To enable the insertion in severely scarred groins, a modification of the deployment technique has been proposed (50).

Clinical Results

Perclose devices have been deployed in over 250,000 patients worldwide. After initial experience using Prostar (48), several uncontrolled studies have investigated the safety and efficacy of the Perclose, Inc. series in patients undergoing diagnostic and interventional catheterization

(51,52). The deployment success rate was 90% (53) (Table 23.1). In a randomized trial, the mean time to hemostasis in the interventional group of 95 patients was 11.0 ± 4.1 minutes and time to ambulation 7.1 ± 7.4 hours (54). Minor complications occurred in 5.3%, major complications in 3.2% and 4% (54,55) (Table 23.1). The relatively high vascular complication rates of 9% with a vascular surgery rate of 2.1% (56) may possibly be reduced after a learning curve of more than 250 cases per user (57).

The largest database for interventional procedures was reported in the STAND-II study (58). A total of 515 patients (90% 8 Fr, 10% 10 Fr sheaths) were randomized to either manual compression or Prostar Plus for immediate sheath removal. In the Prostar group the mean time to hemostasis was 19 minutes, time to standing was 206 minutes, and time to ambulation was 240 minutes; these times were significantly shorter compared with the manual group. However, vascular surgery was 1.2% and groin infection rate was 0.8%, with a total major complication rate of 2.4%.

COMPARISON OF THE FOUR DEVICES

Table 23.1 shows the published data on deployment success rates, time to hemostasis, time to ambulation, and minor and major complications.

Table 23.2 lists the basic differences between these devices. The hole in the artery is not influenced by the VasoSeal and the Duett, thus depending on sheath size only. The classical Vaso-Seal does not insert anything into the arterial lumen, whereas the VasoSeal ES and the Duett use a temporary intraarterial device (J-wire or balloon, respectively). Only the Angio-Seal leaves a part (the anchor) in the artery, which will be resorbed during the following weeks. The tissue track is enlarged by the VasoSeal to 11.5 Fr and by the Perclose device to 21 Fr. The VasoSeal seals the tissue track, whereas Perclose and Angio-Seal devices leave the tissue track open (increased risk of oozing). The Duett seals both the artery and the tissue track.

Table 23.3 gives an overview of which sealing device can be used for which sheath size. For 6

TABLE 23.2. *Differences in mechanisms for achieving hemostasis*

	Arterial puncture site			Tissue track	
	Diameter of the arterial hole	Hemostasis by		Diameter of the tissue track	Hemostasis by
		Intraarterial guidance	Supraarterial closure		
VasoSeal	Depending on sheath size	Temporary J-wire	Collagen (180 mg)	11.5Fr	Collagen
Angio-Seal	8Fr, 6Fr	Resorbable anchor	Collagen (26 mg, 13 mg)	8Fr, 6Fr	—
Duett	Depending on sheath size	Temporary balloon	Procoagulant (thrombin)	Depending on sheath size	Procoagulant (thrombin)
Perclose, Inc.	6Fr/8Fr/10Fr	Guide wire	Suture	21Fr	—

Fr, any of these devices may be used, although immediate post-PTCA sheath removal without a closure device using 6 Fr sheaths and weight adjusted heparin was recently suggested (59). For 7 Fr, VasoSeal, Duett and Perclose devices should be preferred; the Angio-Seal would punch an 8 Fr hole into the "7 Fr" artery, and to date there are no reports on using the 6 Fr Angio-Seal for 7 Fr sheaths. For 8 Fr, all devices are applicable. With 9 Fr sheaths, the Duett and Perclose devices should be preferred, although the 8 Fr Angio-Seal may work as well (42). For 10 Fr, Perclose is the only device to be recommended.

Table 23.4 describes the "ideal" sealing device. Unfortunately, none of the four devices fulfills all of the ideal criteria.

In our catheterization laboratories with many operators, several did not want to experience the rather flat learning curve required for Perclose (59). We have decided to use the Duett as our prevailing sealing device. We based our decision on the Duett's ability to leave no sequelae in the arterial lumen and its ability to simultaneously seal the arterial hole and the tissue track, which becomes increasingly more important with the growing use of GP-IIb/IIIa inhibitors. The major reason for our extensive use of sealing devices is not early ambulation or early discharge (in Germany, the hospitals are predominantly paid by the day and not by procedure) but rather immediate sheath removal. Patients and nurses equally appreciate the fact that the groin has already been "cleared" when the patient is transferred to the ward. Patients stopped on heparin or GP-IIb/IIIa inhibitors are usually ambulated after 6 hours, if intervention occurred in the morning or around noon. The afternoon patients as well as all patients on GP-IIb/IIIa inhibitors are ambulated the next day.

Recently, two new sealing devices have been presented. The DISC-Close-Sure (BioInterventional, Pleasanton, CA) developed a 13 Fr disc for 6 and 7 Fr sheaths as well as a 16 Fr disc

TABLE 23.3. *Sheath size as criteria for choosing a sealing device*

	6Fr	7Fr	8Fr	9Fr	10Fr	11Fr
VasoSeal	+	+	+	—	—	—
Angio-Seal	+	(+)	+	(+)	—	—
Duett	+	+	+	+	—	—
Perclose, Inc.	+	+	+	+	+	—

VasoSeal is recommended up to 8Fr Duett is recommended up to 9Fr; the Perclose series is currently available up to 10Fr.

TABLE 23.4. *Checklist for the "ideal" vascular closure device*

	VasoSeal	Angio-Seal	Duett	Perclose, Inc.
Deployment technique:				
• hole in the artery depends on sheath size only	+	−	+	(+)
• diameter of tissue track is not enlarged by device	−	(+)	+	−
• intraarterial guidance for steerability	(+)	+	+	+
• reaccess after nondeployment	−	−	−	+
• no intraarterial sequelae left	+	−	+	+
• single operator	+	+	+	−
Effectiveness:				
▲ Rapid and complete hemostasis	+	+	+	+
▲ no oozing (tissue track sealing)	+	−	+	−
▲ 100% effective	−	−	−	−
▲ 100% safe	−	−	−	−

for 8 Fr sheaths. X-Site Medical (Blue Pell, PA) presented another suture device as a probably lower-cost alternative to the Perclose series. This X-Site PFC (Percutaneous Femoral Closure) system was recently applied in the first 70 patients in South America.

CONCLUSIONS

With a current application rate of approximately 70,000 applications per month, vascular closure devices have become a substantial tool of invasive cardiology. The four major vascular closure devices for immediate sheath removal after coronary interventions have proven to be comparable regarding deployment success rates, time to hemostasis, and time to ambulation. They all satisfy the needs of the patient and the operator (60). Although some differences may exist regarding local complications (21), none of the devices have shown to reduce major local complications. Prospective randomized studies in patients receiving GP-IIb/IIIa inhibitors, addressing early ambulation (61) and cost/effectiveness aspects are needed. Then, in the words of ZG Turi, "the likelihood of routine arterial sealing of nearly all patients is around the corner" (62).

REFERENCES

1. Krone RJ, Johnson L, Noto T, and the Registry Committee of the Society for Cardiac Angiography and Interventions. Five year trends in cardiac catheterization: a report from the Registry of the Society for Cardiac Angiography and Interventions. *Cathet Cardiovasc Diagn* 1996;39:31–35.
2. Waksman R, Scott NA, Ghazzal ZMB et al. Randomized comparison of flexible versus nonflexible femoral sheaths on patient comfort after angioplasty. *Am Heart J* 1996;131:1076–1078.
3. Bogart DB, Bogart MA, Miller JT, Farrar MW, Barr WK, Montgomery MA. Femoral artery catheterization complications: a study of 503 consecutive patients. *Cathet Cardiovasc Diagn* 1995;34:8–13.
4. Christensen B, Lacarella C, Manion R, Bruhn-Ding B, Meyer S, Wilson R. Sandbags do not prevent complications after catheterization. *Circulation* 1994;90:I-205.
5. Pracyk JB, Wall TC, Longabaugh JP et al. A randomized trial of vascular hemostasis techniques to reduce femoral vascular complications after coronary intervention. *Am J Cardiol* 1998;81:970–976.
6. Resar JR, Prewitt KC, Wolff MR, Blumenthal R, Raqueno JV, Brinker JA. Percutaneous transluminal coronary angioplasty through 6 Fr diagnostic catheters: a feasibility study. *Am Heart J* 1993;125:1591–1596.
7. Cragg AH, Nakagawa N, Smith TP, Berbaum KS. Hematoma formation after diagnostic angiography: effect of catheter size. *J Vasc Interv Radiol* 1991;2:231–233.
8. Waksman R, King III SB, Douglas JS et al. Predictors of groin complications after balloon and new-device coronary intervention. *Am J Cardiol* 1995;75:886–889.
9. Campeau L. Percutaneous radial artery approach for coronary angiography. *Cathet Cardiovasc Diagn* 1989;16:3–7.
10. Kiemenej F, Laarman GJ, Odekerken D, Slagboom T, v.d. Wieken, R. A randomized comparison of percutaneous transluminal coronary angioplasty by the radial, brachial and femoral approaches: The Access Study. *J Am Coll Cardiol* 1997;29:1269–1275.
11. Bertrand ME, Legrand V, Boland J et al. Randomized multicenter comparison of conventional anticoagulation versus antiplatelet therapy in unplanned and elective coronary stenting—the FANTASTIC Study. *Circulation* 1998;98:1597–1603.
12. Leon MB, Baim DS, Popma JJ et al. A clinical trial

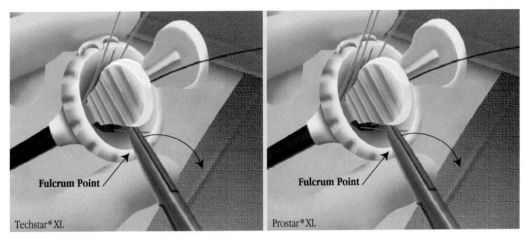

FIG. 23.4. Needle removal.
1. Verify that all needles are present.
2. Remove the posterior needle(s) first.

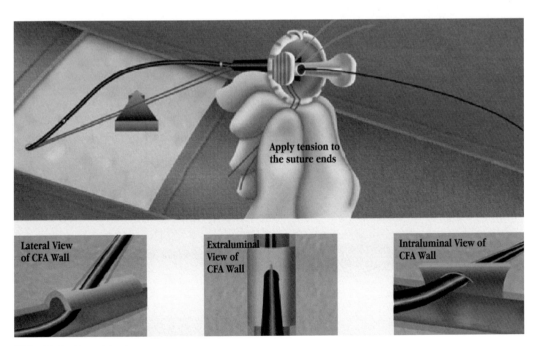

FIG. 23.5. Bowstringing.
1. Sheath should be bent outward away from the operator.
2. Grab the suture adjacent to the sheath and pull the ends through the distal end of the barrel.

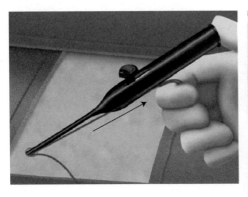

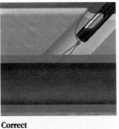

Correct

Incorrect (air knot)

FIG. 23.6. The single-hand knot advancement.
1. To avoid an "air knot," apply tension to the suture while advancing the knot.
2. Tension must be applied to remove slack in the suture while advancing the knot.

Fig. 23.6. A preferred and simpler knot, which is highly recommended over the surgical square knot, is the improved clinch knot (Fig. 23.7). This knot does not require any additional throws over the basic knot. Once mastered, the clinch knot is quicker, simpler, and perhaps stronger and more secure than either the square or surgeon's knots. After the vascular puncture is securely closed, the skin should be thoroughly cleansed and sterilely dressed. The site should be treated like a surgical wound, similar to a permanent pacemaker placement site, utilizing proper surgical technique throughout.

OBJECTIVE RESULTS IN PATIENTS

The outcome in a given individual patient following use of the Perclose device is, for the most part, readily apparent. Failure to achieve control over the arteriotomy is generally obvious, as with any of the available devices used for closure of the access site. Therefore, outcome stud-

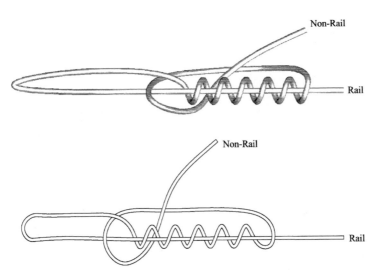

Non-Rail

Rail

Non-Rail

Rail

FIG. 23.7. Improved clinch knot.

ies have been simple in design. Once the devices were shown to be safe and effective in the two principal U.S. trials, STAND I (3) AND STAND II (4), the Food and Drug Administration (FDA) gave approval for their use. Furthermore, the device has received approval for use by trained nonphysician personnel.

TRIALS

Numerous trials involving the use of Perclose devices have been published and are referenced for further reading. Several others are ongoing, or about to begin. A word of caution in interpreting these and other closure device trials is in order. The closure devices carry an associated learning curve. This is not surprising, given the technical nature of these procedures. Some trial results have originated from centers with limited early experience, and others are from centers with more expertise, hence the results have been somewhat varied. In any case, many trials have demonstrated both the safety and efficacy of these devices, as well as their strengths and weaknesses.

THE STAND I AND STAND II TRIALS

The STAND I (sutures to ambulate and discharge) Trial (3) was designed to evaluate the safety and efficacy of suture mediated percutaneous closure of femoral artery access punctures using the 6 Fr TechStar device. The STAND II Trial (4), designed to evaluate the 8 Fr and 10 Fr ProStar Plus devices, was completed in 515 patients by December 1996. STAND I was a prospective multicenter observational study of 200 patients, completed August 1997. STAND II was a multicenter randomized trial to compare results of ProStar use with those of conventional compression. The primary effectiveness endpoint was time to ambulation, with the secondary endpoint being length of hospital stay. The primary safety endpoint was the incidence of major complications within 30 days. The study showed no significant difference in complication rates between conventional treatment (mechanical compression) and Perclose. On the effectiveness side, Perclose patients were

ambulated much sooner than conventionally treated patients in this conservatively designed trial. Investigators were concerned about potential complications with the Perclose device, because it was the first such trial in the U.S. At that time there was not much pretrial experience among the operators from which to draw for the centers involved in the study of the new procedure, and hence the conservative design of the trial. In the time since the early trials, in centers with experienced operators, a significant reduction in time to ambulation has been achieved and has become routine. Time to ambulation has generally been determined by factors other than access-site–related issues. The issue of control over the access site as a factor in determining the length of bed rest for diagnostic and interventional procedures has essentially been removed by use of the Perclose device.

CHANGES IN PATIENT CARE WITH PERCLOSE

After a center has gained expertise in the use of the Perclose device, changes in clinical pathways can safely be made. These changes can result in more efficient use of hospital personnel and resources. Patients can be sent home quickly (generally an hour or so) after diagnostic procedures. Following interventional procedures, times to ambulation and discharge are determined principally by the clinical situation at the interventional target site, rather than by issues related to the vascular access site. For example, following stable peripheral interventions, patients can usually be discharged within a few hours. After stable coronary procedures, such as elective coronary stenting (when an optimal result is attained) patients can routinely be discharged the same day as the procedure. On the other hand, patient's with unstable coronary lesions obviously need to be observed for longer periods of time. An interesting question often arises concerning the practice of leaving sheaths in place after interventions, when the target lesion is potentially unstable. A useful rule of thumb is that if the patient is stable enough to leave the interventional laboratory, the sheath may be pulled, and the site closed with Perclose.

If the clinical situation subsequently deteriorates, the same groin can easily and safely be reaccessed. The efficiencies achievable by use of the Perclose device can be maximized by thoughtful changes in patient clinical pathways. In our hospital, for example, patients proceed to and from the catheterization laboratory via an intake and output unit. The nurses are experienced in helping assess suitability for discharge and this has resulted in appropriately short stays for diagnostic and stable interventional patients.

POTENTIAL COMPLICATIONS

Complications, even very minor ones, following the use of Perclose devices can be minimized to insignificant levels by a combination of appropriate patient selection and careful technique. The device itself is extremely reliable. The vascular wall and suture are remarkably strong. In nearly all cases of complications the cause can be traced to a mistake or a combination of mistakes, including inappropriate case selection and inadequate operator technique. There are, however, some complications that may be potentially more frequent with use of the Perclose device based on several factors. The Perclose procedure is surgical. It results in a small amount of foreign body left in place for a long duration of time (''permanent sutures''). It involves several steps that need to be performed correctly in order to be successful. Complications that might be anticipated include superficial and deep infections, incomplete closure resulting in excessive bleeding, and vascular wall trauma resulting from poor operator technique. Notably rare are complications resulting in limb ischemia. Iliac and aorta trauma also seem to be exceedingly uncommon.

WAYS TO AVOID COMPLICATIONS

First and foremost the Perclose user must be completely familiar with the devices themselves, as well as the way in which the device and suture interact with the vascular wall to achieve hemostasis. Case selection based on the level of experience of the operator is also extremely important. The inexperienced operator (generally including

TABLE 23.5. *Indications and contraindications for beginner level (including the first 20 cases)*

Beginner level, (first 20 cases):
6 Fr TechStar^t
Diagnostic cases.
Common femoral artery
Thin patients.
Little, if any peripheral vascular disease.
Non-tortuous iliac vessel.
Non-anticoagulated patients.
Stable coronary patient.
No previous groin procedures.
Procedures in the Cath Lab only.
Non-diabetic patients.
Femoral angiogram strongly recommended.
Fluoroscopy immediately available.

operators with less than 10 to 20 cases) should begin with diagnostic cases in patients with ideal anatomy. They should continue to use the device in these situations until they feel they have mastered the technique. The operator may then move up to more complicated cases, including more difficult anatomy, low risk interventional cases, and others. Eventually they can take on more challenging cases as experience and technique allow (Tables 23.5, 23.6, and 23.7).

PRACTICAL TIPS

One of the more important ways to avoid complications with the Perclose devices, or with any other access closure device, is to place the femoral puncture in an optimal location (over the femoral head in the common femoral artery)

TABLE 23.6. *Intermediate level: (assumes operator masters all aspects of device use)*

After 20 cases, including the beginner level cases, as well as following:
Stable interventional cases.
8 or 10 French devices.
Some peripheral vascular disease.
Common femoral artery only.
Tortuous iliac vessel.
Stable coronary patient.
Bilateral groin procedures acceptable.
Moderately obese patients.
Diabetic patients.
No recent groin procedures (within the past 3 months).
Fluoroscopy available.
Femoral angiogram strongly recommended.

TABLE 23.7. *Advanced operator level: assumes operator is experienced in 100 or more cases, including several at the intermediate level.*

All of the intermediate level cases and including the following:

Highly anticoagulated patients.
Calcified femoral arteries.
Alternative sites (popliteal, superficial femoral, etc.).
Antegrade punctures (for example, femoral punctures for lower extremity interventions).
Recent groin procedures (including immediate re-stick).
Venous closures.
Procedures outside of the Cath Lab.
Closure following intra-aortic balloon pump.

at a relatively steep angle. Locating the puncture and placing the sheath in this way minimizes the amount of subcutaneous distance through which the device must pass, by permitting the shortest and most direct route between skin and vessel. In the event of failure to completely seal the puncture with the closure device, this technique also permits more effective and direct pressure for complete hemostasis.(5)

CHOOSING THE CORRECT SIZE

For diagnostic cases, the 6 Fr TechStar is appropriate for 4–6 Fr sheaths and for the majority of 7 Fr sheaths as well. The closure device is the correct size when the sheath of the device completely seals the vessel puncture site. If any bleeding is observed around the sheath, the operator should choose the next larger device. Generally speaking, the 8 Fr device works well for interventional cases, using 7 Fr through 9 Fr sheaths and for some intra-aortic balloon pumps. The 10 Fr device works best for 9 Fr sheaths through 11 Fr sheath sizes. When larger than 11 Fr sheaths are anticipated, an 8 or 10 Fr device can be used to preplace the sutures—before dilating the arteriotomy up to larger sizes.

PROBLEMS

In general, when a significant problem arises, before, during, or after use of a Perclose device, the safest course of action is to enlist the help and guidance of a vascular surgeon. Surgical re-

pair is rarely, in fact, needed, but decisions regarding how to proceed to correct the problem are greatly aided by timely consultation. Furthermore, with the surgeon standing by, certain maneuvers—for example, aggressive techniques to free a "stuck device"—can be safely attempted. The techniques that follow should always be employed only after the subsequent positive and negative consequences are carefully considered and anticipated. The overall risks and potential benefits for the patient need to be the foremost factor in the decision making process. In all cases a bolus of antibiotics should be given at the moment a significant problem arises.

WHEN THERE IS DIFFICULTY OBTAINING "MARK"

The operator should use steady and firm coaxial pressure and attempt to obtain marking while rotating the barrel. If no marking is seen, the device should be withdrawn to the position where the barrel end is outside the skin, leaving the sheath remaining well into the vessel. A useful landmark is to withdraw the sheath to the level of the side-rail entry port for the guidewire. The marker port lumen should then be carefully flushed with Heparinized saline. Using a Kelly clamp, the deep subcutaneous tissue should be further spread and dilated. The operator should then reattempt to obtain marking. These steps may be repeated until marking is obtained.

WHEN THERE IS A PRE-EXISTING HEMATOMA

Often the best method available for obtaining hemostasis, when a hematoma, large or small, is present, is use of the Perclose device to secure the arterial puncture site. Very often the hematoma begins to shrink in size noticeably immediately after the Perclose technique is successfully performed. The most important point to remember is that it is imperative to get the Perclose device into ideal position where pulsatile marking is clearly observed.

WHEN THE HANDLE IS DIFFICULT TO PULL (NEEDLE STALL)

Needle stall can result from a variety of factors. It can be seen when excessively tough or calcified vessel wall is encountered. It can also be seen when too much forward pressure is placed on the device (resulting in pinching down of the sheath against the needles), or when one or more of the needles strikes the barrel face. Needle strike of the barrel face can result from the barrel not properly replaced in the locked position, or can result from the operator forcing the device into an angle which can cause the needles to bend away from the target site in the barrel. Needle stall can also occasionally result from excessive suture drag, and occasionally from suture snag. Whatever the cause, the first step should be to attempt to back the needles down by pushing the handle back into position. (Fig. 23.8) The reason for needle stall should then be ascertained prior to another attempt to deploy the needles. In most cases it is very helpful to use a new device. It is important that the operator attempt to deploy the needles very slowly, particularly over the first several millimeters, and especially in arteries which are calcified or fibrous. This will help to give the needles maximum support, and therefore, penetrating power. The device should not be forcibly held against its ''natural lie'' in the vessel and subcutaneous space. Allowing the device to remain as straight as possible maximizes the likelihood that the needles will enter the barrel in the correct position.

WHEN ONE OR MORE NEEDLES DO NOT APPEAR, AFTER THE HANDLE IS FULLY DEPLOYED

Fluoroscopy should be used to try to locate the ''missing needle.'' In most situations, the needle has missed the barrel altogether and is deployed into the subcutaneous space outside the barrel. It is important to remember at this stage not to remove any of the needles which have appeared at the top of the device until all are located and verified to be within the device. Removing any of the needles prior to back-down increases the chance that one or more of the needles will be partially released. This may result in the device being ''trapped'' in the vessel, because the needles can no longer be advanced

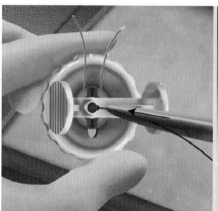 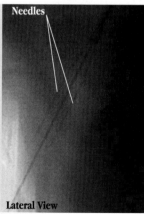 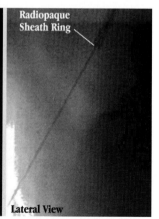

FIG. 23.8. Needle back-down.
1. If needles are not easily deployed, back the needles down into the sheath prior to device removal.
2. Use cine to identify the position of the needle tips, prior to backing down the needles.
3. Use a needle holder to grasp the pull rod a few millimeters proximal to their exit from the device core.
4. Gently feed the pull rod back into the core until the handle snaps into position on the proximal end of the device.
5. Verify that the needle tips are as close as possible to the proximal edge of the radiopaque sheath ring prior to device removal.

or retracted. Back-down should be attempted, and if successful, the device should be withdrawn after a wire is reintroduced. After reintroduction of the wire, the options include replacing the device with a standard sheath or obtaining a new device to close the puncture site.

IF A SUTURE BREAKS

Keeping the sutures well wetted during knot advancement, followed by steady tension on the sutures to advance the knot, will result in adequate closure without suture breakage. Suture breakage usually occurs during the learning phase of the operator's experience. For this reason it is advisable to keep the guidewire in place until the final knot-tightening step, particularly during the operator's first 50 cases, after which the decision to remove the wire without replacing it for knot advancement is a matter of individual preference. Certainly it can be helpful to advance the knots with the wire in place in high-risk cases, so that in the event of suture breakage it is a relatively simple matter to use a new device to place a new set of sutures. In the case of the four-needle devices, the wire can be pulled after one set of sutures is tightened, if desirable.

OOZING

Sometimes even after successful closure of the puncture site in the vessel wall, oozing of blood can be seen from the skin site. The origin of the bleeding is not always apparent, but it most commonly arises from the subcutaneous tissue. Occasionally it may arise from incomplete vessel wall closure. Bleeding from an incomplete closure is more common during an operator's first several cases. Subcutaneous tissue oozing can generally be managed with simple dressing changes, although occasionally gentle manual pressure is needed. Additionally, injection of Lidocaine premixed with Epinephrine into the subcutaneous tissue space can be very helpful. Some operators have also found that subcutaneous sutures can be useful in minimizing bleeding from around the skin edges. If bleeding is apparent immediately after knot tightening is performed, and gentle pressure is not effective in completely stopping the bleeding after a few minutes, the "temporary tamper" device can be used (Fig. 23.9). This device is threaded over the Perclose sutures (which have not yet been trimmed) and the handle of the device turned to apply direct pressure over the vessel puncture site. The device can later be re-

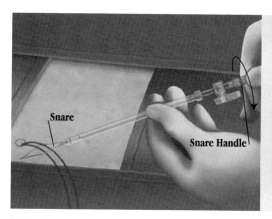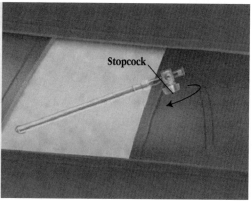

FIG. 23.9. Arterial tamper.
1. Thread exposed suture ends through the *Snare*.
2. Unlock *Snare Handle* by turning it counterclockwise.
3. Pull the suture along with the *Snare* through the arterial tamper.
4. Gently advance over the tensioned suture.
5. Keep *Stopcock* lever facing the patient's right.
6. Secure the arterial tamper by rotating the *Stopcock* lever 90 degrees counterclockwise.
7. Remove arterial tamper after hemostasis is achieved.

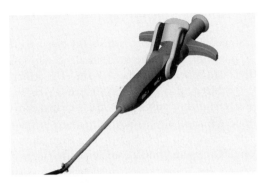

FIG. 23.10. Closer device.

moved, and the sutures trimmed well below the skin level. Antibiotics should always be given when this device is used.

FUTURE DEVICES

The company has introduced a new device called the Closer (Fig. 23.10). This is a very operator- and patient-friendly version of the device, because its profile in the subcutaneous tissue space is much smaller. This advance has allowed easier introduction of the device into proper position by minimizing subcutaneous tissue disruption. Its pathway through the subcutaneous tissue is much smaller, and requires much less preparation. Initial results from its use in Europe have been very favorable with a high degree of success. It is probable that subcutaneous tissue bleeding will be minimized by use of this device. The company has also introduced an automated knot-tying device which further simplifies the overall procedure.

SUMMARY

Patient care is, without doubt, significantly improved with use of the Perclose devices. The devices have the potential to favorably affect patient outcome, particularly among those patients whose pharmacologic regimen and clinical situation result in the need for secure control over the access site. Importantly, the overall experience for the individual patient, whether during a diagnostic procedure, or an interventional pro-

cedure, can be significantly improved by the use of these devices.

REFERENCES

1. Vetter JW, Ribeiro EE, Hinohara T et al. Suture-mediated percutaneous closure of femoral artery access sites in fully anticoagulated patients following coronary interventions. *Circulation* 1994;90(4):901–921.
2. Duda SH, Wikirchen J, Erb M et al. Suture mediated percutaneous closure of antegrade femoral artery access sites in patients who have received full anticoagulation therapy. *Radiology* 1999;21:47–52.
3. Schwarten D, Pinkerton C, Vetter J, Knopf W, Fitzpatrick M, Ho K, St. Acute results of the STAND I Percutaneous Vascular Surgical Device Trial. *Circulation* 1997;96(8): I-137(abst).
4. Baim D, Pinkerton C, Schatz R, Vetter J, Fitzpatrick M, Ho K. Acute results of the STAND II Percutaneous Vascular Surgical Device Trial. *Circulation* 1997;96(8):I-443 (abst).
5. Kim D, Orron D, et al. Role of superficial femoral artery puncture in the development of pseudoaneurysm and arteriovenous fistula complicating percutaneous transfemoral cardiac catheterization. *Cath Cardiovasc Diagn* ;25: 91–97.

SUGGESTED READINGS

1. Gerckens U, Cattelaens N, Muller R, Lampe EG, Grube E. Percutaneous suture closure of the femoral artery access after diagnostic heart catheter examination or coronary intervention; *Dtsch Med Wochenschr*, 1996; 121(48):1487–91.
2. Gerckens U, Cattelaens N, Muller R, Herchenbach M, Staberock M, Grube E. Immediate ambulation following coronary angiography and intervention using a percutaneous closure device (Techstar, Techstar XL): a randomized trial versus manual compression. *Circulation* 1997;96(8): I-137(abst).
3. Morice MC, Lefevre T. Immediate post PTCA percutaneous suture of femoral arteries with the Perclose device: results of high volume users. *J Am Coll Cardiol* 1998; 31(2)[Suppl. A]:1033–104.
4. Gerckens U, Cattelaens N, Muller R, Lampe EG, Grube E. Percutaneous suture of femoral artery access sites after diagnostic heart catheterization and or coronary intervention. Safety and effectiveness of a new arterial suture technique. *Herz* 1998;23(1):27–34.
5. Rickli H, Wetter D, Mayer K, Kiowski W, Sütsch G, Amann FW. Early sheath removal and ambulation Post-PTCA using a percutaneous vascular closure device. An ultrasonographic evaluation. *Am J Cardiol* 1998; 82(7A)[Suppl] 34S (abst).
6. Sharma S, King T, Dangas GCS, Jodhpurwala B, Duvvuri S. Early and safe ambulation after cardiac procedures vascular closure device (Perclose) in high-risk patients. *Am J Cardiol* 1998;82(7A)[Suppl] 108S(abst).
7. Rilling WS, Mewissen MW, Crain MR, Abrar K, Horton MG, Bair DA. Suture mediated closure of the common femoral artery: initial experience with the Perclose device in an interventional radiology practice; *J Vasc Interv Radiol* 1999;10(2)[Suppl]:256.

24

Primary Angioplasty for Acute Myocardial Infarction: The Zwolle Approach to Reperfusion

Felix Zijlstra, on behalf of the Zwolle Myocardial Infarction Study Group

Department of Cardiology, Hospital De Weezenlanden, 8011 JW Zwolle, The Netherlands

Timely restoration of antegrade coronary blood flow in the infarct related artery of a patient with acute myocardial infarction results in myocardial salvage and improved survival (1,2). Intravenous thrombolytic therapy and immediate cardiac catheterization followed by primary angioplasty, if appropriate, are both widely used reperfusion therapies. A recent review of ten randomized trials comparing these two treatment modalities favors primary angioplasty with regard to mortality, reinfarction, and stroke (3). Given the superior safety and efficacy of primary angioplasty, this treatment is now preferred when logistics allow this approach.

As has been shown for angioplasty therapy for stable and unstable angina (4), it is likely that the results of primary angioplasty therapy will be, in part, dependent on the setting in which it is performed, and therefore the results from various hospitals may differ considerably (5). Establishing and maintaining a proficient primary angioplasty program takes great institutional will and effort, and even institutions with a large experience in coronary angioplasty for stable and unstable angina will have something of a learning curve for primary angioplasty (6). The main issues pertinent to the delivery of primary angioplasty therapy will be discussed, following the sequence of events from a patient perspective. Our approach will be described with regard to the prehospital phase, the first 15 in-hospital minutes, initial pharmacological

therapy, angiography, angioplasty, risk stratification, rehabilitation, and secondary prevention.

PREHOSPITAL PHASE

A speedy response and early recognition of acute myocardial infarction by general practitioners and ambulance services are of great importance, mainly for two reasons. First, mortality in the very early hours is substantial, and many patients die before adequate medical help has been sought and delivered (7). Second, although the results of primary angioplasty therapy are less time dependent than the results of thrombolysis (8), in particular during the first few hours, time is muscle. This is not only so from a theoretical perspective, but has been confirmed in a recent study that showed that an increase in median time delay from presentation to first balloon inflation, from 60 to 103 minutes in patients with mainly large anterior infarctions, resulted in a 24% larger enzymatic infarct size and a 4% lower left ventricular ejection fraction measured before hospital discharge (9). Confirmation of the diagnosis of acute myocardial infarction by 12-lead electrocardiography, by either general practitioners or ambulance paramedics, allows a substantial reduction of the time delay to first balloon inflation, because the hospital and the catheterization laboratory can be prepared in advance, and the emergency room and the CCU (with their unavoidable delays) can be skipped on the way to acute angiography. Furthermore, it gives an important opportunity to start the initial pharmacological therapy, and use the transportation time in this regard. A primary angioplasty center must therefore develop additional specific training programs for general practitioners and ambulance services. Excellent communication with these first-line providers of care for patients with acute myocardial infarction is of paramount importance, as this will be among the main factors determining time to therapy.

THE FIRST 15 IN-HOSPITAL MINUTES

If a definitive diagnosis has not been made before arrival at the hospital, it is very important that additional delays are avoided. A limited history and physical examination should be performed and a 12-lead electrocardiogram should be made and interpreted within 5 to 10 minutes (7). Blood tests may be drawn, but results should not be waited for, a chest X-ray is unnecessary. The first responsibility of the emergency room physician is to contact the catheterization laboratory and to get the patient there as soon as possible. Important organizational issues that determine the logistics in this regard are:

1. Who is in charge of patients with suspected cardiac symptoms in the emergency room?
2. Who is in charge of the CCU?
3. What type of nurses are staffing the emergency room?

We have learned that it is a great advantage if:

1. The CCU is run by an interventional cardiologist.
2. The emergency room physicians are supervised by the head of the CCU.
3. The CCU, IC, and emergency room nurses fall within the same organizational unit and therefore know each others work.

Finally, a flexible attitude shared by the catheterization laboratory staff and interventional cardiologist is a prerequisite. They should be prepared to change their program at a moment's notice, drop a nice elective case planned for in-tracoronary ultrasound, multiple stenting, etc., or get out of bed in the middle of the night, to do this job as quickly and proficiently as they can.

INITIAL PHARMACOLOGICAL THERAPY

Adequate pain relief and supplemental oxygen are essential, not only for humanitarian reasons, but in particular because the patient has to endure angiography and angioplasty (7). Aspirin should be given, at least ≥300 mg soluble chewable, but as gastrointestinal symptoms are frequent, we prefer to give 500 mg of aspirin intravenously. Sublingual and intravenous nitroglycerin as well as intravenous beta blockers, unless contraindicated, should be given in an effort to lower oxygen consumption and alleviate myocardial ischemia. High-dose intravenous heparin has been used in an attempt to increase initial patency rates of the infarct related vessel with promising results (10). A larger, randomized study (11) however, showed that a moderate dose of intravenous heparin (10.000–15.000 U) during the angioplasty, without measurements of the activated clotting time, results in a comparable clinical outcome. We therefore give only this moderate dose of intravenous heparin during the procedure; this gives us the additional advantage of being able to remove the arterial sheaths 1 to 3 hours after the procedure. Abciximab and other novel antiplatelet agents as concomitant therapy may be promising, and further data from randomized trials are eagerly waited for (12). Ticlopidine is now used for almost all stented patients (13), and although many patients already receive this drug in the emergency room, it should be realized that its mode of action is rather in days than in hours.

ANGIOGRAPHY

Vascular access can be obtained by either the femoral or brachial approach, but the former is generally preferred. Femoral access allows larger devices if necessary (intra-aortic balloon pump) (14) or transvenous pacing when indicated. The physician can choose between 6 or 7

Fr sheaths and catheters. A low osmolar ionic contrast agent should be used, in particular, to avoid thromboembolic complications (15).

An angiogram of the noninfarcted artery should be performed first to allow identification of multivessel disease and collateral flow into the infarct zone. Contrast ventriculography is only necessary to help determine the infarct artery if this is uncertain based on information of the electrocardiogram and the coronary angiogram, and can usually be skipped. In general, we perform angiography of the infarct artery with an angioplasty guiding catheter, 6 or 7 Fr, so that we can proceed immediately with angioplasty if indicated. During this phase the interventional cardiologist must try to give answers to the following questions:

1. Can I identify the infarct artery with certainty and will I be able to get it open? (If not, ask for help, don't try to be a hero).
2. Consider a conservative approach when there is spontaneous reperfusion, a small myocardial territory at risk, or extensive collateral circulation and think about this: does this patient need bypass surgery; either acutely or following initial stabilization?
3. If the decision to go for angioplasty is taken: Do you need venous access? Temporary pacing? Intra-aortic balloon pumping? In particular, during recanalization of right coronary arteries, bradycardia and hypotension may develop that may necessitate large amounts of intravenous fluids and 0.5 to 2.0 mg atropine or even pressure therapy. The interventional cardiologist who is not prepared to handle these types of complications, but lets him/herself be surprised by these sudden events, may even lose a patient (16).

ANGIOPLASTY

After completion of the angiographic study and with a clear concept on what should be done, the infarct artery should be crossed with a soft or floppy steerable guidewire. After passing the wire it is often possible to have a first impression of the distal vessel following intracoronary nitrates. Balloon sizing should be adequate,

around 1:1 balloon to artery ratio. This mandates repeated bolus doses of intracoronary nitrates in order to avoid serious underestimation of the true arterial size. We perform one or two balloon inflations of 3 to 5 minutes, usually at 8 to 12 atm. Optimal angiographic visualization of the lesion and the distal vessel in multiple projections is necessary, to assess the result and define the need for further balloon inflations or stenting. The operator should strive for an optimal result with <30% residual luminal narrowing and TIMI 3 flow as well as evidence of myocardial reperfusion (17). If a significant residual stenosis remains or if there is intraluminal evidence of dissection, stenting should be considered. If an adequate vessel lumen is evident in multiple angiographic projections, dissections can be left without a stent, provided that reliability of the angiographic result is shown by repeating one or two worst-view projections after 5 to 10 minutes waiting. In selected patients, stenting may be preferable to prevent restenosis and late additional target vessel revascularization (18,19). This is again (see "Initial Pharmacological Therapy") a moment to consider abciximab or other novel antiplatelet drugs (12). The use of thrombolytic therapy should be avoided, because its use, combined with angioplasty, has been associated with increased rates of complications. With rare exceptions, the role of primary angioplasty is to dilate only the infarct artery. Multiple lesions in the infarct vessel can, and sometimes must be, dilated, but dilating a noninfarcted artery during the acute hours jeopardizes too much myocardium. We tend to dilate all significant lesions (DS > 50%) in the main body of the infarct related vessel, with as the only exception, concomitant lesions that seem to carry a very high risk for complications. TIMI 3 flow in the infarct related artery should not be traded for a somewhat less severe distal lesion.

STENTING

The indications for coronary stenting are evolving rapidly. It should be stressed that stenting has so far been shown to be superior to balloon angioplasty only in selected patients (18,19). Our attitude is that an optimal balloon angioplasty result should never be jeopardized just for a somewhat lower rate of target vessel revascularization during the first year after the acute event. In particular, attention should be paid to side branches that may be of more clinical relevance in this setting than with elective angioplasty, the need for long stents to cover the lesion as this predisposes to in-stent restenosis and to the potentially life-threatening consequences of the rare event of subacute stent thrombosis. In our experience, almost all sudden occlusions of infarct arteries after balloon angioplasty occur in-hospital and can usually be managed, but subacute stent thrombosis, although rare, may occur after discharge with sometimes dramatic consequences. All stented patients should be treated with aspirin and ticlopidine for at least 2 to 4 weeks (13).

RISK STRATIFICATION, REHABILITATION, AND SECONDARY PREVENTION

When the care of patients with an acute myocardial infarction is placed into the hands of interventional cardiologists it is crucial that they pay as meticulous attention to further management as to the initial procedure. Therefore, some of the most important aspects are delineated here briefly.

Based on the available clinical data, the angiographic findings, and the 12-lead electrocardiogram (14,17,20), after the primary angioplasty procedure the risk of the individual patient can be estimated reliably, and further management can be tailored accordingly. In high-risk patients, intra-aortic balloon pumping may be considered (7,14). During the first days it is appropriate to assess left ventricular function by echocardiography or radionuclide ventriculography (7). In our approach, most patients have early sheath removal 1 to 3 hours after the primary angioplasty procedure. We give no further intravenous heparin, but we give 2 to 3 days of low molecular weight heparin. ACE-inhibition is given to patients with depressed left ventricular function, and most patients have diet counseling and start with a cholesterol lowering agent (statin) (7). In particular, as patients now are discharged after 3 to 4 days, the outpatient rehabilitation program has become a very important and integral part of infarct patient management, including many aspects of secondary prevention such as smoking cessation, and weight reduction.

In patients with multivessel disease, the need for additional revascularization procedures should be addressed. Signs and symptoms of recurrent ischemia must be carefully sought for during the few in-hospital days and in particular during visits to the outpatient clinic. Dependent on the setting, the general practitioner of the patient may play a central role in this monitoring process. In our setting, conventional planar thallium scintigraphy is often the preferred noninvasive test for restenosis and recurrent ischemia, but our "threshold" for a 6-month follow-up angiogram is very low. Many patients prefer the certainty of angiography over the unavoidable "Bayesian" uncertainties of non-invasive tests.

The most important aspects of primary angioplasty for acute myocardial infarction are summarized in the following ten rules:

1. In suspected MI, initial assessment <15 min: TIME = MUSCLE = LIVES.
2. When diagnosis of MI is confirmed before hospital arrival, go to catheterization laboratory, and not to emergency room or CCU.
3. Do not forget aspirin, heparin, nitrates, and B-blocker.
4. Visualize both coronary arteries with a low osmolar ionic contrast agent.
5. Consider conservative management and acute or elective CABG.
6. Use a balloon and perhaps a stent; forget other techniques.
7. Be sure that somebody looks after the patient when you perform angiography and angioplasty.
8. Beware of, and prepare for, reperfusion arrhythmias, bradycardia, and hypotension.
9. Do not undersize.
10. Stent the plaque, not the vessel.

REFERENCES

1. GUSTO. An international randomised trial comparing four thrombolytic strategies for acute myocardial infarction. *N Eng J Med* 1993;329:673–682.

2. The GUSTO Angiographic Investigators. The effects of tissue plasminogen activator, streptokinase, or both on coronary-artery patency, ventricular function, and survival, after acute myocardial infarction. *N Engl J Med* 1993;329:1615–1622.

3. Weaver WD, Simes RJ, Betriu A et al, for the Primary Coronary Angioplasty vs. Thrombolysis Collaboration Group. Comparison of primary coronary angioplasty and intravenous thrombolytic therapy for acute myocardial infarction: a quantitative overview. *JAMA* 1997; 278:2093–2098.

4. Kimmel SE, Berlin JA, Laskey WK. The relationship between coronary angioplasty procedure volume and major complications. *JAMA* 1996;274:1137–1142.

5. Christian TF, O'Keefe JH, DeWood MA et al. Intercenter variability in outcome for patients treated with direct coronary angioplasty during acute myocardial infarction. *Am Heart J* 1998;135:310–317.

6. Caputo RP, Ho KKL, Stoler RC et al. Effect of continuous quality improvement analysis on the delivery of primary percutaneous transluminal coronary angioplasty for acute myocardial infarction. *Am J Cardiol* 1997;79: 1159–1164.

7. The Task Force on the Management of Acute Myocardial Infarction of the European Society of Cardiology. Acute myocardial infarction: prehospital and in-hospital management. *Eur Heart J* 1996;17:43–63.

8. O'Neill WW, de Boer MJ, Gibbons RJ et al. Lessons from the pooled outcome of the PAMI, ZWOLLE and Mayo Clinic randomized trials of primary angioplasty versus thrombolytic therapy of acute myocardial infarction. *J Invas Cardiol* 1998;10:4A–10A.

9. Liem AL, van 't Hof AWJ, Hoorntje JCA, de Boer MJ, Suryapranata H, Zijlstra F. Influence of treatment delay on infarct size and clinical outcome in patients with acute myocardial infarction treated with primary angioplasty. *J Am Coll Cardiol* (*in press*).

10. Verheugt FWA, Liem AL, Zijlstra F, Marsh RC, Veen G, Bronzwaer JGF. High dose bolus heparin as initial therapy before primary angioplasty for acute myocardial infarction: results of the heparin in early patency (HEAP) pilot study. *J Am Coll Cardiol* 1998;31: 289–293.

11. Liem AL, Zijlstra F, Hoorntje JCA et al. High-dose heparin as pretreatment for primary angioplasty in acute myocardial infarction: the heparin in early patency (HEAP) randomized trial. Submitted.

12. Brener SJ, Barr LA, Burchenal et al. A randomized, placebo-controlled trial of abciximab with primary angioplasty for acute MI. The RAPPORT trial. *Circulation* 1997;96:I-473.

13. Schömig A, Neumann FJ, Kastrati A et al. A randomized comparison of antiplatelet and anticoagulant therapy after the placement of coronary artery stents. *N Engl J Med* 1996;334:1084–1089.

14. Stone GW, Marsalese D, Brodie BR et al. A prospective, randomized evaluation of prophylactic, intraaortic balloon counterpulsation in high-risk patients with acute myocardial infarction treated with primary angioplasty. *J Am Coll Cardiol* 1997;29:1459–1467.

15. Grines CL, Schreiber TL, Savas V et al. A randomized trial of low osmolar ionic versus nonionic contrast media in patients with myocardial infarction or unstable angina undergoing percutaneous transluminal coronary angioplasty. *J Am Coll Cardiol* 1996;27:1381–1386.

16. Gacioch GM, Topol EJ. Sudden paradoxic clinical deterioration during angioplasty of the occluded coronary artery in acute myocardial infarction. *J Am Coll Cardiol* 1989;14:1202–1209.

17. van 't Hof AWJ, Liem AL, Suryapranata H, Hoorntje JCA, de Boer MJ, Zijlstra F. Angiographic assessment of myocardial reperfusion in patients treated with primary angioplasty for acute myocardial infarction. *Circulation* 1998;97:2302–2306.

18. Suryapranata H, van 't Hof AWJ, Hoorntje JCA, de Boer MJ, Zijlstra F. Randomized comparison of coronary stenting with balloon angioplasty in selected patients with acute myocardial infarction. *Circulation* 1998;97:2502–2505.

19. Stone GW. Primary stenting in acute myocardial infarction. The promise and the proof. *Circulation* 1998;97: 2482–2485.

20. van 't Hof AWJ, Liem AL, de Boer MJ, Zijlstra F, on behalf of the Zwolle Myocardial Infarction Study Group. Clinical value of 12-lead electrocardiogram after successful reperfusion therapy for acute myocardial infarction. *Lancet* 1997;350:615–619.

25

Internal Mammary Artery Stenosis

SMH Cardiac Catheterization Laboratory, Mayo Clinic, Rochester, Minnesota 55905

Aortocoronary artery bypass grafting has been performed in the United States for more than 25 years. In 1967 saphenous vein bypass grafting was described, followed a year later by the use of internal mammary artery (IMA) graft (1). Saphenous venous grafts have been shown to have time-dependent attrition so that by 10 years postoperatively, less than 50% of grafts are open and have a normal appearance (2). In contrast, atherosclerosis has been rarely associated with the IMA conduits (3). Several studies at 7 to 10 years have shown patency of IMA grafts to be around 90% (4). Long-term follow-up studies have shown that placement of an IMA, usually to the left anterior descending coronary artery (LAD) in patients undergoing coronary artery bypass surgery, is associated with improvement in the long-term survival (5). The IMA is usually anastomosed to the LAD, but occasionally to the diagonal or an obtuse marginal artery. The distal right coronary artery can be bypassed by right IMA in selected patients. This review of the IMA encompasses the description of IMA stenosis, technical issues with IMA angioplasty, and the results of the studies on IMA interventions.

IMA STENOSIS

Stenosis in IMA grafts may occur at the origin, in the mid portion or at the distal anastomosis with the latter being the most frequent in our experience. The stenoses are usually subtotal, although occlusion can be seen in the mid portion of the graft. The majority of stenoses are probably related to technical issues such as improper handling of the graft and suturing at the distal anastomotic site, because atherosclerosis is extremely uncommon. While infrequent, it is possible that ostial stenosis may occur as the result of unrecognized trauma at the time of diagnostic cardiac catheterization. The typical pathology would appear to be neointimal proliferation rather than atherosclerosis. Typically, patients with stenosis of the IMA graft present within first year after coronary bypass surgery; some patients may present very early postoperatively. In some patients with MIDCAB procedures, immediate surveillance angiography may document a severe stenosis.

As is the case with placement of the saphenous vein grafts, there can be progression of the native coronary arterial disease following IMA placement. This can result in proximal occlusion of the native coronary artery. If the distal disease develops later in the native coronary arteries, then IMA graft can be used as a conduit to reach and treat the distal coronary artery.

IMA GRAFT ANGIOPLASTY

Technical Issues

There are multiple issues related to the treatment of IMA stenosis or to the use of IMA as a conduit to reach and treat the distal native coronary artery disease when there is occlusion of the native coronary artery proximal to the insertion of the IMA (Table 25.1). These include problems with the access to the ostium of the IMA, secure engagement without damping or trauma, tortuosity, the length of equipment re-

TABLE 25.1. *Technical issues*

Problem	Solution
1. Dissection at the ostium: usually as a result of guide trauma	1. Pull the guide back when withdrawing balloon and avoid damping
2. Spasm of IMA	2. Prophylactic nitroglycerin in the graft
3. Tortuosity: common cause of failure of angioplasty in stent delivery	3. Soft wires or hydrophilic guidewire coatings
4. Stenosis in the distal native artery	4. Use short (90-cm) guide catheter and long balloon
5. Pain and heat in the arm and chest with ionic dye injection	5. Use Non ionic or low osmolar dimeric contrast

Care must be taken with the engagement of the ostium. Damping may be a real problem because it can result in arterial damage as well as in the inability to visualize the anatomy. In general, we use the smallest catheters possible, i.e., 6 or 7 Fr, and may also require placement of side holes.

Tortuosity (Fig. 25.1) and the length of the IMA may also be problematic. We usually use a short guiding catheter and a very soft guidewire. Great care must be taken to avoid subintimal passage, which can result in the occlusion of the IMA (Fig. 25.2). When the proximal native coronary artery is occluded and then the IMA graft occludes during manipulation there is the potential for serious morbidity.

quired to reach the stenosis to be treated, and the potential for complications.

The left IMA can be approached through the femoral route in majority of cases. The right IMA is more difficult because of the angulation involved. For the right IMA, a right-arm approach may be preferable. An ipsilateral-arm approach may also be useful in the presence of severe subclavian artery tortuosity or stenosis (6). This approach is also helpful if proper seating with the guide cannot be done from the femoral route. The IMA can be engaged with an IMA guide or a right Judkins guide.

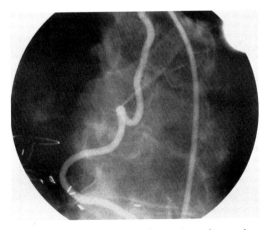

FIG. 25.1. Left anterior oblique view of a moderately tortuous left internal mammary artery (LIMA) to the LAD which can pose problems for interventional cardiology.

Results of the Published Studies

As evident from Table 25.2, IMA graft angioplasty can be achieved with high success rates and low complications. In a small study published by this institution, the angioplasty was successful in 10 out of 11 patients, there was one late death, and all survivors showed functional improvement (7). In the largest study published to date on IMA graft interventions, 86 patients underwent 96 PTCAs of IMA grafts (8). There were 81% males and the patients' mean age was 59 years. Procedural success was obtained in 94.3%. Multilesion PTCA was performed in 74% patients. Major in-hospital complications were limited to one Q-wave myocardial infarction. At a mean follow-up of 20.5 months, there were three late myocardial infarctions, four repeat coronary artery bypass operations, and four late deaths. Actuarial survival at 1 and 5 years was 95% and 92.3% respectively. Event-free survival at 1 and 5 years was 88% and 82% respectively. No angiographic follow-up is mentioned to comment on the restenosis rates. The other studies done on IMA angioplasty show results similar to those in Table 25.2 (6–17). In another study, 68 consecutive patients over a 9-year period underwent angioplasty of IMA (9). The procedural success was achieved in 88%. The median graft age was 9 months. The unsuccessful procedures were due to excessive vessel tortuosity in five patients, major dissection in

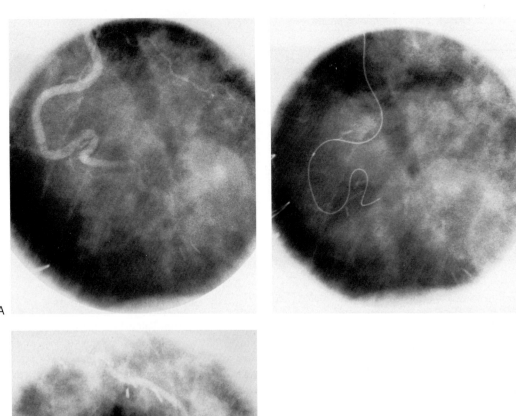

A

B

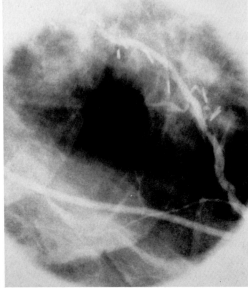

C

FIG. 25.2. A: Left anterior oblique of a very tortuous LIMA graft to the middle LAD. **B:** Even a soft wire and small balloon have trouble negotiating the tortuosity. **C:** Following attempt at passage, a dissection and stenosis are apparent.

two, and inability to dilate in one patient. A study from Japan has reported low success rates of IMA graft angioplasty (10). The angioplasty success in their series of 46 patients (48 lesions) was 73%. Proper anticipation of the problems as listed in Table 25.1 can reduce the complication rates and consequently increase the success rates further; however, given the size and the relative

inflexibility even of the current stent designs, stent delivery may be difficult. There are no series with stents reported on IMA graft intervention to date. Inclusion of the stents in the treatment armamentarium may reduce the dissections and further increase the success. The limitations of the studies published so far are (a) small numbers of patients, (b) incomplete

TABLE 25.2. *Results of IMA graft angioplasty*

Authors	Year	Patient number	Success	Complications	Follow-up
Douglas et al. (11)	1983	1	0	Dissection	Elective CABG
Kereiakas et al. (12)	1984	1	1	—	Asymptomatic at 6 months
Dorros et al. (6)	1986	7	6	Dissection	No clinical recurrence
Pinkerton et al. (13)	1987	7	7	—	Asymptomatic
Shimshak et al. (14)	1988	26	24	Spasm, dissection in 3	1/8 Restenosis
Hill et al. (15)	1989	11	9	—	8 of 9 asymptomatic
Bell et al. (7)	1989	7	7	—	—
Dimas et al. (16)	1991	31	28	2 Dissections	1/7 restenosis
Shimshak et al. (8)	1991	86	81	1 QMI	4 Late deaths 3 late MI
Popma et al. (17)	1992	20	16	—	2/20 restenosis 2 CABG
Hearne et al. (9)	1995	68	60	2 Dissections	19% restenosis
Ishizaka et al. (10)	1995	46	34	1 Spasm	30% restenosis

CABG, coronary artery bypass surgery; QMI, Q-wave myocardial infarction.

angiographic follow-up, and (c) confounding effects on the clinical outcome of the associated progression of the vein graft and native artery disease.

Complications of IMA Angioplasty

The complications of IMA angioplasty are no different from angioplasty during vein graft interventions, with the distinct exception of distal embolization and lower restenosis. The former is a result of low incidence of atherosclerosis in the IMA graft. As mentioned earlier, IMA grafts may be prone to catheter-induced dissection and this may result in significant complications. The most common cause of failure of IMA graft angioplasty is tortuosity of the IMA graft, which is graded as mild, moderate, and severe (14). Mild tortuosity is defined as an isolated curve or series of curves in the graft <90 degrees, moderate tortuosity when the bends make an angle between 90 and 150 degrees, and severe tortuosity is when the graft produced a series of angles in the graft of more than 150 degrees or an isolated turn of 360 degrees. In the majority of IMA graft angioplasty the tortuosity is mild to moderate and does not affect the outcome. Severe tortuosity is associated with technical failure (14) (See Fig. 25.1). A potential complication is rupture of the distal anastomosis in the early postoperative period if dilatation is performed. Although we have not seen that, we avoid oversizing the balloon in this setting and

perform repeat test injection frequently to document the result of treatment.

Restenosis

The restenosis rates following IMA angioplasty have been reported to be lower than those following vein graft intervention. The inherent limitation of the small number and incomplete angiographic follow-up (<25%) should be highlighted. In the study previously mentioned (9), the angiographic follow-up was obtained in 78% of the successful procedures in 68 patients. The restenosis rate in that study was 19%. A subanalysis by the lesion site revealed a restenosis rate of 15% at the distal anastomotic site (6/40) and 43% (3/7) in the body of the graft. Ishizaka et al. (10) reported a restenosis rate of 30% in 34 patients who underwent IMA angioplasty (86% follow-up angiography rate). The majority of the lesions were at the distal anastomotic site. Among the variables studied the only significant predictor for restenosis was percent diameter stenosis of the recipient vessel. The influence of improvement in technology and introduction of stents on IMA graft intervention is not clear as yet.

CURRENT RECOMMENDATIONS

The results of IMA graft intervention are excellent. Angiographic evaluation of IMA should be considered if the patient presents with recurrent ischemia after aortocoronary bypass surgery. This is especially true if the recurrence of symptoms occurs within the first few days of surgery. Coronary interventions at this time are associated with excellent short- and long-term outcomes. High restenosis rates and atheroembolism, which are frequent complications of treating old vein grafts, are less of a concern with IMA graft angioplasty. Continued development of more flexible, lower profile, trackable devices should make these procedures even safer.

REFERENCES

1. Green GE, Stertzer SH, Reppert EH. Coronary arterial bypass grafts. *Ann Thorac Surg* 1968;5:443–450.
2. Bourassa MG, Fisher LD, Campeau L, Gillespie MJ, McConney M, Lesperance J. Long term fate of bypass grafts: the Coronary Artery Surgery Study (CASS) and Montreal Heart Institute experiences. *Circulation* 1985; 72[Suppl V]: V-71–78.
3. Kay HR, Korns ME, Flemma RJ, Tector AJ, Lepley D Jr. Atherosclerosis of the internal mammary artery. *Ann Thorac Surg* 1976;21:504–507.
4. Loop FD, Lytle BW, Cosgrove DM et al. Influence of the internal mammary artery graft on 10-year survival and other cardiac events. *N Engl J Med* 1986;314:1–6.
5. Cameron A, Davis KB, Green G, Schaff HV. Coronary bypass surgery with internal thoracic artery grafts—effects on survival over a 15-year period. *N Engl J Med* 1996;334:216–219.
6. Dorros G, Lewin RF. The brachial artery method to transluminal internal mammary artery angioplasty. *Cathet Cardiovasc Diagn* 1986;12:341–346.
7. Bell MR, Holmes DR Jr, Vlietstra RE, Bresnehan DR. Percutaneous transluminal angioplasty left internal mammary artery grafts: two years' experience with a femoral approach. *Br Heart J* 1989;61:417–420.
8. Shimshak TM, Rutherford BD, McConahay DR, Giorgi LV, Johnson WL, Ligon RW. PTCA of internal mammary artery (IMA) grafts-procedural results and late follow-up. *Circulation* 1991;84[Suppl II]:2345.
9. Hearne SE, Wilson JS, Harrington J et al. Angiographic and clinical follow-up after internal mammary artery graft angioplasty: A 9-year experience. *J Am Coll Cardiol* 1995;25[Suppl A]:139A.
10. Ishizaka N, Ishizaka Y, Ikari Y et al. Initial and subsequent angiographic outcome of percutaneous transluminal angioplasty performed on internal mammary artery grafts. *Br Heart J* 1995;74:615–19.
11. Douglas JS Jr, Gruentzig AR, King SB III et al. Percutaneous transluminal coronary angioplasty in patients with prior coronary bypass surgery. *J Am Coll Cardiol* 1983; 2:745–754.
12. Kereiakas DJ, George B, Stertzer SH, Myler RK. Percutaneous transluminal angioplasty of left internal mammary artery grafts. *Am J Cardiol* 1984;55:1215–1216.
13. Pinkerton CA, Slack J, Orr CM, VanTassel JW. Percutaneous transluminal involving internal mammary artery bypass grafts: a femoral approach. *Cathet Cardiovasc Diagn* 1987;13:414–418.
14. Shimshak TM, Giorgi LV, Johnson WL et al. Application of percutaneous transluminal coronary angioplasty to the internal mammary artery graft. *J Am Coll Cardiol* 1988;12:1205–1214.
15. Hill DM, McAuley BJ, Sheehan DJ, Simpson JB, Selmon MR, Anderson ET. Percutaneous transluminal angioplasty of internal mammary artery bypass grafts. *J Am Coll Cardiol* 1989;13:221A.
16. Dimas AP, Arora RR, Whitlow PL et al. Percutaneous transluminal angioplasty involving internal mammary artery grafts. *Am Heart J* 1991;122:423–429.
17. Popma JL, Cooke RH, Leon MB et al. Immediate procedural and long term clinical results of internal mammary artery angioplasty. *Am J Cardiol* 1992;69:1237–1239.

26

Transradial Approach for Coronary Angioplasty and Stenting

Ferdinand Kiemeneij

Amsterdam Department of Interventional Cardiology, Onze Lieve Vrouwe Gasthuis, 1090 HM Amsterdam, The Netherlands

BACKGROUND

At present PTCA is commonly performed using 8 Fr guiding catheters. The use of these large-bore guiding catheters, in conjunction with anticoagulant and antiplatelet drugs, may contribute to frequent and severe entry-site-related complications such as bleeding, pseudoaneurysms, arteriovenous fistula, nerve damage, and arterial occlusion. Low-profile, rapid-exchange balloon catheters facilitate the use of miniaturized guiding catheters, while advantages of over-the-wire systems are still maintained; free guidewire movement and ability to exchange balloons of different diameters, with maintenance of distal access. Performance of 6 Fr guiding catheters with regard to contrast delivery, pressure monitoring, and backup support is adequate (1) and pressure damping by the guiding catheter is less frequently encountered, as compared to 8 Fr guiding catheters. With these down-sized guiding catheters, arterial puncture holes also become smaller, with reduced bleeding complications, shorter hemostasis time and early ambulation. Another potential advantage of 6 Fr guiding catheters is the possibility to select smaller arteries, such as the brachial or radial artery, as entry sites for PTCA. Safety of transradial coronary angioplasty is mainly determined by the favorable anatomical relations of the radial artery to its surrounding structures. No major veins or nerves are located near the radial artery, minimizing the chance of related injury

of these structures. Because of the superficial course of the artery, hemostasis can be obtained easily by local compression. Thrombotic or traumatic artery occlusion does not endanger the viability of the hand if adequate collateral blood supply by the ulnar artery is present. Campeau performed transradial diagnostic heart catheterization in 100 patients with 5 Fr catheters (2). Additional potential advantages of this approach are based on the immediate mobilization of the patient, increasing patient comfort. Early ambulation allows cost-effective and efficient use of cardiology beds and resources, an important factor in many cost-limited health care systems.

In a search for increased safety, efficiency, and patient comfort the transradial approach was adapted for coronary angioplasty and stenting after the first 6 Fr guiding catheters became commercially available.

THE TECHNIQUE

Patient Selection

Patients with good pulsating radial arteries and with adequate collateral connections with the ulnar artery, as demonstrated by the Allen test, are suitable for transradial coronary angioplasty. The Allen test is performed by compressing both radial and ulnar arteries. The hand will become pale. If the normal color of the hand reappears within 10 seconds after release of pressure of the ulnar artery, while pressure is

TABLE 26.1. *Exclusion criteria*

Absence of radial artery pulsation
Negative Allen test
(Expected) need for intraaortic balloon pumping
(Expected) need for right heart catheterization
LIMA angiography
Intended kissing stent techniques if 6 Fr guiding catheters are used
Intended use of devices, incompatible with the used catheter size

LIMA, left internal mammary artery.

TABLE 26.2. *Suitable guiding catheter characteristics*

Optimal support
Optimal coaxiality
Ability for deep intubation
Atraumatic tip
Stiff shaft to prevent kinking and collapse
Flexible curve to allow smooth passage of rigid systems increased ease of cannulation

maintained over the radial artery, collaterals are present; the Allen test is positive (Table 26.1).

PROCEDURE

The arm of the patient needs to rest on an arm support. The easiest way is to place a board partially under the patient's mattress, in such a way that the extending part of that board parallels the table. The advantage to this of preparation is the normal position of the operator in relation to the patient and to the X-ray tube.

The skin is infiltrated with 2 to 4 cc xylocaine 2%.

The course of the radial artery is palpated, followed by puncture as distal as possible, but at least 1 cm proximal to the styloid process. This prevents perforation of the *retinaculum flexorum* and puncture of a small superficial branch of the radial artery. In addition, this allows successive, more proximal attempts in case of a first failure. Through the needle a spasmolytic cocktail can be injected, followed by introduction of a guidewire. At present, the spasmolytic cocktail used in our clinic consists of verapamil 5 mg and nitroglycerin 200 micrograms, diluted in 10 cc saline. During early experience, 300 cm wires are recommended, because initially more guiding catheter exchanges will be performed. This prevents need for reintroduction of the wire over potentially difficult anatomy, reducing procedural and fluoroscopy times. The size of the guidewire depends of the size of the needle used for puncture. A small skin incision is made to allow passage of the sheath. A long (23–25 cm) sheath is recommended to prevent radial artery spasm and to reduce discomfort.

The guiding catheter choice is of paramount importance (Table 26.2).

At present, special guiding catheters have been designed for transradial coronary cannulation. The Kimny Radial shape (Boston Scientific Scimed/Schneider Worldwide) is a multipurpose catheter for right coronary artery (RCA), left coronary artery (LCA) and vein bypass graft (VBG) cannulation (Fig 26.1). Examples of dedicated catheters for the LCA and RCA are the (MUTA™) curves. Also, "femoral" shapes can be used (Table 26.3).

In general, it is advised to advance the guiding catheter over the guidewire. Before removing the wire, the catheter tip should point towards left coronary sinus for LCA-angioplasty and the right coronary sinus for RCA-angioplasty.

New generation balloon catheters are compatible with 6 Fr guiding catheters up to 5.0 mm. Kissing balloon techniques are feasible with most types of balloon catheters in combination

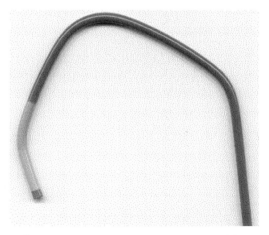

FIG. 26.1. Kimny Radial Shape Guiding Catheter.

TABLE 26.3. *Recommended curves*

LCA	Kimny Radial
	MUTA left (Boston Scientific Scimed)
	Extra backup
	Amplatz left
	Multipurpose
	Judkins left
RCA	Kimny Radial
	MUTA right
	Multipurpose
	Amplatz left
	Judkins right
LCA and RCA	Kimny Radial
	Multipurpose
VBG	Kimny radial
	Multipurpose
	Judkins right

LCA, left coronary artery; RCA, right coronary artery; MUTA, ; VBG, vein bypass graft.

with new generation (≥0.064-in.) 6 Fr guiding catheters. Many intravascular ultrasound transducers are 6 Fr compatible. Via 7 Fr catheters, small rotational atherectomy burrs can be used (burr size up to 1.5 mm). However, visualization will still be problematic, since the burr will completely obliterate the catheter lumen.

A low profile and a free choice of balloon catheters together with the potential to use only one balloon for a stent procedure are the main advantages of unsheathed and unmounted coronary stents. At present, the operator has to make a choice from a wide variety of premounted unsheathed stent systems.

However, a bare stent may shear off the balloon catheter if friction is encountered between the stent and the guiding catheter, or at tortuous coronary segments, or at irregularities in coronary artery wall. Once this occurs, it will be very difficult, or even impossible, to pull back the stent in the small 6 Fr guiding catheter lumen. As a consequence, the stent may embolize in the coronary artery or in the systemic circulation, with potentially hazardous sequelae.

Selection of the proper guiding catheter is of paramount importance in the prevention of stent loss. The proper guiding catheter should have smooth curves, good back-up properties and

should be coaxially aligned with the coronary artery (Fig. 26.2).

One of the potentials of a 6 Fr guiding catheter is the ability to engage the coronary artery deeply (Fig. 26.3). In fact, the catheter may serve

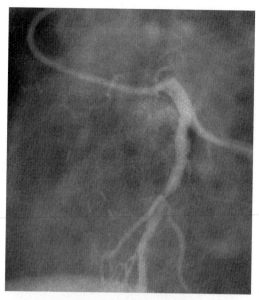

A

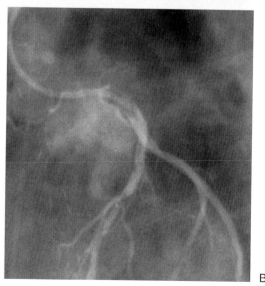

B

FIG. 26.2. A: Suboptimal guiding catheter (Judkins left) characteristics: Substantial shearing forces caused by sharp secondary curve in combination with 90-degree angle between tip and left main. **B:** Coaxiality improved with Amplatz left curve.

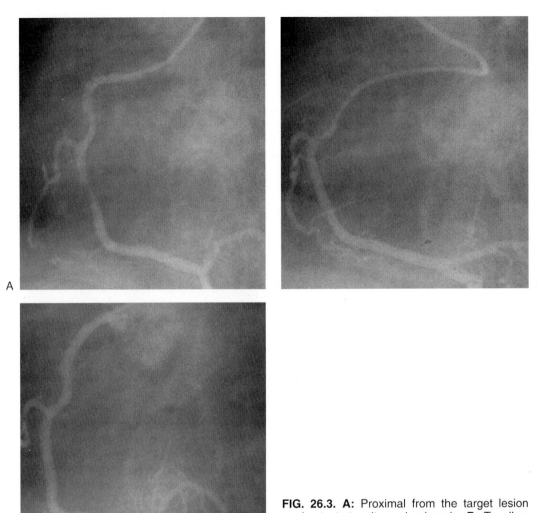

FIG. 26.3. A: Proximal from the target lesion moderate tortuosity and sclerosis. B: To allow safe passage of the stent across the proximal segment, the guiding catheter is deeply intubated C: Good result after stenting; no proximal guiding catheter induced damage.

as a protecting sheath, to prevent the stent from slipping off the balloon in tortuous or diseased segments.

This maneuver has an intrinsic risk for damaging the coronary artery, especially if the catheter is stiff. The ideal guiding catheter should be flexible distally and should be provided with an atraumatic soft tip. Safety of deep intubation is improved by advancing the guiding catheter over the balloon catheter-shaft.

A bare stent may become captured at the edge of the target lesion, especially if this lesion is irregular, calcified, and/or severe. Therefore, proper predilation increases safety of the procedure. Efforts should be directed towards achievement of smooth contours of the target segment.

With the latest generation of low-profile balloon catheters, the stent may easily slip off the balloon, especially if the balloon and stent are improperly prepared.

The deflated balloon profile can be increased by using this balloon for predilatation.

After predilatation, the balloon should be

cleaned with saline or alcohol to remove the lubricating agent, blood clots, and contrast. Also, a noncoated balloon can be selected at the start of the procedure. The stent can be crimped tightly on the balloon at zero intraballoon pressure. To prevent the balloon lumen from becoming obstructed by the crimping process, the balloon should contain the intracoronary guidewire. After crimping, proper fixation of the stent should be evaluated. The leading edge of the stent, especially, should be tightly wrapped over the balloon. In addition, the stent should be inspected for any irregularities before it is advanced on the guiding catheter.

If, despite proper precautions, stent dislodgment from the balloon occurs, it is important to prevent uncontrolled stent loss in the coronary or systemic circulation. If the stent and balloon are already in an intracoronary position and the stent retrieval cannot be attempted, sometimes there is no other option than to expand the stent partially in or proximal to the target lesion, after which a second attempt can be undertaken under optimized circumstances.

Preferably, however, all attempts should be directed towards retrieval of the stent into the guiding catheter.

Since this is may at times be an impossible task, attempts to retrieve the stent should be undertaken at a safe site in the systemic circulation.

The safest method is to retrieve the guiding catheter, balloon catheter, and stent back into the radial artery by keeping these structures in an unchanged relation to each other, while keeping the intracoronary wire distal from the target lesion.

Once in the radial artery, the stent-loaded balloon can be retrieved back into the guiding catheter. If this succeeds, the procedure can be redone after having solved the problem(s) related to inability to deliver the stent. If the stent is going to slip off the balloon, the stent can be expanded in the radial artery. If the stent has already dislodged from the balloon, attempts should be directed towards retrieval of the stent, by using snares or other retrieval devices.

Following the procedure the sheath can be removed immediately, followed by radial artery compression and application of a pressure bandage for approximately 4 hours. The patient is free to mobilize.

EARLY EXPERIENCE WITH TRANSRADIAL CORONARY ANGIOPLASTY

In 1992 the first patients were treated via the radial artery in our center.

In the transradial PTCA feasibility study (3), safety and efficacy of this technique was reported by our group on 100 patients.

Then the Access study (4), was designed: a randomized comparison between transradial, transbrachial, and transfemoral PTCA with 6 Fr guiding catheters in 900 patients. Primary endpoints were entry site and angioplasty related. Successful coronary cannulation was achieved in 279 (93.0%), 287 (95.7%) and in 299 (99.7%) patients randomized to radial (R), brachial (B), and femoral (F) approaches. PTCA success was achieved in 91.7%, 90.7% and 90.7% (p = not significant [ns]). Successful PTCA with an uneventful 1-month follow-up was achieved in 88.0%, 87.7% and 90.0% (p = ns). No major entry site complications were encountered after transradial PTCA, where as seven patients (2.3%) in the brachial and six (2.0%) in the femoral group (p = .035) had major complications. Transradial PTCA led to asymptomatic loss of radial pulsation in nine patients (3%). Procedural (R: 40 ± 24 min; B:39 ± 25 min; F:38 ± 24 min) and fluoroscopy times (R: 13 ± 11 min; B: 12 ± 10 min; F: 11 ± 10 min) were similar in the three respective groups as were number of guiding and balloon catheters and length of hospital stay (1.5 ± 2.5, 1.8 .± 3.8 and 1.8 ± 4.2 days).

Another feasibility study was completed in 100 patients who were selected for transradial coronary stent implantation (5). The purpose of this study was to evaluate feasibility and safety of implantation of unsheathed Palmaz-Schatz (Johnson and Johnson International Systems, Warren, NJ) coronary stents via the radial artery. In 100 consecutive patients, stent implantation was attempted for 122 lesions, distributed in 104 vessels. Immediately after stent implantation and final angiography, the introducer sheath was withdrawn, followed by intense anticoagulation and mobilization. Successful stent implantation via the radial artery was achieved in 96 patients. Procedural success and an uncomplicated clinical course was achieved in 93 patients (93%). A major bleeding was encountered in one patient (1%) in a time when severe bleeding complications following transfemoral stenting were common.

The finding that patients with an optimal stent result following a transradial procedure had no cardiac and entry site related complications in the first 24 hours, brought us the conviction that coronary stenting on an outpatient basis in a carefully selected group of patients is feasible and safe (6).

Patients selected for Palmaz-Schatz stent implantation, were adequately adjusted on Coumadin (Du Pont Pharmaceuticals, Wilmington, DE). At an INR >2.5, stenting was performed via the radial approach. Based on preprocedural, postprocedural, and procedural criteria, considering clinical status, procedural course and outcome, absence of predictors for stent occlusion, and of events during 4 to 6 hours observation, patients were considered candidates for same-day discharge. Heparin was administered only during the procedure. Immediately after the procedure, the arterial sheath was removed. Patients were mobilized and were discharged with a pressure dressing over the puncture site.

Between May 1994 and July 1995, 188 patients underwent Palmaz-Schatz coronary stent implantation via the radial artery. Of these, 88 remained hospitalized for various reasons. In 100 outpatients (Canadian Cardiovascular Society class III and IV; $n = 90$ [90%]) 125 stents were implanted to cover 110 lesions. No cardiac or bleeding events were encountered within 24 hours. During 2 weeks follow-up, one patient was readmitted (day 4) because of a bleeding abdominal aortic aneurysm, requiring surgery. One patient was readmitted with subacute thrombosis 2 weeks after discharge and one patient was readmitted with angina and anemia, which was treated with blood transfusions. At 1-month follow-up, no complications were observed.

Today, outpatient coronary stenting has been established as a routine procedure. In a carefully designed study, outpatient treatment is expanded to balloon angioplasty.

LIMITATIONS OF THE TECHNIQUE

Puncture and Cannulation Problems

The small size of the radial artery makes establishment of arterial access more difficult, when compared to the femoral technique. Attention has to be focused on prevention of pain and discomfort during sheath introduction, catheter manipulation, hemostasis, and during recovery. Radial spasm and local hematoma formation may prohibit arterial access, after an unsuccessful attempt to puncture the vessel. Unexpected abnormal anatomy (e.g., abnormal take-off from the brachial artery, tortuous brachial or subclavian arteries and obstructed or kinked vessels) may lead to failed coronary artery cannulation.

Radial Artery Spasm

Radial artery spasm is the most frequent complication of transradial coronary cannulation. The muscular artery, predominantly of α-adrenergic function is one of the most spasm prone arteries in the human body (7). Spasm is induced by circulating norepinephrine. Therefore the occurrence of spasm also inversely relates to the operator experience. All factors contributing to patient discomfort (anxiety, pain, long procedure duration) add to the incidence of spasm.

However, with adequate precautions such as the use of an appropriate arterial-access kit, long introducer sheaths, exchange guidewires, adequate guiding catheter selection, and proper spasmolytic and analgesic medication, radial artery spasm and discomfort can be minimized.

Limited Angioplasty Tools

Finally, 6 Fr guiding catheters are not compatible with atherectomy devices, but the use of 7 Fr guiding catheters allow a wide range of angioplasty tools. Of course, introduction of these larger guiding catheters requires larger radial arteries. However, a wide range of coronary pathology can be addressed with a broad spectrum of balloons and stents. Via 7 Fr guiding catheters, small-burred rotational atherectomy devices can be used. New IVUS catheters are 6 Fr compatible.

The medical industry is continuously being challenged to down-size its angioplasty equipment. In combination with the improved quality of 6 and 7 Fr guiding catheters, the interventionalists armamentarium will continue to increase.

Learning Curve

Compared to the transfemoral approach, the transradial technique is technically more demanding for several reasons: (a) the greater difficulty of cannulating the small radial artery, (b) occurrence of radial artery spasm, (c) unfamiliarity with arm vasculature, and (d) the different orientation of guiding catheters toward the coronary ostia. For physicians accustomed to working with 8 Fr guiding catheters only, handling characteristics of 6 Fr guiding catheters may give rise to additional problems. Therefore, a learning curve exists when starting with the procedure. The slope of the learning curve will depend on several factors, such as operator motivation, operator experience with arm procedures and/or 6 Fr guiding catheters, patient selection, and patient load. The level of training for the physicians and nursing staff is obviously of paramount importance to the achievement of success. Finally the catheterization laboratory should be well equipped.

Radial Artery Occlusion

We evaluated the incidence of radial artery occlusion and its consequences in 563 patients after transradial PTCA or stenting at discharge and at 1 month by physical examination. A two-dimensional and Doppler ultrasound study was performed in all patients with clinical evidence of radial artery occlusion. Presence of claudication was evaluated by opening and closing the hand 50 times.

At discharge, 30 patients (5.3%) had evidence of radial artery occlusion. At 1 month, 14 patients (46.6%) showed evidence of spontaneous recanalization. Thus, a persistent occlusion was found in 16 patients (2.8%). No ischemia of the hand could be provoked in these patients.

Based on our experience, we consider radial artery cannulation as a low-risk entry site, even if postprocedural radial artery patency is absent. The occurrence of radial artery occlusion is a subclinical event.

Since the incidence of early postprocedural radial artery occlusions approximates 5%, the presence of well-developed collaterals with the ulnar artery is a prerequisite for a safe transradial PTCA.

PROMISES OF THE TRANSRADIAL APPROACH

It is our experience that the transradial approach for coronary angioplasty is associated with some major advantages compared to the traditional approach. Similar positive findings are being reported from those centers throughout Europe, the United States, Canada, and Asia which had adapted the radial approach as a routine technique (8–19).

During 5 years of experience, the technique has indeed proven to be feasible, effective, and safe in terms of dramatically reducing the risk for major entry-site-related complications. The sheath can be withdrawn immediately following PTCA, even under full heparinization. No manpower, but a simple compression bandage is required to obtain hemostasis. The value of simple and safe hemostasis has to be considered in the light of the large number of patients treated with some form of anticoagulant or antiplatelet regimen for stable and unstable coronary syndromes.

The freedom of the patient to mobilize immediately after the procedure is highly appreciated since this brings more comfort compared to forced and prolonged bed rest. Older patients with back aches particularly prefer the early ambulation.

This early ambulation allows short hospitalization times and even treatment on an outpatient basis.

The near elimination of bleeding complications, the effective use of nursing and medical staff, the early ambulation, and the short hospitalization, all contribute to significant cost savings.

And last, but not least, the vast majority of patients prefer the radial approach.

Technical problems are presently being solved; guiding catheters are getting better. The largest internal diameter at present is 0.068 in. Also, more dedicated guiding curves are being developed. New-generation 7 Fr guiding catheters, in combination with lower profile interventional tools, will allow performance of more complex cases such as atherectomy, kissing stent techniques, and so on.

More attention is currently focused on the development of comfortable and effective hemostasis devices.

To enjoy these advantages, invasive cardiologists require only some retraining: a worthwhile investment.

Training programs are currently being refined; they include live demonstrations, proctorships, CD-ROMs, and manuals. Even on the Internet (http://www.radialforce.org), the most updated information on all the aspects the technique is presented for interested physicians.

Finally, it is important to train young cardiologists in this technique. Personally, I think that the transradial approach will take over from the femoral technique.

REFERENCES

1. Urban P, Moles VP, Pande AK. Percutaneous coronary angioplasty through six French guiding catheters. *J Invas Cardiol* 1992;4:336–338.
2. Campeau L. Percutaneous radial artery approach for coronary angiography. *Cathet Cardiovasc Diagn* 1989;16:3–7.
3. Kiemeneij F, Laarman GJ. Transradial artery coronary angioplasty. *Am Heart J* 1995;129:1–7.
4. Kiemeneij F, Laarman GJ, Odekerken D, Slagboom T, van der Wieken R. A randomized comparison of percutaneous transluminal coronary angioplasty by the radial, brachial and femoral approaches: The Access study. *J Am Coll Cardiol* 1997;29:1269–1275.
5. Kiemeneij F, Laarman GJ. Transradial artery Palmaz-Schatz coronary stent implantation: results of a single center feasibility study. *Am Heart J* 1995;130:14–21.
6. Kiemeneij F, Laarman GJ, Slagboom T, van der Wieken R. Outpatient coronary stent implantation. *J Am Coll Cardiol* 1997;29:323–327.
7. He GW, Yang CQ. Characteristics of adrenoreceptors in the human radial artery: clinical implications. *J Cardiovasc Thorac Surg* 1998;115:1136–1141.
8. Stella P, Kiemeneij F, Laarman GJ, Slagboom T, Odekerken D. Incidence and outcome of radial artery occlusion following transradial artery coronary angioplasty. *Cathet Cardiovasc Diagn* 1997;40:156–158.
9. Mick MJ Transradial approach for coronary angiography. *J Invas Cardiol* 1996;8[Suppl. D]:9D–12D.
10. Chatelain P, Keighley C, Urban P et al. Management of coronary restenosis via the radial artery: an elegant approach to the Achilles' heel of PTCA. *J Invas Cardiol* 1997;9:177–180.
11. Tift Mann J III, Cubeddu G, Schneider JE, Arrowood M. Right radial access for PTCA: a prospective study demonstrates reduced complications and hospital charges. *J Invas Cardiol* 1996;8[Suppl D]:40D–44D.
12. Lotan C, Hasin Y, Mosseri M, Rozenman Y, Admon D, Nassar H, Gotsman MS. Transradial approach for coronary angiography and angioplasty. *Am J Cardiol* 1995;76:164–167.
13. Wu CJ, Lo PH, Chang KC, Fu M, Lau KW, Hung JS. Transradial coronary an angiography and angioplasty in Chinese patients. *Cathet Cardiovasc Diagn* 1997;40:159–163.
14. Barbeau GR, Carrier G, Ferland S, Létourneau L, Gleeton O, Larivière MM. Right transradial approach for coronary procedures: preliminary results. *J Invas Cardiol* 1996;8[Suppl D]:19D–21D.
15. Louvard Y, Bradai R, Pezzano M, Harvey R, Lardoux M, Morice MC. Transradial complex coronary angioplasty: the influence of a single operator's experience. In: *Eighth Complex Coronary Angioplasty Course* 1997;647–649.
16. Fajadet J, Brunel P, Jordan C, Cassagneau B, Marco J. Transradial coronary stenting a passing fad or widespread use in the future? In: *Eighth Complex Coronary Angioplasty Course* 1997;247–257.
17. Tift Mann J III, Cubeddu G, Schneider JE et al. Clinical evaluation of current stent deployment techniques. *J Invas Cardiol* 1996;8[Suppl D]:30D–35D.
18. El-Shiekh RA, Burket MW, Mouhaffel A, Moore JA, Cooper CJ. U.S. experience of transradial coronary stenting utilizing Palmaz-Schatz stents. *Cathet Cardiovasc Diagn* 1997;40:166–169.
19. Chatelain P, Arceo A, Rombout E, Verin V, Urban P. New device for compression of the radial artery after diagnostic and interventional cardiac procedures. *Cathet Cardiovasc Diagn* 1997;40:297–300.

27

Treatment of Closure and Threatened Closure

Jane A. Leopold and *Alice K. Jacobs

*Department of Cardiology, Boston Medical Center, and *Cardiac Catheterization Laboratory and Interventional Cardiology, Boston University Medical Center, Section of Cardiology, Boston, Massachusetts 02118*

Acute or threatened vessel closure remains a significant complication of percutaneous coronary revascularization that is often associated with adverse clinical outcomes. Abrupt closure complicates 2% to 8.3% of coronary angioplasty procedures (although the actual incidence during the routine use of intracoronary stents is difficult to assess) and may result in myocardial infarction, emergency coronary artery bypass surgery, or death (1–3). Abrupt closure is recognized as the acute occlusion of the target vessel during or following percutaneous intervention, characterized by Thrombolysis in Myocardial Infarction IIIB trial (TIMI) grade 0 to 2 flow in the artery (4). Clinically, patients experience recurrent angina with ischemic electrocardiographic changes, and rarely, hypotension or ventricular arrhythmias (1,3,5). The timing of abrupt closure following percutaneous coronary revascularization has been best studied following balloon angioplasty. In the majority of procedures, abrupt closure occurs within the first 30 minutes after initial vessel dilation. It has been reported that 57% to 84% of out-of-laboratory abrupt closure occurs within 6 hours of the first balloon inflation and has been temporally associated with discontinuation of anticoagulation, platelet transfusion, or hypotension secondary to noncardiac causes (1,3,6–8). Threatened closure is defined as the angiographic presence of a dissection or thrombus formation following PTCA despite the presence of TIMI grade 3 flow. Threatened closure places the vessel at increased risk of abrupt closure (4).

INCIDENCE OF ABRUPT CLOSURE

Review of the National Heart Lung and Blood Institute (NHLBI) PTCA 1977 to 1981 and 1985 to 1986 Registries reveals that the incidence of abrupt closure complicating coronary balloon angioplasty, 4.5% and 4.9%, respectively, had remained relatively unchanged over time; however, patients included in the second registry tended to be older, with diminished left ventricular function, higher rates of multivessel disease, previous myocardial infarction, and previous coronary bypass surgery when compared to patients in the first registry (9–11). Whereas the rates of myocardial infarction and death remained similar between registries, the rate of emergency bypass surgery was significantly decreased, 5.8% versus 3.5%, respectively, suggesting an improved ability to effectively treat abrupt closure with nonsurgical options. The Multivessel Angioplasty Prognosis Study (MAPS) compared clinical and procedural outcomes in patients treated during 1986 to 1987 and in 1991. There was a significant reduction in total complications (8.0% versus 3.5%, respectively) as well as a decrease in bypass surgery (5.5% versus 1.0%, respectively) between groups. Importantly, 25% of patients were treated with second-generation devices in addition to balloon angioplasty (12). These observations suggest that bailout techniques have improved over time, resulting in a reduction in the adverse sequelae associated with abrupt closure. In fact, in the new device era, the incidence of abrupt closure complicating percutaneous coronary intervention in one center significantly decreased from 4.9% to 1.8% (13). It is important to note, however, that with the exception of stents, nonballoon devices such as directional, rotational, and laser atherectomy do not appear to be associated with a reduced incidence of abrupt closure (14–16).

CONSEQUENCES OF ABRUPT CLOSURE

Abrupt closure is associated with major ischemic complications resulting in myocardial infarction, need for surgical revascularization, and death. Review of the NHLBI Registries reveals that 58% of myocardial infarctions, 48% of coronary bypass procedures, and 33% of deaths occurred in the 6.8% of patients who experienced abrupt closure during coronary angioplasty. Of note, in the 1985 to 1986 Registry, rates of death, late infarction, and coronary surgery remained increased up to 2 years after hospitalization for the initial event in patients with coronary occlusion when compared to those patients with uneventful procedures (11,17).

MECHANISM OF ABRUPT CLOSURE

Balloon dilatation of a coronary artery results in denudation of the endothelium, often with significant intimal fissuring. The media is often disrupted locally; however, extensive interruption of this layer may produce obstructive dissection flaps or intramural hematomas. Exposure of the subendothelium stimulates platelet deposition and activation with formation of thrombin (18). This, in turn, mediates occlusive thrombus formation which may occur either alone or as the result of blood stasis produced by the release of platelet- and endothelium-derived vasoactive factors and loss of endothelial-derived relaxant factors (19). Abrupt vessel closure may then result from elastic recoil, coronary vasospasm, dissection (Fig. 27.1), and/or intracoronary thrombosis, pathophysiologic processes which accompany the therapeutic injury delivered with balloon angioplasty.

Angiographically, vessel wall dissection is recognized by curvilinear or spiral-shaped fill-ing defects or extraluminal extravasation of contrast material (20). In contrast, thrombus may be visualized as a progressively enlarging or mobile, intraluminal lucency surrounded by contrast (6). For lesions with uncertain angiographic profiles, including contrast staining, haziness, or the appearance of a filling defect, intravascular ultrasound or angioscopy may facilitate lesion evaluation (21). For example, in vessels evaluated with intravascular ultrasound or angioscopy, intimal dissection was present in 50% to 80% of vessels following coronary angioplasty (21,22); however, it was those vessels with significant intimal and medial disruption that created a "flap," or with compromise of the lumen, that were more susceptible to thrombus formation and abrupt closure. Intraluminal thrombus has been detected in up to 44% of patients with abrupt closure, often superimposed on medial dissection flaps (2,5,23), (Fig. 27.2). Among patients undergoing unplanned stent placement, thrombosis is the most likely mechanism of abrupt closure, because dissections covered by stents rarely become obstructive except at the proximal and distal stent borders.

RISK FACTORS FOR ABRUPT CLOSURE

An increased risk of acute closure complicating coronary intervention is predicted by certain clinical, morphologic, and angiographic characteristics. For example, retrospective analyses have shown that female gender, diabetes mellitus, unstable angina, and acute myocardial infarction are clinical predictors of abrupt closure. Lesion morphologic characteristics including dissection, lesion length, branch point stenoses, angle >45 degrees, total occlusion, presence of thrombus, and right coronary artery lesion location also increase the risk of abrupt closure. In fact, the preprocedural presence of thrombus increases the risk for abrupt closure up to ninefold (23). Postprocedural characteristics including residual stenosis >35%, transstenotic gradient ≥20 mm Hg, and residual thrombus, or dissection predict acute, or subacute vessel closure (1–3,11,24–26). The factors most frequently associated with abrupt vessel closure during percu-

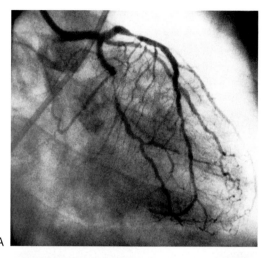

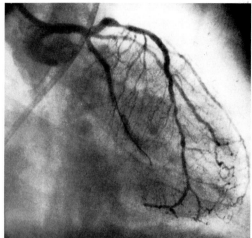

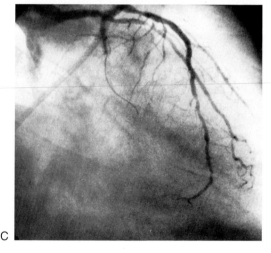

FIG. 27.1. A: Preprocedure single-frame cineangiogram in right anterior oblique caudal projection revealing tubular stenosis in the left circumflex obtuse marginal artery. **B:** Single-frame cineangiogram in the right anterior oblique caudal projection following balloon inflation revealing grade 1 TIMI flow and contrast staining around the wire. **C:** Single-frame cineangiogram in the right anterior oblique caudal projection following repeat balloon dilatation revealing abrupt closure and grade 0 TIMI flow.

taneous coronary intervention are listed in Table 27.1.

PREVENTION OF ABRUPT CLOSURE

Although certain clinical, angiographic, and procedural factors increase the risk of abrupt closure complicating coronary revascularization, the integration of these factors and the prospective prediction of risk in a specific patient remains difficult. Therefore, careful attention to several preventive strategies in both low- and high-risk patients may serve to limit the incidence of abrupt closure and improve patient outcome. In general, preventive strategies are limited to pharmacologic therapy and procedural technique (Table 27.2).

Pharmacologic approaches to prevent abrupt closure have centered on resolution of intracoronary thrombi prior to the procedure as well as suppression of thrombus formation and platelet aggregation at the angioplasty site. The efficacy of antiplatelet agents in reducing the ischemic complications associated with coronary angioplasty has been well established in several randomized trials which noted a decrease in the incidence of periprocedural Q-wave myocardial infarction (27) and of abrupt closure (28) in patients receiving aspirin and dipyridamole therapy versus placebo.

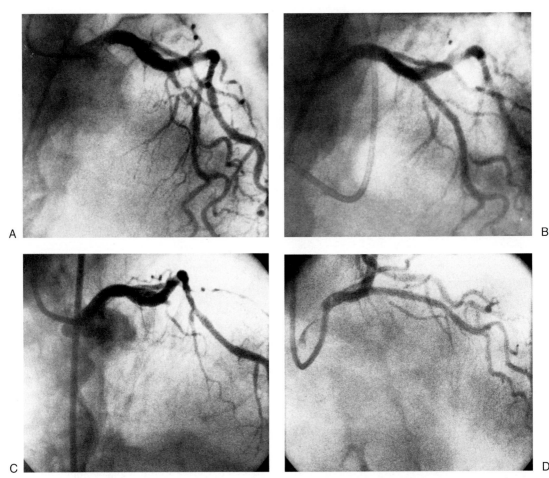

FIG. 27.2. A: Preprocedure single-frame cineangiogram in right anterior oblique cranial projection revealing a significant stenosis with thrombus in the mid left anterior descending artery. **B:** Postprocedure single-frame cineangiogram in right anterior oblique cranial projection following placement of a 3.0-mm intracoronary stent. **C:** Single-frame cineangiogram in right anterior oblique cranial projection revealing abrupt closure and total occlusion of the proximal left anterior descending artery. **D:** Postprocedure single-frame cineangiogram in right anterior oblique cranial projection following repeat dilatation with a 3.5-mm balloon and treatment with a IIb/IIIa receptor antagonist.

Observational data concerning the use of heparin in the prevention of abrupt vessel closure prior to, during, and following coronary angioplasty procedures have been obtained. Heparin has been reported to reduce angiographically visible intracoronary thrombi, to improve procedural success, and reduce abrupt closure (29) when given for several days prior to the procedure. Systemic heparin is universally administered during coronary intervention and the intensity of anticoagulation as measured by the activated clotting time is inversely proportional to the risk of abrupt closure (30). Furthermore, activated clotting times above 300 seconds are associated with low rates of periprocedural ischemic complications (31). In contrast, randomized trials have failed to demonstrate a reduction in ischemic complications in patients treated with heparin for 12 to 24 hours postprocedure compared to patients receiving no aspirin following an uncomplicated angioplasty procedure (32). However, the temporal relationship be-

TABLE 27.1. *Factors associated with abrupt vessel closure*

Clinical
  Unstable angina
  Female gender
  Acute myocardial infarction
  High surgical risk
Angiographic
  Intraluminal thrombus
  ACC/AHA lesion score
  Multivessel disease
  Multiple stenoses in same vessel
  Lesion length >10 mm
  Angulated lesion (>45 degrees)
  Lesion at branch point
  Excessive proximal tortuosity
  Ostial right coronary lesion
  Degenerated saphenous vein graft
  Preprocedure stenosis 90% to 99%
  Intimal dissection
  Postprocedure stenosis >35%
  Postprocedure gradient >20 mm Hg
  Prolonged heparin infusion

tween abrupt vessel closure and discontinuation of heparin therapy suggests that heparin may be effective in prevention of acute vessel closure in selected patients.

The role of intracoronary thrombolytic therapy in the prevention of abrupt closure complicating coronary angioplasty remains unclear and one randomized trial failed to demonstrate the efficacy of intracoronary urokinase in this setting (33). Currently, intracoronary thrombolytic therapy has limited use. However, the efficacy of platelet glycoprotein IIb/IIIa receptor antagonists during coronary intervention has been clearly shown to reduce ischemic complications

TABLE 27.2. *Strategies to prevent abrupt vessel closure*

Pharmacologic
  Periprocedural antiplatelet therapy
  Adequate heparin
  Glycoprotein IIb/IIIa receptor antagonists
  Intracoronary thrombolytic therapy
  Thrombin inhibitors
Mechanical
  Appropriate balloon sizing
  Long balloons (angulated lesions)
  Gradual and prolonged balloon inflation
  Predilatation with small balloon
  Noncompliant balloon material
Thoughtful predilatation strategy

associated with these procedures in multiple clinical settings, even when intracoronary stents are used (34–36).

Certain technical procedural strategies may influence the incidence of abrupt vessel closure. For example, appropriate balloon to artery sizing has been shown to decrease the incidence of coronary dissection (37–38). Similarly, it has been suggested that the use of long balloons (particularly in angulated lesions), noncompliant balloons (39), gradual and prolonged balloon inflation (40), and predilatation with undersized balloons (in large vessels) (41) may reduce the incidence of coronary dissection and subsequent abrupt closure.

MANAGEMENT OF ABRUPT CLOSURE

Overall management is directed toward treatment of intracoronary thrombus, dissection flaps and spasm in an effort to restore flow (Fig. 27.3). This is most easily and successfully accomplished when abrupt vessel closure occurs during the procedure. In contrast, when abrupt closure occurs out-of-lab following the procedure, the incidence of major complications (myocardial infarction) increases (11).

Pharmacologic Management

The experience using pharmacologic agents as the sole therapeutic modality in the management of abrupt closure has offered limited results. Therefore, several treatment protocols designed to manage acute and threatened closure in the cardiac catheterization laboratory have used pharmacologic compounds as adjunctive agents to mechanical intervention to successfully restore vessel patency. These strategies combine the use of novel pharmacologic therapies that effectively target pathophysiologic mechanisms associated with acute vessel closure, such as coronary vasospasm and intracoronary thrombus formation resulting from intimal dissection, with percutaneous revascularization to achieve vessel patency.

Vasodilators

Although refractory coronary vasospasm alone is rarely the etiology of abrupt closure,

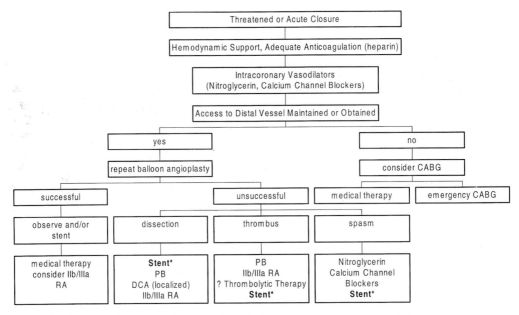

FIG. 27.3. Suggested approach to the treatment of threatened or acute vessel closure during percutaneous coronary intervention. PB, perfusion balloon; RA, receptor antagonists.

coronary vasospasm with subsequent flow reduction and thrombus formation are often associated with vessel wall dissection. The intracoronary administration of vasodilators with antiplatelet properties, such as nitroglycerin (42), has been reported to relieve vasospasm and restore flow in several isolated cases; however, most operators have used nitroglycerin as a bridge to other therapies. Similarly, the calcium channel blockers (43) verapamil and diltiazem, when administered via an intracoronary route, have been used successfully as adjunctive agents to treat vasospasm. The use of these agents is often limited by their hypotensive and, in the case of the calcium channel blockers, A-V nodal blocking property effects.

Heparin

At present, there have been no compelling data to support the administration of additional intravenous or intracoronary heparin to achieve supratherapeutic activated clotting time(s) in the setting of acute or threatened vessel closure. It appears to be more important that the activated

clotting time is maintained in the therapeutic range ($\geq$300) during percutaneous revascularization and it has been shown that there is a significant inverse relationship between the degree of anticoagulation during angioplasty and the risk of abrupt closure (30). In the event of acute or threatened vessel closure, the activated clotting time must be checked frequently, because the clotting cascade has been activated and heparin may be rapidly consumed during the time that vessel patency has been compromised.

Thrombolytic Agents

The use of thrombolytic agents for abrupt closure remains controversial, because these compounds have been used as adjuncts to repeat balloon dilatation in the setting of acute closure with variable success rates. Whereas some studies have failed to demonstrate a benefit with the use of thrombolytic agents, others have cited a 65% to 90% procedural success rate with a reduction in adverse clinical sequelae (44–46). For example, the intracoronary administration of 100,000 to 250,000 U of urokinase following balloon dilatation complicated by reaccumulation of intracoronary thrombus was reported to restore vessel patency in 94% of patients treated with limited adverse sequelae (44). In contrast, a similar group of patients were treated with intracoronary t-PA following coronary angioplasty complicated by acute vessel closure; approximately 50% experienced acute vessel reocclusion within 24 to 36 hours (45). More recently, the TAUSA (Thrombolysis and Angioplasty in Unstable Angina) Trials established a negative effect for the use of thrombolytic therapies as an adjunct to coronary angioplasty in the presence of thrombus (47). These observations may, in fact, reflect the procoagulant effects of some thrombolytic agents and suggest that the additional use of antiplatelet agents or thrombin inhibitors may reestablish a role for thrombolytics in the management of abrupt vessel closure.

Glycoprotein IIb/IIIa Receptor Antagonists

The presence of platelet-rich thrombi at the site of acute closure suggests that the administration of glycoprotein IIb/IIIa receptor inhibitor compounds may restore vessel patency. In an animal model, the glycoprotein IIb/IIIa receptor antagonist abciximab promoted platelet desegregation in an immature thrombus (48). Glycoprotein IIb/IIIa receptor antagonists additionally modulate shear-induced platelet activation and release of mediators of vessel tone by activated platelets, which inhibits coronary vasoconstriction in the distal vessel. Whereas the beneficial effects of glycoprotein IIb/IIIa agents in the prevention of acute ischemic complications have been readily demonstrated, there is a paucity of studies evaluating the efficacy of these agents when used as a ''bailout'' therapy for acute or threatened closure, despite the current frequency of this approach (49). Contemporary practice supports the use of glycoprotein IIb/IIIa inhibitors for acute or threatened closure; with the advent of newer agents with shorter half-lives, glycoprotein IIb/IIIa inhibitor compounds may be extended to patients with abrupt closure who were previously excluded from therapy.

MECHANICAL TREATMENT CORONARY ANGIOPLASTY

Repeat Coronary Angioplasty

Vessel patency may be restored successfully utilizing a conventional balloon catheter; however, this strategy is only variably successful with patency rates of 35% to 87% reported (3,5,11,50). Repeat dilatation allows the operator to attempt to ''tack up'' a dissection flap with repeat inflations. It has been suggested that the same balloon or a slightly oversized balloon (0.5 mm larger than vessel diameter) be used and inflations be done at low pressures (i.e., 1 to 2 atmospheres) (2,3,5). Whereas this procedure may not be well tolerated for long periods of time due to prolonged ischemia, repeat angioplasty may adequately serve as a bridge to a more definitive therapy.

PERFUSION BALLOON CATHETERS

The advent of perfusion balloons has increased the success of catheter-based therapies for acute or threatened closure. These catheters are designed to maintain 40 to 60 ml/min of blood flow to the distal vessel (51) while the balloon is inflated across an area of dissection. Prolonged inflation time achieved with a perfusion balloon may promote ''tacking up'' of a dissection flap or thrombus compression. When used for threatened or acute vessel closure, perfusion balloons have a success rate between 41% and 100% (52–54). The duration of balloon inflation, which is limited by ischemia (55,56), appears to influence procedural success rate. Some operators have suggested that inflation time between 10 and 20 minutes improves angiographic and clinical outcomes whereas others have indicated that inflation time of several hours may be required (52,57). The long-term clinical follow-up of patients who experienced abrupt closure and were treated with perfusion balloons revealed that only 16% of patients required coronary bypass surgery to restore vessel patency (54).

Perfusion balloon catheters have several disadvantages that must be considered as well.

Since they rely on intrinsic blood pressure to maintain perfusion, they are of limited use in patients with systemic hypotension. In addition, these catheters have a higher profile than most balloon catheters and may not easily traverse tortuous or calcified vessels. Furthermore, long, spiral dissections may not be covered adequately by these balloons and if the balloon covers a large side branch, inflation time will be limited by ischemia (52). When compared to immediate coronary stent placement for abrupt closure, perfusion balloon alone resulted in a more favorable outcome, prior to use of current stent deployment techniques and antiplatelet therapy (58).

The perfusion balloon should be placed over the guidewire that is distal to the site of the dissection. The balloon should be positioned to span the dissection or luminal disruption. Once placed, a small injection of contrast may be used to document the adequacy of distal flow and intraluminal position of the catheter. To further enhance blood flow, following balloon inflation, the guidewire may be removed and the guiding catheter backed out of the ostium to promote passive perfusion.

Directional Coronary Atherectomy

Directional coronary atherectomy (DCA) as a salvage therapy for abrupt closure complicating coronary angioplasty has been employed with success rates reported from 80% to 88% in small series of patients (59). DCA offers the ability to resect obstructive intimal flaps and dissections, remove thrombus, and provide a larger residual lumen following conventional balloon dilatation. There are several disadvantages to this strategy that may limit its practical applications in this setting. DCA equipment requires sheath and guide up-sizing and operator familiarity with the device, and is of limited usefulness in tortuous vessels, distal segments, and small caliber vessels. Furthermore, DCA may only be used in vessels in which the intimal flap may be captured in the length of the catheter housing. In addition, aggressive cutting is accompanied by the risk of coronary perforation, a risk that is increased in relation to the length and depth of the dissection. DCA remains a viable option

when a dissection is refractory to balloon angioplasty, and coronary stent placement or bypass surgery are not viable options.

Coronary Artery Stents

Coronary artery stents represent a significant advancement in the management of abrupt and threatened closure. By serving as a luminal scaffold, stents readily secure dissection flaps, prevent significant elastic recoil and preserve vessel geometry (60,61). In turn, stents have greatly reduced the need for emergency coronary surgery following failed angioplasty. There are a number of first-and second-generation stents currently available in the United States, each with its own design profile. Until recently, the Gianturco-Roubin (Cook, Inc., Bloomington, IN) and the Palmaz-Schatz (Johnson & Johnson International Systems, Warren, NJ) stents were the only FDA-approved stents for the treatment of abrupt closure. To date, there are approximately ten different stents available in the United States and many more in Europe. Although each stent offers a unique design profile, the majority of data collected on the efficacy of stenting for abrupt or threatened closure results from the use of only a few stents.

Use of the initial Gianturco-Roubin stent in the treatment of acute or threatened vessel closure after coronary angioplasty resulted in an improvement in vessel diameter stenosis from 63% $\pm$ 25% to 15% $\pm$ 14% and a reduction in major adverse cardiac events. However, an 8.7% incidence of subacute stent thrombosis occurred 5.2 $\pm$ 6.2 days postprocedure. Interestingly, the reported restenosis rate of 39% was similar to that seen with coronary angioplasty (62). The NHLBI/NACI Registry used reported on patients treated with second-generation Gianturco-Roubin stents used for suboptimal angioplasty results, abrupt closure, or other type of technical failure. Major in-hospital events occurred in 9.7% of patients, including death in 1.7%, Q-wave myocardial infarction in 3.1%, and emergency coronary surgery in 6%. Abrupt closure of a stented segment occurred in 3.1% of patients at a mean of 3.9 days. At 1-year follow-up, percutaneous reintervention of the stented segment occurred in 20.4 % of the patients who received an unplanned stent after new device use or balloon angioplasty, compared with 26.2% in the planned stent group (63).

Studies documenting the use of the Palmaz-Schatz stent for acute or threatened closure demonstrate superb efficacy when compared to pre-stent-era therapies. In 301 patients who received a stent for abrupt closure, at 4 weeks, cardiac mortality was 1.3%, nonfatal infarction was 4.0%, and 1% of patients required surgical revascularization. Further, 6.3% of patients needed repeat coronary angioplasty. It is interesting to note that all of these events occurred in 21 patients who developed subacute stent thrombosis (64), which had been shown to be higher when stents were placed for threatened or abrupt closure than in the elective setting (65,66). These data must be interpreted with caution, however, Because these studies were done prior to the advent of optimal anticoagulation regimens and high-pressure postdeployment inflations.

The ACS Multi-Link stent (Guidant Inc., Santa Clara, CA) has a tubular design with multiple rings connected with multiple links to enhance hoop strength, while allowing sufficient longitudinal flexibility. Initial and follow-up outcomes were evaluated in 70 patients who had the stent placed in an unplanned manner for indications including abrupt vessel closure. In-hospital mortality was 1.4%, myocardial infarction occurred in 2.9%, and subacute stent thrombosis in 1.4%. Stenting immediately improved the minimum lumen diameter from 0.97 mm $\pm$ 0.41 mm to 2.72 mm $\pm$ 0.31 mm, but at 6 months it had decreased to 1.89 mm $\pm$ 0.44 mm. Angiographic restenosis occurred in 16.4% and target vessel revascularization was required in 8.7% (67).

The experience with the Gianturco-Roubin, Palmaz-Schatz, and Multi-Link stents has been extended to other stents that are currently available for use. These newer stents have small profiles for improved delivery; most allow access to side branches and are available in a wider variety of diameters and lengths. In addition, whereas some stents are self-expanding, others are mounted on high-pressure balloons to achieve stent deployment and postdilatation in a single step. The availability of numerous stent designs significantly increases the ability to successfully treat abrupt or threatened closure without surgical intervention.

When deploying stents for the treatment of acute or threatened vessel closure, several factors should be considered. In the setting of thrombus, it is important to maintain normal (TIMI grade 3) blood flow and to consider use of adjunctive agents such as a IIb/IIIa platelet receptor antagonist. It is noteworthy that stents are no longer considered contraindicated in the presence of thrombus. In the setting of dissection, the entire dissection should be covered and often this requires multiple views or intravascular ultrasound imaging to define the distal and proximal dissection edge. Stents are usually deployed from distal to proximal vessel location, using appropriately sized smaller stents in distal vessels. Rarely, the dissection flap will continue to protrude through the stent struts and will require additional deployment of a stent within a stent. When a large dissection flap is noted, use of stents with a high surface area is desirable. Although use of multiple stents often results in an excellent angiographic result, data concerning the subacute and long-term efficacy of this strategy are limited.

Coronary Artery Bypass Surgery

Emergency coronary artery bypass grafting remains an option to restore vessel patency after attempts at percutaneous revascularization have failed. In fact, there are certain instances where it is the preferred method of revascularization in the setting of abrupt closure. These scenarios include (a) patients who continue to manifest refractory myocardial ischemia where percutaneous revascularization has failed to restore flow to the vessel, (b) selected patients with high-risk anatomic features such as left main occlusion or compromise, and (c) those patients in whom the initial angioplasty site appears to be severely disrupted or unstable, despite adequate restoration of flow (68,69). Rates of death and Q-wave infarction are consistently higher in patients who undergo coronary surgery in an emergency setting rather than as an elective procedure. In addition, surgical mortality rates have been reported from 0% to 19% with rates of perioperative infarction from 18% to as high as 57% (70,71). Predictors of poor outcome following emergency surgery include multivessel disease, presence of hemodynamic instability, angina, and decreased left ventricular function (72). Despite the increased rates of myocardial infarction and death, the long-term outcome for patients with abrupt closure treated with emergency coronary surgery is good, with 5 year survival rates greater than 90% reported (70,73).

SUMMARY

Abrupt or threatened closure during or following percutaneous revascularization procedures remains a serious complication which is often associated with adverse clinical sequelae. Although the rates of abrupt closure have remained essentially unchanged over time, using contemporary techniques of stent deployment, the rate of abrupt closure following stent placement is lower than the rate associated with nonstent procedures. Furthermore, significant advances in techniques, adjunctive pharmacologic agents, and devices have resulted in more effective management strategies and improved outcomes following abrupt closure. Therefore, percutaneous revascularization may be offered to patients with a higher clinical and angiographic risk profile. Concomitantly, rates of emergency coronary surgery have diminished, suggesting that failed coronary angioplasty may be managed adequately with coronary artery stents in the majority of patients. These observations suggest that further improvements in adjunctive therapies and coronary stents may continue to reduce the rates of adverse sequelae associated with abrupt vessel closure.

REFERENCES

1. Simpfendorfer C, Belardi J, Bellamy G, Galan K, Franco I, Hollman J. Frequency, management, and follow-up of patients with acute coronary occlusions after percutaneous coronary angioplasty. *Am J Cardiol* 1987;59: 267–269.
2. Lincoff AM, Popma JJ, Ellis SG, Topol EJ. Abrupt vessel closure complicating coronary angioplasty: clinical, angiographic and therapeutic profile. *J Am Coll Cardiol* 1992;926–935.
3. de Feyter PJ, van den Brand M, Laarman GH, van Domburd R, Serruys PW, Surypranata H. Acute coronary artery occlusion during and after percutaneous transluminal coronary angioplasty. frequency, prediction, clinical course, management, and follow-up. *Circulation* 1991;83:927–936.
4. Lincoff AM, Topol EJ. Intracoronary stenting compared with conventional therapy for abrupt vessel closure complicating coronary angioplasty: a matched case control study. *J Am Coll Cardiol* 1992;21:866–875.
5. Sinclair IN, McCabe CH, Sipperly ME, Baim DS. Predictors, therapeutic options, and long-term outcome of abrupt reclosure. *Am J Cardiol* 1988;61:61G–66G.
6. Goldbaum T, DeSciascio G, Cowley MJ, Vetrovec GW. Early occlusion following successful coronary angioplasty: clinical and angiographic observations. *Cathet Cardiovasc Diagn* 1989;17:22–27.
7. Gabliani G, Deligonul U, Kern MJ, Vandermael M. Acute coronary occlusion occurring after successful percutaneous transluminal coronary angioplasty: temporal relationship to discontinuation of anticoagulation. *Am Heart J* 1988;116:696–700.
8. Gutowski T, Kauffman G, Lacy C. Abrupt vessel closure following platelet transfusion post-PTCA. *Cathet Cardiovasc Diagn* 1991;23:282–285.
9. Holmes DR, Holubkov R, Vliestra RE et al. Comparisons of complications during percutaneous transluminal coronary angioplasty from 1977 to 1981 and from 1985 to 1986: the National Heart, Lung, and Blood Institute percutaneous transluminal coronary angioplasty registry. *J Am Coll Cardiol* 1988;12:1149–1155.
10. Cowley MJ, Darros G, Kelsey SF, Van Raden M, Detre KM. Emergency coronary bypass surgery after coronary angioplasty: the National Heart, Lung, and Blood Institute's Percutaneous transluminal coronary angioplasty registry experience. *Am J Cardiol* 1984;53:22C–26C.
11. Detre KM, Holmes DR Jr, Holubkov R et al., and coinvestigators of the NHLBI PTCA Registry. Incidence and consequences of periprocedural occlusion. The 1985–1986 National Heart, Lung, and Blood Institute percutaneous transluminal coronary angioplasty registry. *Circulation* 1990;82:739–750.
12. Ellis SG, Cowley, MJ, Whitlow PL et al., for the Multivessel Angioplasty Prognosis Study (MAPS) group. *J Am Coll Cardiol* 1995;25:1137–1142.
13. Kuntz RE, Piana R, Pomerantz RM, Carrozza J, Fishman R, Manwour M et al. Changing incidence and management of abrupt closure following coronary intervention in the new device era. *Cathet Cardiovasc Diagn* 1992;27:183–190.
14. Topol EJ, Leya F, Pinkerton CA et al. A comparison of directional atherectomy with coronary angioplasty in patients with coronary artery disease. *N Engl J Med* 1993;329:221–227.
15. Safian RD, Nizai KA, Strzelecki M et al. Detailed angiographic analysis of high-speed mechanical rotational atherectomy in human coronary arteries. *Circulation* 1993;88:961–968.
16. Prelack MB, Athasiadis A, Voelker W, Baumbach A, Karsch KR. Acute closure during coronary excimer laser angioplasty and conventional balloon dilation. A comparison of management outcome and predictor. *Eur Heart J* 1993;14:195–204.

17. Detre KM, Holubkov R, Kelsey S et al. One-year follow up results of the 1985–1986 National Heart, Lung, and Blood Institute's percutaneous transluminal coronary angioplasty registry. *Circulation* 1989;80:421–428.

18. Losordo DW, Rosenfield K, Pieczek A et al. How does angioplasty work? Serial analysis of human iliac arteries after percutaneous transluminal coronary angioplasty: a quantitative arteriographic analysis. *Circulation* 1988; 78:1323–1334.

19. Fischell TA, Derby G, Tse TM, Stadius ML. Coronary artery vasoconstriction routinely occurs after percutaneous transluminal coronary angioplasty: a quantitative arteriographic analysis. *Circulation* 1988;78:1323–1334.

20. Huber MS, Mooney JF, Madison J, Mooney MR. Use of a morphologic classification to predict clinical outcome after dissection from coronary angioplasty. *Am J Cardiol* 1991;68:467–471.

21. Honye J, Mahon DJ, Jain A et al. Morphologic effects of coronary balloon angioplasty in vivo assessed by intravascular ultrasound imaging. *Circulation* 1992;85: 1012–1025.

22. Davidson CJ, Sheikh KH, Kisslo KB et al. Intracoronary ultrasound evaluation of interventional technologies. *Am J Cardiol* 1991;68:1305–1309.

23. Mabin TA, Holmes DR, Smith HC et al. Intracoronary thrombus: role in coronary occlusion complicating percutaneous transluminal coronary angioplasty. *J Am Coll Cardiol* 1985;5:198–202.

24. Ellis SG, Roubin GS, King SB III et al. Angiographic and clinical predictors of acute closure after native vessel coronary angioplasty. *Circulation* 1988;77:327–329.

25. Myler RK, Shaw RE, Stertzer SH et al. Lesion morphology and coronary angioplasty: current experience and analysis. *J Am Coll Cardiol* 1992;19:1641–1652.

26. Ellis SG, Topol EJ. Results of percutaneous transluminal coronary angioplasty of high-risk angulated stenoses. *Am J Cardiol* 1990;66:932–937.

27. Schwartz L, Bourassa MG, Lesperance J et al. Aspirin and dipyridamole in the prevention of restenosis after percutaneous transluminal coronary angioplasty. *N Engl J Med* 1988;318:1714.

28. Lembo NJ, Black AJR, Roubin GS et al. Effect of pretreatment with aspirin versus aspirin plus dipyridamole on the frequency and type of acute complications of percutaneous transluminal coronary angioplasty. *Am J Cardiol* 1990;65:422–426.

29. Laskey MAL, Deutsch E, Hirshfeld JW, Kussmaul WG, Barnathan E, Laskey WK. Influence of heparin therapy on percutaneous transluminal coronary angioplasty outcome in patients with coronary arterial thrombus. *Am J Cardiol* 1990;65:179.

30. Narins CR, Hilegass WB Jr., Nelson CL et al. Relation between activated clotting time during angioplasty and abrupt closure. *Circulation* 1996;93:667–671.

31. Ogilby JD, Kopelman HA, Klein LW, Agarwal JB. Adequate heparinization during PTCA: assessment using activated clotting times. *Cathet Cardiovascular Diagn* 1989;18:306.

32. Ellis SG, Roubin GS, Wilentz J, Douglas JS, King SB. Effect of 18–24 hours heparin administration for prevention of restenosis after uncomplicated coronary angioplasty. *Am Heart J* 1989;127:777.

33. McGarry TF, Gottlieb RS, Morganroth J et al. The relationship of anticoagulation level and complications after successful percutaneous transluminal coronary angioplasty. *Am Heart J* 1992;123:1445.

34. The EPIC Investigators. Use of a monoclonal antibody directed against the platelet glycoprotein IIb/IIIa receptor in high-risk coronary angioplasty. The EPIC Investigation. *N Engl J Med* 1994;330:956–961.

35. The Epilog Investigators. Platelet glycoprotein IIb/IIIa receptor blockade and low-dose heparin during percutaneous coronary revascularization. *N Engl J Med* 1997; 336:1689–1696.

36. The EPISTENT Investigators. Randomised placebo-controlled and balloon angioplasty-controlled trial to assess safety of coronary stenting with use of platelet glycoprotein-IIb/IIIa blockade. *Lancet* 1998;352:87–92.

37. Roubin GS, Douglas JS, King SB et al. Influence of balloon size on initial success, acute complications, and restenosis after percutaneous transluminal coronary angioplasty. A prospective randomized study. *Circulation* 1988;78:557.

38. Nichols AB, Smith R, Berke AD, Shlofmitz RA, Powers ER: Importance of balloon size in coronary angioplasty. *J Am Coll Cardiol* 1989;13:1094.

39. Mooney MR, Mooney JF, Longe TF. Brandenburg RO. Effect of balloon material on coronary angioplasty. *Am Heart J* 1992;69:1481.

40. Tenaglia AN, Quigley PJ, Kereiakes DJ et al. Coronary angioplasty performed with gradual and prolonged inflation using a perfusion balloon catheter: procedural success and restenosis rate. *Am Heart J* 1992;124:585.

41. Banka VS, Kochar GS, Maniet AR, Voci G. Progressive coronary dilation: an angioplasty technique that creates controlled arterial injury and reduces complications. *Am Heart J* 1993;125:61.

42. Kern MJ, Eilen SD. Coronary vasospasm complicating PTCA. *Am Heart J* 1985;109:1098–1101.

43. Pomerantz RM, Kuntz RE, Diver DJ, Safian RD, Baim DS. Intracoronary verapamil for the treatment of distal microvascular coronary artery spasm following PTCA. *Cathet Cardiovasc Diagn* 1991;24:83–285.

44. Shieman G, Cohen BM, Kozina J et al. Intracoronary urokinase for intracoronary thrombus accumulation complicating percutaneous transluminal coronary angioplasty in acute ischemic syndromes. *Circulation* 1990;82:2052–2060.

45. Gulba DC, Caniel WG, Rudiger S et al. Role of thrombolysis and thrombin in patients with acute coronary occlusion during percutaneous transluminal coronary angioplasty. *J Am Coll Card* 1990;16:563–568.

46. Verna E, Repett S, Boscarini M, Onofri M, Qing LG, Binaghi G. Management of complicated coronary angioplasty by intracoronary urokinase and immediate reangioplasty. *Cathet Cardiovasc Diagn* 1990;19:116–122.

47. Ambrose JA, Almedia OD, Sharma SK et al., for the TAUSA Investigators. Adjunctive thrombolytic therapy during angioplasty for ischemic rest angina. Results of the TAUSA Trial. *Circulation* 1994;90:69–77.

48. Gold HK, Garabdian HD, Dinsmore RE. Restoration of coronary flow in myocardial infarction by intravenous chimeric 7E3 antibody without exogenous plasminogen activators: observations in animals and humans. *Circulation* 1997;95:1755–1759.

49. Muhlestein JB, Karagounis LA, Treehan S, Anderson JL. "Rescue" utilization of abciximab for the dissolution of coronary thrombus developing as a complication

of coronary angioplasty. *J Am Coll Cardiol* 1997;30: 1729–1734.

50. Marquis JR, Schwartz L, Aldridge H, Majid P, Henderson M, Matuschinsky E. Acute coronary artery occlusion during percutaneous transluminal coronary angioplasty treated by redilation of the occluded segment. *J Am Coll Cardiol* 1984;4:1268–1271.

51. Quigley PJ, Hinohara T, Phillips HR et al. Myocardial protection during coronary angioplasty with an autoperfusion balloon catheter in humans. *Circulation* 1988;78: 1128–1134.

52. van der Linden LP, Bakx ALM, Sedney MI, Buis B, Bruschke AVG. Prolonged dilation with an autoperfusion balloon catheter for refractory acute occlusion related to percutaneous transluminal coronary angioplasty. *J Am Coll Cardiol* 1993;22:1016–1023.

53. Leitschuh ML, Mills RM Jr, Jacobs AK, Ruocco NA Jr, LaRosa D, Faxon DP. Outcome after major dissection during coronary angioplasty using the perfusion balloon catheter. *Am J Cardiol* 1991;67:1056–1060.

54. Landau C, Jacobs AK, Currier JW, Leitschuh ML, Ryan TJ, Faxon DP. Long-term clinical follow-up of patients successfully treated with a perfusion balloon catheter for coronary angioplasty-induced dissections or abrupt closure. *Am J Cardiol* 1994;74:733–735.

55. Simonton CA, Kowalchuk GH, Austin WK. Preservation of regional myocardial function during coronary angioplasty with an autoperfusion balloon catheter: a case report. *Cathet Cardiovasc Diagn* 1991;22:28–34.

56. Campbell CA, Rezkall S, Kloner RA, Turi ZG. The autoperfusion balloon angioplasty catheter limits myocardial ischemia and necrosis during prolonged balloon inflations. *J Am Coll Cardiol* 1989;14:1045–1050.

57. Seggewiss H, Gleichmann U, Fassbender D, Vogt J, Mannebach H, Minami K. Therapy for acute vascular complications in percutaneous transluminal coronary angioplasty with the autoperfusion balloon catheter. *Eur Heart J* 1992;13:1649–1657.

58. de Munick ED, den Heijer P, van Dijk RB, Crijins HJGM, Twisk SP, Lip KI. Autoperfusion balloon versus stent for acute or threatened closure during percutaneous transluminal coronary angioplasty. *Am J Cardiol* 1994; 74:1002–1005.

59. McKeever LS, Marek JC, Kerwin PM, Cahill JM, Barr LA, Enger EL. Bail-out directional atherectomy for abrupt coronary artery occlusion following conventional angioplasty. *Cathet Cardiovasc Diagn* 1993;[Suppl 1]: 31–36.

60. Fischman DL, Savage MP, Leon MB et al. Effect of intracoronary stenting on intimal dissection after balloon angioplasty: results of quantitative and qualitative analysis. *J Am Coll Cardiol* 1991;18:1445–1451.

61. Hearn JA, King SB III, Douglas JS, Carlin SF, Lembo NJ, Ghazzal ZMB. Clinical and angiographic outcomes after coronary stenting for acute or threatened closure after percutaneous transluminal coronary angioplasty: initial results with a balloon expandable, stainless steel design. *Circulation* 1993;88:2086–2096.

62. George BS, Voorhoees WD III, Roubin GS et al. Multicenter investigation of coronary stenting to treat acute or threatened closure after percutaneous transluminal coronary angioplasty: clinical and angiographic outcomes. *J Am Coll Cardiol* 1993;22:135–143.

63. Dean LS, George CJ, Holmes DR Jr. et al. The use of the Gianturco-Roubin intracoronary stent: the New Approaches to Coronary Intervention (NACI) registry experience. *Am J Cardiol* 1997;80:89K–98K.

64. Schomig A, Kastrati A, Mudra H et al. Four-year experience with Palmaz-Schatz stenting in coronary angioplasty complicated by dissection with threatened or present vessel closure. *Circulation* 1994;90:2716–2724.

65. Fischman DL, Leon MB, Baim DS et al., for the Stent Restenosis Study Investigators. A randomized comparison of coronary-stent placement and balloon angioplasty in the treatment of coronary artery disease. *N Eng J Med* 1994;331:496–501.

66. Serruys PW, de Jaegere P, Kiemeneij F et al., for the BENESTENT Study Group. A comparison of balloon-expandable-stent implantation with balloon angioplasty in patients with coronary artery disease. *N Engl J Med* 1994;331:489–495.

67. Nakano Y, Nakagawa Y, Yokoi H et al. Initial and follow-up results of the ACS Multi-Link stent: a single center experience. *Cathet Cardiovasc Diagn* 1998;45: 368–374.

68. Murphy DA, Craver JM, Jones EL et al. Surgical management of acute myocardial ischemia following percutaneous transluminal coronary angioplasty: role of the intra-aortic balloon pump. *J Thorac Cardiovasc Surg* 1984;87:332–339.

69. Phillips SJ, Kongtahworn C, Zeff RH et al. Disrupted coronary artery caused by angioplasty: supportive and surgical considerations. *Ann Thorac Surg* 1989;47: 880–883.

70. Buffet P, Danchin N, Villemot JP et al. Early and long-term outcome after emergency coronary artery bypass surgery after failed coronary angioplasty. *Circulation* 1991;84[Suppl 3]:III-254–259.

71. Reul GJ, Cooley DA, Hallman GL et al. Coronary artery bypass for unsuccessful percutaneous transluminal coronary angioplasty. *J Thorac Cardiovasc Surg* 1984;88: 685–694.

72. Naunheim KS, Fiore AC, Fagan DC et al. Emergency coronary artery bypass grafting for failed angioplasty: risk factors and outcome. *Ann Thorac Surg* 1989;47: 816–823.

73. Lazar HL, Haan CK. Determinants of myocardial infarction following emergency grafting after failed coronary angioplasty. *Ann Thorac Surg* 1994;57:1295–1299.

28

Coronary Arterial Perforation: Prediction, Diagnosis, Management, and Prevention

Fengqi Liu, Raimund Erbel, Michael Haude, and Junbo Ge

Division of Internal Medicine, Department of Cardiology,
University-Gesamthochschule-Essen, D-45122 Essen, Germany

Acute coronary arterial perforation following coronary angioplasty can be life-threatening. Even 20 years after the introduction of percutaneous transluminal coronary angioplasty (PTCA) with numerous technical improvements of PTCA and many other devices, coronary perforation remains one of the most challenging events. Coronary artery perforation occurs in about 0.5% of PTCA cases (1–8). The new intravascular devices, such as laser, various atherectomy techniques, and stenting, have been proven more effective for gaining better lumen diameters, but have been reported to perforate coronary arteries more frequently (3–8). An understanding of the mechanisms of coronary perforation is essential for prevention, prompt diagnosis, and active management.

DEFINITION AND CLASSIFICATION

Coronary artery perforation is defined as a persistent extravascular collection of contrast medium beyond the vessel wall with well-defined tears (6–9). It is useful to classify coronary artery perforation (Table 28.1) taking into account morphological criteria.

Type I is a more common form of perforation which is limited to the media or adventitial layer of the vessel wall, producing a focal ulcerated crate and or mushroom appearance angiographically (Fig. 28.1). This is most commonly caused by guidewire or atherectomy devices that create a broad-based inlet into the sealed chan-

nel. The clinical course is usually benign, but type I perforation may result in delayed tamponade and therefore it requires careful clinical vigilance for 24 to 48 hours after intervention (10,11).

The distinguishing angiographic feature of a type II perforation is the limited extravasation, producing patchy blushing or staining within the myocardium or pericardium. The patient's situation is relatively stable and at low risk (12) (Fig. 28.2).

Type III perforation is described as persistent extravasation, with streaming of contrast across the lesion, representing a more serious complication. The clinical course is dependent on whether the perforation is directed into the pericardial space (type IIIA) (Fig. 28.3), an adjacent vascular structure, or ventricular cavity (type IIIB) (Fig. 28.4) (13–16). The clinical sequelae of type III perforation vary widely (Table 28.2) (17). The type IIIA perforation into the pericardium represents an urgent event and is almost uniformly associated with acute tamponade requiring emergency pericardiocentesis, often followed by surgery. Although the patients' situations may be stable in some type IIIB cases, perforation with fistula formation between the coronary artery and ventricles and cardiac veins may result in overt angina or reocclusion due to "steal" phenomenon, or congestive heart failure from left-to-right shunting (15).

Thus, the angiographic differentiation of coronary artery perforations serves to distinguish

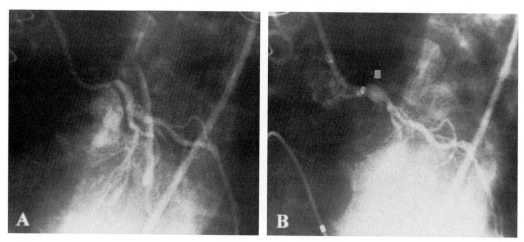

FIG. 28.1. Type I perforation (pseudoaneurysm) due to the "reaming effect" of multiple, angulated attack angles with rotational atherectomy of an ostial left main lesion. **A:** "Protected" left main lesion; retrograde filling of a graft to the first diagonal branch is seen. **B:** Resulting "overdone" aneurysmal dilation within the left main artery after rotational atherectomy. (From ref. 18, with permission.)

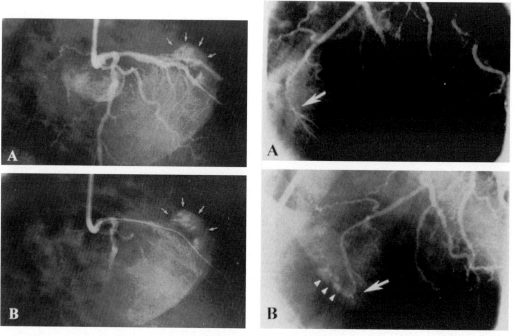

FIG. 28.2. Type II perforation after PTCA. **A:** Subepicardial deposit of contrast medium (arrows) in left anterior descending artery. **B:** After the runoff of the contrast medium the deposit can still be seen clearly (From ref. 12, with permission.)

FIG. 28.3. Type IIIA perforation. **A:** Initial angiogram illustrating the target lesion within the small left posterolateral of the circumflex artery. **B:** Resultant perforation into the pericardium after PTCA with oversized balloon. (From ref. 18, with permission.)

TABLE 28.1. *Angiographic classification of coronary artery perforation*

Classification	Description	Clinical sequelae
Type I	Extraluminal crater without extravation	Risk, if late (gradual) tamponade
Type II	Pericardial or myocardial blush without contrast jet extravation	Relatively stable; low risk
Type III	Extravation through frank (≥ 1 mm) perforation	High risk with increased morbidity and mortality
Subtype		
A	Directed toward the pericardium	Acute tamponade risk
		More benign course; possible fistula formation
B	Directed toward the myocardium	

From ref. 7 (modified), with permission.

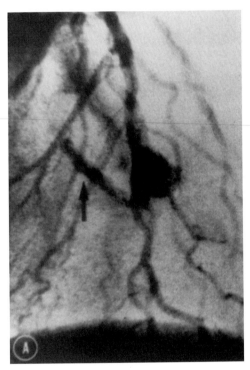 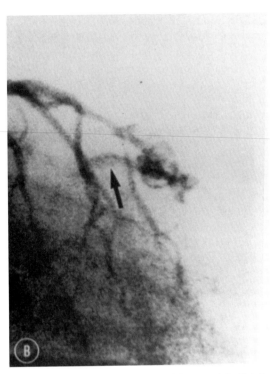

FIG. 28.4. Type IIIB perforation. False aneurysm and left anterior descending-right ventricle fistula (arrows) are seen in left (**A**) and right (**B**) anterior oblique views. (From ref. 16, with permission.)

TABLE 28.2. *Clinical outcome after coronary artery perforation*

Series	Devices	No. perforation (incidence %)	In-hospital complications (%)		
			CABG	AMI	Death
Ajluni (1994)	All (except stent)	35 (0.4)	37	26	5.6
Ellis (1994)	All (except stent)	62 (0.5)	24	26	0
Bittl (1993)	ELCA	23 (3.0)	34.7	4.3	9
Holmes (1994)	ELCA	36 (1.3)	36.1	16.7	4.8
Cohen (1994)	ROTA	22 (0.7)	41	45.5	9
Flood (1994)	All	19 (0.7)	33	5.6	5.9

ELCA, excimer laser coronary angioplasty; ROTA, rotational atherectomy; CABG, coronary artery bypass grafting; AMI, acute myocardial infarction. From ref. 17, with permission.

benign from far more serious lesions, and may predict late prognosis, such as type II perforation, whereas the natural history of type I lesions includes late tamponade. Type III perforation has a relatively high morbidity, mandating prompt recognition and management (18).

INCIDENCE OF CORONARY PERFORATION

The reported incidences of coronary artery perforation during intervention varies with different devices and different studies (Tables 28.3–28.6) (19–33). Conventional balloon angioplasty (PTCA) generally has a low rate of perforation. In a collection of over 20,000 cases of PTCA the incidence of perforation was about 0.1% (7,22,25,28). Excimer laser coronary angioplasty has a perforation rate of about 2%. Directional and rotational atherectomy is accompanied with perforation in about 0.5% to 2.0% of cases.

The introduction of high-pressure angioplasty for coronary stent implantation has reduced the rate of subacute thrombosis significantly. In the beginning, Colombo et. al. suggested not only to use high pressure but also to use larger balloons (34). This resulted in unexpected rate of coronary perforations in the first series of four in 359 patients (1.1%). Since that time other authors also observed coronary perforations and changed their technique to high-pressure only (Table 28.7). Particularly ratio of more than 1.3 between the balloon and coronary artery. Micrometer seem to be dangerous.

The use of high-pressure balloon angioplasty alone without stenting has not increased the number of coronary perforations, as reported by Hering et al. (37). Therefore it seems to be as if high-pressure stenting has a unique mechanism by which perforation can occur. Possibly the stent struts are perforating the vessel wall or a transection of the arterial wall occurs.

MECHANISMS OF PERFORATION AND STRATEGY FOR PREVENTION

Coronary angioplasty is invasive in nature and produces "reasonable" injury levels for thera-peutic purposes. But such an injury is difficult to be kept under "control." The tear of atheromatous intima may extend into media and adventitia. By a variety of mechanisms, vessel perforation results from an uncontrolled exaggeration of such injury, or as a direct result of the angioplastic devices (38). Coronary artery perforation has been reported with the use of all intravascular devices.

While the exaggerated injury-producing perforation remains largely unpredictable, an awareness of the clinical arena within which this event may occur can heighten the operator's vigilance and influence therapeutic response time. The risk of perforation begins with the very first step of an intracoronary intervention. From the moment of insertion of the guidewire, through its removal at the end of the intervention, careful attention to technique, coronary anatomy, and equipment selection is mandated to enhance procedural results and minimize perforation risk (18).

Guidewire Perforation

The perforation of a coronary artery may happen when the guidewire is advanced with too much force. The likelihood of vessel perforation is higher when stiffer wires are used. The availability of new design guidewires with altered transition-free corewire-to-tip properties has improved the ability to cross lesions within an angulated side branch using softer wires, thus avoiding the need of a stiffer wires. Nonetheless, a stiffer guidewire is often necessary to get through lesions such as an extremely angulated segment, or total occlusions. When using a stiffer wire, the operator should always maintain a high level of concentration to assure the wire remains intraluminal.

Coronary perforation can be reduced through a variety of mechanisms in the setting of a chronic total occlusion. First, use a stiffer wire only after failing to cross the lesion with a softer wire. Often the inability to cross a total occlusion relates largely not to the properties of the wire, but rather to inadequate guiding catheter backup. If a wire cannot be placed, switch to a catheter that provides better passive backup, such as an

TABLE 28.3. *Incidence of perforation after percutaneous coronary intervention*

Series	N	Perforation (%)						
		All devices	PTCA	DCA	ROTA	TEC	ELCA	Stent
Ajluni (1994)	8932	0.4	0.1	0.3	0	1.3	2.0	0
Ellis (1994)	12,900	0.5	0.1	0.7	1.3	2.1	1.9	—
Flood (1994)	2426	0.7	0.6	0.3	0.4	0	1.7	0.2
Lansky (1994)	708	2.0	—	3.2	—	2.0	1.7	1.1

PTCA, percutaneous transluminal coronary angioplasty; ELCA, excimer laser coronary angioplasty; DCA, directional coronary atherectomy; ROTA, rotational atherectomy; TEC, transluminal extraction endarterectomy catheter. From ref. 17, with permission.

TABLE 28.4. *Incidence of coronary artery perforation after PTCA*

Series	Patients (n)	Perforation (n)	Incidence (%)
Cowley (1984)	3079	3	0.1
Gonzalez-Santos (1985)	150	4	2.7
Jungbluth (1988)	1000	1	0.5
Greene (1991)	1214	1	0.1
Bittl (1992)	958	2	0.1
Nilsson (1993)	2478	3	0.1
Ellis (1994)	9080	14	0.1

TABLE 28.5. *Incidence of coronary artery perforation after ELCA*

Series	Patients (n)	Perforation (n)	Incidence (%)
Haase (1991)	1139	12	1.1
Holmes (1992)	2025	32	1.6
Bittl (1992)	764	23	3.0
Ghazzal (1992)	206	3.0	1.5
Ellis (1994)	900	17	1.9

TABLE 28.6. *Incidence of coronary artery perforation after DCA*

Series	Patients (n)	Perforation (n)	Incidence (%)
Vlietstra (1989)	480	1	0.2
Johnson (1992)	463	5	1.1
Vetter (1992)	1041	14	1.3
Ellis (1994)	1715	12	0.7

TABLE 28.7. *Incidence of coronary artery perforation after stent*

Series	Patients (n)	Perforation (n)	Incidence (%)
Flood (1994) (22)	2426	5	0.2
Colombo (1995) (34)	359	4	1.1
Fukutomi (1996) (35)	4779	67	1.4
Kasper (1997) (36)	13,722	15	0.1

Amplatz- or hockey-stick-curve catheter is recommended. Achieve active backup by deep seating or "Amplatzing" the guide catheter into the ostium of the artery to avoid the need for a stiffer wire. A softer guidewire can be supported or "rigidified" by advancing the balloon catheter around a proximal bend or to the tip of the wire (18). If crossing the target lesion does ultimately require a stiffer wire, the stiffer wire may be exchanged with a softer wire through the lumen of a balloon catheter or exchange catheter in order to prevent further risk of perforation to the distal segments.

Secondly, be sure that the wire remains within the vessel lumen to avoid perforation. If angioplasty is carried over a misdirected guidewire, type III perforation will occur. Observing the free movement of the distal bend of the wire can help to localize the wire within the distal vessel lumen. Injection of contrast may be necessary to confirm the wire position. This is especially important before advancing a balloon or other devices over the wire. It has been observed that a guidewire perforates the vessel wall because the wire is not fixed while introducing a balloon into the target lesion. A distal wire band may be helpful, too.

Using contralateral injection of contrast media can be helpful in visualizing the positioning of the guidewire within the lumen of the distal part of the coronary artery. This has been observed to be helpful when laser wires are used for recanalization, as suggested by Serruys et al. (39). In case of laser recanalization, the guidewires often leave the vessel lumen. Due to the nature of the occluded vessel, this is usually not accompanied by the risk of a cardiac tamponade (40). Because the search for the true way into the distal lumen is difficult, this side-effect is not called perforation.

The possibility of crossing an occluded vessel was significantly improved when new hydrophilic wires were introduced (Choice Extra Support Choice, Boston Scientific, Minneapolis, MN; Waterston; and Radifocus Guide M, Terumo Corp., Tokyo, Japan) (41). The wires are not only passing occluded or severely stenosed vessels but can also be pushed into the far end of a coronary artery. This very distal positioning of the guidewire must be avoided, because it increases the risk of perforation, as many operators have observed. Follow-up of patients in whom this hydrophilic wire has been used is important. It is also important to take into account the risk of late tamponade, which may occur when very small arteries have been perforated. The transition to very distal parts of the artery is particularly hazardous when the balloon is exchanged and the operator tries to keep the guidewire in position, and when the new balloon is advanced. Therefore, these hydrophilic wires should be used only in a special indication. If a floppy wire is present, it is helpful to exchange the extra support wire. Hydrophilic wires with flexible tips seem to be less dangerous.

An operator should not start angioplasty until convinced that the wire is within the lumen of the artery.

Balloon Induced Perforation

Balloon-associated perforation includes the following mechanisms: balloon oversizing and balloon rupture (Fig. 28.5). The risk of balloon rupture is directly related to the catheter design. Excessive inflation pressure and calcified lesions are the most common causes of balloon rupture. The rated and actual mean burst pressures are available and indicated for every balloon and usually run between 6 and 14 atm. Knowledge of balloon material characteristics and the specific rupture profile of the balloon is imperative to avoid coronary perforation following balloon rupture. Using the lowest pressure necessary to induce a significant change in the lesion diameter, or selection of a balloon that will allow a higher inflation pressure when a calcified or hard lesion is present, may minimize the risk of balloon-induced coronary perforation (18).

Balloon rupture, particularly in calcified lesions is not rare. Also, self-mounted stents can induce balloon damage leading to balloon rupture. This occurrence usually has no deleterious effects, because the contrast material is injected into the coronary artery lumen. If the balloon is attached to the vessel wall, however, a thin hole can lead to coronary vessel dissection and extravasation of contrast and blood. During the inflation of the balloon the patient has heavy chest

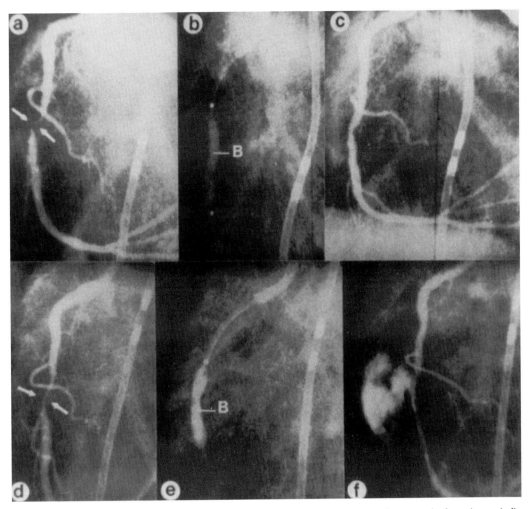

FIG. 28.5. Balloon oversizing induced perforation. Right coronary arteriograms before (**a** and **d**), during (**b** and **e**), and after (**c** and **f**) percutaneous transluminal coronary angioplasty (PTCA). **a:** A discrete severe narrowing is present (arrows). **b:** The stenosis was dilated by a 3-mm Grüntzig balloon (**B**) catheter. **c:** Mild residual narrowing remained after the first PTCA procedure. **d:** The previous area was again severely narrowed (arrows) 3 months after the first PTCA procedure. **e:** The narrowing was dilated by a 3.7 mm balloon (**B**) catheter. **f:** Arteriography after PTCA showed leakage of contrast material into the epicardial tissues. The diameter of the inflated balloon (*e*) is larger than that of the pacing catheter and thus exceeds the diameter of the nonstenotic arterial lumen (From ref. 13, with permission.)

pain which persists after balloon deflation. Visibility of calcium by fluoroscopy should increase the operator's awareness of this possible complication.

Device Oversizing

Oversizing devices to the diameter of the target vessel substantially increases the risk of coronary artery perforation (7,20). Oversized balloons or other devices can cause overstretching, deep tearing, and disruption of the vessel wall. Device-to-artery ratio ($\geq$1.2 for balloon, and $\geq$0.8 for other new devices) are associated with higher a frequency of coronary perforation. Carefully matching the device size and vessel diameter can generally help to avoid this pitfall. Sometimes it is difficult to determine the normal vessel diameter in a diffuse lesion or a total occlusion. Information from intravascular ultrasound imaging is very helpful in defining vessel dimensions in such a situation. Catheters with both imaging and therapeutic capability have the potential to enhance the efficacy and safety of coronary intervention (42).

A properly sized, compliant balloon may become oversized when inflation pressure is increased beyond nominal pressure. Conservative balloon sizing, attention to the balloon compliance characteristics, and frequent comparison of the inflating balloon size to the vessel size can minimize the risk of perforation. On-line quantitative coronary angiography may also be helpful.

High-risk lesions, such as tight, diffuse, bifurcation, or angulated lesions, or total occlusion, may be best approached beginning with a smaller device size and a gradual, stepwise serial increase in subsequent device sizes, or a gradual increment of pressure during balloon inflation. A balloon-to-artery ratio of 1.0 for PTCA, and device-to-artery ratio of 0.5–0.6 for laser and rotational atherectomy devices are recommended to reduce the possibility of perforation (17). When laser, rotational atherectomy, or transluminal extraction catheters are used, it may be prudent to achieve further lumen enlargement by adjunctive balloon dilation rather than increasing device size.

Other Mechanisms

New interventional devices that alter the integrity of the vessel structure may also lead to perforation by tissue removal (directional atherectomy), pulverization (rotational atherectomy), or ablation (laser). These new technologies afford new mechanisms of vessel perforation related to direct vessel-cutting injury, leading more often to more severe (type III) perforation. Studies have indicated higher incidences of coronary perforation with these new devices than with conventional balloon catheter (7). Directional atherectomy devices cut into adventitia in up to 30% of the cases (43,44), and an oblique or angulated cut may increase the likelihood of even deeper cutting. For example, aortoostial lesions or angulated bifurcation lesions expose a fold within the cutting window. A perforation can be caused when the cutting across the apex of the fold is performed.

Ellis and coworkers have defined predictors of perforation, including stenosis angulation, proximal tortuosity, calcified lesion, and small initial lumen (45). In face of the danger of coronary perforation, the concept of "the bigger the better" may be accepted with caution. Special attention should be paid to the above-mentioned high-risk lesions.

On the other hand, the high-speed rotational atherectomy device induces vessel perforation more frequently along the outer curve of a bend of the coronary artery (43). Assuring coaxial positioning of the device with respect to the target vessel may minimize this cutting in angulated passages. Careful navigation of any lesions extending around a bend can also reduce the risk of perforation. Any strong push may induce a Dotter effect, particularly with larger burr sizes. In this situation, excessively high temperatures can result from reduced lubrication and increased wall contact.

The guidewire of the rotational coronary angioplasty system is a monofilament steal wire with a flexible tip. It is important to use the brake on the housing of the Rotablator system (Heart Technologies Inc., Bellevue, WA) to avoid wire spinning during activation of the pneumatic turbine. If the brake is opened, the wire has to be stationary when the system is advanced. Particularly dangerous are wires that have only a very short flexible tip. The use of a 2- or 3-cm floppy end is helpful to avoid vessel wall perforation.

Laser angioplasty devices vaporize atheromatous plaque by direct thermal injury or by breaking molecular bonds. Maintaining a coaxial angle of attack and keeping the laser catheter within the center of the vessel lumen can reduce the risk of ablation of normal vessel wall. Laser energy of proper wavelengths may be absorbed preferentially by atheroma as opposed to frequencies within the natural absorption spectrum of normal vessel wall, and thus may minimize the damage of normal wall and the perforation risk (9).

CLINICAL FEATURES AND DIAGNOSIS

The patient's prognosis depends on rapid diagnosis and active treatment. It is of great importance to be able to recognize the clinical characteristics of acute arterial perforation.

Symptoms

Depending on history, location of stenosis, collateral supply, devices, and techniques employed, symptoms after coronary perforation vary. Patients complain of chest pain of various severity (from dull to moderate and severe) and related anxiety, dizziness, nausea, and vomiting. In some cases the patients feel no pain at all. An injection of contrast medium just before further procedures is considered important in avoiding enlargement of an existing perforation.

Angiographic Characteristics

Angiography is the most important and decisive method in the recognition of acute coronary perforation (see "Definition and Classification"). The first angiographic sign is extravasation of contrast material outside of the vessel wall. In some cases localized subepicardial hematoma develops following perforation (type I). The extravasation hematoma is limited around the broken artery and sometimes may cause acute myocardial ischemia by compressing the vessel. In other cases contrast may cause staining within the myocardium or pericardium (type II). In more severe cases (type IIIA) a free leakage of contrast medium into the pericardial space, that frequently leads to cardiac tamponade, can be detected by angiography. There may be a formation of fistula between the coronary artery and ventricular cavity (type IIIB).

The ruptured vessel wall can be visualized by intravascular ultrasound, but this spatial orientation is sometimes limited. Most important is the diagnosis of extramural hematoma leading to vessel wall compression, which can be detected by angiography only indirectly (46,47). By angiography, distal coronary spasm is usually suggested as the mechanism of luminal narrowing after angioplasty in the distal vessel segment.

Injection of nitroglycerin is ineffective in this situation and may lead to further luminal narrowing. Only additional stenting in the distal vessel segment can stop the progression of luminal narrowing (47).

Hemodynamical Changes

Patients hemodynamics may be stable or may change drastically after coronary perforation. When tamponade develops, heart rate increases and systolic arterial pressure falls, while the central venous pressure increases. Most often the initial event is a drop in heart rate and blood pressure, accompanying the patient's new onset of chest pain and anxiety. Cardiac arrest may follow. On the other hand, in benign cases the perforation is small and not complicated by tamponade or myocardial ischemia.

Echocardiographic Signs

Echocardiography should be performed at the first sign of perforation, if possible. Echocardiography has great value in the diagnosis and management of patients with perforation, especially in the presence of suspected pericardial hemorrhage and cardiac tamponade. The right ventricular and atrial free wall collapse in tamponade during diastole. This abnormal appearance can be detected even before major changes in systemic blood pressure and disappears after pericardiocentesis. That means that echocardiographic signs of tamponade are early findings preceding overt clinical signs of tamponade, an early warning that may prompt the decision to initiate therapy before the deterioration of hemodynamics. It is important to take into account that in case of thrombosis of the blood in the pericardial space, the typical echo-free space may not be present. Hemodynamics are helpful in this situation.

Electrocardiographic Signs

In acute coronary perforation, electrocardiographic changes are mainly associated with myocardial ischemia (e.g., ST-segment elevation or arrhythmia) but not exclusively.

The diagnosis of acute coronary arterial perforation can be readily established through angiography and echocardiography, together with a new chest pain, hemodynamic changes, and ECG abnormality. However, sometimes perforation and subsequent pericardial tamponade may not occur until a few hours or days later after angioplasty (10,11). It is recommended that patients in whom a deep dissection is suspected should be observed closely in coronary intensive care units. Repeat angiography is useful in the diagnosis of delayed perforation. More important, however, is monitoring of heart rate, blood pressure, right atrial and pulmonary pressure, and cardiac output. Increase in right atrial pressure with constant or reduced pulmonary pressure should call for echocardiography to rule out any development of pericardial effusion.

MANAGEMENT OF PERFORATION AND THE CLINICAL SEQUELAE

Coronary artery perforation may be managed nonoperatively or operatively. The decision is made according to the clinical condition. Generally, patients with localized perforation or perforation caused by guidewires are usually stable and may be treated conservatively. In contrast, perforation caused by balloon, atherectomy devices, or laser may result in hemopericardium and hemodynamic collapse, which mandates immediate intervention. Regardless of the causes, initial management should focus on sealing the perforation nonoperatively and stabilizing the patient hemodynamically. In any type of coronary perforation, cardiac surgeons should be notified immediately and the operating room prepared for possible emergency surgery.

Nonoperative Management

Prolonged Balloon Inflation or Implantation of Graft Stent

To stabilize a patient, it is important to use the first available balloon, cross the perforation side, and inflate the balloon to block the further extravasation of blood. The most important problem with this approach is the development of myocardial ischemia. If perforation is induced by a guidewire, a small balloon pushed to the distal end of the coronary artery can be inflated with low pressure and can block further extravasation of blood. Particularly in recanalized coronary arteries, the blocking of the artery by a balloon will not induce ischemia.

Once the patient is stabilized and/or ischemia develops, the balloon should be exchanged with a coronary perfusion catheter. Erbel et al. developed the coronary perfusion catheter to improve the ischemia tolerance of the heart (48). They have suggested the use of such catheters for treatment of coronary perforation. Subsequently, perfusion catheters have been successfully used for the treatment of perforation and large dissections. A perfusion balloon should be immediately positioned at the site of contrast extravasation and inflated to 2–6 atm for at least 10 minutes (17). If sealing is not complete, further low-pressure inflation is performed for a longer time period. No more heparin should be given. In order to get an effective autoperfusion via the balloon, the systemic pressure has to be in the range of 80–120 mm Hg. The higher the pressure, the better the perfusion. Thus, fluid has to be given, not only to prevent tamponade but also to increase flow in the autoperfusion catheter.

If the combination of wall wrapping and autoperfusion balloon is not effective and extravasation continues after balloon deflation, stent implantation can be done (if it was not done previously). It was demonstrated in our laboratory that such stent implantation can stop the blood extravasation. Rarely is stent-in-stent implantation necessary. More recently, stents covered with vein allografts or polytetrafluoroethylene (PTFE) membrane have been successfully used to stop bleeding after coronary perforation (49). This new, membrane-covered Graft-Jostent (Jomed Co., Germany) looks promising as an easy and rapid approach to the management of perforation (Fig. 28.6). Because the Graft Jostent is not as easily crimped as a conventional stent, high pressure is needed to inflate the stent completely. High-pressure balloons, such as the Activa noncomplaint balloon (Boston Scientific, USA), are used. This stent consists of an inner

29

Treatment of Unprotected Left Main Stenoses

Stephen G. Ellis

Sones Cardiac Catheterization Laboratories, Department of Cardiology,
The Cleveland Clinic Foundation, Cleveland, Ohio 44195-5066; Department of Medicine,
Ohio State University, Columbus, Ohio 43210

OVERVIEW

Coronary artery bypass surgery remains the accepted therapy for patients with unprotected left main coronary stenoses, based upon demonstrated benefit relative to medical therapy and due to the 5%–15% risk of sudden cardiac death in the first year after percutaneous treatment in this setting (1). However, in certain circumstances percutaneous treatment may be quite appropriate. These situations generally fall into two categories: (a) surgically high-risk or inoperable patients; and (b) the low-risk patient with good ventricular function who strongly desires not to have bypass surgery.

We believe that it has been convincingly demonstrated that stenting and directional atherectomy are superior to balloon angioplasty in the unprotected left main setting (1–3). The choice between stenting and directional atherectomy should be made based upon operator experience and the anatomy to be treated. The use of stents to treat distal bifurcation lesions, provided both the left anterior descending coronary artery (LAD) and circumflex need to be treated, is technically challenging and may be associated with a higher risk of late complications. Therefore, we believe directional atherectomy is preferred in this setting. Conversely, with ostial and midshaft, left main lesions, stenting is generally preferred because it is quicker and simpler. Technical details and clinical results of stenting and directional atherectomy in this setting are shown

in Table 29.1. Patients are divided into those with ≥40% and <40% left ventricular ejection fraction because left ventricular function appears to greatly influence the risk of cardiac death in the event of restenosis (1,4).

It should be understood of course, that these procedures should be performed only by operators and laboratories that have extensive experience in performing complex coronary procedures, and after full disclosure of the risks and benefits to the patient.

HEMODYNAMIC SUPPORT

Patients with well preserved left ventricular function and a widely patent right coronary artery can tolerate relatively brief (<1–2 minutes) periods of left main coronary ischemia remarkably well. It is generally prudent however, to place an intraaortic balloon pump if there is any question about the patient's capacity to tolerate ischemia. Although not absolutely necessary, placement of a Swan-Ganz catheter to monitor pulmonary pressures is often useful.

For patients with severely impaired left ventricular function, or if a complex procedure with prolonged ischemia in the setting of an occluded right coronary artery is anticipated, use of percutaneous cardiopulmonary support should be considered.

GENERAL CONSIDERATIONS

Generally speaking, the principles guiding the technical approach in this setting are that it must

TABLE 29.1. *ULTIMA registry data*

Lesion location	Non-distal	Non-distal	Distal	Distal	Distal	Distal
Device	stent	stent	DCA	DCA	stent	stent
LVEF (%)	≥40	<40	≥40	<40	≥40	<40
n	51	11	26	6	40	18
Age (yrs)	60 ± 14	64 ± 17	65 ± 10	77 ± 10	66 ± 11	68 ± 17
Male (%)	51	64	81	83	70	67
Rest/progressive angina (%)	29	55	27	17	43	50
Inoperable (%)	6	27	0	17	13	33
RCA occluded (%)	7	27	0	0	3	0
IABP (%)	14	46	69	100	23	44
% stenosis pre (QCA)	64 ± 13	63 ± 14	64 ± 13	67 ± 18	65 ± 14	77 ± 9
% stenosis post (QCA)	2 ± 11	12 ± 13	13 ± 12	19 ± 19	7 ± 12	17 ± 15
Reference diameter (mm)	4.0 ± 0.7	4.2 ± 0.9	3.9 ± 0.7	4.0 ± 0.7	4.2 ± 0.8	4.3 ± 0.8
# of stents	1.01	1.73	—	—	1.23	1.17
In-hospital:						
Cardiac death (%)	0	18	0	33	2.5	5.6
Non-cardiac death (%)	2.0	0	0	0	0	5.6
Emerg CABG (%)	0	0	0	0	0	0
Non-fatal QMI (%)	0	11	0	0	0	0
After discharge						
Restenosis (%)	21	33	20	67	5	57
Death ≤1 yr (%)	7	38	8	0	8	2

DCA, directional coronary atherectomy; IABP, intraaortic balloon pump; LVEF, left ventricular ejection fraction; QCA, quantitative coronary angiography; QMI, Q–wave-myocardial infarction; RCA, right coronary artery.

minimize the duration of ischemia and provide a nearly perfect anatomic result. A guide catheter should be chosen to provide very adequate support and yet not occlude the coronary ostium. The guidewire must be stiff enough to provide adequate support. The angiographic presence of moderate or extensive calcium should prompt consideration of rotational atherectomy, with strong consideration of technical aspects to minimize the production of the ''slow flow'' state. Some experienced operators prefer to use intravascular ultrasound (IVUS) to enhance the likelihood of obtaining a technically superb result.

It should go without saying that an angiographic ''working view'' must be found that shows the relevant anatomic details in a nonforeshortened view. For ostial lesions, particular attention must be paid to radiographic markers providing clues to the actual location of the ostium. A relevant speck of calcium appropriately located is probably the best marker.

Often when the left main is diffusely narrowed it is difficult to decide what to use for a reference diameter. Bear in mind the normal left main artery averages 5 mm in diameter and tapers about 20% at its distal aspect. Therefore, under most circumstances a 4.0-mm result should be the absolute minimum accepted.

To minimize the risk of complications, strong consideration should be given to the use of glycoprotein IIb/IIIa inhibitors, although in the ULTIMA registry (1) their usage was infrequent.

TECHNICAL ASPECTS OF STENTING

A stent should be chosen that provides excellent radial support. Coil stents should be avoided. Although not absolutely necessary, a somewhat radiopaque stent is preferable so that it may be placed most precisely. Although any of several stents may be used, we and others have found the Johnson & Johnson (Warren, NJ) Crown and biliary stents to be quite acceptable if the approach is straightforward. For these lesions, and especially more complicated lesions, the AVE GFX (Arterial Vascular Engineering, Division of Medtronic, Santa Rosa, CA) and the NIR Royale (Scimed, Maple Grove, MN) are ideal, if of appropriate length. The length of the stent must be chosen carefully for optimal positioning. A stent placed too far into the aorta may prevent access in the future, and one placed too distally may make access to the circumflex or LAD difficult.

Pretreatment of the lesion with balloon dilatation or rotational atherectomy is mandatory to prevent the operator from having to struggle with stent delivery. Balloon dilatation and burring time should be kept to a minimum.

Stent delivery in the unprotected left main stenosis is similar to stenting of other sites, other than the need to be especially careful about location and to keep ischemia brief. There must be no question about the adequacy of deployment—to ensure adequate deployment, use high-pressure inflation, IVUS, or both.

Another somewhat unique aspect of stenting in the unprotected left main is dealing with the distal bifurcation, if it is diseased. Most operators in the ULTIMA registry used a single stent in this setting, typically placing it into the proximal LAD and "jailing" the left circumflex. On three occasions the circumflex closed, producing an infarct, one of which was fatal. However, the "T" or "Y" stent approach remains rather awkward, certainly increases the duration of ischemia, and may predispose to restenosis. Therefore, the author prefers either to use directional atherectomy alone or in combination with stenting (treating the smaller of the LAD or circumflex with directional atherectomy if possible), when treating a distal bifurcation lesion in the unprotected left main setting.

TECHNICAL ASPECTS OF DIRECTIONAL ATHERECTOMY

Given the declining use of directional atherectomy, the author has some reservations about recommending directional atherectomy in the unprotected left main setting. The operator should be extremely experienced with this technique before entertaining the idea of using it for this problem.

Guide catheter choice is extremely important. Although newer cutters will fit through a 9 Fr guide catheter, the author prefers 10 Fr guide catheters for stability and support. He has found that advancing the cutter out of a 9 Fr guide catheter typically opens the curve and deflects the guide catheter inferiorly. Clearly, the guide catheter must fit atraumatically and coaxially

with the left main (although some upward angulation is allowed).

Guidewire choice is also important. Generally firm or extra support wires are preferred for stability and easing the passage of the cutter. Care should be taken that the wire can be placed into a position distally in the coronary without trauma.

Due to the need to minimize the duration of ischemia, the initial use of a 6 Fr cutter is often appropriate. During the first series of cuts only a few should be made before withdrawing the cutter. Cuts can then be made circumferentially. The cutter can then be up sized to a 7 Fr GTO (Guidant Inc. Santa Clara, CA) or 7 Fr Graft cutter as determined by the apparent normal vessel diameter.

FOLLOW-UP

Proper arrangements of the patient follow-up in the unprotected left main setting are extremely important. The risk of sudden cardiac death must not be underestimated. Patients should be instructed to return to their interventional cardiologist immediately if they begin to experience fatigue, shortness of breath, or angina. Even without these symptoms they should have repeat angiography at 2 to 3 months after treatment. Patients with depressed left ventricular function should be watched especially carefully, because they appear to be at greatest risk. Follow-up angiography at 6 months is also advisable. The risk of sudden death appears to abate after 9 to 12 months.

REFERENCES

1. Ellis SG, Tamai H, Nobuyoshi M et al. Contemporary percutaneous treatment of unprotected left main coronary stenoses—initial results from a multicenter registry analysis 1994–96. *Circulation* 1997;96:3867–3872.
2. O'Keefe JH, Hartzler GO, Rutherford BD et al. Left main coronary angioplasty: early and late results of 127 acute and elective procedures. *Am J Cardiol* 1989;64:144–147.
3. Kosuga K, Tamai H, Kawashima A et al. Initial and long-term results of elective angioplasty in unprotected left main coronary artery. *J Am Coll Cardiol* 1998;31:101A.
4. Ellis S, Nobuyoshi M, Tamai H, Plokker T, Park S-J, Suzuki T. Correlates of cardiac death early after hospital discharge in patients who have undergone percutaneous treatment of unprotected left main stenoses—what are the lessons? *J Am Coll Cardiol* 1998;31:214A.

30

Diabetes and Coronary Heart Disease

Steven P. Marso

Department of Cardiology, The Cleveland Clinic Foundation, Cleveland, Ohio 44195-5066

Diabetes mellitus is a common chronic disease affecting 8% of the adult world population. Its prevalence in the United States has increased over the past 40 years and continues to do so, especially in older patients. This has lead to an increasing financial burden and medical resource utilization such that over 15% of the US healthcare budget is now spent on the care of diabetic patients (1). Diabetes, whether type I or II, is a potent risk factor for atherosclerotic vascular disease and cardiovascular mortality continues to be the leading cause of death for diabetics. Although there have been great strides in the field of cardiovascular medicine in recent years, little progress has been made in narrowing the gap between diabetic and nondiabetic cardiovascular outcomes.

Diabetes is a spectrum ranging from absolute insulin deficiency and lean body mass to insulin resistance and obesity. However, diabetes has traditionally been categorized into two types. Type I diabetes is relatively uncommon, affecting predominantly Northern Europeans. It strikes in childhood and is characterized by an autoimmune destruction of the pancreatic beta cells, resulting in an absolute insulin deficiency. Type II or non-insulin-dependent diabetes accounts for greater than 90% of all cases. It affects men and women equally and occurs in patients who are usually overweight, older than 40 years of age, and are often hypertensive. The hallmark for type II diabetes is marked insulin resistance.

INSULIN RESISTANCE

Insulin resistance (IR) is a state in which increasing endogenous insulin levels are required to maintain euglycemia. This precedes the onset of overt hyperglycemia by many years (Fig. 30.1). Beta cells of the pancreas eventually fail to produce adequate levels of circulating insulin, leading to increasing glucose levels, overt diabetes, and the need for therapeutic intervention. Many factors contribute to the development of IR, including increasing age, genetics, and obesity. IR is involved in the development of dyslipidemia and atherosclerosis, and antedates the development of hypertension. In fact, lean normotensive offspring of patients with hypertension have markedly decreased insulin sensitivity. The IR state is an important marker for cardiovascular risk and may provide important prognostic information.

GLYCEMIC CONTROL

There are convincing data from the Diabetes Control and Complications Trial (DCCT) that improved glycemic control is associated with decreased rates of microvascular complications such as retinopathy, nephropathy, and neuropathy for type I diabetes (2). Data from the United Kingdom Diabetes Prospective Diabetes Study (UKPDS 33) confirmed that intensive treatment of type II diabetes was associated with a decrease in microvascular complications (3). Although there was a trend for fewer nonfatal myocardial infarctions in the intensively treated group in UKPDS 33, there was not an improved survival for this group of patients.

COMPLICATIONS FROM DIABETES

Diabetes leads to retinopathy, nephropathy, neuropathy (microvascular complications), cor-

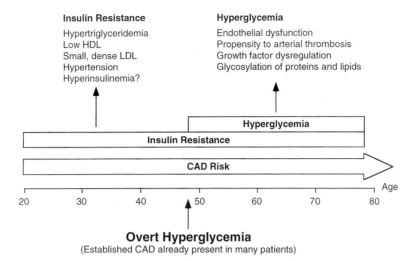

FIG. 30.1. Schematic representation of the proatherogenic characteristics of insulin resistance. Insulin resistance precedes the development of overt hyperglycemia by many years. The insulin-resistant state and hyperglycemia act in concert to promote atherosclerosis. (Adopted with permission from Topol EJ, Aronson D, Rayfield EJ. *Diabetes.* Philadelphia: Lippincott, Williams & Wilkins, 1998: [Ch.7]187).

onary heart disease (CHD), peripheral, and cerebrovascular disease (macrovascular complications). As a result, diabetes is associated with premature morbidity and mortality in millions of patients worldwide. Diabetic nephropathy is present in 30% to 40% of type I and 10% of type II patients and is the leading cause of end-stage renal disease (ESRD) in the United States. There is now compelling data linking the development of diabetic nephropathy to both fatal and nonfatal cardiovascular events. Microalbuminuria, defined as 30 to 250 mg of proteinuria in 24 hours, is an important identifier of early nephropathy and of those patients at increased risk for cardiovascular events including death. Treatment with angiotensin-converting enzyme (ACE) inhibitors and aggressive glycemic control slows the progression of proteinuria and decreases the development of ESRD.

CORONARY HEART DISEASE AND DIABETES

Diabetes is a potent risk factor for the development of atherosclerotic heart disease for both men and women. During the latency period, there is a prolonged period of glucose intoler-

ance, insulin resistance, and atherogenic milieu, increasing the risk of developing CHD (Fig. 30.1). Data from the multi-national WHO survey demonstrated a prevalence of CHD in diabetics to be from 26% to 35% with higher rates in women and older patients. Importantly, diabetes amplifies known coronary risk factors and greatly increases the cardiac risk for women. As a result, diabetes essentially erases the cardioprotective effects of being female.

Although diabetes leads to a spectrum of vascular complications, fatal events are 70 times more likely from cardiovascular events compared with other vascular complications (4). In fact, complications from cardiovascular disease accounts for over 80% all deaths in diabetic patients (1). The annual mortality rate for diabetic patients is 5.4%, nearly twice that of nondiabetics, leading to a decreased life expectancy of 5 to 10 years. The risk of death from coronary heart disease is increased nearly twofold for diabetic women compared with diabetic men (5).

DIABETES AND ASSOCIATED CO-MORBIDITIES

During a 7-year follow-up period, Haffner et al. recently demonstrated the rate of a first-time myocardial infarction for diabetics was nearly six times greater compared with nondiabetics (20.2% versus 3.5%). The reinfarction rate for diabetics was also higher compared with nondiabetics (45% versus 18.8%) (6). Given the increased early hazard for a first-time infarction for diabetics (a rate that parallels the reinfarction rate for nondiabetics), aggressive medical therapy including antiplatelet and lipid lowering agents in this cohort of patients seems warranted. Daily aspirin therapy may be efficacious in diabetics without known CHD. This position is also supported by the American Diabetes Association's recent position statement. Additionally, aggressive lipid management with a target LDL level <100 mg/dL may also confer benefit for this group of diabetics.

In addition to the potent atherogenic effects of diabetes mellitus, patients with type II diabetes also have a higher cardiac risk profile than nondiabetics. In fact, diabetes as a lone risk factor only accounts for half of the increased mortality seen in diabetic patients. Diabetics in the Framingham Study were twice as likely to have additional coronary risk factors compared with nondiabetics. The observations seen in MRFIT, that additional risk factors added additional (perhaps multiplicative) risk, are very important (Fig. 30.2). Men with lone diabetes had an absolute risk of CHD death of 25 per 10,000 patient years. This increased to 47 per 10,000 with the addition of one risk factor and to 78 per 10,000 person years with three additional risk factors (7). Thus, diabetics with increasing number of

risk factors represent a unique group with escalating cardiovascular risk.

DIABETIC DYSLIPIDEMIA

Although there are many metabolic abnormalities linked with diabetes that result in abnormal lipoprotein levels, the level of glycemic control is the key factor for lipid levels in type I diabetes. Lipid levels in type II diabetes are dependent on a complex relationship between hyperglycemia and insulin resistance. The lipoprotein profile in type II diabetes is typified by a 50% to 100% increase in triglyceride levels, normal to modestly elevated LDL levels, and 25% to 30% reduction in HDL. Overproduction, when coupled with inadequate lipoprotein lipase activity, leads to increased serum levels of LDL. LDL levels are usually normal in diabetic patients under adequate glycemic control. However, the LDL particle is more atherogenic given its propensity for glycosylation and oxidation. Whether an elevated serum triglyceride levels is an independent risk factor for coronary artery disease (CAD) in the nondiabetic population is controversial. There is increasing evidence from prospective studies that an elevated triglyceride level is a risk factor for CAD in diabetic patients. However, there are no data to suggest that reduction of serum triglycerides in isolation improves cardiovascular outcome. Low HDL levels in diabetics are tightly linked with CAD risk.

An initial nonpharmacologic approach to control lipids is warranted in diabetics. The guide-

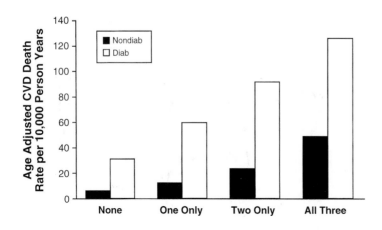

FIG. 30.2. Age-adjusted CHD death rates by the presence of number of risk factors for men screened for MRFIT, with and without diabetes at baseline. Risk factors included hypertension, hyperlipidemia and cigarette smoking. (Adopted with permission from ref. 7.)

lines from the American Diabetes Association are similar to NCEP with the exception that the ADA emphasizes the importance of triglycerides. This includes weight loss, adapting to a low-fat diet, physical exercise, and improved glycemic control. Intensive insulin therapy in type I diabetes results in a decreased microvascular complication rate and normalization of lipoprotein abnormalities. Improved glycemic control, irrespective of mode, improves, but not necessarily normalizes, the lipoprotein abnormalities in type II diabetes. A 20% to 40% reduction in triglycerides can be expected with optimal glucose control. If, after 6 months, nonpharmacologic treatment and optimal glucose control fails to result in improved lipid levels (target LDL level <100mg/dL), antilipid drug therapy is warranted. HMG CoA reductase inhibitors are the first-line agents in diabetic patients with elevated LDL cholesterol. They generally reduce LDL by 30%, triglycerides by 10% to 20%, and have little effect on HDL. Importantly, they do not adversely alter glycemic control. The 4S trial demonstrated a marked reduction in 6-year CHD event rates for diabetics receiving simvastatin compared with placebo (Fig. 30.3) (8). Fibric-acid derivatives (gemfibrozil) and bile-acid resins markedly decrease serum triglyceride levels. Nicotinic acid markedly reduces TG levels, modestly reduces LDL, likely increases HDL, and often worsens glycemic control.

ACUTE CORONARY SYNDROMES AND DIABETES MELLITUS

Although the prevalence of diabetes is 8% in the adult population, nearly 20–30% of patients presenting with acute coronary syndromes are diabetic and they account for over 50% of all cardiovascular mortality. The natural history of diabetic patients, following acute myocardial infarction, was well documented in the prefibrinolytic era. The in-hospital mortality rate was 1.5 to 2 times greater in diabetics. The excess in-hospital mortality is likely related to the increased incidence of congestive heart failure, multivessel disease, and associated comorbidities in this group of patients. Similarly, diabetics seem to have increased rates of reinfarction, infarct extension, and recurrent ischemia compared with nondiabetics. There is no convincing evidence that diabetic patients have larger myocardial infarctions or increased incidence of fatal ventricular arrhythmias.

Diabetic patients likely present with a higher incidence of subclinical cardiomyopathy than do nondiabetics, which likely results in increased

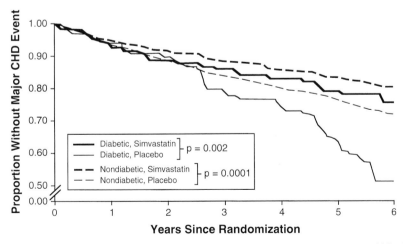

FIG. 30.3. Kaplan-Meier event free survival for diabetic and nondiabetic patients within the 4S trial. (Adopted with permission from Pyorala K, Pedersen T, Kjekshus J, et al., for the 4S Group. Cholesterol lowering with simvastatin improves progress of diabetic patients with coronary heart disease. A subgroup analysis of the Scandinavian Simvastatin Survival Study. *Diabetes Care* 1997;20[4]:68).

short-term mortality following an acute myocardial infarction. Data from the GUSTO and TAMI investigators suggest that diabetics have a decreased ejection fraction and decreased compensatory response of the noninfarcted LV segments compared with nondiabetics (9,10). In addition to left ventricular systolic abnormalities, diastolic dysfunction occurs in 27% to 69% of asymptomatic diabetic patients. Furthermore, diabetic patients have decreased coronary flow reserve when compared to nondiabetics. Diabetics with microvascular complications have been shown to have a further reduction in coronary flow reserve (11). The abnormalities of endothelium-dependent coronary vasodilation is likely due to multiple factors including hyperglycemia, increased generation of free radicals, and the presence of advanced glycosylation end products which deactivate nitric oxide. All of these likely contribute to the decreased contractile reserve seen in the diabetic population.

PHARMACOLOGIC TREATMENT FOR ACUTE MYOCARDIAL INFARCTION

Diabetics derive mortality benefit from fibrinolytic therapy following an ST-segment elevation myocardial infarction; however, they continue to have a nearly twofold increase in short-term mortality compared with nondiabetics. Data from the Fibrinolytic Therapy Trialists (FTT) group, analyzing over 45,000 patients, demonstrated improved 35-day mortality rates for diabetics receiving fibrinolytic therapy (13.6% versus 17.3%) (12). These findings suggest that diabetics derive at least as much benefit (perhaps even greater) from fibrinolytic therapy than nondiabetics. Based on pooled data from the fibrinolytic trials of more than 83,000 patients, diabetics continue to have increased 30-day mortality rates (11.6% versus 7.1%) compared with nondiabetics. Insulin-treated patients have the highest short-term mortality of 13.5%, compared with 10.4% for non-insulin-treated patients. Further supporting the effectiveness of fibrinolytic therapy, the 90-minute patency rates (TIMI grade 3 flow) from the GUSTO-I angiographic substudy demonstrated that diabetics had similar rates of infarct artery patency follow-

ing fibrinolytic therapy as nondiabetics (40.3% and 37.6%, $p = 0.7$) respectively.

The initial theoretical concern for giving fibrinolytic therapy to diabetics with evidence of proliferative retinopathy has not been substantiated in the literature. In fact, there is only a single case report in which fibrinolytic therapy resulted in retinal hemorrhage, which ultimately resolved in 3 weeks (13). Given the paucity of supportive data, proliferate retinopathy can no longer be considered a contraindication to fibrinolytic therapy in diabetic patients.

Data from the GUSTO-I database suggest that diabetics have both high-risk clinical and angiographic characteristics. The 1-year mortality rate was 60% greater for diabetics (14.5% versus 8.9%) (Fig. 30.4). They tended to be older, more often female, and present with an anterior-wall myocardial infarction. Furthermore, they received fibrinolytics an average of 20 minutes later than nondiabetics. Diabetics were also more likely to have any stroke (1.9% versus 1.4%) with insulin-treated patients having the greatest overall risk of 2.7%. Interestingly, these strokes were not more often hemorrhagic.

Although diabetics have increased events following fibrinolytic therapy, it is not a key determinant of outcome. Lee et al. characterized the important clinical variables in determining survival at 30 days in the GUSTO-I trial (14). The single most important predictor of death was age. In patients less than 45 years old, the 30-day mortality rate was 1.1% compared with a 20.5% mortality for people greater than 75 years old. Age combined with a low systolic blood pressure, higher Killip class, tachycardia, and anterior myocardial infarction accounted for 90% of the prognostic information. Diabetes had a similar predictive power, as did time to treatment with fibrinolytics, or current smoking.

CATHETER-BASED REPERFUSION OR FIBRINOLYSIS

There is a paucity of data concerning the outcome of diabetics following primary angioplasty. Similar to the GUSTO data, the PAMI trial demonstrated increased in-hospital mortality rates for diabetics compared with nondiabet-

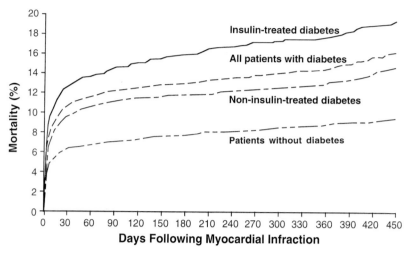

FIG. 30.4. Kaplan-Meier estimates of cumulative mortality for diabetics following acute myocardial infarction. Data is from the GUSTO-I trial. (Adopted with permission from ref. 10).

ics by univariate analysis (10% versus 3.8%, $p = .048$) respectively (15). The difference in mortality was driven by a disproportionate increase in mortality for the t-PA-treated diabetics. Primary PTCA was associated with a decreased short-term mortality compared with fibrinolytic therapy (0% versus 20.8%, $p = .01$). Given these suggestive data, the higher angiographic and clinical risk profile, and the increased rate of future adverse clinical events for diabetics, this author favors a catheter-based reperfusion strategy approach for diabetics. Unfortunately, primary catheter-based reperfusion remains limited to centers equipped for rapid assessment, triage, and timely mechanical reperfusion. At many centers, this is limited to daytime hours. What remains quite clear is prompt restoration of TIMI 3 flow whether via fibrinolysis or catheter-based therapy improves survival. Therefore, the decision process of choosing the reperfusion strategy should not delay instituting therapy, and if the catheterization laboratory cannot be rapidly mobilized for any reason, then fibrinolytic therapy is warranted even at centers generally accustomed to primary intervention.

RESCUE PTCA

Important insights for diabetics undergoing percutaneous coronary intervention (PCI) fol-

lowing fibrinolysis were made by Woodfield et al. from the GUSTO-I angiograpic substudy (16). Diabetics underwent PTCA more often following fibrinolysis within the first 30-days compared with nondiabetics (39% versus 33.8%). They also had a marked increase risk of death following failed rescue angioplasty. Unfortunately, rescue angioplasty failed more often in diabetics (22% versus 11%) and resulted in a 21.7% mortality rate following any rescue PTCA compared with a 9.3% mortality rate for nondiabetics ($p = .02$). Diabetics and nondiabetics had similar survival rates following successful rescue PTCA.

ANTIPLATELET THERAPY

There are now compelling data that antiplatelet agents are effective in the secondary prevention of cardiovascular events. The Antiplatelet Trialists group has convincingly demonstrated that antiplatelet therapy significantly reduces the incidence of nonfatal myocardial infarction, stroke, or vascular deaths in patients at high risk. Substudy analysis of the Antiplatelet Trialists data demonstrated a significant benefit in diabetic patients. There were 38 events prevented for 1,000 diabetic patients treated with antiplatelet therapy ($p < .002$) (17). Antiplatelet therapy was effective in diabetics with either an acute or prior myocardial infarction (38 and 36 events prevented for 1,000 patients treated, $p < .00001$) respectively.

The choice of the most appropriate oral antiplatelet agent, the optimal dose, and optimal duration of therapy remains unclear. There seems to be no additional benefit for high-dose aspirin (1000 milligrams) compared with a midrange dose of 75 to 325 mg per day. Data from ISIS II did not show a benefit in diabetic patients treated with 160 milligrams of aspirin following acute myocardial infarction (18). However, in data from the Early Treatment Diabetic Retinopathy Study (ETDRS) there was a trend for a daily dose of 650 mg of aspirin to reduce vascular events in a 5-year follow-up period (18.8% versus 20.4%) (19). Although there are not convincing prospective data for the optimal dose of aspirin therapy, 325 mg of aspirin therapy indefinitely would seem reasonable given the available literature.

Whether aspirin, or other more potent oral antiplatelet inhibitors, provides maximal benefit remains controversial. The Clopidogrel versus Aspirin in Patients at Risk of Ischaemic Events (CAPRIE) trial recently demonstrated improved event-free survival from ischemic stroke, myocardial infarction, or vascular deaths in patients with known atherosclerotic vascular disease. There was a relative-risk reduction of 8.7% in favor of the clopidogrel-treated group (20). Patients were treated with long-term clopidogrel 75 mg per day or 325 milligrams of aspirin daily. Reportedly the effects of clopidogrel were evenly distributed among the subgroups analyzed. Compared with ticlopidine, clopidogrel has an improved side-effect profile. With the recent association of thrombotic thrombocytopenic purpura with ticlopidine, clopidogrel will likely become the drug of choice for patients intolerant of aspirin.

The role of platelet glycoprotein IIb/IIIa inhibition in the treatment of acute coronary syndromes is currently evolving. The PRISM-PLUS study recently randomized 1,915 patients with either unstable angina or non-Q-wave myocardial infarction (MI) to receive either tirofiban and heparin, tirofiban alone, or heparin alone (21). There was an overall benefit with regard to the composite endpoint of death, nonfatal myocardial infarction, or recurrent ischemia at 7 days for the tirofiban and heparin group versus the heparin only group (12.9% versus 17.9%; $p = .004$). Although underpowered to demonstrate significance, subgroup analysis of this trial demonstrated improved event-free survival for patients with diabetes treated with tirofiban and heparin versus heparin group (14.8 % versus 21.8%) respectively.

The ACE Inhibitor Myocardial Infarction Collaborative Group combined the individual data from 100,000 patients enrolled in large-scale clinical trials in which ACE inhibitor treatment was started within 36 hours of acute myocardial infarction (22). There were 5,012 diabetic patients in this analysis. There was a trend for improved survival in diabetics treated early with ACE inhibitors, the magnitude of which (17.3 lives saved per 1000 patients treated, $p = .2$) appeared greater than that seen in nondiabetics. ACE inhibitor therapy is, without question, indicated in diabetic patients following acute myocardial infarction with nephropathy, congestive heart failure and hypertension, and after anterior-wall myocardial infarctions. The ideal time to initiate ACE inhibitor therapy is less clear. Forty percent of the 30-day survival benefit in the ACE collaborative group was seen in the first 24 hours, an additional 45% was seen from days 2 to 7. These data suggest that early initiation of ACE inhibitors in diabetic patients may well be advantageous.

ACE inhibitors have also been shown to be beneficial in patients with diabetic nephropathy and hypertension. Recent data from the ABCD and FACET trials suggest that ACE inhibitors should be considered as first-line agents for diabetics with hypertension (23,24). Patients receiving calcium channel blockers in both the ABCD and FACET trials had a greater risk of developing cardiovascular endpoints. It is unclear from these two trials whether the results were driven solely by the beneficial effects of ACE inhibitors or whether calcium channel blockers are additionally detrimental. Given these findings and their well-known protective renal effects, ACE inhibitors should be considered first-line agents in diabetics with hypertension.

There is often a reluctance to initiating beta-blockade in diabetic patients, given the inhibitory effect on the autonomic response to hypoglycemia. However, there is increasing evidence that beta-blockers may reduce mortality and re-infarction in diabetics. Recent data from Gottlieb et al. included over 200,000 patients who received beta-blocker therapy postmyocardial infarction (25). They demonstrated a marked 40% reduction in mortality for patients receiving beta-blockers following myocardial infarction. There were 59,445 diabetic patients within this analysis. There was a 17% 2-year mortality rate for diabetic patients receiving beta-blockers compared with a 26.6% rate for diabetics not receiving beta-blockers (relative risk 0.64; 95% confidence limits 0.60 to 0.69). In their analysis, only 31% of diabetic patients received beta-blocker therapy following infarction. Similar data was found in diabetics with known coronary artery disease from a substudy analysis within the Bezafibrate Infarction Prevention (BIP) Trial (26). There were 2,723 non-insulin-dependent diabetics, of which 911 were receiving long-term beta-blocker therapy. There was a 44% reduction in the 3-year mortality rate for diabetics receiving beta-blockers (14.0% versus 7.8%, $p < .001$). Given the high risk for future clinical events in diabetic patients, triple therapy (anti-platelet, beta-blockers, and ACE inhibitors) seems to be a prudent pharmacologic regimen, although this needs to be validated in a prospective randomized fashion.

The importance of tight glycemic control following acute myocardial infarction remains unknown. However, data from the DIGAMI study suggests that an insulin-glucose infusion followed by multiple-dose subcutaneous insulin regimen for diabetic patients improves the 12-month mortality rate when compared with conventional treatment for diabetic patients (27). This study randomized 620 diabetic patients to receive either conventional therapy or insulin-glucose infusion followed by a multiple-dose subcutaneous insulin regimen for 3 months or more. There was a 29% relative reduction in mortality for the active treatment group com-

pared with the conventional group (18.6% versus 26.1%, $p = .027$) respectively.

Although the results of the DIGAMI trial demonstrated a marked survival benefit for diabetics who were managed with an aggressive peri-infarction insulin regimen, the results have not been widely adopted and the mechanism for improved survival remains controversial. Whether these patients derived the enhanced survival benefit from improved glycemic control or from withdrawal of sulfonylurea agents is currently not clear. Sulfonylurea agents exert their hypoglycemic effects by inhibiting the ATP-sensitive potassium (K_{ATP}) channels in the beta-cells of the pancreas. Unfortunately, cardiac myocytes are abundantly populated with K_{ATP} channels and the current generation of sulfonylurea agents are not tissue-selective in binding to these channels. The role of K_{ATP} channels in cardiac myocytes remains poorly understood. However, opening of these channels may play an important role in ischemic preconditioning and myocardial excitability during episodes of ischemia. There is increasing evidence that is-chemic preconditioning is an important mechanism in the intact human heart. Whether sulfonylurea agents contribute significantly to increased cardiovascular events via this mechanism remains to be determined. Nevertheless there are newer pharmacologic alternatives for clinicians now, such as metformin and troglitazone. These agents improve glycemic control and have no known effect on K_{ATP} channels.

SUMMARY OF MEDICAL MANAGEMENT

It is now clear that diabetes is associated with adverse cardiovascular events. Several aspects of diabetes management deserve further mention. It is well documented now that improved glycemic control improves microvascular complications. In the UKPDS 33 trial, a decrease in the HbA_{1c} from 7.9% to 7.0% was associated with 25% risk reduction in microvascular complications. There is still uncertainty about whether improved glycemic control is associated with improved cardiovascular events. Aggressive lipid management is also warranted in diabetics. A target LDL cholesterol rate of less than 100 mg/dL, even in patients without known CAD, seems prudent given their increased risk of a first-time myocardial infarction. Whether aggressive control of triglycerides is warranted is unknown. ACE inhibitors are first-line agents for diabetics with hypertension, decreased LV function, or evidence of diabetic nephropathy (regardless of history of increased blood pressure). Finally, long-term treatment with antiplatelet agents following a coronary event is also important in the secondary prevention strategy of diabetics.

PERCUTANEOUS CORONARY INTERVENTIONS AND DIABETES MELLITUS

There will be an estimated 750,000 PCIs done in the United States alone in 1999 and over 70% of these will likely involve at least one intracoronary stent. In many busy interventional laboratories, 15% to 25 % of these interventions will be on diabetic patients. Given the increasing incidence of both type I and type II diabetes, there will be an increasing demand on cardiologists to appropriately risk-stratify and triage diabetic patients to medical, percutaneous, or surgical therapy. Although many of these patients will undergo bypass surgery, there will also be an increasing number of diabetics undergoing percutaneous coronary interventions, many of whom will have complex coronary lesions. Diabetics have been consistently shown to have a multitude of comorbidities and a higher clinical and angiographic risk profile than their nondiabetic counterparts. Not surprising, this has led to higher short- and long-term adverse cardiac events following PCI when compared with nondiabetic patients. This has led many to reevaluate the role of percutaneous revascularization as an initial revascularization strategy for diabetics with multivessel disease.

INCREASED BASELINE RISK FOR DIABETICS UNDERGOING PCI

Diabetic patients requiring percutaneous revascularization have a higher cardiac risk profile when compared to nondiabetics. Stein et al. provided important insights into the baseline risk of diabetic patients undergoing a first-time PCI. This analysis included over 10,000 patients, 11% of which were diabetic (28). Although diabetes is a potent risk factor for atherosclerotic coronary artery disease, diabetics presented for initial revascularization procedures more than 2 years later than nondiabetics, were more often female, and had a higher Canadian Classification of unstable angina. They were also more likely to have had a prior myocardial infarction, have a history of congestive heart failure and hypertension, be heavier, and have an elevated serum creatinine. In this study, insulin-treated diabetics were more likely to have a greater number of high-risk baseline characteristics than non-insulin-treated diabetics.

OUTCOME FOLLOWING PERCUTANEOUS CORONARY REVASCULARIZATION

Although diabetes has been associated with increased short-term events in the present era, recent data from the EPISTENT trial would suggest that stenting and abciximab improves both short and intermediate-term outcomes. Early data from the NHLBI registry reported by Kip et al. would suggest an early hazard for diabetic patients (29). In this registry, there was a 3.2% in-hospital mortality rate for diabetics compared with a more conventional in-hospital mortality rate of 0.5% for nondiabetics (Odds Ratio 6.7; 95% CI 2.98,15.1). Furthermore, the rate of in-hospital death, myocardial infarction, or need for emergency bypass surgery was considerably higher for diabetic patients (11.0% versus 6.7%; Odds Ratio 1.74; 95% CI 1.1,2.6). The excessive in-hospital death rate among diabetic patients was primarily driven by a disproportionately high in-hospital death rate of 8.3% for diabetic females. There was a similarly high rate of 30-day composite events (death, MI, revascularization) for diabetics treated with stent and placebo in the recent EPISTENT trial. However, the addition of abciximab markedly improved the 30-day safety profile of percutaneous revascularization for diabetics. There was a greater than 50%

reduction in the event rates for the stent-abciximab group compared with the stent-placebo group(5.8% versus 12.1%, $p = .035$). In fact, the 30-day rate rates for abciximab-treated diabetics was similar to nondiabetics (5.3% versus 6.3%) respectively (30).

Diabetics have consistently been shown to have higher clinical and angiographic restenosis rates following balloon angioplasty. This was first demonstrated in the initial report from the NHLBI registry. The angiographic restenosis rate in diabetic patients was 47% compared with 32% for nondiabetics (31). Subsequent studies have reported restenosis rates ranging from 49% to 71% for diabetic patients.

Disease progression contributes significantly to the increased event rates seen in diabetics following PCI. Data from Stein showed that, by 5 years, the mortality rate was 12% for diabetics compared with 7% for nondiabetics. Diabetics had a nearly twofold increase in postprocedural myocardial infarction rate (19% versus 11%, $p < .0001$) and a marked increase in composite event-rates (MI, CABG, or PTCA) (64% versus 47%, $p < .001$) (28).

Data from Kip et al. clearly demonstrate the increased risk of long-term cardiovascular events for diabetics undergoing conventional balloon angioplasty. First, diabetics with multivessel disease are at considerable risk for both short- and long-term mortality (29). The 9-year death rate for diabetic patients was nearly double than that for nondiabetics (35.9% versus 17.9%). Unlike Stein's data, the mortality curves separate early, such that there was a 30-day mortality rate of 3.6% for diabetics compared with 0.7% for nondiabetics. The increased 30-day mortality rate was primarily driven by diabetic patients with multivessel disease. The 9-year mortality rate for diabetics with three-vessel disease was 51.3% compared with 25.1% for nondiabetics with three-vessel disease. The 9-year mortality rate was 36.9% for diabetics with two-vessel disease compared with 21.3% for nondiabetics with two-vessel disease. Diabetics with single-vessel disease had an overall 24.3% mortality rate compared with 12.9% for nondiabetics with single-vessel disease (Fig. 30.5).

Restenosis in diabetics follows a similar time course and does not seem to be associated with a more malignant clinical presentation. However, late-progression of adverse clinical events is

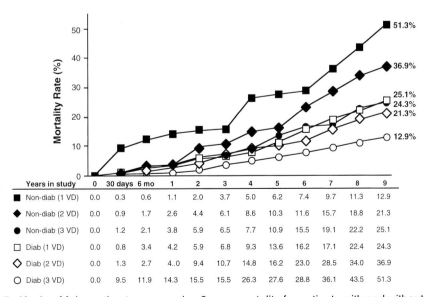

FIG. 30.5. Kaplan-Meier estimates comparing 9-year mortality for patients with and without diabetes stratified the number of diseased vessels. Non-diab, nondiabetic; Diab, diabetic; VD, vessel disease. (Adopted with permission from ref. 29).

clearly evident in diabetic patients. Identifying angiographic and clinical covariates associated with adverse clinical outcomes in diabetics has been the object of many clinical studies. However, to date there has not been an identification of modifiable predictors in diabetic patients. Multivariate predictors of outcome from Kip's analysis included age (in fact diabetics aged less than 60 had an excellent long-term survival of 93%), history of congestive heart failure, insulin treatment, and extent of coronary artery disease. Insulin-treated diabetics were more often female, had a longer duration of diabetes, and were more likely to have diabetic nephropathy and decreased LV function.

The problem with identification of diabetic-dependent predictors of outcome following percutaneous coronary revascularization in the current literature is that investigators, to date, have done a poor job of tracking important diabetic-dependent covariates such as complications from diabetes (e.g., retinopathy, nephropathy, duration of diabetes, mode of therapy, and glycemic control). Furthermore, angiography is likely insensitive in adequately assessing atherosclerotic burden in diabetics.

Proteinuria is a marker for diabetic nephropathy and perhaps a surrogate marker for atherosclerosis. There have been a number of longitudinal studies linking microalbuminuria and increased mortality in maturity-onset diabetes. We recently analyzed the 2-year event rates in over 2,700 patients who underwent percutaneous coronary revascularization. Similar to other data, diabetics had an increased 2-year mortality compared with nondiabetics (13.5% versus 7.3%, $p < .001$). The increased mortality rate in the diabetic group was primarily driven by diabetics with evidence of proteinuria on random screening urinalysis. Nonproteinuric diabetics and nondiabetics had a similar 2-year survival rates (Fig. 30.6) (32). Interestingly, insulin dependence was not a significant predictor by univariate analysis in these data. Proteinuria is not only an important predictor following percutaneous coronary intervention but also following isolated coronary artery bypass grafting (CABG). Likely, proteinuria is a marker of advanced atherosclerosis and is associated with microvascular disease. It clearly predicts adverse clinical events in diabetic patients. If the diabetic story continues to evolve in the future, clinical investigators will need to commit time and resources to tracking diabetic dependent covariates in registries and randomized controlled trials.

THE STENT ERA

Coronary artery stenting has been demonstrated to decrease the rate of target-vessel revascularization in many situations. Although there are conflicting data concerning the angiographic and clinical outcomes of diabetics following stenting, there are increasing data that stenting improves outcome for diabetics compared with PTCA (33–36).

In data from Van Belle et al., diabetics who underwent balloon angioplasty had a nearly two-fold increase in 6-month angiographic restenosis rates compared with nondiabetics (63% versus 36% $p = .0002$) (33). In these data, stenting significantly reduced angiographic restenosis rates for diabetics compared with balloon angioplasty (63% versus 25%, respectively). Surprisingly, in this report diabetics had similar restenosis rates compared with nondiabetics following stenting (25% versus 27%, respectively). As in the balloon angioplasty data, stenting achieved similar acute gain in diabetics and nondiabetics; however, the late loss rates among both groups were nearly identical (0.77 mm versus 0.79 mm). Furthermore, there was only a 2% rate of late vessel occlusion in the stented diabetic group compared with a 14% in the PTCA-diabetic group.

Whether the decreased rates of angiographic restenosis following stenting in diabetics translates into clinical benefit has not been definitively demonstrated. Data from the GUSTO IIb database would suggest that stenting in diabetics improves clinical outcome. Over 2,365 patients underwent percutaneous coronary intervention during follow-up in the GUSTO IIb trial (1632 nondiabetic-PTCA, 310 nondiabetic-stent, 369 diabetic-PTCA, 54 diabetic-stent). The 6-month adverse-event rate (death, MI need for repeat revascularization) was significantly greater in

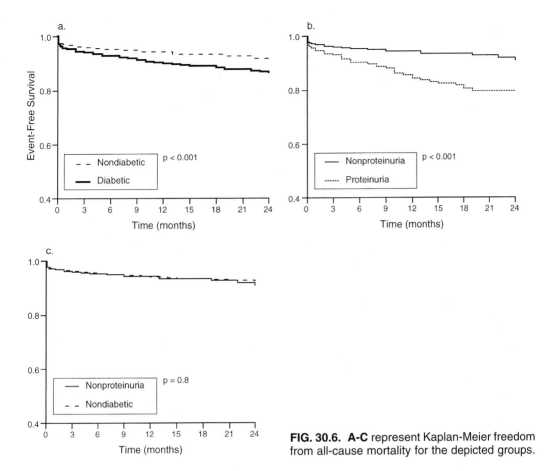

FIG. 30.6. A-C represent Kaplan-Meier freedom from all-cause mortality for the depicted groups.

diabetics compared with nondiabetics (29% versus 24%, respectively, $p = .009$). The increased event rates were primarily seen in the diabetic-PTCA group. There was a 31.4% event rate compared with a 24.6% rate for the nondiabetic-PTCA group ($p = .009$). Interestingly, there was essentially no difference between the diabetic and nondiabetic patients undergoing stenting (19.3% versus 21%, $p = .8$) (37).

Although it appears that stenting improves outcome for diabetics, they still have higher angiographic restenosis rates following stenting (without abciximab) than nondiabetics. Carroza et al. combined data from three large stent trials involving over 5,900 patients and demonstrated that diabetics were significantly more likely to have a higher target-lesion revascularization (TVR) rates when compared with nondiabetics (15% versus 10%, $p = .001$) respectively (38).

Previous analysis comparing stenting among diabetics were most likely underpowered to demonstrate a significant difference with nondiabetics.

Data from the EPISTENT trial provide compelling data that abciximab administration with stenting further improves the clinical and angiographic events in diabetic patients. There were 2,399 (491 of which were diabetic) patients randomized to receive either conventional angioplasty with abciximab, stent-placebo, or stent-abciximab. The 6-month death, myocardial infarction, and target-vessel-revascularization rates for diabetic patients were 25.2%, 23.4%, and 13% for the stent-placebo, balloon-abciximab, and stent-abciximab groups, respectively ($p = .005$). The reduction in 6-month events were not only driven by a reduction in large postprocedural myocardial infarctions (6.2% stent-

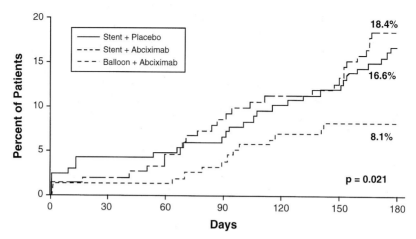

FIG. 30.7. Kaplan-Meier probability curves for target-vessel revascularization for the diabetic patients in the EPISTENT trial.

abciximab versus 11% stent-placebo) but also by a significant 51% relative reduction in the 6-month target-vessel revascularization rate. The 6-month TVR rate for the stent-abciximab group was 8.1% (lower than the 8.8% 6-month TVR nondiabetic rate in the stent-abciximab group) compared with 16.6% and 18.4% for the stent-placebo and balloon-abciximab groups, respectively (p = .02) (Fig. 30.7). The beneficial effect of stenting and abciximab in diabetics was further supported by the results of the diabetic angiographic substudy. There was a marked 67% increase in the net gain for the diabetic stent-abciximab group, compared with the stent-placebo group (0.85 millimeters versus 0.51 millimeters, p = .003). This translated into a significant 41% reduction in the late loss index for the stent-abciximab-treated group (0.64 for the stent-placebo group and 0.38 for the stent-abciximab group, p = .039) (39). These data provide compelling evidence that stenting with abciximab should be considered in all stent-eligible diabetics undergoing percutaneous coronary revascularization.

PCI COMPARED WITH CABG

A great deal of attention was drawn to the initial revascularization strategy of treated diabetics with multivessel disease following the BARI trial. Prior to the publication of BARI in June of 1996, the NHLBI issued a clinical alert to physicians concluding that CABG should be the preferred revascularization strategy for treated diabetics with multivessel disease requiring a first-time coronary revascularization procedure (40). This was based on the BARI trial, which demonstrated a 5-year survival benefit for treated diabetics following CABG compared with PTCA (80.6% versus 65.5%, p = .003) (41). The striking benefit of CABG appeared to be confined to patients with more than three significant lesions. The 5-year survival rate was similar for nondiabetics and diet controlled diabetics following either CABG or PTCA (91.4% versus 91.1%).

Drawing definitive conclusions regarding the optimal revascularization strategy from the current literature for patients is problematic. Firstly, the BARI registry found no difference in unadjusted survival for treated diabetics undergoing CABG compared with PTCA (14.9% versus 14.4%). Secondly, the nine major randomized trials comparing bypass surgery with percutaneous revascularization strategies effectively excluded over 95% of potential revascularization candidates. Thirdly, during the often long follow-up times in these trials, technological developments can occur so rapidly that by the end of the study, the revascularization approaches being studied may well have become outdate. What seems clear, given the current data, is that patients undergoing surgery consistently have improved anginal symptoms and require fewer revascularization procedures in follow-up.

The choice of which diabetics should undergo an initial percutaneous revascularization procedure and which should undergo surgical revascularization is often a difficult decision for the cardiologist. Unfortunately, there are limited prospective data available and virtually no recent data utilizing stenting and abciximab as a percutaneous revascularization strategy and aggressive arterial revascularization as a surgical strategy. Figure 30.8 depicts a suggested revascularization algorithm for diabetics who are both clinically and angiographically eligible for either percutaneous or surgical revascularization.

Whether diabetic patients with a proximal LAD stenosis should be managed by percutaneous or surgical revascularization is also unclear. These patients have a great deal of myocardium at jeopardy, which places them in a higher risk

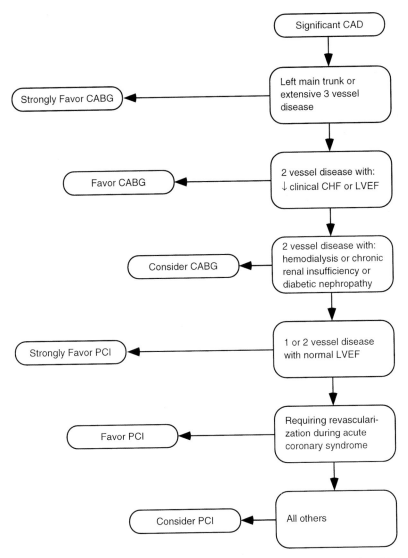

FIG. 30.8. Suggested revascularization strategy algorithm for diabetics eligible for either percutaneous or surgical revascularization requiring a first-time coronary revascularization procedure.

category. In the stent and abciximab era, however, the likelihood of procedural success and long-term vessel patency is exceedingly high. On the other hand, it was precisely this subgroup of patients that benefited with a LIMA to the LAD in the BARI trial. Of course a surgical revascularization carries with it significant morbidity. With the recent advances in minimally invasive bypass surgery, surgical revascularization is gaining more appeal to both the cardiologist and patient. However, the intermediate- and long-term vessel patency rates for minimally invasive bypass surgery needs further investigation before this becomes the preferred surgical revascularization strategy.

FUTURE PERSPECTIVE

Although clinical and angiographic restenosis rates have improved for diabetic patients with stenting and glycoprotein IIb/IIIa inhibition, instent restenosis remains a considerable problem. The only promising therapy on the immediate horizon is radiation therapy. Initial reports from the SCRIPPS trial were especially favorable for diabetic patients. However, the number of diabetic patients was much too small to support conclusions regarding the efficacy of brachytherapy for diabetics. In addition to restenosis, many diabetics are not candidates for either conventional surgical or percutaneous revascularization strategies, given diffuse atherosclerosis and resultant poor target-vessels disease. Therapies currently under investigation which may prove beneficial include laser therapy such as percutaneous myocardial revascularization (PMR) or transmyocardial revascularization (TMR). Another promising mode of revascularization is angiogenesis with vascular endothelial growth factors such as fibroblast growth factor (FGF) or vascular endothelial growth factor (VEGF), although worsening of diabetic retinopathy remains as a concern with the use of either agent.

REFERENCES

1. Harris MI, Hadden WC, Knowler WC, Bennet PH. Prevalence of diabetes and impaired glucose tolerance and plasma glucose levels in U.S. population aged 20–74 yr. *Diabetes* 1987;36:523–534.
2. DCCT Research Group. The effect of intensive treatment of diabetes on the development and progression of long-term complications in insulin-dependent diabetes mellitus. The Diabetes Control and Complications Trial Research Group. *New Engl J Med* 1993;329:977–986.
3. United Kingdom Prospective Diabetes Study (UKPDS) Group. Intensive blood-glucose control with sulfonylureas or insulin compared with conventional treatment and risk of complications in patients with type II diabetes (UKPDS 33). *Lancet* 1998;352:837–853.
4. Turner R, Cull C, Holman R. United Kingdom Prospective Diabetes Study 17: a 9-year update of a randomized, controlled trial on the effect of improved metabolic control on complications in non-insulin-dependent diabetes mellitus. *Ann Intern Med* 1996;124:136–145.
5. Wingard DL, E. B-C. Heart Disease and Diabetes. Diabetes in America. Vol. NIH. Washington, DC: U.S. Department of Health and Human Services, 1995; Publication no. 95-1468. 429–448.
6. Haffner SM, Lehto S, Ronnemaa T, Pyorala K, Laakso M. Mortality from coronary heart disease in subjects with type II diabetes and in nondiabetic subjects with and without prior myocardial infarction. *N Engl J Med* 1998;339:229–234.
7. Stamler J, Vaccaro O, Neaton JD, D. W. Diabetes, other risk factors and 12-year cardiovascular mortality for men screened in the multiple risk factor intervention trial. *Diabetes Care* 1993;16:434–444.
8. Bloomgarden ZT. Cardiovascular disease and diabetes: issues raised at The European Association for the Study of Diabetes annual meeting [news]. *Diabetes Care* 1996; 19:187–190.
9. Granger CB, Califf RM, Young S et al. Outcome of patients with diabetes mellitus and acute myocardial infarction treated with thrombolytic agents. The Thrombolysis and Angioplasty in Myocardial Infarction (TAMI) Study Group. *J Am Coll Cardiol* 1993;21:920–925.
10. Mak KH, Moliterno DJ, Granger CB et al. Influence of diabetes mellitus on clinical outcome in the thrombolytic era of acute myocardial infarction. GUSTO-I Investigators. Global utilization of streptokinase and tissue plasminogen activator for occluded coronary arteries. *J Am Coll Cardiol* 1997;30:171–179.
11. Akasaka T, Yoshida K, Hozumi T et al. Retinopathy identifies marked restriction of coronary flow reserve in patients with diabetes mellitus. *J Am Coll Cardiol* 1997;30:935–941.
12. Fibrinolytic Therapy Trialists' (FTT) Collaborative Group. Indications for fibrinolytic therapy in suspected acute myocardial infarction: collaborative overview of early mortality and major morbidity results from all randomised trials of more than 1000 patients. [published erratum appears in Lancet 1994 Mar 19; 343(8899): 742]. *Lancet* 1994;343:311–322.
13. Caramelli B, Tranchesi B Jr, Gebara OC, de Sa LC, Pileggi FJ. Retinal haemorrhage after thrombolytic therapy [Letter]. *Lancet* 1991;337:1356–1357.
14. Lee KL, Woodlief LH, Topol EJ et al. Predictors of 30-day mortality in the era of reperfusion for acute myocardial infarction. Results from an international trial of 41,021 patients. GUSTO-I Investigators. *Circulation* 1995;91:1659–1668.

15. Stone GW, Grines CL, Browne KF et al. Predictors of in-hospital and 6-month outcome after acute myocardial infarction in the reperfusion era: the Primary Angioplasty in Myocardial Infarction (PAMI) trail. *J Am Coll Cardiol* 1995;25:370–377.

16. Woodfield SL, Lundergan CF, Reiner JS et al. Angiographic findings and outcome in diabetic patients treated with thrombolytic therapy for acute myocardial infarction: the GUSTO-I experience. *J Am Coll Cardiol* 1996; 28:1661–1669.

17. Antiplatelet Trialists' Collaboration. Collaborative overview of randomised trials of antiplatelet therapy—I: prevention of death, myocardial infarction, and stroke by prolonged antiplatelet therapy in various categories of patients. *BMJ* 1994;308:81–106.

18. ISIS-2 (Second International Study of Infarct Survival) Collaborative Group Randomized trial of intravenous streptokinase, oral aspirin, both, or neither among 17,187 cases of suspected acute myocardial infarction: ISIS-2. *Lancet* 1988;2:349–360.

19. ETDRS Investigators. Aspirin effects on mortality and morbidity in patients with diabetes mellitus. Early Treatment Diabetic Retinopathy Study report 14. *JAMA* 1992; 268:1292–1300.

20. CAPRIE investigators. A randomised, blinded, trial of clopidogrel versus aspirin in patients at risk of ischaemic events (CAPRIE). CAPRIE Steering Committee. *Lancet* 1996;348:1329–1339.

21. Platelet Receptor Inhibition in Ischemic Syndrome Management in Patients Limited by Unstable Signs and Symptoms (PRISM-PLUS) Study Investigators. Inhibition of the platelet glycoprotein IIb/IIIa receptor with tirofiban in unstable angina and non-Q-wave myocardial infarction. *N Engl J Med* 1998;338:1488–1497.

22. ACE Inhibitor Myocardial Infarction Collaborative Group. Indications for ACE inhibitors in the early treatment of acute myocardial infarction: systematic overview of individual data from 100,000 patients in randomized trials. *Circulation* 1998;97:2202–2212.

23. Estacio RO, Jeffers BW, Hiatt WR, Biggerstaff SL, Gifford N, Schrier RW. The effect of nisoldipine as compared with enalapril on cardiovascular outcomes in patients with non-insulin-dependent diabetes and hypertension. *N Engl J Med* 1998;338:645–652.

24. Tatti P, Pahor M, Byington RP et al. Outcome results of the Fosinopril Versus Amlodipine Cardiovascular Events Randomized Trial (FACET) in patients with hypertension and NIDDM. *Diabetes Care* 1998;21:597–603.

25. Gottlieb SS, McCarter RJ, Vogel RA. Effect of beta-blockade on mortality among high-risk and low-risk patients after myocardial infarction. *N Engl J Med* 1998; 339:489–497.

26. Jonas M, Reicher-Reiss H, Boyko V et al. Usefulness of beta-blocker therapy in patients with non-insulin-dependent diabetes mellitus and coronary artery disease. Bezafibrate Infarction Prevention (BIP) Study Group. *Am J Cardiol* 1996;77:1273–1277.

27. Malmberg K, Ryden L, Efendic S et al. Randomized trial of insulin-glucose infusion followed by subcutaneous insulin treatment in diabetic patients with acute myocardial infarction (DIGAMI study): effects on mortality at 1 year. *J Am Coll Cardiol* 1995;26:57–65.

28. Stein B, Weintraub WS, Gebhart SP et al. Influence of diabetes mellitus on early and late outcome after percutaneous transluminal coronary angioplasty. *Circulation* 1995;91:979–989.

29. Kip KE, Faxon DP, Detre KM, Yeh W, Kelsey SF, Currier JW. Coronary angioplasty in diabetic patients. The National Heart, Lung, and Blood Institute Percutaneous Transluminal Coronary Angioplasty Registry. *Circulation* 1996;94:1818–1825.

30. The EPISTENT Investigators. Evaluation of platelet IIb/IIIa inhibitor for stenting. Randomised placebo-controlled and balloon-angioplasty-controlled trial to assess safety of coronary stenting with use of platelet glycoprotein-IIb/IIIa blockade. *Lancet* 1998;352:87–92.

31. Holmes DR Jr, Vlietstra RE, Smith HC et al. Restenosis after percutaneous transluminal coronary angioplasty (PTCA): a report from the PTCA Registry of the National Heart, Lung, and Blood Institute. *Am J Cardiol* 1984;53:77C–81C.

32. Marso SP, Ellis SG, Tuzcu M, et al. The importance of proteinuria as a determinant of mortality following percutaneous coronary revascularization in diabetics. *J Am Coll Cardiol* 1999;33:1269–1277.

33. Van Belle E, Bauters C, Hubert E et al. Restenosis rates in diabetic patients: a comparison of coronary stenting and balloon angioplasty in native coronary vessels [see comments]. *Circulation* 1997;96:1454–1460.

34. Carrozza JP Jr, Kuntz RE, Fishman RF, Baim DS. Restenosis after arterial injury caused by coronary stenting in patients with diabetes mellitus. *Annals of Internal Medicine* 1993;118:344–349.

35. Foley JB, Penn IM, Brown RI et al. Safety, success, and restenosis after elective coronary implantation of the Palmaz-Schatz stent in 100 patients at a single center. *Am Heart J* 1993;125:686–694.

36. Ellis SG, Savage M, Fischman D et al. Restenosis after placement of Palmaz-Schatz stents in native coronary arteries. Initial results of a multicenter experience. *Circulation* 1992;86:1836–1844.

37. Marso SP, Ellis SG, Bhatt DL, Sapp SK, Emanuelsson H, Topol EJ. The stenting in diabetics debate: insight from the large GUSTO IIb experience with extended follow-up. *Circulation* 1998;98:397A.

38. Carrozza JP, Ho KK, Neimann D, Kuntz RE, DE C. Diabetes mellitus is associated with adverse 6-month angiographic and clinical outcome following coronary stenting. *Circulation* 1998;98:399A.

39. Marso SP, Tanguay JF, Bhatt DL, Kleiman NS, Hammoud T, EJ T. Optimizing the percutaneous coronary interventional strategy for diabetics—The EPISTENT Experience. *Circulation* 1998;98:400A.

40. NHLI BARI clinical alert on diabetics treated with angioplasty. *Circulation* 1995;92.

41. The Bypass Angioplasty Revascularization Investigation (BARI) Investigators. Comparison of coronary bypass surgery with angioplasty in patients with multivessel disease. *New Engl J Med* 1996;335:217–225.

SECTION III

Adjunctive Therapies

31

Heparin: How Much in Patients Undergoing Percutaneous Coronary Intervention?

Craig R. Narins

Division of Cardiology, New Mexico Heart Institute, Albuquerque, New Mexico 87106

Because arterial injury at the site of percutaneous transluminal coronary intervention (PTCI) serves as a potent stimulus for thrombus formation, anticoagulant and antiplatelet agents are administered routinely during the procedure to reduce the likelihood of acute thrombotic complications. While randomized controlled trials have demonstrated significant reductions in thrombotic events in conjunction with a variety of antiplatelet agents, including aspirin, ticlopidine, and platelet glycoprotein (GP) IIb/IIIa receptor antagonists (1–4), information regarding the importance and proper dosing of heparin during PTCI, especially in the new-device era, remains less precise. During the early experience with balloon angioplasty, heparin was typically administered via an empirically derived, fixed-dosing schedule, and the degree of anticoagulation was not monitored. Over the past decade, the activated clotting time (ACT) assay has entered into widespread use as a means to monitor and more precisely titrate the degree of heparin anticoagulation during angioplasty. Using ACT, the importance of heparin therapy during balloon angioplasty has been established through demonstration of an inverse relationship between the degree of heparin anticoagulation during the procedure and the risk of abrupt vessel closure and its attendant clinical sequelae. (5,6).

Despite the demonstrated importance of heparin therapy during stand-alone balloon angioplasty, the proper degree of anticoagulation during new-device angioplasty and coronary stent implantation has been poorly studied. Of even greater importance, the emergence of platelet GP IIb/IIIa receptor antagonists has placed even more importance on the precise dosing and monitoring of the degree of anticoagulation, given the striking association among potent platelet inhibitor therapy, excess heparin administration, and hemorrhagic complications. This chapter focuses on the principles and techniques essential to the monitoring of heparin therapy during PTCI, review data regarding the benefits and risks of heparin anticoagulation during balloon angioplasty, and, while data regarding the proper use of heparin continues to emerge, provide practical guidelines for the dosing of heparin in the current new-device, GP IIb/IIIa receptor antagonist era.

ACTIVATED CLOTTING TIME

Early practitioners of balloon angioplasty typically administered standard doses of heparin during the procedure (e.g., 10,000 to 15,000 U prior to the intervention, with subsequent boluses at various intervals) primarily as a means of preventing the formation of blood clots on the indwelling angioplasty equipment, but also as a potential strategy to reduce ischemic complications during the procedure. With the arrival of the ACT assay in the catheterization laboratory in the late 1980s, it became apparent that administration of a standard bolus of heparin to all patients prior to angioplasty did not result consistently in therapeutic anticoagulation. For example, it was reported by Dougherty et al. (7) that, following a standard 10,000-U bolus of heparin in a series of patients undergoing angioplasty, ACT (measured with the Hemotec device [Medtronic, Englewood, Co]) was less than 250 seconds in 58% of individuals studied.

Technical Aspects

ACT has emerged as the preferred assay to determine the degree of anticoagulation during PTCI. The test, first described by Hattersly in 1966, measures the time required for whole blood to clot in a test tube when exposed to a procoagulant material. Two commercially available, automated ACT devices are currently in widespread use: the Hemochron (International Technidyne Corporation, Edison, NJ) and the HemoTec systems. It is critical to recognize that, because these two devices utilize different reagents and measurement techniques, they yield disparate ACT values when exposed to identical samples of blood (8).

Avendaño and Ferguson (9) performed a detailed comparison of the ACT values obtained from the Hemochron and HemoTec systems on 311 paired samples of blood from 113 patients undergoing angioplasty. Within this population, the Hemochron ACT was consistently and significantly greater than the value obtained via the HemoTec device. Although wide interindividual variability existed, the mean ACT was a mean of 11 ± 23 seconds greater with the Hemochron device prior to heparin therapy (125 seconds versus 114 seconds), and a mean of 100 ± 86 seconds greater after heparin administration (414 seconds versus 314 seconds). Using linear regression analysis, the relationship between the two devices within this population fit the equation:

HemoTec ACT

$$= 47 + 0.63 \text{ (Hemochron ACT)}$$

Thus, although both systems yield ACT values that correlate in a linear fashion with heparin concentration, the absolute values obtained from these devices differ markedly. The operator,

therefore, must adjust the target ACT based on the particular measurement system in use.

ACT Versus Activated Partial Thromboplastin Time

ACT, akin to the more widely used activated partial thromboplastin time (aPTT) assay, primarily assesses the degree of inhibition of the intrinsic pathway of the coagulation cascade. However, the ACT assay is associated with several practical advantages relative to the aPTT for the monitoring of heparin therapy during PTCI. From a technical standpoint, the devices currently available to measure ACT are easily operated by catheterization laboratory personnel without the need for specialized training. The ACT assay can be performed at the bedside, thus allowing rapid turnaround time. Furthermore, relative to aPTT as performed in a centralized laboratory, ACT is a far less expensive test to run (10).

The most important attribute of the ACT assay, which makes this test ideal for monitoring anticoagulation during PTCI, is its ability to maintain accuracy when high concentrations of heparin are used. In contrast, the relatively large doses of heparin that are required during PTCI and cardiopulmonary bypass typically exceed the measurement limits of the aPTT assay. For example, in a series of 18 patients who had received continuous infusions of heparin for more than 24 hours immediately prior to percutaneous transluminal coronary angioplasty (PTCA), Grill et al. (11) measured a mean ($\pm$ standard deviation) baseline PTT of 69 ± 18 seconds, which corresponded to a mean ACT (Hemochron system) of 169 ± 17 seconds. Following the administration of an additional 10,000 U of heparin prior to the initial balloon inflation, aPTT was unmeasurable in all patients (greater than 180 seconds), whereas mean ACT was in the therapeutic range at 381 ± 57 seconds. While several investigators have reported a good correlation between ACT and aPTT at lower heparin concentrations, Reiner et al. (12) suggested that, for the purpose of monitoring heparin therapy postintervention, at ACT values of less than 225 seconds, ACT is less sensitive than aPTT in predicting the degree of anticoagulation.

ACT and Various Anticoagulants

The ACT assay responds quite differently to the various anticoagulants used during PTCI. As discussed, ACT responds in a linear fashion to increasing serum concentrations of heparin. Interestingly, however, ACT is not a sensitive assay by which to monitor anticoagulation with low-molecular-weight heparin (LMWH). Greiber et al. (13) measured both ACT and anti–factor Xa levels (which reflects LMWH concentration in blood) in a group of patients treated with LMWH (35-IU per kilogram bolus of dalteparin followed by a 10-IU per kilogram per hour infusion) during hemodialysis. Despite consistently therapeutic levels of anti–factor Xa activity, no sustained increase in ACT was detected in response to LMWH. The authors postulated that, because the low-molecular-weight subfraction has a more specific effect on antithrombin III than unfractionated heparin, with less influence on the activities of platelets and intrinsic pathway components including factors IX and XI, its effects on broad-based anticoagulation assays such as ACT are minimal.

In contrast to the situation with LMWH, ACT is a sensitive assay to gauge the degree of anticoagulation elicited by the direct thrombin inhibitor hirulog. In a study of 211 patients treated with escalating doses of hirulog, Topol et al. (14) demonstrated a linear dose–response curve of both the ACT and aPTT assays.

ACT and IIb/IIIa Antagonists

The influence of the platelet GP IIb/IIIa receptor antagonist abciximab on ACT among patients enrolled in the EPIC trial was investigated by Moliterno et al. (15).Using linear regression modeling and adjusting for patient weight, the predicted maximal procedural ACT was determined to be 34.2 seconds greater in patients receiving abciximab in conjunction with heparin compared with patients who were randomized

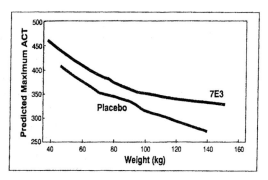

FIG. 31.1. Maximum ACT in subjects receiving the platelet GP IIb/IIIa receptor antagonist abciximab (7E3) or placebo in the EPIC trial. (From ref. 15, with permission.)

to receive heparin and placebo (Fig. 31.1). When examined by type of monitoring device, ACT was a mean of 43 seconds greater in abciximab-treated patients when measured with the Hemochron assay, and 21 seconds greater with the HemoTec system. In a separate *in vitro* experiment, Ammar et al. (16) determined that abciximab, when added to nonheparinized blood, did not prolong ACT. However, when the blood sample was first pretreated with heparin, ACT was significantly prolonged (by a mean of 34 seconds) by the addition of abciximab. While knowledge of the interaction between abciximab and ACT carries importance in terms of heparin dosing in the clinical setting, it remains uncertain as to whether abciximab possesses true anticoagulant properties in addition to its potent antiplatelet effects. It has been postulated that, because activated platelets contribute to thrombin generation, inhibition of platelet activity by abciximab may reduce overall thrombin generation and hence reduce the tendency of whole blood to clot, as reflected by ACT.

Arterial Versus Venous ACT

The variability of the ACT assay when two duplicate samples (obtained from the same vascular site) are run has been shown to be less than 10% (17). A variety of investigators have compared relative ACT values derived from simultaneously obtained samples of venous and arterial blood; however, these studies have yielded disparate conclusions regarding the relative influence of sampling site. In a study of 48 patients undergoing PTCI, by Peseola et al., venous ACT was slightly but consistently greater (by approximately 25 to 35 seconds) than the arterial ACT on serial samples obtained up to 60 minutes following the initial heparin bolus. Similarly, in a study of 115 patients undergoing PTCA, the venous ACT exceeded the arterial value by 10% to 20% in 55% of instances; however, substantial variation between simultaneous arterial and venous samples was not infrequent, with 20% differing by 50 seconds or more. In contrast, among 40 patients studied by Rath and Bennett (17), who underwent serial paired arterial and venous ACT measurements over a 60-minute period, ACT of the arterial sample exceeded that of the venous sample in 70% of instances. Because the majority of interventions at our institution are currently performed without insertion of a venous sheath, arterial ACTs are typically followed. However, as is evident from the previously mentioned studies, in instances in which both arterial and venous access sites are available, it may be preferable to consistently monitor either the arterial or venous ACT during the procedure, as alternation of sampling sites may result in substantial variability in ACT.

Kerensky et al. (18) examined in detail the influence of site of heparin administration and timing of sampling on ACT. Among patients undergoing angioplasty, when heparin was administered into the ascending aorta via the guide catheter, ACT gradually increased and then reached a plateau by 60 seconds. In contrast, when heparin was administered through the femoral arterial sheath, there was an early "overshoot" in venous ACT, which did not plateau until approximately 5 minutes following the bolus. Despite the more rapid equilibration of the heparin effect available with central aortic administration, this mode of delivery typically entails patient discomfort (burning sensation in the chest) and carries a small but finite risk of injection of air bubbles into the central circulation. Peripheral intravenous administration of heparin boluses stands as the preferred site of delivery at our institution, and the blood sample

for ACT determination is obtained 2 to 5 minutes following the bolus.

CLINICAL EXPERIENCES
Cardiopulmonary Bypass

Given its ability to accurately reflect the degree of anticoagulation with large doses of heparin, ACT first entered into broad clinical use in the mid-1970s as a means to monitor heparin anticoagulation and its reversal with protamine during cardiopulmonary bypass. Bull and colleagues (19) demonstrated the potential importance of individualizing heparin therapy via ACT monitoring by establishing the inability of a variety of commonly used standard heparin protocols to result in safe levels of anticoagulation (empirically defined as ACTs of 300 to 600 seconds). Other investigators demonstrated significant reductions in hemorrhagic complications during and after cardiopulmonary bypass in patients who underwent ACT-guided as opposed to empiric heparin administration. In an attempt to establish a safe-threshold ACT value above which thrombus formation did not occur in the cardiopulmonary bypass circuit, Young et al. (20) determined ACT values in nine rhesus monkeys during 2 hours of cardiopulmonary bypass. Fibrin monomers were detected during the first 30 minutes of bypass in six of nine animals, and in five of these six, ACT was less than 400 seconds. Interestingly, based primarily on the results of this small observational animal study, a threshold ACT of more than 400 seconds gained general acceptance as the appropriate target during cardiopulmonary bypass.

Heparin Dosing during PTCA

ACT monitoring during coronary angioplasty first emerged in the mid-to-late 1980s. Based on the surgical experience, recommended target ACT levels for balloon angioplasty were empirically set at 300 or 350 seconds by various authors. The first systematic study of the relationship between the degree of heparin anticoagulation as assessed by ACT and acute complications during angioplasty was undertaken by

Ferguson and colleagues (5) at the Texas Heart Institute. These investigators retrospectively compared ACT values between 103 patients who experienced major procedural complications (defined as death or emergency or urgent bypass surgery) and 400 patients with uncomplicated angioplasties. It was found that patients who experienced a complication were significantly more likely to have had an ACT (Hemo-Tec) of less than 250 seconds at the onset of the procedure than were patients who underwent uncomplicated PTCA (61% versus 27%, $p < .0001$). Furthermore, complications occurred in *all* patients with final (immediate post-procedure) ACTs less than 250 seconds, but in only 0.3% with a final ACT greater than 300 seconds.

Harrington et al., using data available from the CAVEAT study, demonstrated a significant relationship between a higher "ACT index" (defined as the minimum procedural ACT adjusted by the total heparin dose administered, body weight, and procedure length) and procedural success in patients undergoing either balloon angioplasty or directional coronary atherectomy. The ACT index was likewise associated with a reduced incidence of ischemic complications, including myocardial infarction, emergency bypass surgery, abrupt vessel closure, or postintervention thrombus.

In attempt to (a) further support a relationship between the degree of heparin anticoagulation and abrupt closure during balloon angioplasty and (b) establish an optimal target ACT value for angioplasty, investigators from Duke University (6) compared Hemochron ACT values between 62 patients with documented abrupt closure and 124 matched controls who did not experience abrupt closure. Relative to the control population, patients who developed abrupt closure had significantly lower ACTs at the time of initial balloon inflation (350 seconds versus 380 seconds, $p = .004$) and minimum intraprocedural ACTs (345 seconds versus 370 seconds, $p = .014$). Among this population, a strong inverse linear relationship existed between ACT and the probability of abrupt closure, such that no threshold ACT was evident above which a further increase in the degree of anticoagulation

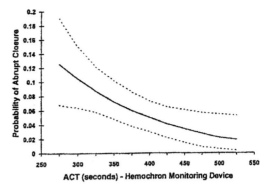

FIG. 31.2. The probability of abrupt closure (with 95% confidence intervals) as a function of the initial procedural ACT. (From ref. 6, with permission.)

would not be associated with a further reduction in the probability of abrupt closure (Fig. 31.2).

Whereas the risk of abrupt closure appears to fall with progressive increases in ACT, evidence likewise exists to suggest that the incidence of bleeding complications rises as the level of heparin anticoagulation is increased. Among 438 patients undergoing elective or urgent angioplasty, Hillegass et al. (21) found maximum in-laboratory ACT to be a significant independent predictor of procedurally related bleeding complications. Similarly, in a retrospective analysis of 5,042 patients who underwent balloon or new-device angioplasty at Emory University (22), total intraprocedural heparin dose emerged as a significant independent predictor for vascular complications, although ACT values were not reported.

Continuation of Heparin Postprocedure

The role of continued intravenous heparin therapy following successful balloon angioplasty remains uncertain. McGarry et al. (23), in an observational report of 363 patients who received a heparin infusion for 18 to 24 hours following successful angioplasty, noted a four-fold increase in abrupt closure rates prior to hospital discharge in patients who did not achieve an aPTT value of greater than or equal to three times control while receiving heparin. Ellis et al. (24), however, in a randomized trial of an 18- to 24-hour heparin infusion following PTCA (goal aPTT of 1.5 to 2.5 times control), did not observe a difference in postprocedure abrupt closure rates between heparin and placebo-treated patients (1.8% versus 2.4%, respectively). Heparin administration was, however, associated with a twofold increase in major bleeding events (8.2% versus 3.9%). The lack of acute benefit of postprocedural heparin has been supported by two additional randomized trials (25,26), and, because a prolonged heparin infusion delays arterial sheath removal, this approach has been associated with an increased risk of vascular complications. While the risks of routine heparin therapy following successful angioplasty appear to outweigh any potential benefits, the utility of postprocedural heparin when a suboptimal angiographic result persists following PTCI remains less certain.

HEPARIN DOSING WITH GP IIB/IIIA RECEPTOR ANTAGONIST THERAPY

In the EPIC trial, administration of abciximab in conjunction with standard-dose heparin (target ACT of 300 to 350 seconds) and aspirin resulted in a 35% relative reduction in short-term (30-day) ischemic complications relative to treatment with heparin and aspirin alone in high-risk patients undergoing either balloon angioplasty or directional atherectomy (3). While associated with this dramatic reduction in thrombotic complications, the benefits of abciximab administration in this study population were ameliorated by a threefold increase in major bleeding complications (10.6% in patients treated with abciximab bolus plus 12-hour infusion versus 3.3% in the placebo group, $p <$ .001). On logistic regression analysis, the maximum in-laboratory ACT served as one of several significant independent predictors of bleeding events (Table 31.1) (27).

In light of the substantial increase in bleeding complications associated with abciximab in EPIC, the EPILOG study attempted to determine if the incidence of hemorrhagic events could be reduced via improved heparin dosing and earlier

TABLE 31.1. *Factors associated with bleeding and/or vascular complications in the EPIC trial*

Abciximab therapy
Acute myocardial infarction at enrollment
High baseline hematocrit
Procedural length
Heavier weight
Female gender
Maximum in-laboratory ACT
Sheath size
Older age

From ref. 27, with permission.

vascular sheath removal, without compromising treatment efficacy (4). In EPILOG, 2,792 high- and low-risk patients undergoing coronary angioplasty were randomized to one of three treatment arms: (a) abciximab bolus and 12-hour infusion with standard dose heparin (100-U per kilogram bolus), (b) abciximab bolus/infusion with low dose heparin (70 U per kilogram), or (c) placebo plus standard heparin. In addition, contrary to the EPIC trial protocol, which mandated a 12-hour heparin infusion with similarly delayed sheath removal following the intervention, no further heparin was administered following angioplasty in EPILOG, and the arterial sheath was removed during the abciximab infusion (as soon as ACT fell below an acceptable threshold).

Compared with placebo, patients in EPILOG who received abciximab and low-dose heparin experienced a reduction in the composite 6-month endpoint of death, myocardial infarction, or repeat revascularization (25.8% versus 22.8%, $p =$ .034) and, surprisingly, a trend toward *reduced* major bleeding complications (3.1% versus 1.8%). The results of this trial emphasize the critical importance of reduced heparin administration and early sheath removal when abciximab is used. Since the publication of the EPILOG trial, many practitioners at the Cleveland Clinic have continued to reduce the dose of heparin used in conjunction with abciximab, administering initial heparin boluses in the 50- to 70-U per kilogram range, with a goal procedural ACT of 220 to 250 seconds.

Although the efficacy of abciximab administration as a ''bailout'' therapy remains unproved, this agent is occasionally administered in the midst of a complicated angioplasty procedure after large doses of heparin have already been given. Because of the profound association between abciximab, high ACT, and bleeding complications, Kereiakes et al. (28) have proposed a strategy of protamine administration to partially reverse heparin's effects when abciximab is administered on a ''rescue'' basis. Among a group of ten patients (none of whom were insulin-dependent diabetics), an average of 20 mg of protamine was given immediately following the abciximab bolus, resulting in a reduction in mean ACT from 378 to 221 seconds. No ischemic or major bleeding complications occurred in this small cohort.

HEPARIN DOSING DURING STENT IMPLANTATION

Whereas the incidence of abrupt vessel closure typically ranged from 4% to 8% among studies performed in the pre-stent era, with approximately half of these patients requiring emergency bypass surgery, the availability of coronary stents has dramatically improved the safety of PTCI. For example, in the BENESTENT-II trial, which randomized 827 patients to heparin-coated stent implantation or balloon angioplasty, among patients in the stent arm the angiographic success rate was 99%, emergency bypass surgery was required in 0.7%, and subacute stent thrombosis occurred in only 0.2%. While no systematic evaluation of the relationship between ACT and ischemic complications during stent implantation has been performed, given the reduced rate of such events in patients treated with stents, it would be expected that the incremental value of heparin in preventing thrombotic events during planned stent implantation would be decreased relative to balloon angioplasty. However, given the inverse relationship between ACT and abrupt closure during balloon angioplasty, it would be reasonable to assume that adequate heparin therapy in conjunction with a strategy of optimal balloon dilatation would reduce the need for bailout stent deployment.

ANTICOAGULATION IN PATIENTS WITH HEPARIN-INDUCED THROMBOCYTOPENIA

Heparin-induced thrombocytopenia (HIT) is an uncommon but potentially devastating immunologically mediated complication of heparin therapy. This idiosyncratic syndrome results from the development of an IgG antibody that recognizes the circulating heparin–platelet factor-4 complex, and leads to the development of simultaneous thrombocytopenia and platelet activation. HIT is associated with an estimated 30% to 50% risk of clinically manifest thrombotic events, and the occurrence of such events heralds a mortality rate of approximately 30% (29). In patients with a documented history of HIT, the management of anticoagulation during PTCI remains problematic. Several alternative pharmacotherapeutic agents to unfractionated heparin have been isolated or developed, but large-scale safety and efficacy data are currently lacking, and the availability of most agents for commercial use in the United States remains restricted.

Of foremost importance, when a patient with prior HIT comes to coronary angiography or intervention, it is essential that heparin is eliminated from all flush solutions and that it not be added to the radiographic contrast material. In addition, platelet transfusions are contraindicated in the setting of ongoing HIT, as hemorrhagic complications are uncommon and transfusions may precipitate arterial thrombosis.

Among potential alternatives to heparin, three agents appear to hold promise for use during coronary intervention in patients with a history of HIT (Table 31.2). The direct thrombin inhibitor hirudin and its synthetic analogue hirulog do not cross-react with the HIT antibody, and the efficacy of these agents during PTCA has been demonstrated. The relative safety of hirudin in the setting of HIT was suggested by a preliminary report of 82 affected patients who were treated with this agent. Refludin, a form of hirudin, has recently become approved and is commercially available for treatment of patients with HIT. Argatroban (Novastatin, Texas Biotech-

TABLE 31.2. *Potential anticoagulants for coronary intervention in patients with heparin-induced thrombocytopenia*

Anticoagulant with HIT antibody	Primary mechanism	Potential cross-reactivity
Hirudin/hirulog	Direct thrombin inhibition	No
Argatroban	Direct thrombin inhibition	No
Danaproid sodium	Factor Xa inhibition	Yes
Low-molecular-weight heparin	Antithrombin III potentiation	Yes

nology Corp.), a synthetic agent that, similar to hirudin, blocks the catalytic site on thrombin, represents a second anticoagulant that may be efficacious in the setting of HIT. Case reports have suggested the potential safety of this agent during PTCI , and a well-orchestrated, open-label trial of this agent during coronary intervention among patients with HIT is nearing completion. Finally, several experts regard the low-molecular-weight heparinoid danaproid sodium (Orgaron, Orgaron Pharmaceuticals) to be the anticoagulant of choice in patients with ongoing or prior HIT (30). This agent, which is available in the United States on a compassionate-use basis, achieves anticoagulation primarily via inhibition of factor Xa activity (the ACT assay is therefore insensitive to its effects). Because it possesses structural similarities to heparin, however, cross-reactivity with the HIT antibody does occur in an estimated 10% to 20% of patients treated with danaproid sodium.

LMWH, an agent that is currently available, has been used safely in patients with HIT undergoing PTCI. The potential for cross-reactivity is, however, believed to be greater with LMWH than with the three agents discussed earlier. It has been recommended that LMWH be used clinically only if the potential for cross-reactivity is first excluded by an *in vitro* platelet-inhibition assay employing serum from the affected patient. The use of GP IIb/IIIa receptor antagonist therapy either alone or in conjunction with a reduced dose of one of the previously mentioned alternate anticoagulant agents holds intrinsic appeal, but it cannot be recommended given a current lack of clinical data.

CONCLUSIONS AND RECOMMENDATIONS

Based on the clinical and observational trial information currently available, the following practical guidelines have evolved at the Cleveland Clinic as a means to guide heparin dosing during percutaneous coronary revascularization. If the patient is receiving continuous heparin therapy prior to the intervention, the infusion is discontinued on arrival to the catheterization laboratory, and baseline ACT is determined immediately after arterial access is obtained. The heparin dosing strategy is then determined primarily based on whether concomitant GP IIb/IIIa receptor antagonist therapy is to be administered. If abciximab use is planned and baseline ACT is less than 150 seconds, heparin is given in a bolus dose of 50 to 70 U per kilogram body weight, with a target ACT of 220 to 250 seconds (using the Hemochron device). This initial dose is reduced accordingly if baseline ACT is elevated. It is important to recall that abciximab itself will elicit an approximate 20-second (HemoTec) to 40-second (Hemochron) increase in ACT. Thus, if baseline ACT exceeds 200 seconds in patients who have received heparin prior to arrival in the catheterization laboratory, an additional heparin bolus at the start of the intervention may be unnecessary. ACT should be determined approximately 5 minutes after administration of the GP IIb/IIIa receptor antagonist bolus and prior to instrumenting the coronary artery, to ensure adequate anticoagulation.

If GP IIb/IIIa receptor antagonist therapy use is not planned and baseline ACT is not elevated, the initial dose of heparin is increased to 100 U per kilogram body weight. ACT is checked 2 to 5 minutes after the heparin bolus, and a target ACT of more than 350 seconds is maintained, although even higher ACTs may provide additional advantages. Once the target level of anticoagulation has been achieved, additional ACTs are checked on a 30-minutes basis throughout the procedure, and additional heparin boluses are administered as required to maintain ACT in the target range. If abciximab is required on a ''bailout'' basis, ACT is determined. If ACT is below 300, abciximab is administered. If ACT is greater than 300, the need for abciximab is reevaluated. When it is felt by they operator that (a) the potential benefits of abciximab outweigh the potential bleeding risks and (b) risk factors for a protamine reaction are absent (primarily the presence of insulin-requiring diabetes), incremental doses of protamine can be administered following the abciximab bolus to reduce the ACT to below 300 seconds.

Following the intervention, early removal of the arterial sheath is performed whenever possible as a means to reduce vascular access site complications. Serial ACTs are performed on the cardiac ward, and the sheath is removed when ACT has fallen to less than 170 seconds. The sheath can be safely removed while continuing the abciximab infusion. The potential benefits of percutaneous arterial closure devices, which permit sheath removal immediately following the procedure while the patient remains fully anticoagulated, remain to be established.

REFERENCES

1. Schwartz L, Bourassa MG, Lesparance J, et al. Aspirin and dipyridamole in the prevention of restenosis after percutaneous transluminal coronary angioplasty. *N Engl J Med* 1988;318:1714–1719.
2. Bertrand ME, Allain H, LaBlanche JM. Results of a randomized trial of ticlopidine versus placebo for prevention of acute closure and restenosis after coronary angioplasty: The TACT study. *Circulation* 1990; 82[Suppl 3]:190.
3. The EPIC Investigators. Use of a monoclonal antibody directed against the platelet glycoprotein IIb/IIIa receptor in high-risk coronary angioplasty. *N Engl J Med* 1994;330:956–961.
4. The EPILOG Investigators. Platelet glycoprotein IIb/IIIa receptor inhibition with abciximab with lower heparin dosages during percutaneous coronary revascularization. *N Engl J Med* 1997; 336:1689–1696.
5. Ferguson JJ, Dougherty KG, Gaos CM, Bush HS, Marsh KC, Leachman DR. Relation between procedural activated clotting time and outcome after percutaneous transluminal coronary angioplasty. *J Am Coll Cardiol* 1994;23:1061–1065.
6. Narins CR, Hillegass WB, Nelson CL, et al. Relation between activated clotting time during angioplasty and abrupt closure. *Circulation* 1996;93:667–671.
7. Dougherty KG, Gaos CM, Bush HS, Leachman R, Ferguson JJ. Activated clotting time and activated partial thromboplastin times in patients undergoing coronary angioplasty who receive bolus doses of heparin. *Cathet Cardiovasc Rev* 1992;26:260–263.
8. Bowers J, Ferguson JJ III. The use of activated clotting time to monitor heparin therapy during and after interventional procedures. *Clin Cardiol* 1994;17:357–361.
9. Avendano A, Ferguson JJ. Comparison of Hemochron and HemoTec activated coagulation time target values during percutaneous transluminal coronary angioplasty. *J Am Coll Cardiol* 1994;23:907–910.
10. Simko RJ, Tsung FFW, Stanek EJ. Activated clotting time versus activated partial thromboplastin time for therapeutic monitoring of heparin. *Ann Pharmacother* 1995;29:1015–1021.
11. Grill HP, Spero JE, Granato JE. Comparison of activated partial thromboplastin time to activated clotting time for adequacy of heparin anticoagulation just before percutaneous transluminal coronary angioplasty. *Am J Cardiol* 1993;71:1219–1220.
12. Reiner JS, Coyne KS, Lundergan CF, Ross AM. Bedside monitoring of heparin therapy: comparison of activated clotting time to activated partial thromboplastin time. *Cathet Cardiovasc Diagn* 1994;32:49–52.
13. Greiber S, Weber S, Galle J, Bramer P, Schollmeyer P. Activated clotting time is not a sensitive parameter to monitor anticoagulation with low molecular weight heparin in hemodialysis. *Nephron* 1997;76:15–19.
14. Topol EJ, Bonan R, Jewitt D, et al. Use of a direct antithrombin, hirulog, in place of heparin during coronary angioplasty. *Circulation* 1993;87:1622–1629.
15. Moliterno DJ, Califf RM, Aguirre FV, et al. Effect of platelet glycoprotein IIb/IIIa integrin blockade on activated clotting time during percutaneous transluminal coronary angioplasty or directional atherectomy (the EPIC trial). *Am J Cardiol* 1995;75:559–562.
16. Ammar T, Scudder LE, Coller BS. In vitro effects of the platelet glycoprotein IIb/IIIa receptor antagonist c7E3 Fab on the activated clotting time. *Circulation* 1998;95:614–617.
17. Rath B, Bennett DH. Monitoring the effect of heparin by measurement of activated clotting time during and after percutaneous transluminal coronary angioplasty. *Br Heart J* 1990;63:18–21.
18. Kerensky RA, Azar GJ, Bertolet B, Hill JA, Kutcher MA. Venous activated clotting time after intra-arterial heparin: effect of site of administration and timing of sampling. *Cathet Cardiovasc Diagn* 1996;37:151–153.
19. Bull BS, Korpman WM, Huse WM, Briggs BD. Heparin therapy during extracorporeal circulation: I. Problems inherent in existing heparin protocols. *J Thorac Cardiovasc Surg* 1975;69:674–684.
20. Young JA, Kisker CT, Doty DB. Adequate anticoagulation during cardiopulmonary bypass determined by activated clotting time and the appearance of fibrin monomer. *Ann Thorac Surg* 1978;26:231–240.
21. Hillegass WB, Brott BC, Narins CR, et al. Predictors of blood loss and bleeding complications after angioplasty. *J Am Coll Cardiol* 1994;23[Suppl A]:69A.
22. Waksman R, King SB III, Douglas JS, et al. Predictors of groin complications after balloon and new-device coronary intervention. *Am J Cardiol* 1995;75:886–889.
23. McGarry TF, Gottlieb RS, Morganroth J, et al. The relationship of anticoagulation level and complications after successful percutaneous transluminal coronary angioplasty. *Am Heart J* 1992;123:1445–1451.

24. Ellis SG, Roubin GS, Wilentz J, Douglas JS, King SB III. Effect of 18- to 24-hour heparin administration for prevention of restenosis after uncomplicated coronary angioplasty. *Am Heart J* 1989;117:777–782.

25. Moscucci M, Mansour KA, Kent C, et al. Peripheral vascular complications of directional coronary atherectomy and stenting: predictors, management, and outcome. *Am J Cardiol* 1994;74:448–453.

26. Popma JJ, Satler LF, Pichard AD, et al. Vascular complications after balloon and new device angioplasty. *Circulation* 1993;88:1569–1578.

27. Blankenship JC, Hellkamp AS, Aguirre FV, Demko SL, Topol EJ, Califf RM. Vascular access site complications after percutaneous coronary intervention with abcixi-mab in the Evaluation of 7E3 for the Prevention of Ischemic Complications (EPIC) trial. *Am J Cardiol* 1998; 81:36–40.

28. Kereiakes DJ, Broderick TM, Whang DD, Anderson L, Fye D. Partial reversal of heparin anticoagulation by intravenous protamine in abciximab-treated patients undergoing percutaneous intervention. *Am J Cardiol* 1997;82:633–634.

29. Brieger DB, Mak K-H, Kottke-Marchant C, Topol EJ. Heparin-induced thrombocytopenia. *J Am Coll Cardiol* 1998;31:1449–1459.

30. Warkentin TE. Heparin-induced thrombocytopenia: pathogenesis, frequency, avoidance and management. *Drug Saf* 1997;17:325–341.

32

Adjunctive Therapy: ADP Antagonists

David R. Holmes, Jr.

Division of Cardiovascular Diseases and Internal Medicine, Mayo Clinic and Mayo Foundation, Department of Medicine, Mayo Medical School, Rochester, Minnesota 55905

Adjunctive therapy for interventional cardiology has assumed increasing importance as the number of agents has increased and the scientific database has expanded. Some of the adjunctive agents are specifically used in the setting of stent implantation (e.g. ticlopidine or clopidogrel), while others may have more general applications (low molecular weight heparin or IIb/IIIa drugs).

ASPIRIN

Aspirin has been the core of antiplatelet therapy since the beginning of interventional cardiology. All patients should receive it prior to the procedure and indefinitely afterwards, unless there is a contraindication to its use. Schwartz et al. randomized 376 patients undergoing percutaneous transluminal angioplasty to either aspirin and dipyridamole or placebo and found a significant reduction in periprocedural Q-wave myocardial infarction in the aspirin and dipyridamole group (1.6% versus 6.9%, p = .011). White et al. randomized 333 patients to placebo, aspirin, and dipyridamole, or ticlopidine prior to angioplasty and found that the two active treatment groups had significantly fewer complications. Barnathan et al. performed a retrospective analysis of patients taking aspirin alone, aspirin and dipyridamole, or no aspirin. Using multivariate analysis, he found that antiplatelet therapy was associated with improved outcome.

Although early studies evaluated the combination of aspirin and dipyridamole, the latter has not been found to provide incremental benefit over aspirin alone. Accordingly, dipyridamole is no longer used.

The specific dose of aspirin required is not clear. Initial studies utilized high dosage (990 mg per day). Given the frequency of side-effects at higher doses, these are not used. There have been concerns raised about bioavailability and steady-state concentrations. In addition, up to 25% of patients can be classified as "nonresponders." It is preferable to start aspirin 24 hours prior to the procedure. Given the enthusiasm for *ad hoc* dilatation, this may not be feasible. If a patient has not received aspirin within the past 24-hours, four chewable baby aspirin are given at the time of dilatation. During follow-up we traditionally use 325 mg daily. In patients who have an aspirin allergy, we would use an alternative agent, either ticlopidine or clopidogrel, and a IIb/IIIa drug.

TICLOPIDINE

The role of ticlopidine has assumed increasing importance in interventional cardiology since the widespread use of stents. It is a thienopyridine derivative that requires metabolic activation in the liver. It is a noncompetitive and selective antagonist of ADP-induced platelet aggregation. It has been shown to be effective in high-risk patients, including those with cerebrovascular disease and transient ischemic attacks or stroke as well as peripheral vascular or ischemic heart disease. In patients at high risk for stroke, it has been found to be more effective in preventing all course mortality than aspirin.

In the early days of stent use, in an attempt to decrease stent thrombosis, aspirin, low-molecular-weight dextran, dipyridamole, intravenous heparin, and warfarin were all used. This regimen was associated with increased bleeding and long hospital stays. The seminal ISAR trial also found that this regimen was associated with more subacute closure than a combination of aspirin and ticlopidine. Using the aspirin-ticlopidine combination, subsequent randomized trials have documented subacute closure rates of less than 2%.

Ticlopidine is not without risk and has relatively frequent side effects, including diarrhea and rash. The most serious problems are hematologic. It has been associated with a small incidence of thrombotic thrombocytopenia purpura, which has major morbidity including neurologic abnormalities in 75% of patients and mortality of approximately 20%. A more frequent but still significant problem is neutropenia, which can also be life threatening. Early studies of stent patients with ticlopidine continued the treatment for 4 to 6 weeks. Because of the potential for neutropenia, which can occur in approximately 1% of patients treated for more than 2 weeks, serial white blood counts were usually recommended.

The need for these 4 to 6 week ticlopidine courses has since been evaluated. We found that in the era of high-pressure balloon inflation and aspirin-plus-ticlopidine treatment, subacute closure did not occur in any patient after 14 days. Accordingly, we modified our practice to use a 500-mg loading dose of ticlopidine immediately prior to the procedure (along with aspirin), then 250 mg ticlopidine twice a day for 2 weeks only. A total of 827 patients undergoing successful stent placement in 1,061 segments were analyzed. Stents were placed electively in 51% of those patients, for treatment of dissection or abrupt closure in 31%, and for treatment of suboptimal PTCA results in 18%. In this experience, adverse cardiac events within 14 days of stent implantation occurred in 11 patients (1.3%). Between 15 and 30 days there were no cardiovascular deaths, infarctions, coronary surgical operations, or repeat revascularizations. In the group who received ticlopidine for two weeks only, no neutropenia developed in any patient. We concluded that the risk of stent thrombosis after 2 weeks of aspirin and ticlopidine therapy is less than the 1% risk of ticlopidine-induced neutropenia when ticlopidine is continued for more than 2 weeks. One group of patients may need longer treatment with a thienopyridine. This is the group of patients treated with radiation for prevention or treatment of stenosis. In these patients, there may be delayed re-endothelialization of the stented surface. Current protocols call for these patients to be treated with ticlopidine for approximately 6 weeks.

CLOPIDOGREL

A new thienopyridine derivative, clopidogrel, is now available. It has been tested in animal models of platelet-dependent arterial thrombosis and has been found to have a more rapid onset of action than ticlopidine, after an initial loading dose. It was developed to provide a treatment that causes less bone-marrow suppression and fewer other side-effects. The CAPRIE Study of 19,185 patients with atherosclerotic cerebrovascular, peripheral vascular, or coronary artery disease found that 75 mg clopidogrel every day was more effective than 325 mg aspirin in reducing the combined incidence of ischemic stroke, infarction, or vascular death. The rate of severe neutropenia with long-term clopidogrel use was only 0.055%, similar to the rate with aspirin (0.04%). The incidence of severe rash and diarrhea with clopidogrel was less that that reported with ticlopidine.

Because of the improved profile of clopidogrel, it has been tested in observational studies of interventional cardiology patients. From our institution, Berger et al. evaluated 500 conservative stent patients treated with ticlopidine plus aspirin. Subacute closure occurred in 0.2% of clopidogrel-plus-aspirin patients, versus 0.7% in ticlopidine-plus-aspirin patients. The composite endpoint of death, death and myocardial infarction, or CABG or repeat PTCA occurred in 0.8% of the clopidogrel group and 1.6% of the ticlopidine group ($p = .23$). This combination was also evaluated by Moussa in 283 patients compared with 1,406 patients treated with ticlopidine plus aspirin. At 1 month, they found no difference in in-stent thrombosis (1.5% versus 1.4%). The clopidogrel patient group had fewer side effects; neutropenia did not occur in the clopidogrel group.

The specific optimal dosing schedule of clopidogrel remains to be determined. In both of the observational studies above, a loading dose of 300 mg clopidogrel was used. This has been found to provide 80% platelet inhibition in 5 hours. We have followed this loading dose with 75 mg for 14 days—similar to the 14 days of ticlopidine that we used in the past. This has been associated with an excellent outcome, although no randomized trial data exist.

SUMMARY

Antiplatelet agents are essential for the practice of interventional cardiology, both conventional PTCA as well as stent implantation. Aspirin should be given to all patients. In stent patients, there is clear data, from randomized trials, that ticlopidine is required to optimize results. In our practice, when ticlopidine is used, 500 mg is used as a loading dose followed by 250 mg twice a day for 2 weeks. Because of concern about bone-marrow suppression, there is increasing interest in clopidogrel. In observational studies, clopidogrel given as a 300-mg loading dose, followed by 75 mg per day, results in an excellent outcome, at least as good as a ticlopidine outcome, but with fewer side effects.

SUGGESTED READINGS

1. Popma JJ, Bittl JA, Ohman EM et al. Antithrombotic therapy in patients undergoing coronary angioplasty. *Chest* 1998.
2. Schwartz L, Bornassa MG, Lesperance J et al. Aspirin and dipyridamole in the prevention of restenosis after percutaneous transluminal coronary angioplasty. *New Engl J Med* 1988;318:1714–1719.
3. White CW, Chartman B, Lassar TA et al. Antiplatelet agents are effective in reducing the immediate complications of percutaneous transluminal coronary angioplasty. Results of the ticlopidine multicenter trial. *Circulation* 1987;76:IV-400(abst).
4. Barnathan ES, Schwartz JS, Taylor L et al. Aspirin and dipyridamole in the prevention of acute coronary thrombosis complicating coronary angioplasty. *Circulation* 1987;76:125–134.
5. Berger PB, Bell MR, Hasdai D et al. Safety and efficacy of ticlopidine for only two weeks after successful intracoronary stent placement. *Circulation* 1999;99:248–253.
6. Schomig A, Newmann FJ, Kastrati A et al. A randomized comparison of antiplatelet and anticoagulant therapy after the placement of coronary artery stents. *New Engl J Med* 1996;334:1084–1089.
7. Bennett CL. Thrombotic thrombocytopenia purpura. *J Am Coll Cardiol* 1999;33A.
8. Moussa I, Oetgen M, Roubin G et al. The effectiveness of Clopidogrel and aspirin versus ticlopidine and aspirin in preventing stent thrombosis after coronary stent placement. *Circulation* (*in press*).
9. Leon MB, Baim DS, Popma JJ et al. A clinical trial comparing three antithrombotic drug regimens after coronary artery stenting. *New Engl J Med* 1998;339:1665–1671.

33

Glycoprotein IIb/IIIa Antagonists

A. Platelet Glycoprotein IIb/IIIa Receptor Antagonists During Percutaneous Coronary Revascularization

A. Michael Lincoff

Department of Cardiology, Center of the Ohio State University, The Cleveland Clinic Foundation, Cleveland, Ohio 44195-5066

Plaque rupture and vascular thrombosis are key initiating factors in the pathogenesis of ischemic complications of percutaneous coronary revascularization (1,2). The central role of platelet activity in this setting is highlighted by the unequivocal benefit of aspirin in the preventing death or myocardial infarction (MI) among patients undergoing coronary intervention (3). Newer strategies for more potent inhibition of platelet activity at the injured coronary plaque focus on the integrin glycoprotein (GP) IIb/IIIa receptor ($\alpha_{IIb}\beta_3$) on the platelet surface membrane, which binds circulating fibrinogen or von Willebrand factor and cross-links adjacent platelets as the final common pathway to platelet aggregation (4). A new class of pharmacologic compounds directed against GP IIb/IIIa block this receptor, prevent binding of circulating adhesion molecules, and potently inhibit platelet aggregation.

THE AGENTS

Three intravenous GP IIb/IIIa antagonists have undergone large-scale Phase III and Phase IV trial evaluation in the setting of percutaneous coronary revascularization, and all are currently approved by the US Food and Drug Administration (FDA) for clinical use. *Abciximab* (c7E3 Fab, ReoPro, Centocor, Malvern, PA), the first agent of this class, is a human-murine chimeric monoclonal Fab antibody fragment that binds with high affinity and a slow dissociation rate to the GP IIb/IIIa receptor (5,6). Abciximab is cleared rapidly from the plasma, but remains bound to circulating platelets for as long as 21 days (7). Binding of abciximab is not specific for the platelet GP IIb/IIIa receptor; this agent has equal affinity for the vitronectin receptor ($\alpha_v\beta_3$), which appears to play a role in cell adhesion, migration, and proliferation. *Eptifibatide* (Integrilin, COR Therapeutics, South San Francisco, CA), a cyclic heptapeptide based on the Lys-Gly-Asp (KGD) amino acid sequence, is a highly specific, competitive inhibitor of the GP IIb/IIIa complex. Blockade of the receptor by eptifibatide is rapidly reversible, with a plasma half-life in humans of about 2.5 hours (8). *Tirofiban* (Aggrastat, Merck,White House Station, NJ) is a tyrosine-derivative, nonpeptide mimetic inhibitor of GP IIb/IIIa, which also specifically and competitively binds to the receptor in a rapidly reversible fashion (9) and has a short (approximately 1.6 hours) serum half-life. Platelet aggregation is inhibited by all of these agents in a dose-related manner, with nearly complete abolition of platelet thrombosis at levels of receptor occupancy greater than 80% (6). After discontinuation of abciximab, platelet aggregation returns toward baseline over the subsequent 12 to 36 hours (6), while normalization of platelet function occurs much more quickly (over 30 minutes to 4 hours) following discontinuation of the reversible eptifibatide or tirofiban (8,9).

INITIAL PIVOTAL TRIALS OF AGENTS DURING CORONARY INTERVENTION

The EPIC Trial

Proof of concept that GP IIb/IIIa inhibition would diminish ischemic complications of percutaneous coronary revascularization was provided by the first Phase III study of this class of agents, the EPIC (Evaluation of c7E3 Fab for Prevention of Ischemic Complications) trial, leading to the clinical approval of abciximab. This trial evaluated the efficacy of two dosing strategies of abciximab versus placebo among patients considered to be at high risk for coronary intervention on the basis of acute ischemic syndromes or clinical and angiographic characteristics (10). A total of 2,099 patients were enrolled, received aspirin and heparin (10,000 to 12,000 U to maintain an activated clotting time [ACT] greater than 300 to 350 seconds), and were randomized in a double-blind fashion to placebo, abciximab 0.25-mg per kilogram bolus, or abciximab 0.25-mg per kilogram bolus followed by a 10-μg per minute infusion for 12 hours. Heparin infusion was continued, and vascular access sheaths remained in place for the 12-hour duration of study drug.

The primary efficacy endpoint was a composite of death, MI (defined by new Q waves or CK-MB isoenzyme elevation to greater than or equal to three times the control value), urgent repeat revascularization, or stent or balloon pump placement by 30 days following randomization. This composite event rate was reduced from 12.8% among patients receiving placebo to 11.4% among patients receiving the abciximab bolus (10% relative risk reduction, $p = .43$) and to 8.3% among patients receiving the abciximab bolus and 12-hour infusion (35% relative risk

reduction, $p = .008$) (Fig. 33.1, Table 33.1). Although the treatment effect of abciximab was present in all subgroups, certain patients appeared to derived enhanced benefit (11,12). Most notably, among those with unstable angina (postinfarction, rest, or refractory angina with transient ischemic electrocardiographic changes), the composite endpoint rate was decreased by 71% with abciximab; the most serious endpoints of death or MI were reduced by 94% (11.1% in the placebo group versus 0.6% in the abciximab bolus and infusion group; $p < .001$) (11).

The clinical efficacy of abciximab in EPIC was maintained at 6-month and 3-year clinical follow-up (13,14). Moreover, abciximab was associated with a reduction in the need for target-vessel revascularization procedures, from 22.3% among patients receiving placebo to 16.5% among those receiving the bolus and infusion of abciximab (26% relative risk reduction, $p = .007$) at 6 months, a finding that led to speculation that this agent may reduce restenosis following coronary intervention. There was a trend toward decreased mortality by abciximab over 3 years in the overall cohort, with a more marked 60% reduction in late death by abciximab among the 555 highest risk patients who had been enrolled with unstable angina or acute MI (12.7% versus 5.1% in the placebo and abciximab bolus and infusion groups, respectively; $p = .01$).

Hemorrhagic complications were significantly increased by abciximab, raising concerns regarding the potential clinical utility of this form of therapy. Compared with placebo, the bolus and infusion of abciximab resulted in a doubling in the rates of major bleeding (7% versus 14%, $p = .001$) and red blood cell transfusions (7% versus 15%, $p < .001$) (10). Conjunctive heparin therapy appeared to have played a key role in the pathogenesis of bleeding among these patients (15). Heparin dosages in EPIC were not weight adjusted, and a relationship was observed between the risk of bleeding and lighter body weight (and hence, relative "overdosage" of heparin on a per-weight basis). Moreover, major bleeding rates were strongly correlated with total heparin dose and the intensity of anticoagulation (as measured by peak

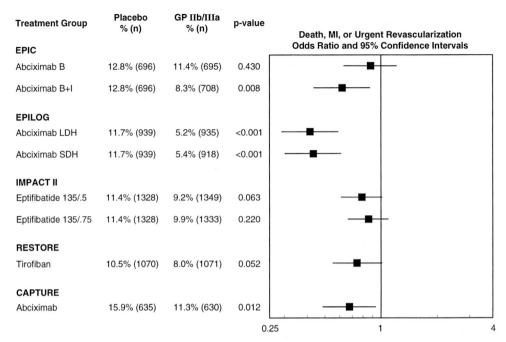

Treatment Group	Placebo % (n)	GP IIb/IIIa % (n)	p-value
EPIC			
Abciximab B	12.8% (696)	11.4% (695)	0.430
Abciximab B+I	12.8% (696)	8.3% (708)	0.008
EPILOG			
Abciximab LDH	11.7% (939)	5.2% (935)	<0.001
Abciximab SDH	11.7% (939)	5.4% (918)	<0.001
IMPACT II			
Eptifibatide 135/.5	11.4% (1328)	9.2% (1349)	0.063
Eptifibatide 135/.75	11.4% (1328)	9.9% (1333)	0.220
RESTORE			
Tirofiban	10.5% (1070)	8.0% (1071)	0.052
CAPTURE			
Abciximab	15.9% (635)	11.3% (630)	0.012

FIG. 33.1. Composite 30-day endpoint (death, MI, or urgent repeat revascularization) event rates for the five initial pivotal trials of GP IIb/IIIa receptor blockade during coronary intervention. RESTORE Trial endpoints listed here are for the published post hoc analysis including only *urgent* repeat revascularization for consistency with the other trials (The prespecified primary composite endpoint of RESTORE included *urgent or elective* repeat revascularization). RESTORE trial endpoints listed here differ from those of the other trials in that only patients with successful crossing of the lesion with the guidewire were included in the efficacy analysis of RESTORE, providing a "treated patient" analysis rather than the "intention-to-treat" analysis utilized in the other studies. B, bolus; B + I, bolus plus infusion; LDH, low-dose, weight-adjusted heparin; MI, myocardial infarction; SDH, standard-dose, weight-adjusted heparin; 135/0.5 and 135/0.75, eptifibatide doses (see text). (Reprinted from Lincoff AM. Trials of platelet glycoprotein IIb/IIIa receptor antagonists during percutaneous coronary revascularization. *Am J Cardiol* 1998;82:36P–42P, with permission.)

ACT) during the interventional procedure. The subsequent pilot PROLOG study suggested that bleeding associated with abciximab might be attenuated by using lower, weight-adjusted doses of heparin as well as by early removal of the vascular sheath (during infusion of abciximab) to eliminate the need for postprocedural heparin infusion (16).

The EPILOG Trial

The EPILOG (Evaluation in PTCA to Improve Long-term Outcome with abciximab GP IIb/IIIa blockade) trial was designed to determine if the clinical benefits of abciximab therapy could be extended to all patients undergoing cor-

onary intervention, regardless of their risk of ischemic complications, and to evaluate whether the incidence of hemorrhagic complications could be reduced without loss of efficacy by weight adjustment or reduction in heparin dose (17). Only the highest risk patients with acute MI or unstable angina with electrocardiographic changes were excluded, based on the profound clinical benefit derived from abciximab among this subgroup in EPIC. Patients received aspirin and were randomized in a double-blind fashion to placebo with standard-dose, weight-adjusted heparin (bolus 100 U per kilogram, adjusted to ACT greater than 300 seconds); abciximab bolus and 12-hour infusion with standard-dose, weight-adjusted heparin; or abciximab bolus and

TABLE 33.1. *Thirty-day efficacy endpoint events in the initial pivotal trials of GP IIb/IIIa blockade during coronary intervention*

	Death (%)	MI (%)	Urgent PCI (%)	Urgent CABG (%)
EPIC trial				
Placebo	1.7	8.6	4.5	3.6
Abciximab bolus	1.3	6.2	3.6	2.3
Abciximab bolus + infusion	1.7	5.2	0.8	2.4
EPILOG trial				
Placebo	0.8	8.7	3.8	1.7
Abciximab + reduced heparin	0.3	3.7	1.2	0.4
Abciximab + standard heparin	0.4	3.8	1.5	0.9
IMPACT II trial				
Placebo	1.1	8.1	2.8	2.8
Eptifibatide 135/0.5 dose	0.5	6.6	2.6	1.6
Eptifibatide 135/0.75 dose	0.8	6.9	2.9	2.0
RESTORE trial[a]				
Placebo	0.7	5.7	4.0	1.4
Tirofiban	0.8	4.2	2.3	1.1
CAPTURE trial				
Placebo	1.3	8.2	4.4	1.7
Abciximab	1.0	4.1	3.1	1.0

[a] RESTORE trial endpoints listed here are for the published post hoc analysis including only *urgent* repeat revascularization for consistency with the other trials. The primary composite endpoint of RESTORE included *urgent or elective* repeat revascularization. RESTORE trial endpoints listed here differ from those of the other trials in that only patients in whom the lesion was successfully crossed with the guidewire were included in the efficacy analysis of RESTORE, providing a "treated patient" analysis rather than the "intention-to-treat" analysis utilized in the other studies.

PCI, percutaneous coronary intervention; CABG, coronary artery bypass graft.

12-hour infusion with low-dose, weight-adjusted heparin (bolus 70 U per kilogram, adjusted to ACT greater than 200 seconds). Postprocedural heparin was discouraged, and vascular sheaths were to be removed within 2 to 6 hours (during the abciximab infusion). Planned enrollment was 4,800 patients, but the trial was terminated at an enrollment of 2,792 patients after an unexpectedly strong clinical benefit was observed at the first interim analysis.

Patients representing a broad spectrum of risk strata and clinical indications for revascularization were enrolled in the trial. The incidence of the primary composite endpoint of death, MI, or urgent revascularization at 30 days was 11.7% in the placebo group, 5.2% in the abciximab with low-dose heparin group (56% relative risk reduction, $p < .0001$), and 5.4% in the abciximab with standard-dose heparin group (54% relative reduction, $p < .0001$) (see Fig. 33.1). Each of the components of the composite endpoint was similarly reduced (see Table 33.1), and the treatment effect of abciximab with either heparin regimen was homogeneous across all patient groups. At 6-month and 1-year follow-up, the suppression of acute ischemic events was maintained without attenuation; in contrast to the findings of EPIC, however, rates of repeat target-vessel revascularization in EPILOG converged after 30 days, indicating no effect of abciximab on the incidence of "clinical restenosis."

Hemorrhagic complications in EPILOG occurred infrequently and were not increased by abciximab therapy. Major bleeding occurred in 3.1%, 2.0%, and 3.5% of patients randomized to placebo, abciximab with low-dose heparin, and abciximab with standard-dose heparin, respectively. When compared with the experience in EPIC, bleeding in EPILOG was reduced in both placebo and abciximab groups, likely as a consequence of weight adjustment and reduction of heparin dosing and early vascular sheath removal. The treatment effect of abciximab in reducing ischemic complications was enhanced in EPILOG compared with EPIC (56% and 35% relative reductions, respectively, in the risk of the primary 30-day efficacy endpoint), suggesting that elimination of excess bleeding permits the full potential benefit of this form of therapy to be realized.

The IMPACT II Trial

The IMPACT II (Integrilin to Minimize Platelet Aggregation and Coronary Thrombosis-II) trial evaluated the peptide inhibitor eptifibatide among 4,010 patients undergoing elective, urgent, or emergency coronary revascularization (18). After receiving aspirin and heparin (bolus 100 U per kilogram, adjusted to achieve an ACT greater than 300 seconds), patients were randomized to placebo, eptifibatide 135 μg per kilogram bolus followed by an infusion of 0.5 μg per kilogram per minute for 20 to 24 hours ("135/0.5 group"), or eptifibatide 135 μg per kilogram bolus followed by an infusion of 0.75 μg per kilogram per minute for 20 to 24 hours ("135/0.75 group"). Postprocedural heparin was discouraged, and vascular sheaths were to be removed within 4 to 6 hours.

The primary composite endpoint of death, MI, urgent revascularization, or stent placement for abrupt closure by 30 days occurred in 11.4% of patients in the placebo group, 9.2% of patients in the 135/0.5 group (19% relative risk reduction, $p = .063$), and 9.9% of patients in the 135/0.75 group (16% relative risk reduction, $p = .22$) (see Fig. 33.1, Table 33.1). Baseline characteristics or risk stratification were not predictive of treatment effect. Over 6 months of follow-up, the differences in death and MI rates observed at 30 days were maintained, although there were no differences in rates of revascularization. An angiographic substudy of approximately 900 patients demonstrated no effect of eptifibatide on angiographic restenosis. Treatment with eptifibatide was not associated with an increased risk of major bleeding or transfusions.

The RESTORE Trial

The RESTORE (Randomized Efficacy Study of Tirofiban for Outcomes and REstenosis) trial tested the nonpeptide GP IIb/IIIa antagonist tirofiban among 2,139 patients undergoing coronary

intervention for unstable angina or acute MI (19). Patients received aspirin and were randomized after successful passage of the guidewire across the target lesion to receive placebo or tirofiban (10 μg per kilogram bolus, then 0.15 μg per kilogram per minute infusion). Because of the rapidly reversible nature of tirofiban binding to the GP IIb/IIIa receptor, the study drug infusion was prolonged to 36 hours to achieve approximately the same duration of platelet inhibition as that obtained with the 12-hour abciximab infusion in EPIC and EPILOG. Heparin was administered with a 10,000-U bolus, adjusted to an ACT of 300 to 400 seconds; postprocedural heparin was discouraged, and sheaths were removed following the procedure.

The primary efficacy endpoint was the composite of death, MI, repeat target-lesion percutaneous revascularization, coronary artery bypass surgery, or stent implantation by 30 days (this endpoint in RESTORE differed slightly from that of EPIC, EPILOG, IMPACT II, and CAPTURE, in that the latter trials considered only *urgent* revascularization of the target or any other vessel). The composite endpoint occurred in 12.2% of patients in the placebo group and in 10.3% of patients in the tirofiban group (16% relative risk reduction, $p = .16$). With a post hoc reclassification of revascularization events to allow comparison with the other trials, the 30-day composite of death, MI, or urgent revascularization was 10.5% for the placebo group and 8.0% in the tirofiban group (24% relative risk reduction, $p = .052$) (see Fig. 33.1, Table 33.1). The trend toward benefit with tirofiban was present regardless of the indication for revascularization. Follow-up over 6 months demonstrated no attenuation in the reduction in death or MI, although no significant differences in rates of target-vessel revascularization were observed. An angiographic substudy of approximately 600 patients demonstrated no effect of tirofiban on angiographic measurements of restenosis. Bleeding complications were not significantly different in the placebo and tirofiban groups (major bleeding in 3.7% and 5.3%, respectively; $p = .096$).

The CAPTURE Trial

CAPTURE (C7E3 Anti Platelet Therapy in Unstable REfractory angina) differed from the four other initial pivotal trials, in that CAPTURE evaluated a strategy of *pretreatment* with abciximab prior to percutaneous revascularization among patients with refractory unstable angina. Patients qualified for enrollment if they had unstable angina with episodes of chest pain and ischemic electrocardiographic changes despite therapy with intravenous heparin and nitroglycerin and had been demonstrated on angiography to have a lesion suitable for coronary angioplasty. All patients received aspirin and were randomized to placebo or abciximab for 18 to 24 hours prior to angioplasty and continued for 1 hour after completion of the procedure (CAPTURE was designed and initiated before the findings of EPIC regarding the importance of a 12-hour postprocedural abciximab infusion were fully appreciated). Heparin was administered, and vascular sheaths remained in place from enrollment throughout the pretreatment phase and until at least 1 hour after angioplasty. Planned sample size was 1,400 patients, but the trial was stopped with 1,266 patients on the basis of efficacy at the third interim analysis.

The primary composite endpoint of death, MI, or urgent revascularization by 30 days occurred in 15.9% of patients in the placebo group and in 11.3% of patients in the abciximab group (29% relative risk reduction, $p = .012$), due primarily to reduction in MI (see Fig. 33.1, Table 33.1). Clinical benefit of abciximab began to accrue during the pretreatment phase before the angioplasty procedure, with the preprocedural MI rate reduced from 2.1% among control patients to 0.6% among those treated with abciximab ($p = .029$). Rates of major bleeding were significantly increased among patients receiving abciximab, from 1.9% to 3.8% (excluding coronary artery bypass graft [CABG]-associated bleeding, $p = .043$). Over 6 months of follow-up, the incidences of death or revascularization were not different among placebo- and abciximab-treated patients. The treatment effect of abciximab on MI rates persisted by 6 months but was some-

what attenuated. Such attenuation over long-term follow-up is in contradistinction to the experience in the other GP IIb/IIIa trials during coronary intervention, and may be related to the severity of the acute ischemic syndrome or to inadequacy of a 1-hour postprocedural abciximab infusion in CAPTURE.

EXTENDING THE INDICATIONS

Primary Angioplasty for Acute MI: The RAPPORT Trial

The role of abciximab therapy among patients undergoing direct or primary angioplasty for acute MI was evaluated in RAPPORT (ReoPro in Acute MI Primary PTCA Organization and Randomization Trial). A total of 483 patients undergoing angioplasty within 12 hours of onset of symptoms were randomized to receive placebo or abciximab (bolus and 12-hour infusion) in addition to aspirin and heparin (100 U per kilogram) (20). The primary endpoint of death, recurrent MI, or any (elective or urgent) repeat target-vessel revascularization by *6 months* was not different in the two treatment groups (28.1% and 28.2% among patients randomized to placebo and abciximab, respectively), owing to the absence of an effect of abciximab therapy on long-term revascularization procedures. The composite endpoint of death, reinfarction, or urgent repeat target-vessel revascularization (comparable to the primary endpoint used in the other trials) was significantly reduced by abciximab from 11.2% to 5.8% at 30 days (48% relative risk reduction, $p = .038$). Hemorrhagic complications were increased by abciximab in RAPPORT (major bleeding rates were 9.5% in the placebo group and 16.6% in the abciximab group, $p = .02$), likely as a result of the relatively high heparin doses and long vascular access sheath dwell times (median, 19 hours).

Elective Stenting: The EPISTENT Trial

The introduction of GP IIb/IIIa receptor blockade into clinical interventional practice was paralleled by the widespread acceptance of elective coronary stenting as a safe and effective means of reducing revascularization rates following percutaneous interventions. All of the initial pivotal studies of GP IIb/IIIa blockade had excluded enrollment of patients undergoing elective stent implantation, reserving the use of stents for "bailout" indications. The EPIS-TENT (Evaluation of Platelet Inhibition in STENTing) trial was designed to evaluate the clinical benefit of abciximab therapy in reducing ischemic complications among patients undergoing elective stent implantation, as well as to assess the clinical efficacy of abciximab (with balloon angioplasty) relative to stenting. Patients were eligible for inclusion if they had at least one target lesion suitable for allocation to either stenting or balloon angioplasty and were not undergoing primary intervention in the setting of acute MI. A total of 2,399 patients were enrolled, treated with aspirin, and randomized to receive stent plus placebo, balloon angioplasty plus abciximab (bolus and 12-hour infusion), or stent plus abciximab. Stent implantation in the balloon angioplasty plus abciximab group was to be reserved for clear "bailout" indications (rather than suboptimal results) and was performed in only 19% of patients randomized to angioplasty. Patients randomized to receive abciximab were treated with the EPILOG low-dose, weight-adjusted heparin regimen (70 U per kilogram bolus, ACT greater than 200 seconds), while those receiving placebo were treated with standard-dose, weight-adjusted heparin (100 U per kilogram, ACT greater than 300 seconds). Ticlopidine was administered following stent placement.

A broad spectrum of patients was enrolled in this study, representing "real world" coronary stenting rather than the ideal or narrow subgroups assessed in previous stent versus balloon angioplasty trials. The primary efficacy composite endpoint of death, MI, or urgent repeat revascularization occurred in 10.8% of patients in the stent plus placebo arm, 6.9% of patients in the balloon plus abciximab arm (36% relative risk reduction, $p = .007$), and 5.3% of patients in the stent plus abciximab arm (51% relative risk reduction, $p < .001$). Compared with stenting alone, adjunctive use of abciximab with stenting reduced the rates of death, MI (particularly Q-wave and large non–Q-wave infarction), and repeat revascularization. Compared with stenting alone, abciximab with balloon angioplasty was associated with equivalent rates of death and revascularization, but greater safety with regard to lower rates of MI. Treatment effect of abciximab was present in all patient subgroups. No increase in hemorrhagic complications (and a trend toward reduced risk for major bleeding) was observed in patients receiving abciximab relative to placebo.

Two principal endpoints were predefined for assessment at 6 months: (a) a composite of death or MI and (b) the incidence of repeat target-vessel revascularization. The incidence of death or MI was 11.4% in the stent plus placebo group, 5.6% in the stent plus abciximab group ($p < .001$), and 7.8% in the PTCA plus abciximab group ($p = .013$), a durable treatment effect maintained since 30 days. Mortality was significantly reduced by stenting compared with percutaneous transluminal coronary angioplasty (PTCA) among patients receiving abciximab (0.5% versus 1.8%, $p = .018$). Rates of repeat target-vessel revascularization (percutaneous or surgical) were 10.6% in the stent plus placebo group, 8.7% in the stent plus abciximab group ($p = .216$), and 15.4% in the PTCA plus abciximab group ($p = .005$). Among stented patients, treatment with abciximab rather than placebo was associated with a nonsignificant trend toward reduced rates of target vessel revascularization (18% relative risk reduction, $p = .215$). In patients with diabetes, repeat target-vessel revascularization rates following stent implantation were significantly reduced by abciximab; stenting alone (with placebo) did not reduce the incidence of subsequent target-vessel revascularization procedures compared with PTCA, whereas the rate of this endpoint was halved by the combination of abciximab and stenting. Findings of an angiographic substudy were concordant with the clinical findings of target-vessel revascularization. Among the overall cohort of patients in the trial, stenting with abciximab was associated with trends toward better angiographic luminal dimensions and significantly better net gain than was stenting with placebo, while patients with diabetes had significant improvements in follow-up minimum luminal diameters and net gain with abciximab instead of placebo with stenting.

Coronary Intervention in Trials of Unstable Angina

Four large-scale trials have assessed GP IIb/IIIa inhibition among patients with unstable angina or non–Q-wave MI in whom percutaneous revascularization was not mandated. In two of these trials, PURSUIT (Platelet glycoprotein IIb/IIIa in Unstable angina: Receptor Suppression Using Integrilin Therapy) and PRISM PLUS (Platelet Receptor Inhibition in Ischemic Syndrome Management in Patients Limited by Unstable Signs and Symptoms), a substantial number of patients underwent early coronary intervention while on study drug infusion, providing important information regarding the efficacy of these agents as preprocedural and postprocedural therapy. In PURSUIT, 9,461 patients were randomized to receive placebo or eptifibatide (180 μg per kilogram bolus, then 2.0 μg per kilogram per minute infusion for 72 to 96 hours) in addition to heparin or aspirin, of whom, 1,228 underwent percutaneous revascularization within the first 72 hours (while receiving study drug) (21). Eptifibatide was associated with a significant reduction in the risk of MI prior to the revascularization procedure (5.5% versus 1.8%, $p < .001$), as well as a significant reduction in the composite endpoint of death or MI by 30 days (16.8% versus 11.8%, 30% relative risk reduction, $p = .01$). In PRISM PLUS, 1,570 patients were treated with placebo or tirofiban (0.4 μg per kilogram per minute for 30 minutes, then 0.1-μg per kilogram per minute infusion for 48 to 96 hours in addition to aspirin and heparin) (22). Catheterization and percutaneous revascularization were encouraged, but were to be deferred for 48 hours, and 475 patients underwent coronary intervention while receiving study drug. During the first 48 hours (before intervention), death or MI rates were reduced from 2.6% to 0.9% by tirofiban in the overall 1,570-patient cohort ($p = .01$); among the 475 patients undergoing intervention, 30-day rates of death or MI were 10.2% and 5.9% in the placebo and tirofiban groups, respectively (42% relative risk reduction, $p = .12$).

SYNTHESIS OF THE RANDOMIZED TRIALS

Efficacy

The consistent finding among over 15,000 patients enrolled in the trials of GP IIb/IIIa receptor blockade during coronary intervention has been that of reduction in the risk of important acute ischemic events by as much as 50% to 60%, unequivocally establishing the clinical efficacy of this class of therapy in this setting (see Fig. 33.1). This treatment effect extends to each of the components of the composite clinical endpoints (death, MI, and emergency revascularization) (see Table 33.1), attesting to the common platelet–thrombus-mediated pathophysiology of these events. The inhibition of acute ischemic events is achieved early, primarily in the first 12 to 48 hours after the revascularization procedure, and is almost invariably maintained without attenuation over long-term (up to 3-year) follow-up.

Improved outcome with this therapy has been apparent in every subgroup of patients tested, and no demographic, clinical, angiographic, or procedural characteristic has been observed that will identify patients who do *not* benefit from GP IIb/IIIa blockade. Patients with acute ischemic syndromes such as unstable angina, however, appear to derive exceptional treatment effect from this class of therapy. Other subsets of patients who are at increased risk for acute ischemic events, such as those requiring bailout stenting (23) or with diabetes (24), also tended to experience a enhanced absolute treatment effect from GP IIb/IIIa inhibition.

Clinical benefit is derived from GP IIb/IIIa blockade irrespective of the technique or modality used for percutaneous coronary revascularization. The EPISTENT trial clearly demonstrated a magnitude of treatment effect with abciximab during elective stenting (absolute risk reduction of 5.5%, relative risk reduction of 51%) that was essentially identical to that obtained with abciximab during balloon angioplasty in EPILOG (absolute risk reduction of 6.4%, relative risk reduction of 56%). Similarly, subgroup analysis of patients in EPIC and EPILOG undergoing directional atherectomy confirmed previous findings that atherectomy patients are at substantially greater risk for ischemic complications than are their counterparts treated with angioplasty, and that the treatment effect of abciximab during atherectomy tended, if anything, to be greater than during balloon angioplasty (25). The decision to utilize these agents during a revascularization procedure thus should not be made contingent on whether balloon angioplasty, stent implantation, or atherectomy is planned.

The influence of GP IIb/IIIa blockade on restenosis remains uncertain. Although a significant reduction by abciximab in long-term target-vessel revascularization rates was observed in the EPIC trial, this treatment effect was not confirmed in the subsequent trials of abciximab during balloon angioplasty. Moreover, angiographic substudies of IMPACT II and RESTORE did not detect an influence of GP IIb/IIIa blockade on angiographic restenosis following angioplasty. In contrast, however, the 6-month findings of EPISTENT suggest that abciximab may inhibit the neointimal hyperplastic component of in-stent restenosis. Target-vessel revascularization rates and angiographic parameters of restenosis trended toward improvement among patients receiving abciximab rather than placebo with stenting. Strikingly, diabetic patients receiving stents, a group in whom increased neointimal hyperplasia has been observed (26,27), had marked and statistically significant improvements in repeat target-vessel revascularization rates and angiographic restenosis with abciximab.

Differences in Efficacy among the GP IIb/IIIa Antagonists

Although all three of the agents tested in large-scale trials (abciximab, eptifibatide, and tirofiban) reduce ischemic risk, there does appear to be heterogeneity among the drugs with regard to the magnitude of treatment effect. The bolus followed by a 12-hour infusion regimen of abciximab was demonstrated to reduce 30-day endpoints by as much as 50% to 60% in the EPILOG, RAPPORT, and EPISTENT trials, while more modest risk reductions on the order of 15% to 25% were achieved with eptifibatide and tirofiban in IMPACT II and RESTORE. Importantly, definitive assessment of the magnitude of the differences among these agents is limited by the lack of direct comparative trials, which are unlikely to ever be performed. Nevertheless, based on indirect comparisons, the differences in treatment effects may be real and clinically relevant. Variability in efficacy may in part be due to the pharmacodynamics of receptor binding. Abciximab dissociates slowly from the GP IIb/IIIa receptor, thus providing gradually diminished inhibition of platelet aggregation for 36 hours or more after termination of drug infusion (6,7); in contrast, platelet aggregation following discontinuation of the rapidly reversible agents (eptifibatide and tirofiban) is normalized within 2 to 4 hours (8,9). Additionally, the nonspecific blockade by abciximab of both the platelet GP IIb/IIIa receptor and the $\alpha_v\beta_3$ vitronectin receptor may provide an advantage over the specific agents, as *ex vivo* experimental studies have suggested that dual-receptor blockade more completely suppresses platelet-mediated thrombin generation than does inhibition of either receptor alone (28).

For eptifibatide, the relatively modest treatment effect in the IMPACT II trial was almost certainly due at least in part to inadequate dosing based on Phase II studies using sodium citrate as an anticoagulant for platelet aggregation studies. Subsequent to IMPACT II, it was observed that the binding of eptifibatide to GP IIb/IIIa was exaggerated in blood anticoagulated by citrate (which chelates calcium) relative to that which would occur at physiologic calcium concentrations (29). Doses of eptifibatide used in IMPACT II thus likely achieved only 30% to 40% inhibition of platelet aggregation *in vivo*. The potential for higher doses of eptifibatide to more effectively reduce ischemic complications is suggested by the greater treatment effect among the subgroup of patients in the PURSUIT trial who underwent early percutaneous coronary revascularization (described previously). Importantly, however, patients undergoing coronary intervention with tirofiban in the PRISM PLUS trial also had a more substantial treatment effect than was seen with the same drug (at essentially the same dose) in RESTORE. Thus, a prolonged duration of treatment (72 hours or more), perhaps with a period of preprocedural therapy, may be required for the rapidly reversible agents to have an optimal effect on reduction of ischemic endpoints.

Safety

The major potential safety issue with this as well as other classes of agents directed against platelet function or coagulation is that of bleeding. The findings of the first trial of this class of therapy, EPIC, highlighted the potential for hemorrhagic risk with these agents. Most bleeding with GP IIb/IIIa antagonists in this and subsequent trials has been at sites of vascular access, although spontaneous gastrointestinal and genitourinary bleeding also occurs; long-term sequelae have been infrequent. Importantly, pooled analysis of the trials indicates that rates of intracranial hemorrhage do *not* appear to be increased. The remarkable improvement in the safety profile of these agents subsequent to the EPIC experience clearly shows that modification of conjunctive anticoagulant therapy with heparin by weight adjustment and dose reduction is the key intervention in abrogating excess bleeding risk. Early removal of vascular sheaths and meticulous care of the access site are also likely important means of avoiding hemorrhage. Bleeding may nevertheless be a concern in certain groups of patients, such as those who receive GP IIb/IIIa blockade as an unplanned or bailout intervention in the setting of full-dose heparinization or those undergoing "rescue" angioplasty for failed reperfusion after full-dose thrombolysis. Partial reversal of heparinization with protamine in the former situation and very careful heparin dose reduction and ACT monitoring in the latter will likely improve the balance between risk and benefit in these patients.

There is often considerable concern on the part of cardiac surgeons regarding the risk of excessive perioperative bleeding among patients who require emergency coronary artery bypass surgery for failed angioplasty after administration of a GP IIb/IIIa inhibitor. These concerns are understandable, given that noncardiologists rarely have substantial direct experience with this new class of agents. In this regard, the rapidly reversible agents eptifibatide and tirofiban present little in the way of perioperative bleeding risk; platelet aggregation and bleeding times return to normal within a few hours following discontinuation of both of these agents, which is the time period required for coronary artery bypass to be performed. For patients treated with abciximab, the ability to neutralize the antiplatelet effect by transfusion of mixed donor platelets (following discontinuation of abciximab infusion) ameliorates most, if not all, of the hemorrhagic risk. Because some data suggest that GP IIb/IIIa blockade may actually be *protective* of platelets during cardiac surgery, with less thrombocytopenia following cardiopulmonary bypass (30), it seems reasonable to defer platelet transfusions if possible until after the cardiopulmonary bypass is completed. Platelet transfusions are also helpful among patients who develop refractory or life-threatening bleeding complications following abciximab therapy.

Thrombocytopenia occurs infrequently following GP IIb/IIIa inhibition, but may be profound (platelet count less than 20,000 mm^{-3}); the excess risk of profound thrombocytopenia associated with abciximab (approximately 0.4% to 1.0%) appears to higher than with eptifibatide or tirofiban. The mechanism of development of thrombocytopenia is unknown. Thrombocytopenia occurring after administration of a GP IIb/IIIa agent can usually be differentiated from that due to the heparin-induced thrombocytopenia syndrome by the early and precipitous onset, generally within the 1 to 24 hours after administration of the GP IIb/IIIa inhibitor (31). There is little evidence of ongoing platelet clearance following discontinuation of the GP IIb/IIIa antagonist, and most patients experience an increase in platelet count of about 20,000 to 30,000 mm^{-3} per day (the rate of bone marrow production). Unlike heparin-induced thrombocytopenia, platelet transfusions are a safe and protective therapy for profound thrombocytopenia with or without serious bleeding induced by GP IIb/IIIa inhibitors. It is thus of critical importance that platelet counts be measured early (within the first 2 to 4 hours) and again approximately 12 hours after administering these agents, in order to detect this rare, potentially life-threatening but manageable complication.

The development of a human antichimeric antibody (HACA) response in approximately 5% to 6% of patients within the first month after receiving abciximab raises the question of safety of readministration of this agent. No antibodies have been observed to develop in response to treatment with eptifibatide or tirofiban. A prospective abciximab readministration registry has found no instances of hypersensitivity or anaphylactic reactions following abciximab readministration, and efficacy of the agent in reducing ischemic complications appears to be similar with readministration as with first-time use (32). Rates of thrombocytopenia following readministration were somewhat higher, however, than those seen with first time administration, although the presence or absence of a positive HACA titer was not predictive of a lack of clinical effectiveness, development of thrombocytopenia, or other sequelae in patients undergoing readministration.

Economics

An important factor that appears to limit the widespread use of these agents is that of cost. Abciximab is expensive to produce, and the average (weight-adjusted) dose (bolus plus 12-hour infusion) of this agent costs approximately $1,400. Prices for eptifibatide and tirofiban are lower, approximately $300 per day, although the optimal duration of therapy for these latter drugs is not defined. Cost–benefit analyses for these agents are difficult to perform, as there exist no widely accepted benchmarks for acceptable cost for prevention of ischemic events other than death. It is important to recognize, however, that drug price does not reflect the true economic cost of these therapies, as the prevention of ischemic events by GP IIb/IIIa blockade translates

into cost savings. In both EPIC and EPILOG, for example, the prevention of ischemic events by abciximab was associated with $600 to $700 cost savings during the hospitalization period (33). In EPIC, cost savings from suppression of ischemic events were offset by the increased incidence of bleeding complications; in contrast, in EPILOG, in which bleeding risk was not increased, the net hospitalization cost per patient for abciximab therapy was only approximately $600. Among the highest risk patients undergoing revascularization for unstable angina in EPIC, abciximab therapy was actually *cost saving*, and thus the "dominant strategy" (11).

RECOMMENDATIONS

Who to Treat

From a scientific standpoint, the extensive body of randomized data with this class of agents indicates that virtually all patients undergoing percutaneous coronary revascularization should receive a GP IIb/IIIa receptor antagonist. In clinical practice, however, these agents are not universally utilized, primarily due to economic considerations. Despite these constraints, it seems imperative to at least provide the marked benefits of this class of therapy to patients who are at elevated risk for periprocedural complications—most importantly those with the acute ischemic syndromes of unstable angina or MI, but also those with complex lesion morphology, extensive myocardium at jeopardy, multivessel or multilesion interventions, or unplanned bailout stent implantation. As stated earlier, the elective use of stents should not be considered as a replacement for GP IIb/IIIa receptor blockade in high-risk patients.

In many centers and countries, abciximab is utilized primarily in an unplanned or bailout fashion as a strategy to reduce overall costs for this agent. Although anecdotal data suggest that abciximab is useful in reversing thrombotic complications of coronary intervention (34), this approach has never been tested in a randomized fashion. It is apparent that bailout abciximab administration does not completely reverse the increased ischemic risk in these complicated patients and that bleeding complications are likely to be relatively high due to full-dose heparinization. Until systematically investigated, such a strategy must therefore be regarded as suboptimal relative to planned or prophylactic use of GP IIb/IIIa receptor blockade. The planned CACHET study will evaluate the efficacy of provisional abciximab therapy superimposed on optimal antithrombin coverage with hirulog instead of heparin.

Which Agent to Use

Aside from the economic considerations, the available data consistently suggest that the current efficacy standard for GP IIb/IIIa blockade during and after percutaneous coronary intervention is abciximab administered as a bolus followed by a 12-hour infusion. A pretreatment regimen of abciximab, as was utilized in CAPTURE, is effective in stabilizing patients prior to coronary revascularization, but offers no clear advantage in stable patients or even in unstable patients for whom revascularization can be immediately performed. Regardless of whether a period of pretreatment with abciximab is used, the 12-hour postprocedural infusion appears to be mandatory for optimal passivation of the revascularized lesion.

For patients presenting with unstable angina or non–Q-wave MI in whom revascularization is not immediately planned, both eptifibatide and tirofiban have been unequivocally shown to improve clinical outcome prior to intervention, following intervention, or in patients treated conservatively without early intervention. Once a course of empiric therapy with eptifibatide or tirofiban has been initiated, it is unclear whether patients would experience substantial incremental benefit by conversion to abciximab during subsequent percutaneous coronary revascularization, as the treatment effects of eptifibatide and tirofiban in PURSUIT and PRISM PLUS were considerable in these patients. If eptifibatide is employed during coronary intervention, the available pharmacodynamic and clinical data

(see previously) strongly suggest that the PURSUIT dose of a 180-μg per kilogram bolus and a 2.0-μg per kilogram per minute infusion be utilized, rather than the lower doses employed in IMPACT II.

Conjunctive Heparin Therapy and Vascular Access Management

The low-dose, weight-adjusted heparin regimen, using an initial bolus of 70 U per kilogram (maximum 7,000 U) adjusted to attain and maintain an ACT greater than 200 seconds, has clearly been shown to be the safest and most effective means of administering heparin when abciximab therapy is planned (Table 33.2).

TABLE 33.2. *Recommended algorithm of low-dose, weight-adjusted heparin administration during therapy with abciximab or other GP IIb/IIIa receptor antagonists during coronary intervention*

1. Heparin initial bolus dose: 70 U/kg (maximum, 7,000 U).
2. Measure ACT after *both* initial heparin bolus and GP IIb/IIIa agent bolus have been administered (as both heparin and GP IIb/IIIa agents influence ACT value).
3. Target ACT is >200 seconds (by Hemochron machine).
4. If ACT is >200 seconds, proceed with coronary intervention.
5. If ACT is <200 seconds, administer additional 20-U/kg heparin boluses, measure ACT after each bolus, and readminister 20-U/kg boluses until ACT is >200 seconds.
6. If patient enters the catheterization laboratory on a preprocedural heparin infusion, modify initial bolus as follows:
   Check ACT after administering GP IIb/IIIa agent, but before heparin bolus.
   If ACT = 150–199 seconds: Initial heparin bolus = 50 U/kg
   If ACT is <150 seconds: Initial heparin bolus = 70 U/kg (≤7,000 U)
7. After the procedure begins, measure ACT every 30 minutes until completed, with 20-U/kg heparin reboluses as necessary to maintain ACT >200 seconds. Alternatively, a heparin infusion at a rate of 7 U/kg/min can be administered during the procedure.
8. Postprocedural heparin is rarely indicated. If postprocedural heparin is desired, do not remove vascular sheath during heparin infusion. Set initial heparin infusion rate at 7 U/kg/h, with adjustment according to activated partial thromboplastin time to maintain a value of 45 to 55 seconds while GP IIb/IIIa infusion is ongoing.

There are no data to suggest that postprocedural heparin provides additional benefit in this setting, even in patients treated for acute ischemic syndromes; vascular access sheaths can typically be removed 2 to 6 hours after the procedure, during the abciximab infusion, once the ACT is less than 175 seconds or the activated partial thromboplastin time is less than 50 seconds. Manual or mechanical groin compression should be maintained for at least 30 minutes, followed by strict bed rest with leg immobilization for 6 to 8 hours after sheath removal. The use of femoral artery closure devices in patients treated with abciximab has not yet been extensively investigated but appears to be promising. Other measures to help reduce bleeding risk at the vascular access site include anterior arterial puncture only (rather than the traditional Seldinger through-and-through technique), avoidance of routine venous sheath placement, and adequate patient sedation and immobilization during periods of strict bed rest.

Optimal heparin dosing during coronary intervention in patients treated with eptifibatide and tirofiban has not been investigated. The higher bleeding rates observed with eptifibatide in PURSUIT as compared with IMPACT II, as well as favorable preliminary experience with high-dose eptifibatide and reduced-dose heparin during coronary intervention in the ongoing Phase II PRIDE study, suggest that intraprocedural heparin doses should be weight adjusted and reduced with eptifibatide and tirofiban in manner similar to that with abciximab.

Finally, many laboratories routinely employ a "standard-dose" weight-adjusted heparin regimen (100-U per kilogram, maximum 10,000-U, initial bolus, adjusted to attain and maintain target ACT greater than 300 seconds) among patients undergoing percutaneous coronary intervention for whom abciximab therapy is *not* planned. With this strategy, bleeding risk may be reduced if abciximab or other GP IIb/IIIa inhibitors are required on a bailout basis, as very high ACT levels (greater than 400 seconds) are usually avoided.

SUMMARY

Platelet GP IIb/IIIa inhibition represents one of the most significant advances in the practice of interventional cardiology. Large-scale randomized, controlled trials have unequivocally demonstrated that these agents reduce the risk of periprocedural ischemic complications by up to 50% to 60% and are efficacious in a broad spectrum of patients undergoing revascularization irrespective of risk profile, clinical indication for revascularization, or interventional technique. This clinical benefit may be achieved without excess bleeding risk by modification of conjunctive heparin dosing. Issues for future study include critical evaluation of the medicoeconomic aspects of this therapy, the effectiveness of these agents when used in an unplanned or bailout fashion, the role of oral GP IIb/IIIa antagonists currently under evaluation in extending the clinical benefit achieved by periprocedural parenteral administration, and the potential for combining GP IIb/IIIa antagonists with novel inhibitors of thrombin or other components of the coagulation cascade.

REFERENCES

1. Steele PM, Chesebro JH, Stanson AW, et al. Balloon angioplasty. Natural history of the pathophysiological response to injury in a pig model. *Circ Res* 1985;57: 105–112.
2. Uchida Y, Hasegawa K, Kawamura K, Shibuya I. Angioscopic observation of the coronary luminal changes induced by percutaneous transluminal coronary angioplasty. *Am Heart J* 1989;117:769–776.
3. Schwartz L, Bourassa MG, Lesperance J, et al. Aspirin and dipyridamole in the prevention of restenosis after percutaneous transluminal coronary angioplasty. *N Engl J Med* 1988;318:1714–1719.
4. Phillips DR, Charo IF, Parise LV, Fitzgerald LA. The platelet membrane glycoprotein IIb/IIIa complex. *Blood* 1988;71:831–843.
5. Coller BS. Blockade of platelet GPIIb/IIIa receptors as an antithrombotic strategy. *Circulation* 1995;92: 2373–2380.
6. Tcheng JE, Ellis SG, George BS, et al. Pharmacodynamics of chimeric glycoprotein IIb/IIIa integrin antiplatelet antibody Fab 7E3 in high-risk coronary angioplasty. *Circulation* 1994;90:1757–1764.
7. Mascelli MA, Lance ET, Damaraju L, Wagner CL, Weisman HF, Jordan RE. Pharmacodynamic profile of short-term abciximab treatment demonstrates prolonged platelet inhibition with gradual recovery from GP IIb/IIIa receptor blockade. *Circulation* 1998;97:1680–1688.
8. Harrington RA, Kleiman NS, Kottke-Marchant K, et al. Immediate and reversible platelet inhibition after intra-

venous administration of a peptide glycoprotein IIb/IIIa inhibitor during percutaneous coronary intervention. *Am J Cardiol* 1995;76:1222–1227.

9. Kereiakes DJ, Kleiman NS, Ambrose J, et al. Randomized, double-blind, placebo-controlled dose-ranging study of tirofiban (MK-383) platelet IIb/IIIa blockade in high risk patients undergoing coronary angioplasty. *J Am Coll Cardiol* 1996;27:536–542.

10. EPIC Investigators. Use of a monoclonal antibody directed against the platelet glycoprotein IIb/IIIa receptor in high-risk coronary angioplasty. *N Engl J Med* 1994; 330:956–961.

11. Lincoff AM, Califf RM, Anderson KM, et al. Evidence for prevention of death and myocardial infarction with platelet membrane glycoprotein IIb/IIIa receptor blockade by c7E3 Fab (abciximab) among patients with unstable angina undergoing percutaneous coronary revascularization. *J Am Coll Cardiol* 1997;30: 149–156.

12. Lefkovits J, Ivanhoe R, Anderson K, Weisman H, Topol EJ. Platelet IIb/IIIa receptor inhibition during PTCA for acute myocardial infarction: insights from the EPIC trial. *Circulation* 1994;90:I-564(abst).

13. Topol EJ, Califf RM, Weisman HS, et al., for the EPIC Investigators. Reduction of clinical restenosis following coronary intervention with early administration of platelet IIb/IIIa integrin blocking antibody. *Lancet* 1994;343: 881–886.

14. Topol EJ, Ferguson JJ, Weisman HF, et al., for the EPIC Investigator Group. Long-term protection from myocardial ischemic events in a randomized trial of brief integrin $\beta 3$ blockade with percutaneous coronary intervention. *JAMA* 1997;278:479–484.

15. Aguirre FV, Topol EJ, Ferguson JJ, et al., for the EPIC Investigators. Bleeding complications with the chimeric antibody to platelet glycoprotein IIb/IIIa integrin in patients undergoing percutaneous coronary intervention. *Circulation* 1995;91:2882–2890.

16. Lincoff AM, Tcheng JE, Califf RM, et al., for the PROLOG Investigators. Standard versus low dose weight-adjusted heparin in patients treated with the platelet glycoprotein IIb/IIIa receptor antibody fragment abciximab (c7E3 Fab) during percutaneous coronary revascularization. *Am J Cardiol* 1997;79:286–291.

17. EPILOG Investigators. Platelet glycoprotein IIb/IIIa blockade with abciximab with low-dose heparin during percutaneous coronary revascularization. *N Engl J Med* 1997;336:1689–1696.

18. IMPACT II Investigators. Randomized placebo-controlled trial of effect of eptifibatide on complications of percutaneous coronary intervention: IMPACT II. *Lancet* 1997;349:1422–1428.

19. RESTORE Investigators. Effects of platelet glycoprotein IIb/IIIa blockade with tirofiban on adverse cardiac events in patients with unstable angina or acute myocardial infarction undergoing coronary angioplasty. *Circulation* 1997;96:1445–1453.

20. Brener SJ, Barr LA, Burchenal JEB, et al., on behalf of the ReoPro and Primary PTCA Organization and Randomized Trial (RAPPORT) Investigators. A randomized, placebo-controlled trial of platelet glycoprotein IIb/IIIa blockade with primary angioplasty for acute myocardial infarction. *Circulation* 1998;98:734–741.

21. PURSUIT Trial Investigators. Inhibition of platelet glycoprotein IIb/IIIa with eptifibatide in patients with acute coronary syndromes. *N Engl J Med* 1998;339:436–443.

22. PRISM PLUS Study Investigators. Inhibition of the platelet glycoprotein IIb/IIIa receptor with tirofiban in unstable angina and non-Q-wave myocardial infarction. *N Engl J Med* 1998;338:1488–1497.

23. Kereiakes DJ, Lincoff AM, Miller DP, et al., for the EPILOG Investigators. Abciximab therapy and unplanned coronary stent deployment. Favorable effects on stent use, clinical outcomes, and bleeding complications. *Circulation* 1998;97:857–864.

24. Kleiman NS, Lincoff AM, Kereiakes DJ, et al., for the EPILOG Investigators. Diabetes mellitus, glycoprotein IIb/IIIa blockade, and heparin. Evidence of a complex interaction in a multicenter trial. *Circulation* 1998;97: 1912–1920.

25. Ghaffari S, Kereiakes DJ, Lincoff AM, et al., for the EPILOG Investigators. Platelet glycoprotein IIb/IIIa receptor blockade with abciximab reduces ischemic complications in patients undergoing directional coronary atherectomy. *Am J Cardiol* 1998;82:7–12.

26. Carrozza JP, Kuntz RE, Fishman RF, Baim DS. Restenosis after arterial injury caused by coronary stenting in patients with diabetes mellitus. *Ann Intern Med* 1993; 118:344–349.

27. Kornowski R, Mintz GS, Kent KM, et al. Increased restenosis in diabetes mellitus after coronary interventions is due to exaggerated intimal hyperplasia. A serial intravascular ultrasound study. *Circulation* 1997;95: 1366–1369.

28. Reverter JC, Beguin S, Kessels H, Kumar R, Hemker HC, Coller BS. Inhibition of platelet-mediated, tissue factor-induced thrombin generation by the mouse/human chimeric 7E3 antibody. *J Clin Invest* 1996;98: 863–874.

29. Phillips DR, Teng W, Arfstent A, et al. Effect of Ca^{2+} on GP IIb-IIIa interactions with Integrilin. Enhanced GP IIb-IIIa binding and inhibition of platelet aggregation by reductions in the concentration of ionized calcium in plasma anticoagulated with citrate. *Circulation* 1997;96:1488–1494.

30. Boehrer JD, Kereiakes DJ, Navetta FI, Califf RM, Topol EJ, for the EPIC investigators. Effects of profound platelet inhibition with c7E3 before coronary angioplasty on complications of coronary bypass surgery. *Am J Cardiol* 1994;74:1166–1170.

31. Berkowitz SD, Harrington RA, Rund MM, Tcheng JE. Acute profound thrombocytopenia after c7E3 Fab (abciximab) therapy. *Circulation* 1997;95:809–813.

32. Tcheng JE, Kereiakes DJ, Braden GA, et al. Safety of abciximab retreatment—final clinical report of the ReoPro Readministration Registry (R3). *Circulation* 1998; 98:I-17(abst).

33. Mark DB, Talley JD, Topol EJ, et al., for the EPIC Investigators. Economic assessment of platelet glycoprotein IIb/IIIa inhibition for prevention of ischemic complications of high-risk coronary angioplasty. *Circulation* 1996;94:629–635.

34. Muhlestein JB, Karagounis LA, Treehan S, Anderson JL. ''Rescue'' utilization of abciximab for the dissolution of coronary thrombus developing as a complication of coronary angioplasty. *J Am Coll Cardiol* 1997;30: 1729–1734.

B. The Role of Oral Platelet Glycoprotein IIb/IIIa Antagonists in the Setting of Percutaneous Coronary Intervention

Steven R. Steinhubl and *Eric J. Topol

*Department of Cardiology/PSMC, Wilford Hall Medical Center, Lackland AFB, Texas 78236-5300; and *Ohio State University School of Medicine and Department of Cardiology, The Cleveland Clinic Foundation, Cleveland, Ohio 44195*

Antiplatelet therapy has been a critical component of adjunctive medical therapy during percutaneous coronary interventions (PCIs) since the inception of this technique over 20 years ago (1). Although in these initial patients the use of aspirin and its 3-day duration of treatment were empiric, subsequent placebo-controlled studies established the importance of early aspirin use in decreasing the risk of thrombotic complications of percutaneous transluminal coronary angioplasty (PTCA) (2). When the results of early experimental models implicated platelets in the pathogenesis of neointimal hyperplasia (3,4), prolonged antiplatelet therapy was evaluated for the prevention of restenosis in a number of clinical trials (2,5–8). Disappointingly, all regimens tested, including aspirin and dipyridamole, ticlopidine, and thromboxane A_2-receptor inhibitors, were found to be ineffective in preventing restenosis. Nonetheless, because of the increased risk of patients undergoing coronary intervention for future thrombotic vascular events, and the proven benefit of antiplatelet therapy in the secondary prevention of these events (9), patients undergoing a percutaneous coronary revascularization (PCI) are typically maintained on chronic aspirin therapy.

The advent of platelet glycoprotein (GP) IIb/IIIa receptor inhibitors has more recently allowed for the reevaluation of the role of antiplatelet therapy in the setting of PCI. Unlike previously available therapies that were able to inhibit only one of many possible mediators of platelet activation, GP IIb/IIIa inhibitors block the final common pathway of platelet aggregation irrespective of the agonist (10). As reviewed

earlier, trials of several parenteral GP IIb/IIIa inhibitors have proven the clinical benefit of antiplatelet protection beyond that provided by aspirin for the reduction of adverse cardiac events associated with PCI (11–15). Because of the requirement for intravenous dosing, treatment with these agents has been limited to only a short duration following the coronary intervention. This limitation potentially prevents maximization of the benefits of complete blockade of platelet aggregation. Indeed, although up to 36-hour infusions of short-acting GP IIb/IIIa antagonists following angioplasty have demonstrated benefit during the infusion, that benefit was lost after completion of the infusion (11,12).

The development of orally active GP IIb/IIIa receptor antagonists allows for the possibility of sustained blockade of platelet aggregation. By maintaining more complete platelet inhibition for several days to weeks following angioplasty, it may be possible to enhance the long-term benefit of these agents—potentially even impacting restenosis. Furthermore, by continuing therapy indefinitely following an intervention, there is the potential for improved secondary prevention of thrombotic vascular events in this high-risk population. This chapter explores the therapeutic potential of these agents in patients undergoing coronary intervention, and evaluates the data currently available regarding their efficacy and safety.

THE ROLE OF PLATELET INHIBITION IN THE PREVENTION OF RESTENOSIS

It is clear that the endothelial disruption and deep arterial injury created during a PCI lead to the local formation of a platelet-rich thrombus (16,17). The presence of a mural thrombus has been confirmed angioscopically early following PTCA with adjunctive heparin and aspirin (18), and organized thrombus has been shown histologically up to 30 days following stenting (19,20). Similarly, angioscopic evaluation of 56 patients within 4 weeks of a myocardial infarction (MI) demonstrated visible thrombus at the culprit lesion in 79% of patients between 2 to 4 weeks following their infarct, despite heparin and aspirin in all patients and thrombolytics in many (21).

The local release of the contents of intracellular platelet granules such as platelet-derived growth factor (PDGF), transforming growth factor-β, and other growth and mitogenic factors has been postulated to play a central role in restenosis, because these growth factors stimulate the migration and proliferation of smooth muscle cells (22). The results of early studies in various animal models supported the hypothesis that the prevention of thrombus formation at the site of intraarterial injury could prevent neointimal hyperplasia. One of the first of these studies evaluated a thrombocytopenic rabbit model of arterial injury (23). In this model, the investigators demonstrated that following balloon injury of a rabbit aorta, neointimal hyperplasia could be significantly suppressed by maintaining a mean platelet count of less than 7,000 per cubic centimeter (normal, 363,000 per cubic centimeter) for up to 28 days using anti-rabbit platelet sera. Other important observations from this study were that thrombocytopenia had to be achieved by the time of balloon injury in order to be effective, and that there was a threshold effect in that rabbits with platelet counts greater than 7,000 per cubic centimeter developed intimal hyperplasia similar to that seen in control animals.

A second animal model investigating the influence of thrombocytopenia on neointimal hyperplasia utilized a rat carotid artery injury model (24). In this study, profound thrombocytopenia was maintained following a single injection of anti-rat platelet antibody given prior to injury for only 24 hours following injury. Platelet accumulation at the injury site appeared to be similar to that of controls, but delayed by 24

to 48 hours (Fig. 33.2). Although there was a significant decrease in neointimal hyperplasia found in the thrombocytopenic animals at days 4 and 7 compared with controls, by day 14 the intimal areas were the same in both groups. Interestingly, in a small group of animals that were maintained thrombocytopenic for 7 days, no intimal thickening was observed.

Agents that inhibit platelet function have also been evaluated in animal models of restenosis. In a chronically instrumented dog model, the severity of neointimal proliferation at 21 days was shown to correlate with the frequency and severity of cyclic coronary blood flow variations—a manifestation of localized platelet thrombus formation and dislodgment—during the 7 days following instrumentation (3). They further demonstrated that continuous therapy with a dual thromboxane A_2 synthetase inhibitor and receptor antagonist and a serotonin S_2 receptor antagonist for 15 days could abolish cyclic flow variations and retard neointimal hyperplasia. Another study evaluated a cyclic peptide that nonselectively inhibits the $\alpha_{IIb}\beta_3$ and $\alpha_v\beta_3$ integrins in a hamster carotid artery model (25). There were three important observations from this study that reinforced the findings from early studies of platelets and restenosis: (a) Platelet inhibition starting prior to the time of injury was necessary to maximize the antiproliferative effects, (b) increasing levels of inhibition of platelet aggregation were associated with a decreasing amount of neointimal formation, and (c) prolonged antiplatelet therapy (greater than 3 days) was necessary to prevent neointima formation.

Despite the role of platelets in restenosis suggested by these animal models, no clinical trials of antiplatelet (2,5,7) or antithrombotic therapies (26,27) in humans have been shown to prevent angiographic restenosis. However, all of these trials were limited by either incomplete platelet inhibition or inadequate duration of therapy. The GP IIb/IIIa inhibitor abciximab is the only agent that has been shown to potentially influence clinical restenosis, although the results have been inconsistent (28,29). Interestingly, not only does abciximab profoundly inhibit platelet aggregation at the time of the procedure, but it also maintains some degree of platelet receptor blockade

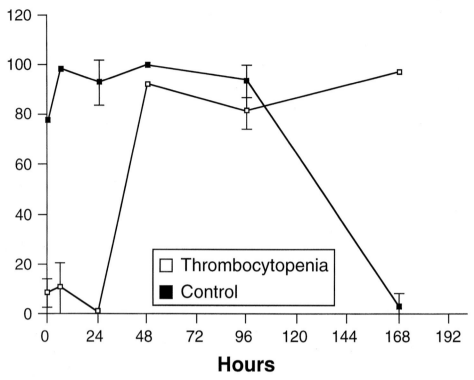

FIG. 33.2. Time-dependent platelet adherence in denuded rat carotid arteries demonstrating that short-term maintenance of profound thrombocytopenia only delays platelet accumulation at the site of injury. (From ref. 24, with permission.)

for up to 8 to 15 days following a standard-bolus and 12-hour infusion (30). This prolonged affect, which among parenteral GP IIb/IIIa antagonists is characteristic of only abciximab, may be central to its influence on clinical restenosis in some patients. However, in the majority of patients, the degree of platelet inhibition maintained beyond 24 hours with abciximab is minimal. On the other hand, prolonged therapy with oral GP IIb/IIIa inhibitors should, for the first time, allow high levels of platelet inhibition to be maintained over many days, and as a consequence could more completely inhibit neointimal formation and prevent restenosis.

LONG-TERM RISK OF ISCHEMIC EVENTS IN PATIENTS FOLLOWING PCI

Patients undergoing a PCI represent a group of individuals at high risk for recurrent vascular events. A number of longitudinal studies of patients undergoing coronary intervention have shown event rates of over 50% in the 10 years following angioplasty (31,32). The first year following an intervention is associated with the highest incidence of adverse cardiac events with the composite of death, MI, or revascularization occurring in nearly one-third of patients in the modern era of PCI (33,34). However, because of the risk for ischemic events in other vascular territories, there is not a plateau in the occurrence of adverse events in the ensuing years. In fact, a consistent increase in cumulative events of 4% to 5% per year has been demonstrated in most studies following the first year after PCI. A report of the 3-year follow-up on patients enrolled in the EPIC (Evaluation of Platelet IIb/IIIa Inhibition for Prevention of Ischemic Complications) trial, in which patients undergoing percutaneous coronary revascularization were randomized to either placebo, an abciximab

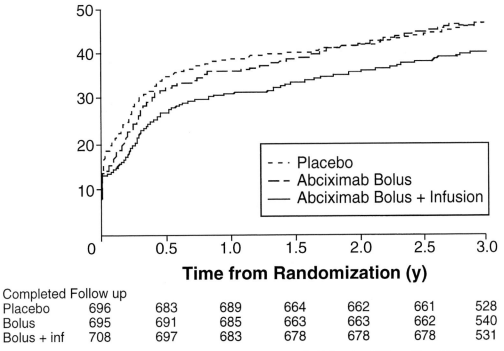

Completed Follow up							
Placebo	696	683	689	664	662	661	528
Bolus	695	691	685	663	663	662	540
Bolus + inf	708	697	683	678	678	678	531

FIG. 33.3. Three-year composite outcome of death, myocardial infarction (*MI*), and need for revascularization among patients undergoing a percutaneous coronary intervention in the EPIC trial, demonstrating an approximately 5% per year event rate following the first year. (From ref. 33, with permission.)

bolus alone, or an abciximab bolus plus a 12-hour infusion, demonstrated a cumulative incidence of 41% to 47% of death, MI, or revascularization, depending on the treatment arm (33) (Fig. 33.3). Similarly, studies following patients after coronary stenting also demonstrated a steadily increasing incidence of adverse events over time (34,35) (Fig. 33.4). Because all of these patients received chronic aspirin therapy following their PCI, it is anticipated that greater antiplatelet protection long-term with oral GP IIb/IIIa antagonists could prevent a substantial percentage of events in this high-risk population.

CLINICAL EXPERIENCE WITH ORAL GP IIb/IIIa ANTAGONISTS

The initial experience with prolonged GP IIb/IIIa inhibition using oral agents in patients undergoing a PCI was first described by Simpfendorfer and colleagues in 1997 (36). This was a randomized, single-blind, placebo-controlled study of xemilofiban in 30 patients with unstable angina undergoing a percutaneous coronary revascularization. Xemilofiban is a prodrug of a nonpeptide mimetic of the tetra peptide RGDF that is readily absorbed and metabolized to its active moiety SC-54701, a potent specific inhibitor of the platelet GP IIb/IIIa. Plasma levels strongly correlate with the degree of inhibition of platelet aggregation, and elimination is primarily through renal excretion.

In this study, 20 patients were randomized to receive xemilofiban as a 35-mg loading dose 1 to 3 hours prior to their procedure, with 16 patients then receiving 25 mg tid and four patients 20 mg tid. All patients also received aspirin. Enrollment in the later group was discontinued early by the sponsor due to severe bleeding events, highlighting one of the major findings of this pilot study. Of the 20 patients randomized to xemilofiban, seven patients were withdrawn

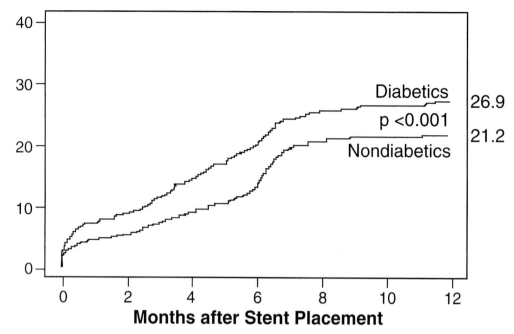

FIG. 33.4. One-year composite outcome of death, myocardial infarction (*MI*), and target-lesion revascularization following successful stent placement in 715 diabetic and 2,839 nondiabetic patients. (From from ref. 34, with permission.)

prior to hospital discharge (four due to bleeding complications). Importantly, two patients had severe bleeding complications: one with gastric bleeding requiring 22 units of packed red blood cells, and a second patient who died following emergency bypass surgery complicated by profuse bleeding requiring 54 U of packed red blood cells. Only ten patients completed their full 30-day course of therapy, and all but one patient reported minor bleeding episodes. Pharmacodynamic studies demonstrated interpatient variability in the degree of platelet inhibition, but the majority of patients achieved early levels of inhibition similar to those achieved with parenteral agents. Platelet inhibition long term was dependent on timing of the test in relation to dosing, with 83% of patients having greater than or equal to 80% inhibition to adenosine diphosphate (ADP) at 2 hours after their morning dose, but with only 36% of patients maintaining this level prior to their morning dose.

A second dose-ranging study of xemilofiban evaluated much lower doses than previously studied: 5 to 20 mg bid for 2 weeks in patients following coronary stenting (37). This placebo-controlled study involved 170 patients, all of whom also received aspirin, with the 51 patients randomized to placebo also receiving ticlopidine. Unlike the initial study, xemilofiban was not started until the morning after the interventional procedure. As expected, a dose response was found in terms of ADP-induced aggregation, with only the 20-mg dose achieving greater than or equal to 80% inhibition of aggregation. Hemorrhagic complications were much rarer in this study, with only three patients discontinuing xemilofiban due to minor bleeding. However, there were two cases of stent thrombosis in xemilofiban-treated patients. Thirty patients enrolled in this study also received abciximab during their procedure at the discretion of the operator. A report of the pharmacodynamics in a subset of these patients demonstrated that the magnitude and duration of platelet inhibition by xemilofiban was enhanced in patients treated with abciximab (38). Unlike patients not receiving abciximab, all doses of xemilofiban achieved greater than or equal to 80% inhibition of plate-

trial. Coronary Artery Restenosis Prevention on Repeated Thromboxane A2-Antagonism Study (CARPORT). *Circulation* 1991;84:1568–1580.

7. White CW, Chaitman B, Knudson ML, Chisholm RJ, and the Ticlopidine Study Group. Antiplatelet agents are effective in reducing the acute ischemic complications of angioplasty but do not prevent restenosis: results from the ticlopidine trial. *Coron Artery Dis* 1991;2: 757–767.

8. Bertrand ME, Allain H, Lablanche JM, on behalf of the investigators of the TACT study. Results of a randomized trial of ticlopidine versus placebo for prevention of acute closure and restenosis after coronary angioplasty (PTCA). The TACT study. *Circulation* 1990;82:III-190.

9. Antiplatelet Trialists' Collaboration. Collaborative overview of randomised trials of antiplatelet therapy—I. Prevention of death, myocardial infarction, and stroke by prolonged antiplatelet therapy in various categories of patients. *BMJ* 1994;308:81–106.

10. Lefkovits J, Plow EF, Topol EJ. Platelet glycoprotein IIb/IIIa receptors in cardiovascular medicine. *N Engl J Med* 1995;332:1553–1559.

11. The IMPACT-II Investigators. Randomised placebo-controlled trial of effect of eptifibatide on complications of percutaneous coronary intervention: IMPACT-II. *Lancet* 1997;349:1422–1428.

12. The RESTORE Investigators. Effects of platelet glycoprotein IIb/IIIa blockade with tirofiban on adverse cardiac events in patients with unstable angina or acute myocardial infarction undergoing coronary angioplasty. *Circulation* 1997;96:1445–1453.

13. The EPISTENT Investigators. Randomised placebo-controlled and balloon-angioplasty-controlled trial to assess safety of coronary stenting with use of platelet glycoprotein-IIb/IIIa blockade. *Lancet* 1998;352: 87–92.

14. The EPILOG Investigators. Platelet glycoprotein IIb/IIIa receptor blockade and low-dose heparin during percutaneous coronary revascularization. *N Engl J Med* 1997;336:1689–1696.

15. The EPIC Investigators. Use of a monoclonal antibody directed against the platelet glycoprotein IIb/IIIa receptor in high-risk coronary angioplasty. *N Engl J Med* 1994;330:956–961.

16. Wilentz JR, Sanborn TA, Haudenschild CC, Valeri CR, Ryan TJ, Faxon DP. Platelet accumulation in experimental angioplasty: Time course and relation to vascular injury. *Circulation* 1987;75:636–642.

17. Lam JYT, Chesebro JH, Steele PM, et al. Deep arterial injury during experimental angioplasty: relation to a positive indium-111-labeled platelet scintigram, quantitative platelet deposition and mural thrombosis. *J Am Coll Cardiol* 1986;8:1380–1386.

18. Yanagida S, Mizuno K, Miyamoto A, et al. Comparison of findings between coronary angiography and angioscopy. *Circulation* 1989;80:II-376.

19. Farb A, Sangiorgi G, Carter AJ, et al. Pathology of acute and chronic coronary stenting in humans. *Circulation* 1999;99:44–52.

20. Komatsu R, Ueda M, Naruko T, Kojima A, Becker AE. Neointimal tissue response at sites of coronary stenting in humans. Macroscopic, histological, and immunohistochemical analysis. *Circulation* 1998;98:224–233.

21. Van Belle E, Lablanche J-M, Bauters C, Renaud N, McFadden EP, Bertrand ME. Coronary angioscopy

findings in the infarct-related vessel within 1 month of acute myocardial infarction. Natural history and the effect of thrombolysis. *Circulation* 1998;97:26–33.

22. LeBreton H, Plow EF, Topol EJ. Role of platelets in restenosis after percutaneous coronary revascularization. *J Am Coll Cardiol* 1996;28:1643–1651.

23. Friedman RF, Stemerman MB, Wenz B, et al. The effect of thrombocytopenia on experimental arteriosclerotic lesion formation in rabbits. *J Clin Invest* 1977;60: 1191–1201.

24. Fingerle J, Johnson R, Clowes AW, Majesky MW, Reidy MA. Role of platelets in smooth muscle cell proliferation and migration after vascular injury in rat carotid artery. *Proc Natl Acad Sci U S A* 1989;86: 8412–8416.

25. Matsuno H, Stassen JM, Vermylen J, Deckmyn H. Inhibition of integrin function by a cyclic RGD-containing peptide prevents neointimal formation. *Circulation* 1994;90:2203–2206.

26. Bittl JA, Strong J, Brinker JA, et al. Treatment with bivalirudin (hirulog) as compared with heparin during PTCA for unstable or post-infarction angina: Hirulog Angioplasty Study Investigators. *N Engl J Med* 1995; 333:764–769.

27. Serruys P, Herrman J, Simon R, et al. A comparison of hirudin with heparin in the prevention of restenosis after PTCA. *N Engl J Med* 1995;333:757–763.

28. Lincoff AM, Tcheng JE, Califf RM, et al. The EPISTENT trial at 6 months: relative and combined effects of abciximab and stenting on reduction of acute ischemic events and late revascularization. *Circulation* 1998;98: I-767(abst).

29. The EPIC Investigators. Randomised trial of coronary intervention with antibody against platelet IIb/IIIa integrin for reduction of clinical restenosis: results at six months. *Lancet* 1994;343:881–886.

30. Mascelli MA, Lance ET, Damaraju L, Wagner CL, Weisman HF, Jordan RE. Pharmacodynamic profile of short-term abciximab treatment demonstrates prolonged platelet inhibition with gradual recovery from GP IIb/IIIa receptor blockade. *Circulation* 1998;97: 1680–1688.

31. Ruygrok PN, de Jaegere PPT, van Domburg RT, van den Brand MJ, Serruys PW, de Feyter PJ. Clinical outcome 10 years after attempted percutaneous transluminal coronary angioplasty in 856 patients. *J Am Coll Cardiol* 1996;27:1669–1677.

32. Kip KE, Faxon DP, Detre KM, Yeh WL, Kelsey SF, Currier JW. Coronary angioplasty in diabetic patients—The National Heart, Lung, and Blood Institute Percutaneous Transluminal Coronary Angioplasty Registry. *Circulation* 1996;94:1818–1825.

33. Topol EJ, Ferguson JJ, Weisman HF, et al. Long-term protection from myocardial ischemic events in a randomized trial of brief integrin $\beta3$ blockade with percutaneous coronary intervention. *JAMA* 1997;278:479–484.

34. Elezi S, Kastrati A, Pache J, et al. Diabetes mellitus and the clinical and angiographic outcome after coronary stent placement. *J Am Coll Cardiol* 1998;32: 1866–1873.

35. Kimura T, Yokoi H, Nakagawa Y, et al. Three year follow-up after implantation of metallic coronary-artery stents. *N Engl J Med* 1996;334:561–566.

36. Simpfendorfer C, Kottke-Marchant K, Lowrie M, et al. First chronic platelet glycoprotein IIb/IIIa integrin

blockade. A randomized, placebo-controlled pilot study of xemilofiban in unstable angina with percutaneous coronary interventions. *Circulation* 1997;96:76–81.

37. Kereiakes DJ, Kleiman N, Ferguson JJ, et al. Sustained platelet glycoprotein IIb/IIIa blockade with oral xemilofiban in 170 patients after coronary stent deployment. *Circulation* 1997;96:1117–1121.

38. Kereiakes DJ, Runyon JP, Kleiman NS, et al. Differential dose-response to oral xemilofiban after antecedent intravenous abciximab administration for complex coronary intervention. *Circulation* 1996;94:906–910.

39. Kereiakes DJ, Kleiman NS, Ferguson JJ, et al. Pharmacodynamic efficacy, clinical safety, and outcomes after prolonged platelet glycoprotein IIb/IIIa receptor blockade with oral xemilofiban. Results of a multicenter, placebo-controlled, randomized trial. *Circulation* 1998;98:1268–1278.

40. Cannon CP, McCabe CH, Borzak S, et al. Randomized trial of an oral platelet glycoprotein IIb/IIIa antagonist, sibrafiban, in patients after an acute coronary syndrome. Results of the TIMI 12 trial. *Circulation* 1998;97:340–349.

41. Coller BS, Scudder LE, Beer J, et al. Monoclonal antibodies to platelet GPIIb/IIIa as antithrombotic agents. *Ann N Y Acad Sci* 1991;614:193–213.

42. Peter K, Schwarz M, Ylanne J, et al. Induction of fibrinogen binding and platelet aggregation as a potential intrinsic property of various glycoprotein IIb/IIIa ($\alpha IIb\beta 3$) inhibitors. *Blood* 1998;92:3240–3249.

43. Catella-Lawson F, Kapoor S, Moretti DT, et al. Chronic oral glycoprotein IIb/IIIa antagonism in patients with unstable coronary syndromes: reduced antiplatelet effect in comparison to patients with stable coronary artery disease. *Circulation* 1998;98:I-251.

44. Mascelli MA, Worley S, Veriabo NJ, et al. Rapid assessment of platelet function with a modified whole-blood aggregometer in percutaneous transluminal coronary angioplasty patients receiving anti-GPIIb/IIIa therapy. *Circulation* 1997;96:3860–3866.

45. Smith JW, Steinhubl SR, Lincoff AM, et al. The rapid platelet function assay (RPFA): an automated and quantitative cartridge-based method. *Circulation* 1999;99:620–625.

46. Gawaz M, Ruf A, Neumann F-J, et al. Effect of glycoprotein IIb/IIa receptor antagonism on platelet membrane glycoproteins after coronary stent placement. *Thromb Haemost* 1998;80:994–1001.

C. Provisional Use of Abciximab During Coronary Angioplasty

Sorin J. Brener

*Department of Medicine, Ohio State University, Columbus, Ohio 43210 and
Department of Cardiology, The Cleveland Clinic Foundation, Cleveland, Ohio 44195-5066*

Platelets play a key role in the development of ischemic complications during and after percutaneous coronary intervention (1,2). They migrate toward, and adhere quickly to, the site of intimal injury caused by device activation. Subsequent platelet activation and the accompanying structural changes herald thrombus formation. In turn, the fresh thrombus is responsible for abrupt vessel closure, side-branch occlusion, or distal embolization with ensuing myocardial ischemia or infarction. Furthermore, residual clot at the lesion site may initiate the process of smooth muscle migration and proliferation, considered an important precursor of restenosis. Patients suffering from these intraprocedural complications have increased mortality, morbidity, and resource utilization (3).

In the last 5 years, the use of potent platelet inhibitors at the level of the glycoprotein IIb/IIIa receptor has dramatically affected the results of coronary intervention. Most of the data were accrued with abciximab (ReoPro, Centocor, Malvern, PA), a chimeric (murine–human) antibody, which binds noncompetitively to this and other integrins on the platelet surface. When given within 60 minutes before first device activation (prophylactic), abciximab reduced the incidence of death, myocardial infarction (MI), and urgent revascularization at 30 days by approximately 45%, translating into five to six events prevented for every 100 patients treated (4–6). This benefit is independent of the demographic, clinical, or angiographic characteristics of the patients. Atheroablation of the coronary plaque, frequently associated with distal embolization and enzymatic evidence of myocardial necrosis, is favorably affected by abciximab use (7,8), as is the implantation of coronary stents (9).

Two major limitations curtail the widespread utilization of abciximab, and other similar agents, for all patients undergoing coronary angioplasty. The first is the high cost of the compound, amounting to approximately $1,350 for a 12-hour infusion. The second is the modest, though significant, incidence of major bleeding. It ranges from 2% to 4% during elective intervention (5) to 12% to 16% after primary angioplasty for acute MI (10). These events are costly, associated with important morbidity, and reduce the net clinical benefit obtained from the prevention of ischemic complications. Reduced heparin dosing, meticulous sheath care, and early removal of the sheath have dramatically reduced the incidence of access site bleeding. Also of concern is the development of antibodies against this chimeric murine–human antibody in 5% to 7% of patients and significant thrombocytopenia in 2% to 4%.

Consequently, many interventional cardiologists have adopted the strategy of utilizing abciximab on a provisional basis in response to important intraprocedural complications. Currently, approximately one-fourth of the use of abciximab in the United States is on a *provisional or rescue* basis, encompassing approximately 15% of all interventional procedures, as assessed by an informal survey of 100 interventional cardiologists in 1998. Overall, abciximab is used in over half of all angioplasty procedures. When given provisionally, abciximab is commenced in response to the occurrence of new intracoronary thrombus, abrupt vessel closure, distal embolization of thrombus or atheromatous material, or large dissections with impending vessel closure or decreased briskness of flow.

The putative benefit of rescue abciximab stems from its ability to rapidly inhibit the platelets accumulated at the site of intimal injury, preventing new thrombus formation on a platelet nidus, and dissolving freshly accumulated thrombus. Because of advantageous kinetics, abciximab displaces fibrinogen from the interconnected platelets. Moreover, abciximab has been shown to inhibit plasminogen-activator inhibi-

tor-1, paving the way for the natural fibrinolytic system to promote further thrombus removal (11). These effects are present both at the epicardial and at the arteriolar level, explaining the improvement in flow briskness, even without additional mechanical interventions.

OBSERVATIONAL STUDIES OF RESCUE ABCIXIMAB: EFFICACY AND SAFETY

There is a remarkable paucity of data regarding this strategy despite the use of abciximab in approximately 50% of all coronary interventions in the United States. Muhlestein et al. (12) reported the first series of 29 patients receiving rescue abciximab in response to newly developed or expanding thrombus during angioplasty. Most procedures were performed in native coronary vessels (left anterior descending, 52%), and 94% of the lesions were ACC/AHA type B/C. The thrombolysis in MI (TIMI) thrombus scale (0–4) was used to compare the size of newly formed thrombus before and after the administration of abciximab (0.25 mg per kilogram bolus, followed by 12-hour infusion at 10 μg per minute). All patients had balloon angioplasty alone, and at least two inflations were performed before and one after abciximab bolus. The interval between first device activation and abciximab bolus is not provided. The main results are shown in Table 33.4. There was significant improvement in the thrombus grade and normalization of flow, with procedural success in 27 of 29 patients (97%). Four patients (14%) experienced transient abrupt closure. At 6 months, there were no deaths, two (7%) suffered an MI, and six (21%) underwent repeat revascularization. Major bleeding occurred in two patients (7%). The authors acknowledged that the very small patient population and the lack of randomization of treatment and of blinding of angiogram interpretation limit the ability to draw firm conclusions regarding the utility of this strategy.

Abizaid et al. (13) and Brener et al. (14) reported two large series of rescue abciximab administration. The former retrospectively compared 41 and 131 patients treated with prophylactic and rescue abciximab, respectively, in

TABLE 33.4. *Angiographic outcome of patients treated with rescue abciximab*

	Pre-PTCA	Pre-Abciximab	Post-Abciximab	p Value
% Stenosis	93 ± 4	57 ± 22	21 ± 16	<.001
Thrombus grade	1.4 ± 1.3	3.0 ± 0.9	0.9 ± 0.9	<.001
TIMI flow grade	2.5 ± 1.0	2.5 ± 0.7	2.9 ± 0.3	.008

PTCA, percutaneous transluminal coronary angioplasty; TIMI, thrombolysis in myocardial infarction flow classification.
Adapted from ref. 12.

a nonrandomized fashion. The main intraprocedural complications leading to abciximab administration were new thrombus formation (26%), severe dissections (24%), "no reflow" (8%), and abrupt closure (3.5%). The main outcomes are listed in Table 33.5. There was a high, statistically similar incidence of non–Q-wave infarction and major bleeding requiring transfusion in both groups. Late revascularization did not appear to be increased in the group receiving rescue abciximab for procedural complications.

In contrast, at our institution, rescue abciximab was associated with less favorable results, when compared with prophylactic administration. We analyzed the outcome of all patients (n = 644) receiving abciximab, either prophylactically (n = 527, 82%) or as rescue intervention (n = 117, 18%) between February 1995 and October 1996 (14). We excluded from the analysis primary or rescue angioplasty patients. The prophylactic group had a significantly higher incidence of unstable angina and a lower incidence of prior revascularization than did the rescue group. All other demographic and clinical parameters were statistically similar. The indica-

tions for rescue abciximab were severe dissections (37%), distal embolization (12%), abrupt closure (12%), new thrombus formation (9%), and high risk for abrupt closure (28%). The latter indication comprised patients with diminished flow, transient abrupt closure, or suboptimal angiographic results. The lesion severity was similar in both groups. The interval between first device activation and abciximab bolus was 61 ± 56 minutes. The important clinical outcomes are outlined in Table 33.6. Of note are the markedly higher rates of non–Q-wave infarction and blood transfusion in the rescue patients. In this group, patients with primarily thrombotic complications (new thrombus, distal embolization) had a similar incidence of non–Q-wave MI as those with primarily mechanical complications (severe dissections, side-branch closure). The direct hospital costs were higher in the rescue group. Obviously, because of lack of randomization and control treatment arm, we could not evaluate whether rescue abciximab prevented ischemic complications, attenuated them, or did not affect the cascade of events that was already in place. The rate of target-vessel revasculariza-

TABLE 33.5. *In-hospital and late clinical outcomes in patients treated with prophylactic and rescue abciximab*

	Prophylactic (n = 41)	Rescue (n = 131)	p Value
In-hospital (%)			
Procedure success	97	97	NS
D/MI/CABG	0	2/2/1	NS
Non–Q-wave MI[a]	18	21	NS
Major bleeding/transfusion	7/7	12/8	NS
Late outcome (%)			
Target-vessel revascularization	8	12	NS

D, death; MI, myocardial infarction; CABG, coronary artery bypass grafting; NS, not significant.
[a] Defined as more than two times upper limit of normal for institution.
Adapted from ref. 13.

TABLE 33.6. *Important clinical endpoints and costs in patients with prophylactic or rescue abciximab administration*

Outcome	Prophylactic (n = 527)	Rescue (n = 117)	p Value
Procedure success (%)	93	89	.10
Composite endpoint (%)[a]	19	34	.0002
Death (%)	2.1	4.3	.18
Q-wave MI (%)	0	1.7	.03
Non–Q-wave MI (%)[b]	7.6	17.9	.0005
Emergency CABG (%)	1.0	0.9	>.95
Urgent repeat PCR (%)	0.4	1.7	>.95
Stroke (%)	0.6	0	>.95
Access site complication (%)	5	5	>.95
Transfusion (%)	7	14	.007
Direct costs ($)[c]	8,275 (6,731–10,669)	10,004 (7,770–14,633)	.004

MI, myocardial infarction; CABG, coronary artery bypass grafting; PCR, percutaneous coronary revascularization.

[a] Composite of death, any infarction, urgent CABG, bleeding/transfusion, or access site complication. More than one endpoint may have occurred in an individual patient.

[b] Defined as more than 30 U CKMB (upper limit of normal is 7 U).

[c] Median (25th and 75th percentiles).

tion at 1 year was 19% and 14.5% ($p > .1$) in the prophylactic and rescue groups, respectively. Any adverse ischemic event occurred in 24.5% and 27.5% in the two groups ($p = .6$).

Despite the different indications for administration of rescue abciximab in the two series, the incidence of non–Q-wave MI and major bleeding requiring transfusion was remarkably similar.

PRACTICAL ASPECTS OF RESCUE ABCIXIMAB ADMINISTRATION

Timing of Abciximab Administration

When compared with randomized trials of prophylactic abciximab for coronary intervention, the high incidence of non–Q-wave infarction in the two large series of rescue abciximab would suggest that the chain of events that led to temporary or permanent myocardial ischemia could not be reversed (completely) by the administration of abciximab. In our analysis, delay to abciximab bolus was not an independent predictor of worse outcome, but most patients received the drug quite late after the beginning of the procedure. It would seem prudent to administer it as soon as important complications occur, while continuing with other mechanical strategies designed to improve flow.

Intensity of Concomitant Anticoagulation

Particularly because the efficacy of rescue abciximab is uncertain, the safety of its use is a major concern. Most patients treated with the drug in this fashion undergo full anticoagulation with heparin at the beginning of the procedure, and it is not anticipated at this time that abciximab will be used. The addition of abciximab further elevates activated clotting time (ACT) by approximately 40 seconds (15). In our series, the mean peak ACT was 346 and 383 seconds, in the prophylactic and rescue groups, respectively. This exaggerated level of anticoagulation prolonged the sheath dwell time by approximately 2 hours and was associated with an almost doubling of major bleeding events. It also may contribute to excessive platelet aggregation via platelet factor 4 release and thromboxane synthesis (16,17). Thus, maintaining an ACT in the high 200s or very low 300s would allow one to administer abciximab on a provisional basis without reaching very high levels of anticoagulation. Alternatively, if the ACT before the abciximab bolus is already very high (greater than 350 seconds), some interventionalists use protamine in small doses to counteract the enhanced anticoagulation after abciximab administration.

In the presence of large amounts of coronary thrombus, urokinase in 250,000-U aliquots may be used after abciximab is given. Theoretically, abciximab prevents urokinase-mediated platelet activation related to release of clot-bound thrombin (18). In my experience with approximately 15 cases, there was significant improvement in flow without exaggerated bleeding. Maintaining relatively low ACTs before and after administration of abciximab is obviously important in limiting the risk of bleeding.

Timing of Sheath Removal

Because rescue abciximab typically results in higher ACTs than during procedures performed with prophylactic or no abciximab, sheath removal is delayed, leading to more access site bleeding and vascular complications. Thus, every effort should be made to shorten sheath dwell time by discontinuing heparin infusion after the completion of the case. Preferably, the sheath should be removed as soon as possible, while abciximab is infused. This strategy has been shown to be safe in two large randomized trials of prophylactic abciximab (5,9). If absolutely needed, heparin can be resumed after sheath removal or termination of abciximab infusion.

FUTURE RESEARCH AND CONCLUSIONS

The data presented here do not clearly establish the role of rescue abciximab in patients with intraprocedural complications. It is possible that in some patients this intervention significantly reduces the incidence of in-hospital ischemic complications, while in others has no effect. The characteristics predicting improved outcome have not been identified. The long-term outcome appears favorable, and comparable with that of patients receiving prophylactic abciximab. This raises the possibility that, while not reversing the immediate results of ischemia, rescue abciximab attenuates some of the consequences of important intraprocedural complications, typically associated with high rates of repeat revascularization. Because of these inconclusive data, a randomized trial (A Multicenter, Open-Label, Randomized Trial comparing Clinical Outcome

with Hirulog and Provisional Abciximab versus Planned Abciximab and Low-Dose Heparin in Patients Undergoing Percutaneous Intervention—CACHET) started enrollment of patients in the fall of 1998. Approximately 5,000 patients will be randomly assigned to abciximab and low-dose heparin or hirulog (synthetic direct thrombin inhibitor) and rescue abciximab for one of the following indications: large dissections, decreased flow in the target vessel, new thrombus, no reflow, side-branch closure, unplanned stenting, or persistent, significant residual stenosis. The main objective of the study is to demonstrate equivalency of the two strategies with respect to the composite of death, infarction, or urgent revascularization at 30 days. Although it does not directly compare abciximab and placebo for patients with intraprocedural complications, this trial will test the two strategies of prophylactic versus provisional abciximab in a large cohort of patients undergoing elective or urgent coronary angioplasty.

Further refinements in the dose of rescue abciximab can be investigated with a new, bedside platelet aggregation test (Accumetrics), which provides platelet IIb/IIIa receptor occupancy within 60 seconds. This information may be particularly helpful in those who may have excessive or insufficient degrees of platelet inhibition and require different dosing regimens.

Meanwhile, specific recommendations regarding the use of rescue abciximab have to be tempered by the lack of adequate information. It appears that rescue abciximab is not as efficacious as its prophylactic administration in the prevention of ischemic complications following percutaneous revascularization. Probably, acute thrombotic complications (without vessel disruption) respond better to rescue abciximab than do mechanical disturbances of flow. Earlier administration of abciximab is more likely to minimize myocardial damage by quickly restoring brisk flow. Importantly, the possibility that abciximab may be used in a provisional fashion should be kept in mind when prescribing the initial anticoagulation regimen, in order to avoid bleeding complications associated with the addition of the antiplatelet agent. Finally, adequate economic analysis of the role of rescue abciximab is important in weighing the relative merits of this strategy.

As usual, it appears that "preventing trouble" works better than "improvisations." The only way to dispel this notion is to compare abciximab with placebo in a randomized fashion in patients with intraprocedural complications.

REFERENCES

1. Pope CF, Ezekowitz MD, Smith EO, et al. Detection of platelet deposition at the site of peripheral balloon angioplasty using indium-111 platelet scintigraphy. *Am J Cardiol.* 1985;55:495–497.
2. Gasperetti CM, Gonias SL, Gimple LW, Powers ER. Platelet activation during coronary angioplasty in humans. *Circulation.* 1993;88:2728–2734.
3. Lincoff A, Topol E. Abrupt vessel closure. In: Topol E. *Textbook of interventional cardiology,* 2nd ed. Philadelphia: WB Saunders, 1994:207.
4. The EPIC Investigators. Use of monoclonal antibody directed against the platelet glycoprotein IIb/IIIa receptor in high-risk coronary angioplasty. *N Engl J Med.* 1994;330:956–961.
5. The EPILOG Investigators. Platelet glycoprotein IIb/IIIa receptor blockade and low-dose heparin during percutaneous coronary revascularization. *N Engl J Med.* 1997;336:1689–1696.
6. The Capture Investigators. Randomized placebo-controlled trial of abciximab before and during coronary intervention in refractory unstable angina: the CAPTURE study. *Lancet.* 1997;349:1429–1435.
7. Braden GA, Applegate RJ, Young TM, Utley LM, Sane DC. ReoPro decreases creatine kinase elevation following rotational atherectomy: evidence for a platelet dependent mechanism. *Circulation.* 1996;94:I-248.
8. Ghaffari S, Kereiakes DJ, Lincoff AM, et al., for the EPILOG Investigators. Platelet glycoprotein IIb/IIIa receptor blockade with abciximab reduces ischemic complications in patients undergoing directional coronary atherectomy. *Am J Cardiol.* 1998;82:7–12.
9. The EPISTENT Investigators. Randomized placebo-controlled and balloon-angioplasty-controlled trial to assess safety of coronary stenting with use of platelet glycoprotein IIb/IIIa blockade. *Lancet.* 1998;352:87–92.
10. Brener SJ, Barr LA, Burchenal JEB, et al., for the RAPPORT Investigators. A randomized, placebo-controlled trial of platelet glycoprotein IIb/IIIa blockade with primary angioplasty for acute myocardial infarction. *Circulation.* 1998 (*in press*).
11. Deng G, Royle G, Seiffert D, Loskutoff DJ. The PAI-I/vitronectin interaction: two cats in a bag? *Thromb Haemost.* 1995;74:66–70.
12. Muhlestein JB, Karagounis LA, Treehan S, Anderson JL. "Rescue" utilization of abciximab for the dissolution of coronary thrombus developing as a complication of coronary angioplasty. *J Am Coll Cardiol.* 1997;30:1729–1734.
13. Abizaid AS, Popma JJ, Clark C, et al. Prophylactic versus rescue ReoPro in patients with complex or complicated coronary intervention. *Am J Cardiol.* 1997;80:48S.
14. Brener SJ, Ellis SG, DeLuca S, Topol EJ. Abciximab in coronary angioplasty—comparison of planned and rescue administration. *J Invest Cardiol.* 1997;9:50C.
15. Moliterno DJ, Califf RM, Aguirre FV, et al. Effect of platelet glycoprotein IIb/IIIa integrin blockade on activated clotting time during percutaneous transluminal coronary angioplasty or directional atherectomy. Evaluation of c7E3 Fab in the Prevention of Ischemic Complications (EPIC) trial. *Am J Cardiol.* 1995;75:559–562.
16. Storck J, Hollger N, Zimmermann RE. The influence of heparin and protamine sulfate on platelet ADP and platelet factor 4 release and the expression of glycoprotein IIb/IIIa. *Haemostasis* 1994;24:358–363.
17. Landolfi R, De Candia E, Rocca B, et al. Effects of unfractionated and low molecular weight heparins on platelet thromboxane biosynthesis "in vivo." *Thromb Haemost.* 1994;72:942–946.
18. Paolini R, Casonato A, Boeri G, et al. Effect of recombinant-tissue plasminogen activator, low molecular weight urokinase and unfractionated heparin on platelet aggregation. *J Med* 1993;24:113–130.

34

Local Drug Delivery: Current Clinical Applications

Steven R. Bailey

Department of Medicine and Radiology, University of Texas Health Science Center at San Antonio, and Cardiac Catheterization Laboratories, University Hospital, San Antonio, Texas 78229-4493

Percutaneous coronary interventions, despite the use of endovascular stents, still have limitations due to early thrombotic events and late neointimal proliferation (1–4). Thrombus formation has been aggressively addressed using new oral and intravenous systemic antiplatelet therapy and improved flow with stents (5–7). Despite these newer therapies, there are still major problems such as acute myocardial ischemia and saphenous vein graft degeneration (8–10). Progressive disease in saphenous vein grafts is often with a friable and thrombotic base that continues to represent a challenging scenario for percutaneous interventions. Local delivery of pharmacologic agents is now possible using catheters specifically designed for regional or site-specific delivery (11,12). These catheters have been developed to allow an increased volume of agent to be infused at a chosen site in an arterial segment. Using the properties of passive diffusion, or active infusion, these catheters will deliver pharmaceuticals or genes into the arterial wall.

Clinical approaches have used the ability of the new catheters to approach this problem in one of three techniques (a) low-pressure diffusion, (b) low-volume infusion, or (c) direct injection into the artery wall or pericardium. Examples of the types of current systems are summarized in Table 34.1.

Though each catheter system has its own unique characteristics, the current delivery systems have equivalent efficiencies of approximately .1 to 1.0% (13) (Table 34.2). While low,

this still represents nearly a 100-fold increase over that seen with systemic administration or infusion through a guide catheter. Identification of a delivery catheter has not been the limiting problem. Instead, the limiting problem has been determining which pharmaceutical agent should be administered and which specific clinical problem we are treating.

THROMBUS AND ACUTE VESSEL CLOSURE

Coronary dissection and thrombus formation, resulting in acute and subacute vessel closure, remain as significant problems (14). The decision of which agents to use for local delivery centers upon those agents with prior FDA approval. The widespread availability of thrombolytic and antiplatelet therapies resulted in the early use of these agents for local administration. The Dispatch catheter (Scimed Life Systems, Maple Grove, MN) was one of the first systems evaluated in the clinical arena as a local administration device for the indication of coronary thrombus. A nondilating catheter that allows antegrade blood flow while the drug infusion was occurring, the Dispatch also offered the opportunity for prolonged administration of agents without causing myocardial ischemia. This catheter was extensively characterized in humans by Camezind et al. (15) in a novel and elegant manner. Using a continuos infusion of tracer that did not have myocardial uptake with rapid clearance

TABLE 34.1. *Catheter systems*

Type	First-generation	Second-generation	Third-generation
Diffusion	Double-balloon (Cordis)	Dispatch (Scimed)	Angiomed (angiomed 6TC)
Infusion	Wollinsky (USCI)	Transport (Scimed)	InfusaSleeve (Localmed)
Direct injection	Direct injection	Iontophoretic balloon	Infiltrator (IVT)

angiomed, Karlsruhe, Germany; Scimed, Scimed Life Systems, Maple Grove, MN; IVT, Interventional Technologies, IUT, San Diego, CA.

(MAG-3) these authors were able to demonstrate that the actual site of administration could be imaged and that the washout from the site could be calculated and standard models applied.

The Dispatch and other catheters have been evaluated in a porcine model for the amount of intramural deposition of urokinase when delivered by different techniques. Table 34.2 summarizes the work of Mitchel et al. (16) in the pig model. Note that there are small but significant differences in the delivery efficiency between the different methods of administration.

The clinical use of these catheters has been reported in over 500 patients to date from registry studies. The earliest studies were those using the first-generation catheters. Table 34.3 reviews the registry studies that have been reported to date.

The administration of urokinase has also been investigated in a single-center investigation by Glazier et al. (17). This study evaluated the use of a hydrogel-coated balloon onto which urokinase had been adsorbed. The investigators immersed the balloon into a solution of urokinase containing 50,000 units per cc. Ninety-five patients were enrolled because of the presence of thrombus angiographically (acute MI = 50; postinfarction angina, $n = 23$; and unstable angina, $n = 22$). Though no deaths or emergency bypass procedures occurred there was a 7.4% incidence of acute complications with no-reflow in 3 patients, distal embolization in 1 patient,

and late vessel closure in 1 patient. The late clinical event rate composed of death, myocardial infarction, and recurrent angina was 30.5%. The results of this study may be due to the fact that thrombolytic therapy increases platelet activation in the setting of acute ischemia and therefore may increase the risk of embolization and late platelet-driven thrombotic events.

This same group (18) utilized the Dispatch catheter in a small pilot series of 13 patients with saphenous vein grafts that averaged 11 years old. This population all had thrombosis or occlusion of aged saphenous and 12 of the 13 patients presented with unstable angina pectoris. These patients underwent infusion of urokinase through a Dispatch catheter (Scimed Life Systems), followed by definitive therapy with a balloon inflation or stent placement.

The Dispatch catheter is a nondilating catheter and the residual stenosis post urokinase infusion was still 50% ± 16%. After definitive therapy, the minimal lesion stenosis fell to 26% ± 15%. Procedural success was 14 of 15 lesions (12 patients). Two patients had transient no-reflow and in patient non-Q-wave myocardial infarction developed. Late clinical events were present in 4 patients with restenosis. A fifth patient with severe three-vessel coronary disease had sudden death at home; this death was not believed to be related to the therapy.

The concept of giving local administration of

TABLE 34.2. *Efficacy of delivery using local delivery catheters*

Treatment	Dose (units)	Units deposited	% delivery
Systemic	1,000,000	4 ± 1	0.0004 ± 0.00004
Guiding catheter	500,000	20 ± 30	0.004 ± 0.003
Roubin infusion cath	150,000	6 ± 5	0.004 ± 0.006
Dispatch	150,000	125 ± 97[a]	0.08 ± 0.06
Hydrogel balloon	700	12 ± 8	1.83 ± 1.29[b]

[a] $p < 0.05$ vs. all other rows; [b] $p \geq 0.05$ vs. all other rows.
(From ref. 16, with permission.)

TABLE 34.3. *Local therapy registries*

Study	No. Patients
Infusasleeve registry	95
Local PAMI	120
EDGE	60
InfusaSleeve registry	95
InfusaSleeve	35
Infiltrator safety study	20
PILOT (D)	18
PILOT (P)	25
Infiltrator Milan	30
VGEF registry	19
Total patients	541

TABLE 34.5. *DUET trial results at 180 days*

	Dispatch ($n = 27$)	Routine ($n = 26$)
Composite	6 (30.7)	2 (9.3)
Death	0	1 (3.8)
Reinfarction	2 (9.1)	0
Stroke	0	1 (3.8)
CABG	1 (5.6)	1 (5.6)
Rehosp	7 (33.2)	3 (14.8)
Re angio	8 (39.6)	3 (14.0)
TVR	4 (19.6)	0
Angina	12 (52.3)	6 (31.6)

CABG, coronary artery bypass graft; Re angio, repeat angioplasty; rehosp, rehospitalization; TVR, target vessel revascularization.

urokinase was explored in more detail in the Dispatch and Urokinase in the Elective treatment of Thrombus [DUET] trial. This randomized, multicenter trial also evaluated the use of the Dispatch catheter in saphenous vein grafts. It was initiated at the same time that intravenous glycoprotein IIb/IIIa antiplatelet therapies were being investigated. This resulted in a limited enrollment of 53 patients. The trial was discontinued early due to an inability to enroll patients, as well as an interim analysis that demonstrated a trend towards more complications during the course of the investigation. As seen in Tables 34.4 and 34.5, patients who had the Dispatch catheter used were more prone to early distal embolization and vascular complications.

We have examined the use of abciximab, using local delivery catheters (19), in a group of patients with angiographically and angioscopically defined thrombus. The abciximab was delivered as 10 mg in 5cc over 5 minutes. An-

gioscopy was performed within 5 minutes after abciximab infusion to confirm the effects of local abciximab infusion (Fig 34.1).

Figure 34.1A is the angiogram from a patient who presented with unstable angina after stent placement. Figure 34.1B is the angioscopic appearance of the thrombus prior to abciximab delivery. Figure 34.1C and 34.1D represent the appearance after local abciximab infusion. This therapy is contrary to conventional wisdom regarding the use of abciximab; however, if local elution of this agent is possible, then the arterial wall can serve as a reservoir for prolonged release of the drug.

RESTENOSES

Local delivery of unfractionated and fractionated heparin has been evaluated. Prior animal models including rat, rabbit, and pig (20–23) have suggested that high-dose systemic heparin could reduce late neointimal hyperplasia.

Clinical studies using heparin therapy, delivered using catheter based systems, have been promising. Lopez-Sendon (24) demonstrated decreased neointimal proliferation at 28 days in a porcine model, after infusion using a double-balloon catheter. Heparin has been demonstrated to diffuse across the entire arterial wall and into the adventitia.

The hypothesis that limiting acute platelet deposition will decrease late restenosis was the basis for the HIPS trial. This trial randomized 250 patients between 5000 units intracoronary heparin and intraluminal heparin using the end-

TABLE 34.4. *DUET trial acute results*

	Dispatch ($n = 27$)	Routine ($n = 26$)
Death	0 (00.0)	0 (00.0)
Reinfarction	1 (3.7)	0 (00.0)
Stroke	0 (00.0)	1 (3.7)
IABP	1 (3.7)	0 (00.0)
CABG	0 (00.0)	0 (00.0)
Stent	6 (22.2)	4 (15.4)
Ischemia	6 (22.2)	1 (3.8)
TVR	2 (7.4)	0 (00.0)
Re angio	2 (7.4)	0 (00.0)
Bleeding	1 (3.7)	0 (00.0)

CABG, coronary artery bypass graft; IABP, intraaortic balloon pump; re angio, repeat angioplasty; TVR, target vessel revascularization.

points, where angiographic stenosis as well as intravascular ultrasound determined plaque volume.

This procedure was very safe with a similar percentage of procedural success of 99.4% versus 100%. The procedural and clinical outcomes are listed in Table 34.6. There were no differences in the late clinical outcomes with respect to revascularization. One patient suffered a Q-wave myocardial infarction and subsequently died in the intramural group, and the incidence of Non-Q myocardial infarctions was no different between the groups (8.8% versus 12.5%). Note that the 6-month revascularization rate is

exceptionally low in both groups. This is consistent with the large vessels that were entered into this study.

The intravascular ultrasound determined vessel volume was 36.4 ± 20.1 mL^3 in the intramural treated group and 44.1 ± 25.1 mL^3 in the intraluminal control group (p not significant).

The limitations of the HIPS trial included the utilization of a low dose of heparin for local administration. It is possible that the study dosage was inadequate to achieve sufficient local therapeutic levels. Animal trials had used equivalent doses ten times higher than those used in this study.

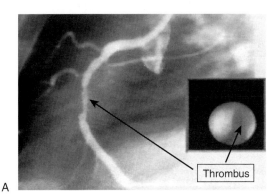

A

Thrombus

Angioscope   IVUS IMAGE

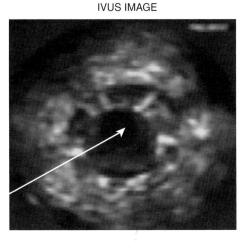

B   PLATELET THROMBUS

FIG. 34.1. A: Baseline image. **B:** Prior to abciximab infusion. *(Figure continues.)*

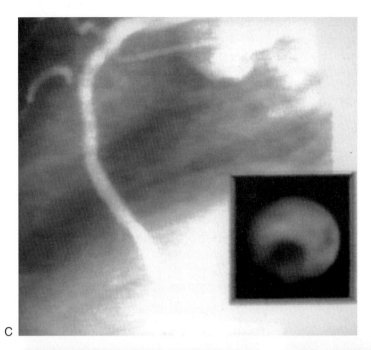

C

FIG. 34.1. *Continued.*
C: Post-abciximab infusion;
D: Post-abciximab infusion.

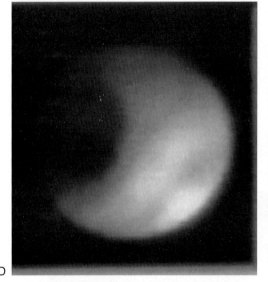

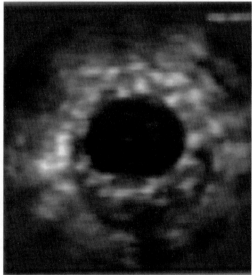

D

Alternatively, this form of therapy may not be effective in preventing late intimal hyperplasia. This finding was predicted by the studies of Edelman et al. who demonstrated that diffusion was not effective in treating the thick arteries found in diseased coronary vessels. They showed that adventitial delivery of heparin was required for suppression of neointimal proliferation.

The use of unfractionated heparin covalently bound to stents was evaluated in the heparin-coated stent study "BENESTENT II" (25) This trial evaluated a novel, covalently bound heparin-coated stent compared to balloon angioplasty. The subacute rate was exceptionally low; however, the rate of restenosis in the stent group was not different than that predicted from the noncoated stent used in the BENESTENT I trial.

TABLE 34.6. *HIPS Trial Procedural Outcomes*

Outcomes	Mural	Luminal
Success (%)	99.4	100
SAT	0	0
MLD (mm)	2.96 ± 0.44	2.96 ± 0.43
MLD FU(mm)	2.11 ± 0.75	2.06 ± 0.58
Stenosis (%)	31.1 ± 19.5	32.3 ± 16.7
Restenosis	12.7	12.7
TLR Free	86.2	90.7
TVF Free	77.0	75.6

Re angio, repeat angioplasty; MLD, minimum lumen diameter; MLD FU, minimum lumen diameter follow up; SAT, subacute thrombosis; TLR, target lesion revascularization; TVR, target vessel revascularization.

This suggests that there is no antiprofliferative effect of the heparin coating. This mirrors data from animal studies that also failed to demonstrate a decrease in neointimal proliferation in a porcine model (26). It is unclear whether higher doses of heparin or noncovalently bound heparin would have decreased the incidence of neointimal proliferation.

The use of low-molecular-weight heparin was evaluated in the animal model by Hong et al. (27). This study utilized the channeled balloon to deliver enoxaparin (10 mg/kg) in a rabbit iliac model. This study demonstrated that acute administration of a single dose of low-molecular-weight heparin was no more effective than control. The combination of acute administration followed by systemic administration was effective in decreasing late neointimal proliferation. Efficacy of delivery was only 0.1%–0.2%. Measurement of systemic anti-Xa levels demonstrated that the majority of the enoxaparin was distributed systemically. It is unclear whether the low rate of local delivery may explain the lack of efficacy or it is simply not an effective agent for neointimal hyperplasia. It is also unclear if the additional injury from the balloon delivery played a role in the late outcomes.

The hypothesis that low-molecular-weight heparin might reduce restenosis has been tested by Kiesz et al. (28) in the Polish Local Delivery in the NIR Stent trial (POLONIA trial). This 100-patient trial utilized low-molecular-weight heparin (enoxaparin) as a single 10-mg dose with 2,500 μ intravenous heparin infused into the artery using the transport balloon prior to stent placement, compared to standard 10,000 μ intravenous heparin. Both the acute outcomes as well as the late clinical and angiographic outcomes were assessed. Vessel site was 2.9 ± 0.4 mm. This trial demonstrated that use of locally delivered enoxaparin was sufficient to avoid the need for systemic heparinization during the procedure. Late loss was significantly less in the local heparin group (0.63 ± 0.48 mm versus 0.83 ± 0.43 mm, $p < .05$). This data is the first study to demonstrate angiographic and clinical success using locally delivery in clinical cardiology.

It is unclear what amount of heparin must be available from local delivery. The only available study with quantitative information is from Mitchel et al. (29) This study demonstrated that the delivery of only 0.5–0.6 units was sufficient to decrease early platelet deposition but it took 30–60 units to attenuate smooth muscle cell proliferation.

Local delivery of glycoprotein IIb/IIIa agents is being considered. The exciting data that clinical events are decreased up to 3 years after systemic administration is encouraging. There is data that supports the use of locally delivered glycoprotein IIb/IIIa agents using stents. The work of Agarwal et al. (30) demonstrated that platelet deposition could be significantly inhibited by a murine antibody to the glycoprotein IIb/IIIa locus is an important finding. The authors found that using polymer-coated stents onto which the AZ1 antibody had been adsorbed inhibited platelet deposition both in vitro and in vivo. The elution curves demonstrated a biexponential curve with an early rapid phase followed by a slow elution such that 40% of the AZ1 antibody was still present at 14 days. Platelet deposition as assessed by actual platelet counts and physiologic parameters such as cyclic flow variation were improved in the coated stent.

Unfortunately, this study did not demonstrate any difference in the late intimal thickness, or the intima to media thickness ratio in the AZ1-coated stent compared to the non-AZT-coated stent. This finding may represent the fact that the stent had an inadequate amount of the glycoprotein IIb/IIIa agent present or, more likely, the fact that a different receptor blockade may be required.

Clinical information regarding the use of other agents such as Taxol (Bristol-Myers Squibb, Wallingford, CT) is not yet available. This agent does have significant promise in the treatment of neointimal proliferation. This agent acts in a different manner than agents that decrease cell proliferation. Taxol and other Taxines interfere with the ability of microtubules. This interferes with the ability of smooth muscle cells to change shape and move into the artery wall. This agent has been demonstrated by Sollott et al. (31) to decrease neointimal hyperplasia in a rat model at 11 days in a dose dependent manner. Subsequent studies have been presented in abstract form that also indicate that this agent can be delivered via stents in a local manner to decrease late neointimal hyperplasia. This therapy has many similarities to the effects of irradiation and may mimic the cytostatic, rather than cytotoxic, agents that have previously been employed. Axel et al. (32) have evaluated the use of Taxol for local infusion using the microporous infusion catheter from Cordis corporation. This agent had both an in vitro effect as well an a significant effect in a thermal injury rabbit carotid model. The decrease in intimal hyperplasia was significantly greater in the treated animals than in the control animals. The neointimal area was $0.21 \pm .16 \text{ mm}^2$ versus $0.36 \pm 0.29 \text{ mm}^2$ in the treated versus the control vessels. Importantly, this decrease was not accompanied by any delay in endothelialization. This differs from the findings seen after irradiation therapy in which the endothelial cell were significantly delayed. In addition the concentrations required to inhibit microtubule cross-linking were tenfold lower than that required to inhibit cell proliferation. These levels are achievable using local delivery techniques. In addition, the use of paclitaxel combined with low dose locally delivery irradiation also appears to have promise as a new therapeutic modality. This technique could potentiate both the microtubular effect as well as the cytotoxic effect of both therapies.

CONCLUSIONS

Local drug delivery of thrombolytic agents such as urokinase has been shown to be safe and effective for the treatment of intracoronary thrombus. The delivery of glycoprotein IIb/IIIa agents is currently being evaluated in the same setting. Early experience suggests that local delivery of these agents may be as effective as systemic delivery. Whether long term benefits will be seen is unclear at this time.

Current techniques of local delivery using conventional doses of heparin have not been shown to decrease restenosis in a prospective randomized trial or to decrease the amount of neointimal hyperplasia. There is evidence that new therapies using cell cycle specific agents such as paclitaxel may inhibit cell proliferation and the production of extracellular matrix.

Current experience indicates that the choice of the delivery system is important to the procedural outcomes as seen in the DUET trial. Careful consideration will need to be given prior to future studies in characterizing the limitations of delivery system and efficiency prior to embarking on future studies of local therapy to decrease neointimal proliferation.

REFERENCES

1. Hoffmann R, Mintz GS, Dussaillant GR et al. Patterns and mechanisms of in-stent restenosis: a serial intravascular ultrasound study. *Circulation* 1996;94(6):1247–1254.
2. Faxon DP, Coats W, Currier J. Remodeling of the coronary artery after vascular injury. *Progress in Cardiovascular Diseases* 1997;40(2):129–140.
3. Kimura T, Kaburagi S, Tamura T et al. Remodeling of human coronary arteries undergoing coronary angioplasty or atherectomy. *Circulation* 1997;96(2):475–483.
4. Kronowski R, Mintz GS, Kent KM et al. Increased restenosis in diabetes mellitus after coronary interventions is due to exaggerated intimal hyperplasia. *Circulation* 1997;95(6):1366–1369.
5. Lefkovits J, Ivanhoe RJ, Califf RM et al. Effects of platelet glycoprotein IIb/IIIa receptor blockade by a chimeric monoclonal antibody (abciximab) on acute and six-month outcomes after percutaneous transluminal coronary angioplasty for acute myocardial infarction. Epic Investigators. *Am J Cardiol* 1996;77:1045–1051.
6. Tcheng JE. Glycoprotein IIb/IIIa receptor inhibitors: putting the EPIC, Impact II, Restore, and Epilog trials into perspective. *Am J Cardiol* 1996;78:35–40.
7. Topol EJ. Prevention of cardiovascular ischemic complications with new platelet glycoprotein IIb/IIIa inhibitors. *Am Heart J* 1995;130:666–672.
8. Bauters C, Isner JM. The biology of restenosis. *Prog Cardiovasc Dis* 1997;40(2):107–116.
9. Mintz GS, Popma JJ, Pichard AD et al. Arterial remodeling after coronary angioplasty. *Circulation* 1996;94(1):35–43.

10. Rogers C, Edelman ER. Endovascular stent design dictates experimental restenosis and thrombosis. *Circulation* 1995;91(12):2995–3001.

11. Bailey, SR. Local drug delivery: current applications. 1997;40(2):183–204.

12. Brieger D, Topol E. Local drug delivery systems and prevention of restenosis. *Cardiovasc Res* 1997;35: 405–413.

13. Edelman ER, Lovich M. Drug delivery models transported to a new level. *Nature Biotechnology* 1998;l6: 136–137.

14. Schieman G, Cohen BM, Kozina J et al. Intracoronary urokinase for intracoronary thrombus accumulation complicating percutaneous intracoronary thrombus accumulation complicating percutaneous transluminal coronary angioplasty in acute in acute ischemic syndromes. *Circulation* 1990;82:2052–2060.

15. Camenzind E, Bakker A, Reijs A et al. Site-specific intracoronary heparin delivery in humans after balloon angioplasty: a radioisotopic assessment of regional pharmacokinetics. *Circulation* 1997;96(l):154–165.

16. Mitchel, JF, Shwedick M, Alberghini TA, Knibbs D, McKay RG. Catheter-based local thrombolysis with urokinase; comparative efficacy of intraluminal clot lysis with conventional urokinase infusion techniques in an in vivo porcine thrombus model. *Cathet Cardiovasc Diagn* 1997;41:293–302.

17. Glazier JJ, Hirst JA, Kernan FJ et al. Site-specific intracoronary thrombolysis with urokinase-coated hydrogel balloons: acute and follow-up studies in 95 patients. *Cathet Cardiovasc Diagn* 1997;41:246–253.

18. Glazier JJ, Kernan FJ, Bauer HH et al. Treatment of thrombotic saphenous vein bypass grafts using local urokinase infusion therapy with the Dispatch catheter. *Cathet Cardiovasc Diagn* 1997;41:261–267.

19. Bailey SR, O'Leary E, Chilton R. Angioscopic evaluation of site-specific administration of ReoPro. *Cathet Cardiovasc Diagn.* 1997;42(2):181–184.

20. Guyton JR, Rosneber RD, Clowes AW, Karnowsky MJ. Inhibition of rat arterial smooth muscle cell proliferation by heparin. *Circ Res* 1980;46:625–634.

21. Clowes AW, Clowes MM. Kinetics of cellular proliferation after arterial injury. II. Inhibition of smooth muscle growth by heparin. *Lab Invest* 1985;52:611–616.

22. Wolinsky H, Thung SN. Use of a perforated catheter to deliver concentrated heparin into the wall of the normal

into the wall of the normal coronary artery. *J Am Coll Cardiol* 1990;15:475–481.

23. Azrin Ma, Mitchel JF, Fram DB et al. Decreased platelet deposition and smooth muscle cell proliferation following intramural heparin delivery with hydrogel-coated balloons. *Circulation* 1994;90:433–441.

24. Lopez-Sandon J, Sobrino N, Bamallo C et al. Locally delivered heparin reduces intimal hyperplasia and lumen stenosis following balloon injury in swine. *Eur Hear J* 1993;14[Suppl]:191(abst).

25. Serruys P, Van Hout B, Bonnier H et al. Randomized comparison of implantation of heparin-coated stents with balloon angioplasty in selected patients with coronary artery disease (Benestent II). *Lancet* 1998; 352(9129):673–681.

26. Hardhammar PA, van Beusekom HM, Emanuelsson HU et al. Reduction in thrombotic events with heparin-coated Palmaz-Schatz stents in normal porcine coronary arteries. *Circulation* 1996;93(3):423–430.

27. Hong MK, Wong SC, Barry JJ, Bramwell O, Tjurmin A, Leon MB. Feasibility and efficacy of locally delivered enoxaparin via the channeled balloon catheter on smooth muscle cell proliferation following balloon injury in rabbits. *Cathet Cardiovasc Diagn* 1997;41: 232–240.

28. Kiesz RS, Buszman P, Martin JL et al. Polish-American Local Lovenox NIR Stent Assessment Study (POLONIA): Final Results. *J Am Coll Cardiol* 1999; 33(2)[Suppl A]:14A(abst).

29. .Mitchel JF, Azrin MA, Fram DB, Laurine MB, McKay RG. Localized delivery of heparin to angioplasty sites with iontophoresis. *Cathet Cardiovasc Diagn* 1997;41: 315–323.

30. Agarwal RK, Ireland DC, Azrin MA, Ezekowitz MD, deBono DP, Gershlick Ah. Antithrombotic potential of polymer-coated stents eluting platelet glycoprotein IIb/IIIa receptor antibody. *Circulation* 1996;94(12): 3311–3317.

31. Sollott SJ, Cheng L, Pauly RR et al. Taxol inhibits neointimal smooth muscle cell accumulation after angioplasty in the rat. *Journal Clinical Investigation* 1995; 95:1869–1876.

32. Axel DI, Kunert W, Goggelmann C et al. Paclitaxel inhibits arterial smooth muscle cell proliferation and migration in vitro and in vivo using local drug delivery. *Circulation* 1997;96(2):636–645.

SECTION IV

Related Issues

35

Quality Management in the Cardiac Catheterization Laboratory

Warren K. Laskey

Division of Cardiology, University of Maryland, Baltimore, Maryland 21201

The modern cardiac catheterization laboratory is an amalgam of complex, highly sophisticated medical and radiologic instrumentation utilized in the diagnosis and management of patients with not only clinically stable but also life-threatening cardiovascular disease. The physicians working within this environment are among the most dedicated, procedure- and detail-oriented individuals within the medical profession. Moreover, the support personnel dedicated to this facility are highly trained, intensely motivated health care professionals providing a continuous and unvarying level of technical and clinical service. As such, the need for a system which maintains optimal performance at all levels is essential. This document will summarize and attempt to justify the key components of a quality improvement program in the "average" interventionally oriented cardiac catheterization laboratory. The components are: clinical proficiency and competency, equipment maintenance and management, fiscal management, radiation safety, and continuing educational programs.

CLINICAL PROFICIENCY AND COMPETENCY

The assessment of clinical proficiency in the catheterization laboratory is based on a composite of cognitive skills, procedural conduct, and clinical judgment. A deficiency in any one element is sufficient to significantly impact clinical outcomes. Therefore, all elements must be con-

sidered. Unfortunately, there is no unique, incontrovertible source that tells one "how to do things correctly." While experience is the *sine qua non* of proficiency, the myriad of techniques and technology preclude rigid delineation of "the right way." There is one incontrovertible bottom line, however: patient outcomes. Patient outcomes are the most important indicators of proficiency and competency in interventional cardiology (1) although arguably the most difficult to accurately quantify (2). The importance of risk-adjustment of crude event frequencies cannot be overstated (3). Therefore, it is essential that careful and complete preprocedural and intraprocedural information be reliably collected, stored, and statistically analyzed. Given that operator (and institutional) outcomes depend on many demographic, clinical, anatomic, and administrative variables, the importance of an adequate information systems infrastructure within the laboratory is mandatory. Without a complete recording of such variables, meaningful statistical analysis of event rates is precluded.

A quality improvement program, with regard to clinical proficiency, cannot succeed in a vacuum. The program must function under the broader rubric of system-level performance which, importantly, should connote a more constructive (in contrast to punitive) context (4). Given this caveat, the emphasis on individual and institutional outcomes is appropriate (1). Operators must be responsible for their actions and the consequences thereof. Algorithms to es-

TABLE 35.1. *Assessment of proficiency in coronary intervention*

	Component	Mode of assessment
Individual	Cognitive	Formal training program (4 years); "board" certification
	Procedural	Risk-adjusted outcomes or cost-effectiveness
	Judgment	"Board" certification; peer recognition
Institutional	Procedural outcomes	Risk-adjusted outcomes; volume-outcome relation; comparison across institutions

timate the likelihood of significant complication (5,6), appropriate device selection (7) and procedural conduct, prompt recognition and management of ischemic complications, and, importantly, the ability to say "no," are hallmarks of an experienced, competent operator. Admittedly, all are hard to measure, but there is little ambiguity when outcomes are either consistently superior (e.g., less than 2% major complication rate) or consistently suboptimal (e.g., more than 5% major complication rate). It is when adverse outcome frequencies fall within the broad gray zone of an average of 3.5 % (95% confidence interval 0.6% to 9.9% for 100 procedures) that the above-outlined approach is recommended. Although the frequencies of signal (adverse) events are likely to change over time as the result of continuing improvements in technology, clinical competence and its assessment will remain the foundation on which a quality management program rests. Table 35.1 summarizes current approaches to the assessment of proficiency in coronary intervention for both individuals and institutions.

EQUIPMENT MAINTENANCE AND MANAGEMENT

Perhaps there is no more intimidating environment within clinical medicine than a modern interventional catheterization laboratory. A summation of sophisticated radiologic, electronic, and increasingly computer-based technology, the laboratory's operating efficiency depends on a rigorous maintenance and troubleshooting program. The cardiac imaging system, a crucial component of every laboratory, must be carefully assessed at frequent intervals in order to detect early signs of a fall-off in performance. Unfortunately, this aspect of quality control is the first to be sacrificed in an era of intensive resource utilization. The inevitable consequence of this approach ("benign" neglect) is X-ray or TV-camera-tube failure with total loss of function. While close attention to cinefilm development and film image quality is advocated by professional groups (8), the reality of catheterization laboratory life precludes close scrutiny of films until the end of the day. Many, if not most, diagnostic and therapeutic decisions are made intraprocedurally as a consequence of the astonishing advances in digital image processing. However, at the present time, there is little expertise and even less information base on the criteria to evaluate system performance and image quality in the "filmless" laboratory.

A program of periodic assessment of system performance and image quality has been recommended by the Society for Cardiac Angiography and Interventions for many years (8–10). Currently, additional programs which will address issues specific to digital imaging systems are under evaluation (11). An outline of the performance characteristics needed to assess radiographic cardiac imaging systems is presented in Table 35.2.

It is important to point out that irrespective of

TABLE 35.2. *Performance characteristics of radiographic imaging systems*

Category	Example
System measures	Image quality Dynamic range Modulation transfer function
Component measures (not inclusive)	Cinefilm sensitometry Cinefilm on-frame optical density Cine and fluoro spatial resolution Cine and fluoro image size accuracy Cine and fluoro contrast resolution Cine and fluoro automatic exposure control

the means of recording the image, i.e., cine versus digital, the assessment of the portion of the imaging chain responsible for image acquisition is independent of the recording medium. As the prevalence of "filmless" facilities increases, this caveat will become increasingly important. The critical role of high-resolution video systems in complex coronary interventional procedures mandates a "front end" which possesses excellent low-contrast, as well as spatial, resolution. The critical roles of X-ray exposure and input dose must also be defined, because they fundamentally affect image quality (the radiation safety aspects will be discussed below). Many X-ray systems are incapable of responding to the radiographic (exposure) challenges of medium- to large-body habitus adults (12). Patient exposure and input dose are clearly linked. However, the decrease in image quality consequent to increased patient exposure must be kept in mind.

Interventional procedures occur in environments of high information density. Physiologic recorders, in the past utilized only for the acquisition and recording of analog signals, are now required to serve as front ends for an increasingly complex universe of data gathering. In order to obviate the need for double or triple entry of demographic, clinical, and ancillary administrative data, these recorders have essentially been transformed into desktop personal computers capable of acquiring and storing data and transmitting it to other sites. Given the critical importance of this data for numerous purposes (such as billing, quality assurance, and report generation), flawless and lossless transmission must take place all the time. As is true with all data stored in electronic format, back-up systems and low cost storage media are essential.

Precautions related to patient safety must always be mentioned. Not only are coronary interventional procedures life-saving; they may also be life-threatening. The operational efficiency of infrequently used pieces of equipment, such as defibrillators, must be tested on a routine basis. Electrical isolation and grounding systems must be regularly assessed. The number of ancillary devices used in coronary intervention, such as Doppler-tipped wires and ultrasound catheters, requires that electrical safety precautions advised in the past (13) may need to be revisited.

FISCAL MANAGEMENT

Effective cost management is a hallmark of the quality of administration of an interventional laboratory. The tremendous growth in device technology and pharmacologic adjunctives over the past decade has led to proportional increases in inventory, cost over-runs when referenced to prior years, and the need for highly sophisticated information systems to track utilization. Coupled with decreasing reimbursement rates, the growth of managed care and capitated programs, and the increase in laboratory utilization (due to more aggressive approaches to the management of ischemic heart disease), the inevitable imbalance between costs and revenues have resulted in creative approaches to cost containment. These approaches range from modification of individual physician behavior to wholesale hospital contracting arrangements in which single vendors supply multiple products across multiple cost centers. Table 35.3 outlines a number of past and presently successful strategies that have resulted in significant cost reduction for the catheterization laboratory.

Not all strategies are equally effective in all environments, because demographics, payer mix, the presence of capitation, and the characteristics of the physician make-up of the laboratory (i.e., geographic full-time versus non-geographic part-time), significantly affect the

TABLE 35.3. *Cost management strategies for the interventional laboratory*

Category	Example
Limiting equipment use	Revenue sharing on cost savings; physician profiling; reduced (simplified) inventory
Reduction of expenditures	"Capitation" programs with vendors;" profit sharing programs with facility; bulk purchasing agreements
Limiting extent of hospitalization	Ad hoc intervention; 23-hour observational units; improved risk stratification

TABLE 35.4. *Cost and resource utilization strategies*

Strategy	Advantage	Disadvantage
(a) "Line-item" approach	Maintain product diversity. Negotiating flexibility.	Costlier than b, c.
(b) "Per procedure" approach (bundling)	Simplifies inventory. Decreased cost/procedure. Allows for incentives.	Decreased choice. May constrain operating style.
(c) "Capitated" approach	Most cost advantageous. Predictable expenditures. Identifies "outliers."	Involves "risk sharing." May be even more constraining than (b).

behavioral homogeneity of a facility's operating philosophy.

Cost-effectiveness programs, much discussed but infrequently applied, require sophisticated data system support (itself a relatively high-cost item). Deciding on clinically relevant outcomes against which to apply cost data is an inexact science. As noted above, outcomes must be risk-adjusted to be meaningful. These adjusted outcomes must then be compared to some relevant standard (which may change over time). Finally, procedural cost in most institutions is a difficult number to define, given the universal practices of cost-shifting and "top-down" accounting. The dynamic nature of many current pricing arrangements between vendors and hospitals renders cost estimates a moving target. As an example, contrast the cost implications of a "line-item approach," "procedural" approach, and "capitated" approach shown in Table 35.4.

It is readily apparent that all models are exquisitely sensitive to small changes in utilization or practice patterns. A practice policy of (near) universal stenting, for example, would translate into a strikingly less cost-effective approach than would the application of stenting in accord with the findings of the DEBATE study (14). Unfortunately, very few facilities subscribe to any but the most rudimentary cost-management approaches (Paul Marshall, personal communication), with the expected strained relationship between hospital administration and physician users.

RADIATION SAFETY

Few areas of the catheterization laboratory are as poorly understood (and therefore, appear as intimidating) as the estimation and clinical significance of exposure to ionizing radiation. A recent membership survey performed by the American College of Cardiology indicated that concerns surrounding exposure to X-rays was a leading factor in the decision not to enter the field of interventional cardiology (15). Quality management in the catheterization laboratory must include: (a) an effective and ongoing educational program in the diagnostic use of X-ray, (b) accurate monitoring and reporting of personnel exposure, and (c) modification of procedural conduct in those cases where exposure levels are of concern. The Society for Cardiac Angiography and Interventions has, appropriately, had a long-standing interest in this area and has taken the lead in the publication of numerous position papers and guidelines (16,17). More recently, the American College of Cardiology, in collaboration with the Society for Cardiac Angiography and Interventions, has examined multiple aspects of radiation safety, particularly the issue of risk (15). These documents should serve as required components of a laboratory's quality assurance program.

The fundamental tenets of reduction in personnel exposure have not changed: reduce the time of exposure, utilize the inverse square law by increasing distance from the source (of scatter), and maintain appropriate shielding. Utilization of these principles in practice remain the easiest, most consistent way to reduce risk. Prior to the interventional era (pre 1980's), the "average" cardiac catheterization procedure necessitated an admixture of fluoroscopy and cineangiography such that 80%–90% of an operator's total exposure per procedure derived from the cine portion and the remainder of the total exposure from the fluoroscopic portion. Coupled with (relatively) higher framing rates at more than 30 fps and the use of smaller fields of view (5 in.), total dose equivalents in excess of 50 mSv/year were not unusual. Currently, improvements in the imaging chain, more efficient X-ray production and shielding, and the diminishing role of cinefilm acquisition translate into the potential for significant reductions in personnel exposure. Of note, however, is the virtual inversion of the above-noted distribution in exposure source: currently 80%–90% of an operator's total exposure during coronary intervention derives from the fluoroscopic portion of the procedure and the remaining 10%–20% from the cineangiographic recording portion. It must be pointed out that while exposures related to fluoroscopy are, on average, one tenth of cine exposures, the duration of use of fluoroscopy during interventional procedures has increased exponentially. Furthermore, modifications in fluoroscopic systems now include stations for higher dose-rates than conventional diagnostic fluoroscopy and an inherent increase in dose during digital imaging at high (greater than 512×512) matrix acquisitions. These caveats should remind the operator that the basic tenets of radiation protection still very much apply in the interventional laboratory.

ONGOING EDUCATION (AS A QUALITY MANAGEMENT TOOL)

Interventional cardiology is perhaps the most dynamic subspecialty within medicine today. Over a 10-year period, improvements in instrumentation, imaging, data recording, and procedural outcomes have proceeded at an astonishing pace. Continuing education for practitioners beyond the level of training programs has become the "norm" for the acquisition of many of these skills. Training programs themselves have grown from a traditional 1-year program in interventional cardiology to, in most formal training programs, 2 years. The development of sub-sub-specialty certification boards in interventional cardiology reflects a burgeoning knowledge base. All of this translates to the need to provide continuing education to all members of the team.

The implementation of new technology without critical evaluation of both the experience in the literature as well as within one's own institution is unacceptable. An organized program of didactic presentations, coupled with cautious early clinical experience, is an ideal mechanism for the introduction of new therapies. These types of programs, in conjunction with attendance at regional or national scientific meetings devoted to the unbiased presentation of new data, provide a solid infrastructure for staff education and personal growth. Continuing education requirements for credentialing purposes are a reality for both physicians and nonphysicians. Attention to this aspect of laboratory quality improvement goes a long way in maintaining both expertise and morale.

REFERENCES

1. Hirshfeld JW Jr, Ellis SG, Faxon DP et al. Recommendations for the assessment and maintenance of proficiency in coronary interventional procedures. *J Am Coll Cardiol* 1998;31:722–743.
2. Ellis SG, Omoigui N, Bittl JA et al Analysis and comparison of operator-specific outcomes in interventional cardiology: from a multicenter database of 4,860 quality-controlled procedures. *Circulation* 1996;93:431–439.
3. Block PC, Peterson EC, Krone R et al Identification of variables needed to risk adjust outcomes of coronary interventions: evidence-based guidelines for efficient data collection. *J Am Coll Cardiol* 1998;32:275–282.
4. Heupler FA, Al-Hani AJ, Dear WE et al Guidelines for continuous quality improvement in the cardiac catheterization laboratory. *Cathet Cardiovasc Diag* 1993;30:191–200.
5. Kimmel SE, Berlin JA, Strom BL, Laskey WK. Development and validation of simplified predictive index for major complications in contemporary percutaneous transluminal coronary angioplasty practice. Registry Committee of the Society for Cardiac Angiography and Interventions. *J Am Coll Cardiol* 1995;26:931–938.
6. Ellis SG. Coronary lesions at increased risk. *Am Heart J* 1995;130:643–646.
7. Baim DS, Detre KM, Kent K. Problems in the development of new devices for coronary intervention: possible role for a multicenter registry. *J Am Coll Cardiol* 1989;14:1389–1392.
8. Sones M. The Society for Cardiac Angiography. *Cathet Cardiovasc Diagn* 1978;4:233–345.
9. Mevin P. Judkins Cardiac Imaging Symposium. Society for Cardiac Angiography and Interventions Annual Scientific Meeting, 1988–1998.
10. Moore RJ. SCA cine imaging standards/guidelines. In: Moore RJ, ed. *Imaging principles of cardiac angiography.* Rockville, MD:, 1990:241–247.
11. Laskey WK, Holmes DR, Kern MJ. Image quality as-

sessment: a timely look. *Cathet Cardiovasc Diagn* (in press).

12. Holmes DR, Wondrow M, Stueve R et al. Variability of radiation output dynamic range in modern cardiac catheterization imaging systems. *Cathet Cardiovasc Diagn* 1998;44:443–448.

13. Judkins MP and the Laboratory Performance Standards Committee of the Society for Cardiac Angiography. Guidelines for electrical safety in the cardiac catheterization laboratory. *Cathet Cardiovasc Diagn* 1984;10:299–301.

14. Serruys PW, di Mario C, Pick J et al, for the DEBATE Study Group. Prognostic value of intracoronary flow velocity and diameter stenosis in assessing the short-and long-term outcomes of coronary balloon angioplasty. *Circulation* 1997;96:3369–3377.

15. Limacher MC, Douglas PA, Germano G et al Radiation safety in the practice of cardiology. *J Am Coll Cardiol* 1998;31:892–913.

16. Society for Cardiac Angiography Laboratory Performance Standards Committee. Guidelines for radiation protection in the cardiac catheterization laboratory. *Cathet Cardiovasc Diagn* 1984;10:87–92.

17. Johnson LW, Moore RJ, Balter S. Review of radiation safety in the cardiac catheterization laboratory. *Cathet Cardiovasc Diagn* 1992;25:186–194.

SECTION V

Summary and Future Directions

36

Summary and Future Directions

David R. Holmes, Jr.

Division of Cardiovascular Diseases and Internal Medicine, Mayo Clinic and Mayo Foundation, Department of Medicine, Mayo Medical School, Rochester, Minnesota 55905

The major advances in interventional cardiology continue as new technology is developed, tested, and brought to the clinical arena, and as new patient groups are treated. These advances have led to the significant increase in procedural volume so that currently, the number of percutaneous treatment procedures exceeds the number of coronary bypass surgical operations.

We have tried to explore the practice of interventional cardiology in this book, with descriptions of the clinical experience with specific stents and specific devices such as Doppler flow velocity, pressure wires, and intravascular ultrasound. These later devices allow us to access the physiology and the anatomy behind the angiogram so that we can make intelligent decisions about what to treat and then decide when we have done enough. We have explored new technology such as the use of radiation to either treat or prevent restenosis.

One of the most important goals of the text was to bring the technology to bear on specific angiographic and clinical subsets of patients. These are the problem areas which face the interventional cardiologist daily in his or her practice. These are the patients with adverse lesion morphology, bifurcation disease, chronic total occlusion, severe calcification, ostial lesions, and vein graft disease, to name but a few. These are the subsets which are associated with increased potential for complications or decreased success rates, or both. We have brought true expert opinions to bear on how to approach these subsets.

Often, the approach selection was not based on a randomized trial but instead on clinical experience and registry data. These sources are essential for the myriad of subsets that we face daily.

We have also dealt with the complications which can inevitably occur. The majority of these, like coronary perforation, are rare in current practice, but they can result in marked increases in morbidity and even mortality. In some patients, we can solve these complications; in others, the optimal solution remains to be determined.

Finally, the field of adjunctive therapy is burgeoning. New agents such as glycoprotein IIb/IIIa drugs have been intensively studied and now occupy a central position in the field of interventional cardiology. Adjunctive therapy remains the focus of great interest so that we can optimize the outcome after we have treated the lesion mechanically.

Questions linger in regard to a number of issues, including: positioning new devices for optimal use, matching the specific device to specific lesions, prevention and treatment of restenosis, identification of vulnerable plaques, the role of new imaging modalities, and the optimal use of adjunctive therapy. To answer questions like these—and to optimize patient care—will require continued investigation of the ideas and issues discussed in this book. The importance of this investigation characterizes the greatest challenges—and greatest rewards—of interventional cardiology.

Subject Index

Numbers followed by the letter *f* indicate figures; numbers followed by the letter *t* indicate tables.

DATE DUE

GAYLORD   #3523PI   Printed in USA